Human Retrovirology

Human Retrovirology

Edited by Mariana Warne

hayle
medical

New York

Hayle Medical,
750 Third Avenue, 9th Floor,
New York, NY 10017, USA

Visit us on the World Wide Web at:
www.haylemedical.com

ISBN: 978-1-63241-657-5

Cataloging-in-Publication Data

Human retrovirology / edited by Mariana Warne.
   p. cm.
Includes bibliographical references and index.
ISBN 978-1-63241-657-5
1. Retroviruses. 2. Retrovirus infections. 3. Medical microbiology. I. Warne, Mariana.
QR414.5 .H86 2019
616.918 8--dc23

Table of Contents

Preface

The purpose of the book is to provide a glimpse into the dynamics and to present opinions and studies of some of the scientists engaged in the development of new ideas in the field from very different standpoints. This book will prove useful to students and researchers owing to its high content quality.

The type of RNA viruses which insert a copy of their genome into the DNA of the host cells that they invade, and consequently change the genome of, are called retroviruses. After entering the host cell's cytoplasm, the retroviruses use their own reverse transcriptase enzyme to produce DNA from their RNA genome. The study of retroviruses and the diseases caused by them, is called retrovirology. Retroviruses, including Mouse mammary and Rous sarcoma virus can cause diseases, like tumor and cancer. The transmission of retroviruses can be airborne, from cell-to-cell, or through fluids. Antiretroviral drugs are the common medications used for treating the infection caused by retroviruses. This book elucidates the concepts and innovative models around prospective developments with respect to human retrovirology. It includes some of the vital pieces of work being conducted across the world, on various topics related to human retrovirology. This book will help new researchers by foregrounding their knowledge in this branch.

At the end, I would like to appreciate all the efforts made by the authors in completing their chapters professionally. I express my deepest gratitude to all of them for contributing to this book by sharing their valuable works. A special thanks to my family and friends for their constant support in this journey.

Editor

Moloney leukemia virus 10 (MOV10) inhibits the degradation of APOBEC3G through interference with the Vif-mediated ubiquitin–proteasome pathway

Cancan Chen[1,2,3], Xiaocao Ma[1,2], Qifei Hu[1,2], Xinghua Li[4], Feng Huang[1,2], Junsong Zhang[1,2], Ting Pan[1,2], Jinyu Xia[4], Chao Liu[1,2]* and Hui Zhang[1,2]

Abstract

Background: MOV10 protein has ATP-dependent 5′–3′ RNA helicase activity and belongs to the UPF1p superfamily. It can inhibit human immunodeficiency virus type 1 (HIV-1) replication at multiple stages and interact with apolipoprotein-B-mRNA-editing enzyme catalytic polypeptide-like 3G (APOBEC3G or A3G), a member of the cytidine deaminase family that exerts potent inhibitory effects against HIV-1 infection. However, HIV-1-encoded virion infectivity factor (Vif) protein specifically mediates the degradation of A3G via the ubiquitin–proteasome system (UPS).

Results: We demonstrate that MOV10 counteracts Vif-mediated degradation of A3G by inhibiting the assembly of the Vif-CBF-β-Cullin 5-ElonginB-ElonginC complex. Through interference with UPS, MOV10 enhances the level of A3G in HIV-1-infected cells and virions, and synergistically inhibits the replication and infectivity of HIV-1. In addition, the DEAG-box of MOV10 is required for inhibition of Vif-mediated A3G degradation as the DEAG-box mutant significantly loses this ability.

Conclusions: Our results demonstrate a novel mechanism involved in the anti-HIV-1 function of MOV10. Given that both MOV10 and A3G belong to the interferon antiviral system, their synergistic inhibition of HIV-1 suggests that these proteins may play complicated roles in antiviral functions.

Keywords: MOV10, A3G, Vif, HIV-1, Ubiquitin–proteasome system (UPS)

Background

Cellular apolipoprotein-B-mRNA-editing enzyme catalytic polypeptide-like 3G (APOBEC3G or A3G) is a potent antiviral host factor that can be packaged into HIV-1 virions and induces a C–U conversion in the newly synthesized minus-stranded viral DNA, thereby triggering the breakage of viral DNA or generating G-to-A hypermutations that result in a premature stop codon or mutated viral protein [1–5]. HIV-1 virion infectivity factor (Vif) can effectively counteract the antiviral

activity of A3G by inducing its degradation through the ubiquitin–proteasome system (UPS) [6–10]. Vif interacts with A3G through its N-terminal domain and has a SOCS-box motif within its C-terminal domain, which includes a BC-box and Cullin-box and interacts with Cullin 5, ElonginB, and ElonginC to form an E3 ubiquitin ligase complex and subsequently mediate the ubiquitination of A3G. CBF-β can bind with Vif directly and facilitate the degradation of A3G. Moreover, CBF-β can increase the stability of HIV-1 Vif and promote assembly of Vif-Cullin 5-E3-ubiquitin-ligase complex; however, ElonginB and ElonginC facilitate the binding of CBF-β with Vif [11–16].

MOV10 is originally identified in the MOV-10 mouse strain, which carries the Moloney murine leukemia

---

*Correspondence: liuchao9@mail.sysu.edu.cn
[1] Institute of Human Virology, Zhongshan School of Medicine, Sun Yat-sen University, Guangzhou 510080, China
Full list of author information is available at the end of the article

virus. It is a member of the UPF1p family and has ATP-dependent 5′–3′ RNA helicase activity [17, 18]. MOV10 has complicated functions and features. For example, MOV10 is found to interact with Argonaute proteins and plays a role in microRNA (miRNA)-mediated regulation [19, 20]. MOV10 is also involved in polycomb-mediated repression of the tumor-suppressor INK4a [21]. Moreover, it has been reported that MOV10 is a type I interferon stimulated gene and several reports have indicated that this protein has broad antiretroviral activity against various viruses, such as HIV-1, murine leukemia virus (MLV), and equine infectious anemia virus (EIAV) [22–25]. Its inhibitory effect on LINE-1 retrotransposition has also been investigated [26, 27]. MOV10 can also be packaged into HIV-1 particles and affects HIV-1 replication at multiple stages [22, 28–30]. MOV10 expresses in varieties of human cells. And according to the data from GEO profile, we found that the expression profile of MOV10 is in moderate or high level in CD4 + T cells and monocytes (https://www.ncbi.nlm.nih.gov/geoprofiles, GEO Profiles ID: 89710126, 106167926, 52933168, 51070326).

Recently, several studies have reported that MOV10 interacts with A3G and both of these proteins are located in P-bodies and can be induced by interferon-α [23, 29, 31]. Based on the similar features of MOV10 and A3G, a research group has studied the possible relationship between these two restriction factors in HIV-1 infection [29]. They co-expressed MOV10 with A3G, but failed to find any functional synergistic effects on viral replication. Conversely, after knocking down endogenous MOV10 by siRNA in the presence of A3G, they did not find any significant impact on HIV-1 infectivity. Nevertheless, they detected the possible synergy of these two inhibitors in the absence of HIV-1 Vif protein. Given that MOV10 can bind with A3G, we hypothesize that MOV10 may affect the process of Vif-mediated degradation of A3G.

Thus, in this study, we aim to elucidate the correlations between MOV10 and A3G in the presence of Vif, which could occur during natural infection by HIV-1. Our findings provide important insights into the role of MOV10 in Vif-mediated A3G degradation and the mechanism

through which MOV10 mediates the functional assembly of the Vif-CBF-β-Cullin 5-ElonginB-ElonginC complex to affect the Vif-medicated ubiquitin–proteasome pathway.

Results

MOV10 counteracts Vif-mediated degradation of A3G by interfering with the ubiquitin–proteasome pathway

In order to examine the relationships among MOV10, A3G, and Vif, we co-transfected MOV10-FLAG-, A3G-HA-, and Vif-HA-expressing plasmids into 293T cells, and then evaluated the expression levels of A3G and Vif. Interestingly, significant increases in A3G and Vif protein expression were observed in cells overexpressing MOV10 (Fig. 1a). To confirm this phenomenon, we analyzed changes in expression of A3G and Vif in the presence of different levels of MOV10. We found that the enhancement of A3G and Vif expression was correlated with the level of MOV10 (Fig. 1b). We also observed the same phenotype by depleting endogenous MOV10 with MOV10-specific siRNA (Fig. 1c) [32]. To exclude the possibility of off-target effects of siRNA, a restoration experiment was conducted. Co-transfection of rMOV10-FLAG-expressing plasmid, a MOV10 construct that is resistant to siRNA-targeting, with the MOV10-specific siRNA restored the expression of A3G (Fig. 1d), indicating that MOV10-specific siRNA does not have off-target effects.

To further validate this phenotype, a similar experiment was performed in H9 cells infected with wild-type HIV-1. MOV10-knockdown H9 cells were constructed by the infection of MOV10-specific shRNA-expressing lentivirus. The cells were then infected with wild-type HIV-1 viruses. The culture supernatants were collected at different days after infection, and HIV-1 p24 was detected by ELISA kit. After culture for 12 days, HIV-1 p24-positive cells were sorted by flow cytometry (Fig. 2). In these HIV-1 p24-positive cells, the expression of endogenous A3G was significantly down-regulated by endogenous MOV10 depletion. HIV-1 replication and the expression of Gag protein were also enhanced by the depletion of MOV10 (Fig. 2d). The results demonstrate that MOV10 and A3G synergistically inhibit the replication of HIV-1.

(See figure on next page.)
Fig. 1 MOV10 counteracts Vif-mediated degradation of A3G. **a, b** MOV10 overexpression inhibits Vif-mediated A3G degradation. Human 293T cells were transfected with pcDNA3.1-A3G-HA (0.8 µg), pcDNA3.1-Vif-HA (0.5 µg), and pcDNA3.1-MOV10-FLAG (1.5 µg) (**a**) or different amounts of pcDNA3.1-MOV10-FLAG (from 0.5 to 2 µg) (**b**). Then, cells were collected and lysed at 48 h, and analyzed by western blotting with anti-HA, anti-FLAG, and anti-GAPDH antibodies. **c, d** The effect of MOV10 depletion on Vif-mediated degradation of A3G. Cells were transfected with pcDNA3.1-A3G-HA (0.8 µg), pcDNA3.1-Vif-HA (0.5 µg), MOV10-specific siRNA (50 nM) (**c**) and/or siRNA-resistant MOV10 construct (rMOV10-FLAG) (0.4 µg) (**d**). After 48 h, cells were collected and analyzed by western blotting assay with anti-HA, anti-FLAG, anti-MOV10 and anti-GAPDH antibodies. Empty vector pcDNA3.1 was used in each transfection to normalize DNA amounts. Values in **a–d** represent percentages of A3G or MOV10 normalized against GAPDH and compared with control. The bar graphs represent the average expression of A3G with different treatment and relative to the A3G-only reaction control (set to 100%). All the data represent mean ± SD from three independent experiments. Statistical significance was determined using t test: *p ≤ 0.05; **p ≤ 0.01; ***p ≤ 0.001

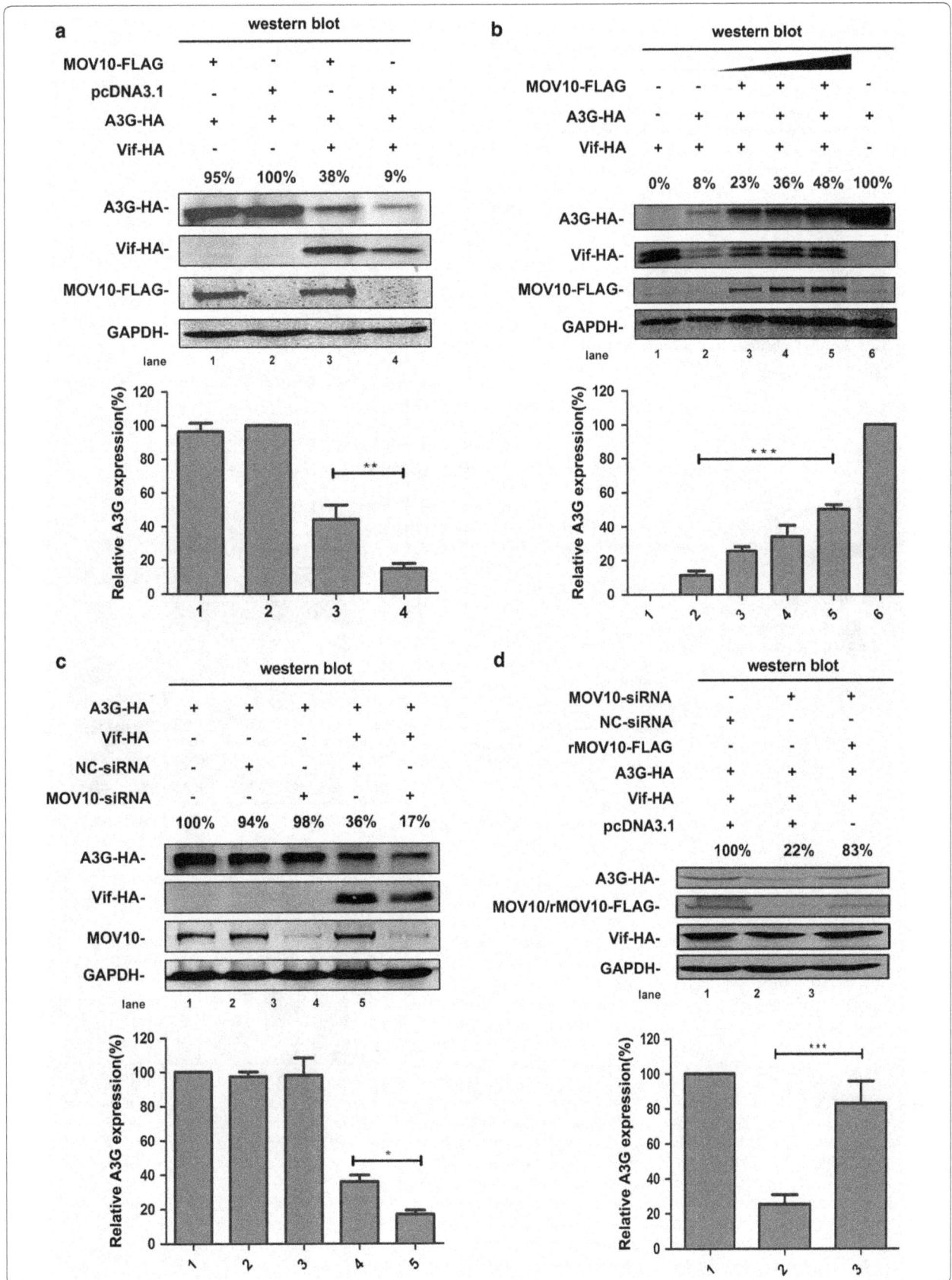

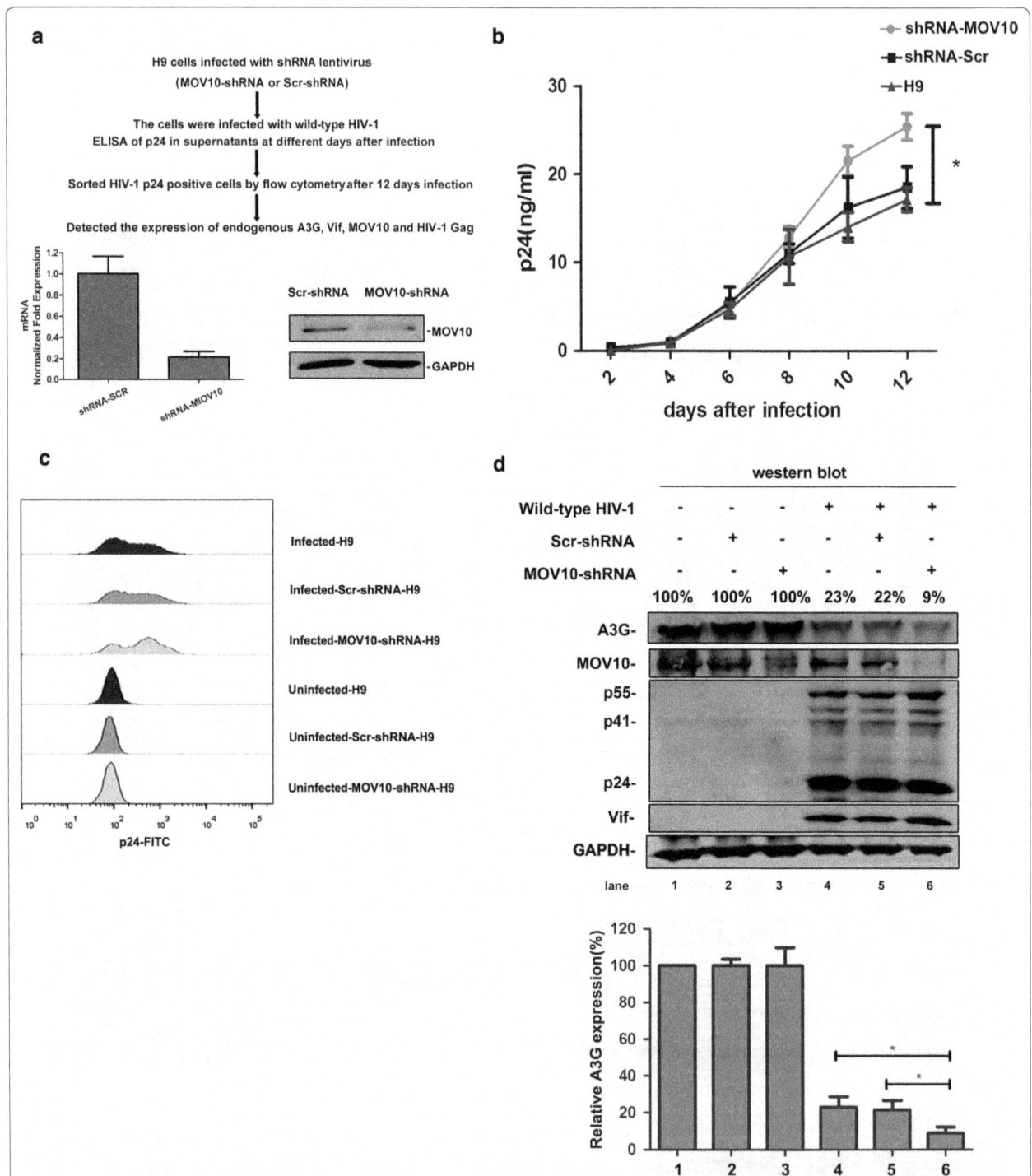

Fig. 2 MOV10 protects A3G from Vif-mediated degradation in wild-type HIV-1. **a** H9 cells were infected with pLKO.1-MOV10-shRNA or pLKO.1-Scr-shRNA lentivirus for 8 h and then selected with puromycin for 2 weeks. MOV10-knockdown H9 cells and control cells were infected with wild-type HIV-1 for 3 h and cultured with fresh medium for 12 days. The culture supernatants were collected at the indicated time points. Then HIV-1 p24 was detected using HIV-1 p24 ELISA kit at different time points (**b**). And at 12th day, these cells were analyzed by flow cytometer (**c**). HIV-1 p24 positive H9 cells were sorted and detected by western blotting with anti-MOV10, anti-A3G, anti-Vif, anti-HIV-1 p24, and anti-GAPDH antibodies (**d**). Values in **d** represent percentages of A3G or MOV10 normalized against GAPDH and compared with control. The *bar graphs in* **d** represent the average expression of A3G with different treatment and relative to the A3G-only reaction control (set to 100%). Data in **a**, **b**, and **d** represent mean ± SD from three independent experiments. *, statistically significant, $p \leq 0.05$ (*t* test). All the results are representative of at least three independent experiments

Moloney leukemia virus 10 (MOV10) inhibits the degradation of APOBEC3G through interference...

5

Considering the relationships between Vif/A3G and the ubiquitin–proteasome pathway [6–8, 10, 33], we evaluated the effects of MOV10 on the expression levels of A3G and Vif in the presence of the proteasome inhibitor MG132. After treatment with MG132 for 16 h, the expression levels of A3G and Vif were not affected by MOV10 overexpression (Fig. 3a). Further study showed that MOV10 could decrease the ubiquitination of A3G directly (Fig. 3b). Taken together, these data indicate that MOV10 can protect A3G from Vif-mediated degradation by interfering with the ubiquitin–proteasome pathway.

MOV10 affects the assembly of the Vif-CBF-β-Cullin 5-ElonginB-ElonginC complex

Previous studies have reported that A3G can bind with Vif (Fig. 4a) [10]. And, A3G protein contains two domains: the N-terminal domain is responsible for encapsidation and the C-terminal domain is responsible for deamination activity [34, 35]. Only the N-terminal domain of A3G can bind with Vif and the binding initiates the degradation process of A3G [36]. Because A3G can also interact with MOV10 (Fig. 4b) [20], the interaction of Vif with A3G may be affected by MOV10. To this end, we investigated the effects of MOV10 on the interaction between Vif and A3G in the presence of MG132. Human 293T cells were transfected with MOV10-FLAG-, A3G-HA-, and Vif-FLAG-expressing plasmids and then treated with MG132 for 16 h. However, we did not detect any changes in the levels of Vif-FLAG in the A3G-HA-immunoprecipitated samples with or without MOV10 (Fig. 4c). These results suggest that MOV10 does not affect the binding of Vif with A3G and therefore it may interfere with other steps in the A3G degradation process.

The interaction of Vif with CBF-β, Cullin 5, ElonginB, and ElonginC can facilitate the formation of a ubiquitin ligase complex, which is required for Vif to induce the degradation of A3G [11–13, 37, 38]. Therefore, we next examined

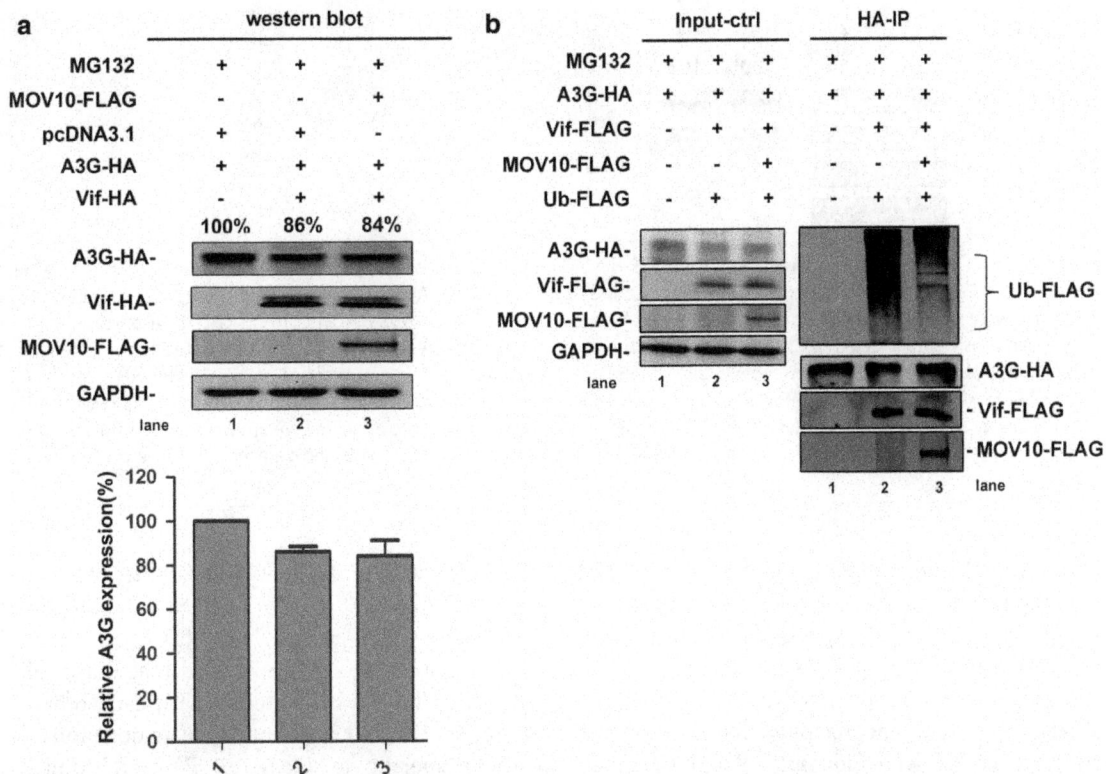

Fig. 3 MOV10 prevents A3G from Vif-induced degradation by decreasing the ubiquitination of A3G. **a** Human 293T cells were transfected with pcDNA3.1-A3G-HA (0.8 μg), pcDNA3.1-Vif-HA (0.5 μg), and pcDNA3.1-MOV10-FLAG (1.5 μg) and then treated with MG132 (4 μM) for 16 h. Lysed cells were collected at 48 h and detected by western blotting with anti-HA, anti-FLAG, and anti-GAPDH antibodies. **b** 293T cells were transfected with pcDNA3.1-A3G-HA (2 μg), pcDNA3.1-Vif-FLAG (1.25 μg), pcDNA3.1-MOV10-FLAG (2.5 μg), and pcDNA3.1-Ub-FLAG (3 μg). Cells were treated with MG132 (4 μM) for 16 h and analyzed by co-immunoprecipitation with anti-HA agarose beads. And then, samples were detected by western-blotting using anti-HA, anti-FLAG, and anti-GAPDH. Values in **a** represent percentages of A3G normalized against GAPDH and compared with control. The *bar graphs in* **a** represent the average expression of A3G with different treatment and relative to the A3G-only reaction control (set to 100%). Data in **a** represent mean ± SD from three independent experiments. Empty vector pcDNA3.1 was used to equalize DNA amounts in each transfection. Data in **a** and **b** are representative of at least three independent experiments

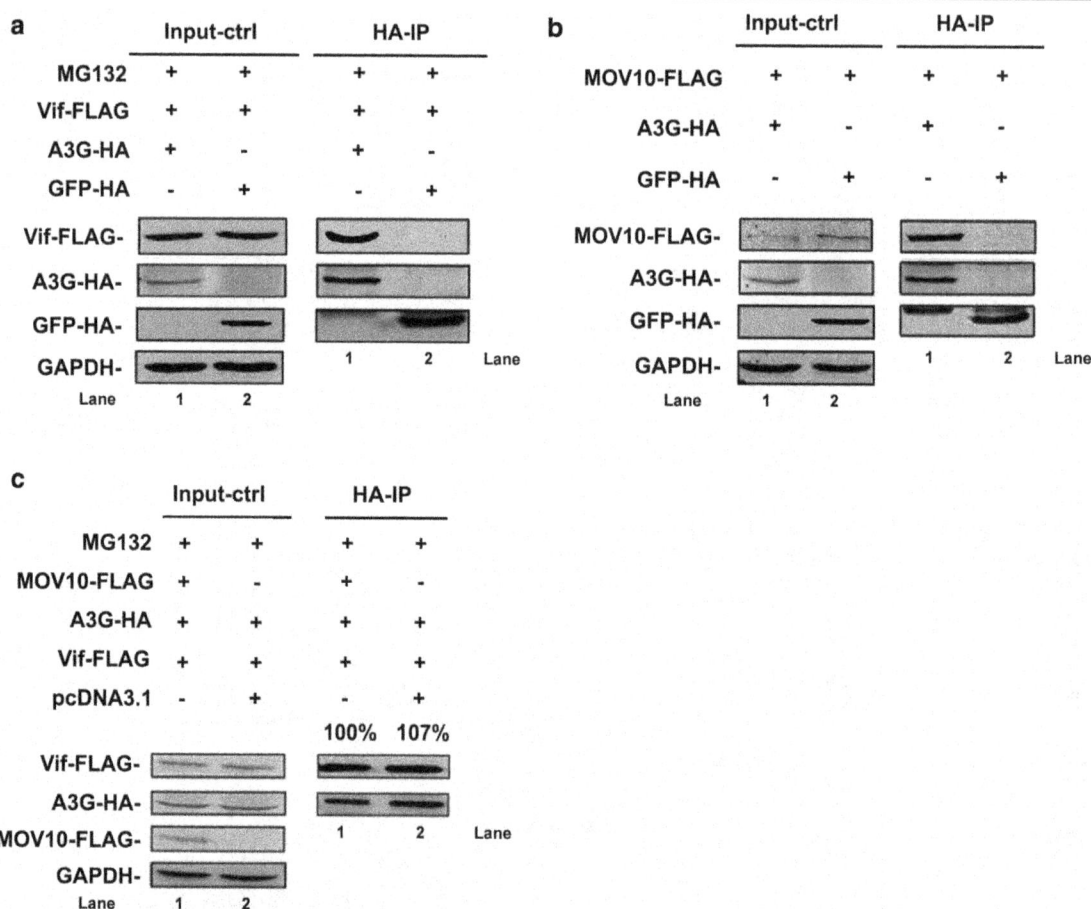

Fig. 4 MOV10 has no influence on the binding of A3G with Vif. **a**, **b** A3G interacts with Vif or MOV10 effectively. **a** Human 293T cells were transfected with 2 μg of pcDNA3.1-A3G-HA (pcDNA3.1-GFP-HA as a control) and 1 μg of pcDNA3.1-Vif-FLAG and then treated with MG132 for 16 h. **b** Human 293T cells were transfected with 1 μg of pcDNA3.1-Vif-FLAG and 2 μg of pcDNA3.1-A3G-HA or pcDNA3.1-GFP-HA. **a**, **b** lysates from these transfected cell samples were subjected to co-immunoprecipitation analysis using anti-HA agarose beads and then detected by western blotting. **c** The effect of MOV10 on the interaction between A3G and Vif. 293T cells were transfected with 2 μg of pcDNA3.1-A3G-HA together with 1 μg of pcDNA3.1-Vif-FLAG, and 2 μg of pcDNA3.1-MOV10-FLAG and then treated with MG132 (4 μM) for 16 h. Samples were immunoprecipitated with anti-HA agarose beads and analyzed by western blotting. Empty vector pcDNA3.1 was used to equalize DNA amounts in each transfection. Values in **c** represent portions of Vif-FLAG normalized against A3G-HA relative to control values. Data in **a**, **b**, and **c** are representative of at least three independent experiments

the effects of MOV10 on the interaction between Vif and different components in the complex. We transfected Vif-HA- and MOV10-FLAG-expressing plasmids with pcDNA3.1-ElonginB-FLAG, pcDNA3.1-ElonginC-FLAG, pcDNA3.1-Cullin 5-FLAG, or pcDNA3.1-CBF-β-FLAG into 293T cells. After immunoprecipitation, we found that the interactions of Vif with ElonginB, ElonginC, Cullin 5, and CBF-β significantly decreased when MOV10 was overexpressed (Fig. 5a–d), indicating that MOV10 affects Vif-ElonginB, Vif-ElonginC, Vif-Cullin 5, and Vif-CBF-β interactions during the assembly of the Vif-CBF-β-Cullin 5-ElonginB-ElonginC complex.

According to the above results, we suspected that MOV10 could interact with ElonginB, ElonginC, Cullin 5, or CBF-β. To test this hypothesis, we co-transfected

293T cells with pcDNA3.1-MOV10-HA plus pcDNA3.1-ElonginB-FLAG, pcDNA3.1-ElonginC-FLAG, pcDNA3.1-Cullin 5-FLAG or pcDNA3.1-CBF-β-FLAG. Previous study has demonstrated that ElonginC, ElonginB, and Cullin 5 can interact with each other [39]. To eliminate the influence of these endogenous proteins, siRNAs specific to *ElonginB*, *ElonginC*, and *Cullin 5* mRNA were also co-transfected into cells at the same time (Fig. 6a). After immunoprecipitation and western blotting, significant binding was found between MOV10 and ElonginC or Cullin 5 (Fig. 6c, d). To further confirm the binding, we detected the interaction between MOV10-HA and endogenous ElonginC or Cullin 5. As shown in the Fig. 6f, g, the same phenomenon was observed. After treatment with an RNase mixture,

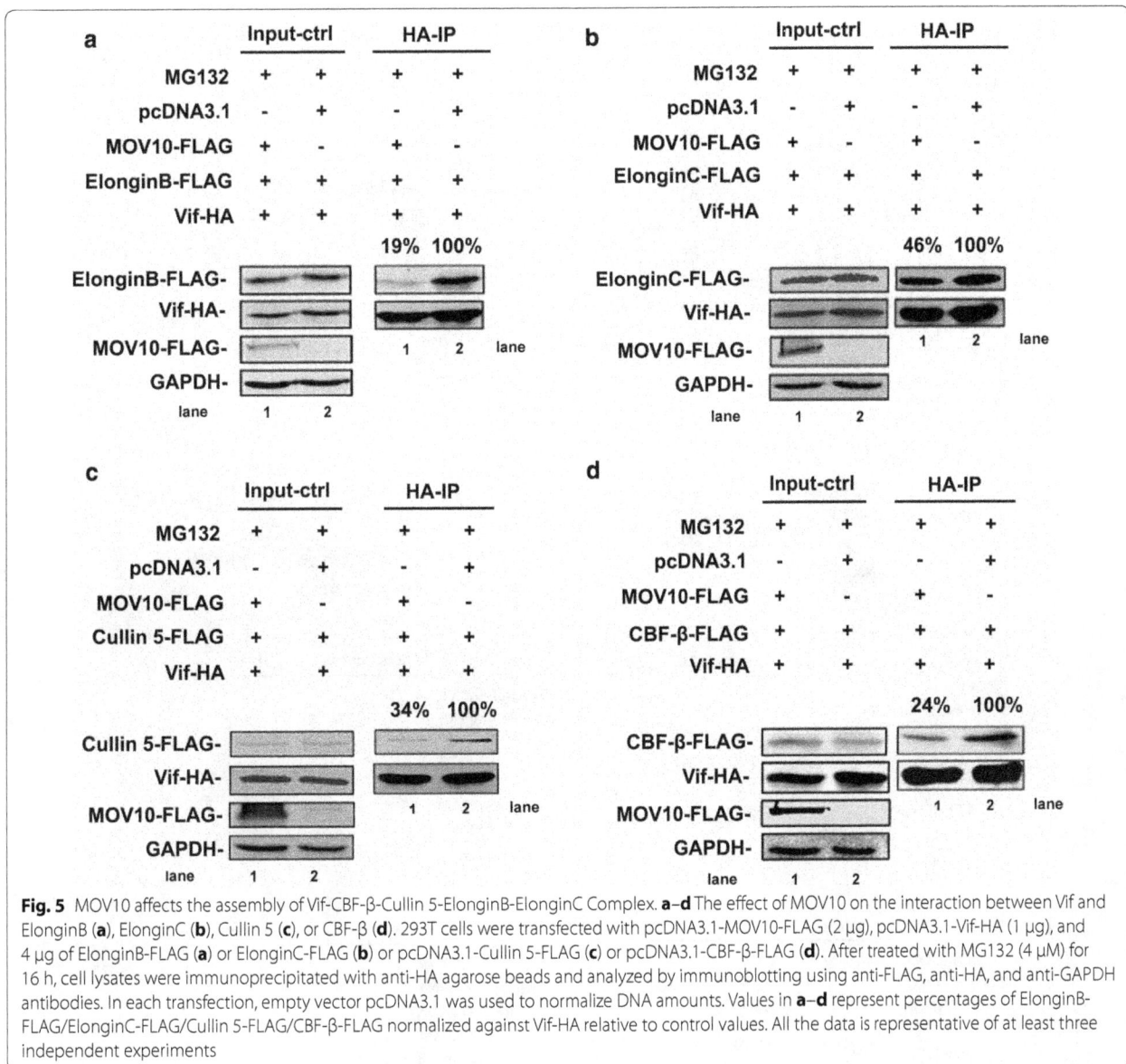

Fig. 5 MOV10 affects the assembly of Vif-CBF-β-Cullin 5-ElonginB-ElonginC Complex. **a–d** The effect of MOV10 on the interaction between Vif and ElonginB (**a**), ElonginC (**b**), Cullin 5 (**c**), or CBF-β (**d**). 293T cells were transfected with pcDNA3.1-MOV10-FLAG (2 µg), pcDNA3.1-Vif-HA (1 µg), and 4 µg of ElonginB-FLAG (**a**) or ElonginC-FLAG (**b**) or pcDNA3.1-Cullin 5-FLAG (**c**) or pcDNA3.1-CBF-β-FLAG (**d**). After treated with MG132 (4 µM) for 16 h, cell lysates were immunoprecipitated with anti-HA agarose beads and analyzed by immunoblotting using anti-FLAG, anti-HA, and anti-GAPDH antibodies. In each transfection, empty vector pcDNA3.1 was used to normalize DNA amounts. Values in **a–d** represent percentages of ElonginB-FLAG/ElonginC-FLAG/Cullin 5-FLAG/CBF-β-FLAG normalized against Vif-HA relative to control values. All the data is representative of at least three independent experiments

we found that the binding of MOV10 with Cullin 5 was partially dependent on RNA, whereas the interaction between MOV10 and ElonginC was not (Fig. 6h, i). However, the interaction between MOV10 and ElonginB or CBF-β was not detected (Fig. 6b, e).

The helicase activity center of MOV10 is required for its inhibitory effects on Vif-mediated A3G degradation

MOV10 contains a DEAG-box (D-E-A-G = Asp-Glu-Ala-Gly) motif and the DEAG-box mutant impairs the helicase activity of MOV10 [18, 28]. To examine whether the DEAG-box motif was required for the effects of MOV10 on Vif-mediated degradation of A3G, we used a MOV10-DEAG mutant (a point mutation in the DEAG-box motif, from DEAG to DQAG) to repeat the experiment shown as Fig. 1a [18, 22, 23, 32, 40]. Compared with wild-type MOV10, the MOV10-DEAG mutant almost lost the ability to prevent the degradation of A3G mediated by Vif (Fig. 7a), suggesting that the DEAG-box motif is involved in regulating this inhibitory effects of MOV10. To confirm this conclusion, we further detected the binding of the MOV10-DEAG mutant with ElonginC or Cullin 5. Compared with wild-type MOV10, the bindings of MOV10-DEAG mutant with ElonginC or Cullin 5 decreased significantly (Fig. 7b, c), suggesting that the DEAG-box motif of MOV10 plays an important role in the interaction between MOV10 with ElonginC or Cullin 5.

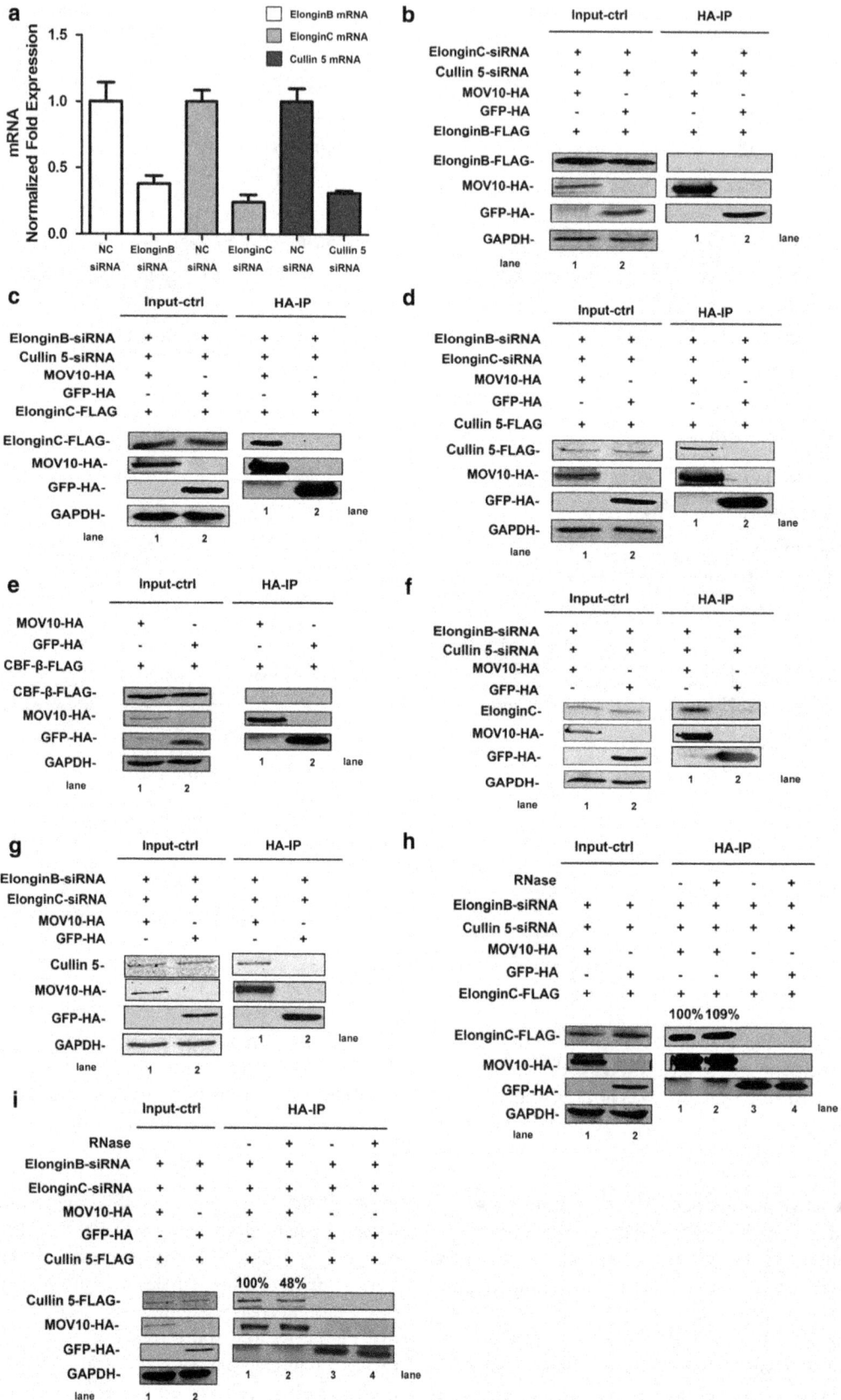

(See figure on previous page.)

Fig. 6 MOV10 binds with ElonginC or Cullin 5. **a** The knockdown efficiency of siElonginB, siElonginC and siCullin 5. 293T cells were transfected with siElonginB, siElonginC or siCullin 5, after 48 h, the cells were collected and detected with qRT-PCR. Data in A represents mean ± SD (*error bars*). **b–i** Co-immunoprecipitated analysis of the interaction between MOV10 and ElonginB (**b**), ElonginC (**c**, **f**, **h**), Cullin 5 (**d**, **g**, **i**), or CBF-β (**e**). pcDNA3.1-ElonginB-FLAG plus siElonginC and siCullin 5 (**b**), pcDNA3.1-ElonginC-FLAG plus siElonginB and siCullin 5 (**c**, **h**), pcDNA3.1-Cullin 5-FLAG plus siElonginB and siEloingC (**d**, **i**) or pcDNA3.1-CBF-β-FLAG (**e**) was transfected into 293T cells with pcDNA3.1-MOV10-HA or pcDNA3.1-GFP-HA. 293T cells were transfected with pcDNA3.1-MOV10-HA (pcDNA3.1-GFP-HA as a control) plus siElonginB and siCullin 5 (**f**) or siElonginB and siEloingC (**g**). After 48 h, the cells were collected and immunoprecipitated with anti-HA agarose beads (**b–i**). The samples in **h** and **i** were treated with RNase mixture. And then, immunoprecipitated samples were analyzed by immunoblotting with anti-FLAG, anti-HA, anti-GAPDH, anti-MOV10, anti-ElonginC, and anti-Cullin 5 antibodies. Empty vector pcDNA3.1 was used to equalize DNA amounts in each transfection. Values in **h** and **i** represent portions of ElonginC-FLAG/Cullin 5-FLAG normalized against MOV10-HA and compared with control. Data in **a–i** is representative of at least three independent experiments

MOV10 counteracts Vif-mediated A3G degradation in the context of HIV-1 replication

All of the above experiments were performed in the context of lack of other HIV-1 proteins. To verify whether the effect of MOV10 on Vif-mediated A3G degradation could be observed in the context of HIV-1 replication, we used two types of HIV-1 pNL4-3ΔEnv-GFP clones. Human 293T cells were transfected with pNL4-3ΔEnv-GFP-ΔVif, pcDNA3.1-Vif-HA, pcDNA3.1-A3G-HA, and different amounts of MOV10-FLAG-expressing plasmid. Consistent with Fig. 1b, the expression levels of A3G and Vif were correlated with the expression levels of MOV10 in the presence of other HIV-1 proteins (Fig. 8a). Moreover, the same results were observed when we co-transfected 293T cells with pNL4-3ΔEnv-GFP, pcDNA3.1-A3G-HA, and different amounts of pcDNA3.1-MOV10-FLAG (Fig. 8b). To further confirm this, we examined the effect of MOV10 depletion on Vif-mediated A3G degradation in the context of HIV-1 replication. The same phenotypes as shown in Fig. 1c were recapitulated by *MOV10*-specific siRNAs (Fig. 8c, d). These data indicate that MOV10 can inhibit Vif-mediated degradation of A3G in the context of HIV-1 replication.

MOV10 increases the quantity of A3G in HIV-1 virions by protecting A3G from Vif-mediated degradation

As noted above, we demonstrated that MOV10 could increase the quantity of A3G by interfering with the proteasome pathway in virus-producing cells. Given that A3G can be packaged into HIV-1 virions and exert anti-HIV-1 activity [2, 35, 41–44]. We next evaluated the effects of MOV10 on the quantity of A3G in HIV-1 virions. We co-transfected 293T cells with pNL4-3ΔEnv-GFP, pcDNA3.1-A3G-HA, and pcDNA3.1-MOV10-FLAG, subsequently collected the supernatants and cells of each sample. Interestingly, although MOV10 enhanced A3G levels in cell lysates, the quantity of A3G was also increased in the supernatant viral particles (Fig. 9a). To further confirm this, the A3G levels were analyzed in virus-producing cells and viral particles following

depletion of endogenous MOV10 with *MOV10*-specific siRNAs. MOV10 knockdown could reduce the quantity of A3G in both virus producing cells and viral particles (Fig. 9b). Previous studies showed that MOV10 can be packaged into virions and affects HIV-1 replication at multiple stages. Here, we overexpressed MOV10 in a dose-dependent manner, and we found that there was a synergy between the packaging levels of MOV10 and A3G (Fig. 9c). Taken together, these results demonstrate that MOV10 increases the quantity of A3G in HIV-1 virions by interfering with the Vif-mediated ubiquitin–proteasome pathway.

Furthermore, to explore the potential synergistic effect of MOV10 and A3G on the infectivity of the newly-produced virions, NL4-3-ΔEnv-GFP and NL4-3-ΔEnv-GFP-ΔVif particles were produced with increasing amounts of MOV10 in either the presence or absence of A3G. After normalization for HIV-1 p24, TZM-bl cells were infected with these viral particles and then the infectivity of viruses was determined (Fig. 10a, b). For NL4-3-ΔEnv-GFP-ΔVif particles, compared with the group of single MOV10 or A3G treatment, the inhibitory effect of MOV10 or MOV10-DEAG mutant plus A3G group was equal to the effect of single A3G treatment group. And, the depletion of endogenous MOV10 with siRNA in the presence of A3G also has no impact on HIV-1 infectivity. It is consistent with previous study that co-expression of MOV10 did not enhance the inhibitory effect of A3G on the infectivity of ΔVif HIV-1 (Fig. 10a) [29]. However, for NL4-3-ΔEnv-GFP particles, the fold reductions in infectivity at various amounts of MOV10 were different in the presence or absence of A3G and endogenous MOV10 was helpful for A3G to decrease the infectivity of HIV-1. But, MOV10-DEAG mutant lost its ability to help A3G decrease the infectivity of HIV-1 (Fig. 10b). This data further confirms that DEAG-box motif of MOV10 plays an important role in protecting A3G from Vif-mediated degradation. These results indicate that the inhibitory effect of A3G on the infectivity of HIV-1 can be synergistically enhanced by MOV10.

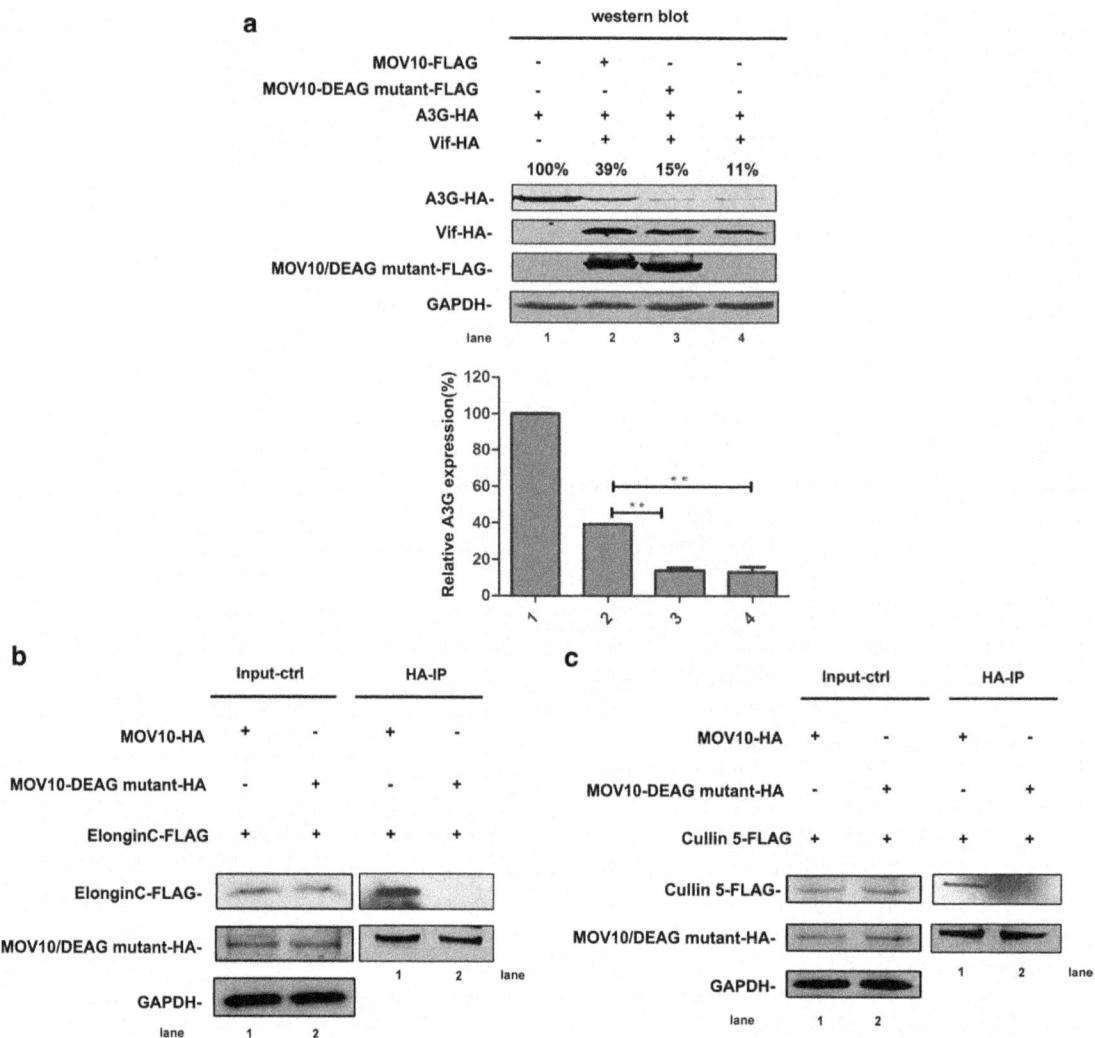

Fig. 7 The DEAG-box motif of MOV10 is required for the binding of MOV10 with ElonginC or Cullin 5. **a** The effect of MOV10-DEAG mutant on Vif-mediated A3G degradation. 293T cells were transfected with 0.4 μg of pcDNA3.1-Vif-HA, 0.8 μg of pcDNA3.1-A3G-HA, and 1.5 μg of pcDNA3.1-MOV10-FLAG or pcDNA3.1-MOV10-DEAG-mutant-FLAG as indicated. After 48 h, cell lysates were detected by western blotting assay with anti-HA, anti-FLAG, and anti-GAPDH antibodies. Values represent portions of A3G-HA normalized against GAPDH and compared with control. **b**, **c** Co-immunoprecipitated analysis of the interaction between MOV10-DEAG mutant and ElonginC or Cullin 5. Human 293T cells were transfected with 2 μg of pcDNA3.1-MOV10-HA or pcDNA3.1-MOV10-DEAG-HA and 6 μg of pcDNA3.1-ElonginC-FLAG or pcDNA3.1-Cullin 5-FLAG. After 24 h, MG132 were added in the transfected cells for 16 h. Then, the cells were collected for co-immunoprecipitation analysis with anti-HA agarose beads and detected by western blotting with anti-HA, anti-FLAG, and anti-GAPDH antibodies. In each transfection, empty vector pcDNA3.1 was used to equalize DNA amounts. Values in **a** represent percentages of A3G-HA normalized against GAPDH relative to control. The *bar graphs* in **a** represent the average expression of A3G with different treatments and relative to the A3G-only reaction control (set to 100%). Data in **a** represent mean ± SD from three independent experiments. Statistical significance was determined using t test: **$p \leq 0.01$. All the data in **a**, **b**, and **c** is representative of at least three independent experiments

Discussion

In this report, we studied the relationship between MOV10 and A3G in the presence of HIV-1 Vif. Interestingly, we observed that MOV10 increased the levels of A3G and Vif in a concentration-dependent manner. The phenomenon is consistent with the previous study that the expression levels of A3G and Vif can be increased simultaneously in the presence of the proteasome inhibitor MG132 [45, 46]. Vif is an E3 ubiquitin ligase substrate receptor that interacts with host factors ElonginB, ElonginC, Cullin 5, and CBF-β to form an E3 ubiquitin ligase complex, which results in the polyubiquitylation of both Vif and A3G. And then, the Vif-A3G complex can be degraded together via the ubiquitin–proteasome system

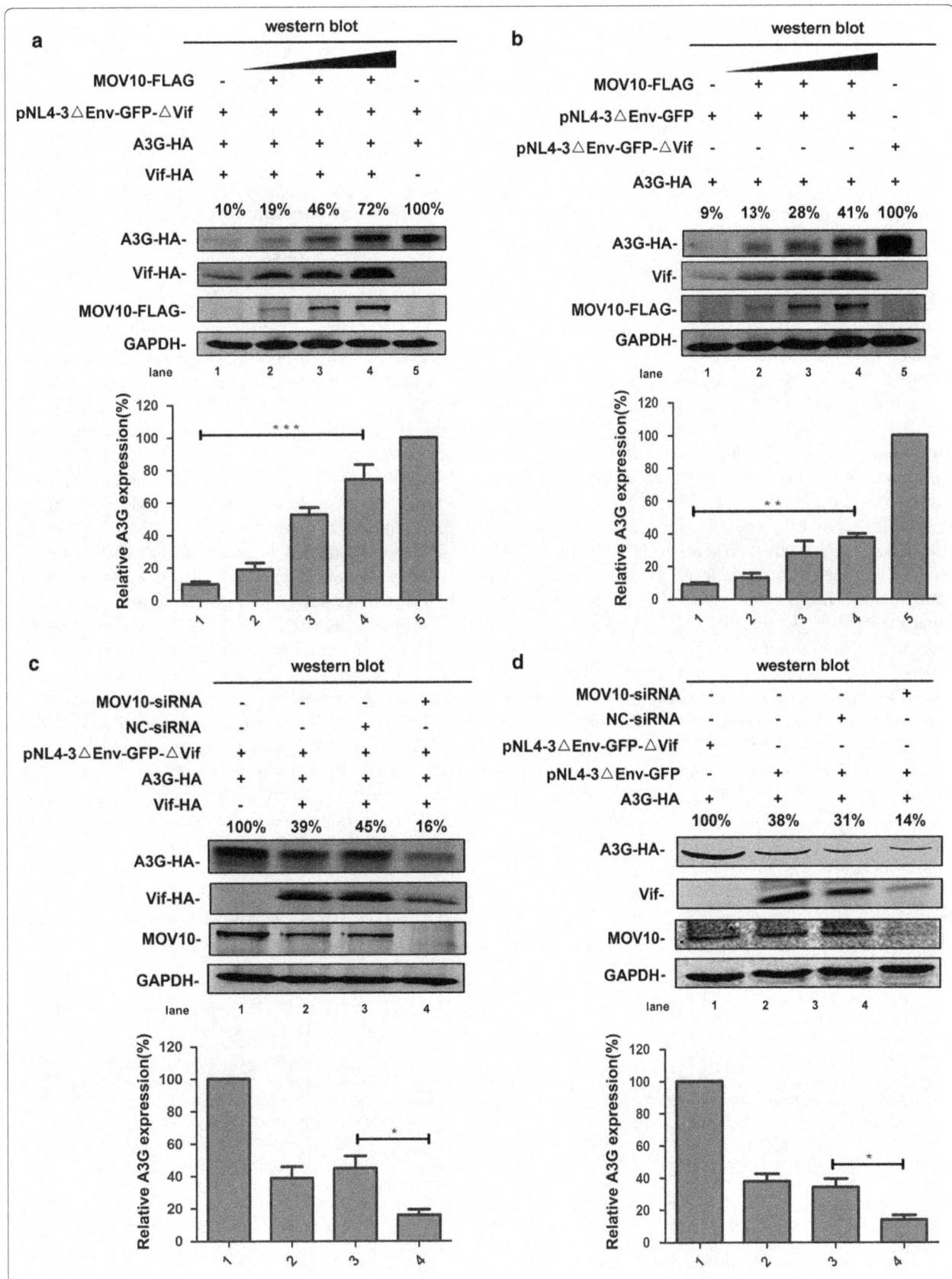

(See figure on previous page.)

Fig. 8 MOV10 reduces A3G proteasomal degradation significantly in the context of HIV-1 replication. **a, b** Overexpression of MOV10 inhibits Vif-induced A3G degradation in the context of HIV-1 replication. Human 293T cells were transfected with 0.8 μg of pcDNA3.1-A3G-HA, different amounts of pcDNA3.1-MOV10-FLAG (from 0.5 μg to 2 μg), 0.5 μg of pcDNA3.1-Vif-HA, 1 μg of pNL4-3ΔEnv-GFP-ΔVif (**a**) and/or 1 μg of pNL4-3ΔEnv-GFP (**b**) as indicated. Then, cells were collected at 48 h for western blotting assay with anti-FLAG, anti-HA, anti-Vif, and anti-GAPDH antibodies. **c, d** The effect of MOV10 depletion on the proteasomal degradation of A3G in the context of other HIV-1 proteins. 293T cells were transfected with pcDNA3.1-A3G-HA (0.8 μg), pcDNA3.1-Vif-HA (0.5 μg), *MOV10*-specific siRNA (or negative control-siRNA), 1 μg of pNL4-3ΔEnv-GFP-ΔVif (**c**) and/or 1 μg of pNL4-3ΔEnv-GFP (**d**). Cell lysates were detected by immunoblotting with anti-HA, anti-FLAG, anti-MOV10, anti-Vif, and anti-GAPDH antibodies. The *bar graphs* represent the average expression of A3G with different treatment and relative to the A3G-only reaction control (set to 100%). Data in **a–d** represent mean ± SD from three independent experiments. Statistical significance was determined using *t* test: *$p \leq 0.05$; **$p \leq 0.01$; ***$p \leq 0.001$. Empty vector pcDNA3.1 was used to equalize DNA amounts in each transfection. Values in **a–d** represent portions of A3G-HA normalized against GAPDH and compared with control. Each data is representative of at least three independent experiments

[6, 12, 28, 37, 47, 48]. HIV-1 Vif has at least 4 conserved motifs, which are required for interactions with host proteins. The HCCH motif can bind to Cullin 5, the BC-box motif (144-SLQYLA-149) binds to ElonginC, 101-DVMK-104 binds to ElonginB, and 88-EW-89 is crucial for binding with CBF-β [38, 49–51]. Through a series of co-immunoprecipitation analyses, we found that MOV10 can disrupt the interaction of Vif with ElonginB, ElonginC, Cullin 5, or CBF-β and then decrease the ubiquitination of A3G. Finally, the degradations of A3G and Vif are blocked and their expression levels in cells are increased subsequently. These results suggest that MOV10 functions to mediate assembly of the Vif-CBF-β-ElonginB-ElonginC-Cullin 5 complex.

Previous studies have shown that Cullin 5 functions as a scaffold protein for the *E3 ubiquitin ligase* [52, 53] ubiquitin–proteasome . ElonginB, ElonginC, and CBF-β are adaptor proteins that function to maintain this complex. Moreover, Vif acts as a substrate acceptor to modulate the degradation of A3G [52, 54]. Therefore, reduced binding of Vif with Cullin 5 could affect the complex assembly efficiency. Moreover, researchers have verified the interactions between the different components of the complex. The binding of Cullin 5 to Vif enhances the stability of the Vif-CBF-β interaction [55]. Conversely, CBF-β is also crucial for the binding of Vif with Cullin 5, ElonginB,

and ElonginC [37, 56, 57]. ElonginB and ElonginC play important roles in the interaction between Vif and CBF-β [16]. To clarify the mechanisms through which MOV10 disrupts the assembly of the Vif-CBF-β-ElonginB-ElonginC-Cullin 5 complex, we examined whether there were direct interactions between MOV10 and different components of the CBF-β-Cullin 5-ElonginB-ElonginC complex. The results demonstrate that MOV10 can bind with ElonginC or Cullin 5 and that binding between MOV10 and Cullin 5 is partially dependent on RNA. Our own study and previous studies have shown that MOV10 usually interacts with numerous RNA-associated proteins, such as AGO1/2, A3G, and HIV-1 Rev [20, 32]. Thus, it is not surprising that MOV10 interacts with Cullin 5 in an RNA-dependent manner. Accordingly, significant decreases in the binding of Vif with ElonginB, ElonginC, Cullin 5, and CBF-β were observed when MOV10 was overexpressed. For the inhibitory effects of MOV10 on the binding of Vif with ElonginB or CBF-β, the interactions of MOV10 with ElonginC, Cullin 5, and Vif may induce structural changes in the Vif-CBF-β-ElonginB-ElonginC-Cullin 5 complex, subsequently disrupting the interactions between Vif and ElonginB and between Vif and CBF-β. Several studies have shown that DEAG-box motif of MOV10 is crucial for its helicase activity [18, 28]. In our report, we also explored the

(See figure on next page.)

Fig. 9 MOV10 increases the quantity of A3G in HIV-1 virions. **a** Overexpression of MOV10 increases the quantity of A3G in virions. Human 293T cells were transfected with 0.8 μg of pcDNA3.1-A3G-HA, 1.5 μg of pcDNA3.1-MOV10-FLAG, 1 μg of pNL4-3ΔEnv-GFP or pNL4-3ΔEnv-GFP-ΔVif as indicated. **b** The effect of endogenous MOV10 knockdown on Vif-induced A3G degradation in HIV-1 virions. Cells were transfected with 0.8 μg of pcDNA3.1-A3G-HA, 50 nM of *MOV10*-specific siRNA (or negative control siRNA), and 1 μg of pNL4-3ΔEnv-GFP or pNL4-3ΔEnv-GFP-ΔVif. **c** MOV10 can be packaged into HIV-1 virions and its packaging level increases with the survival level of A3G. 293T cells were transfected with 0.8 μg of pcDNA3.1-A3G-HA, different amounts of pcDNA3.1-MOV10-FLAG (from 0.5 to 1.5 μg), 1 μg of pNL4-3ΔEnv-GFP or pNL4-3ΔEnv-GFP-ΔVif. **a, b** and **c** After 48 h, cell pellets and supernatants were collected respectively. Cell pellets were lysed and subjected to immunoblotting with anti-HA, anti-FLAG, anti-MOV10, anti-Vif, and anti-GAPDH antibodies. VLPs were collected from filtered supernatants by ultracentrifugation. The pelleted VLPs were lysed and detected by western blotting with anti-HA, anti-FLAG, and anti-p24 antibodies. The *bar graphs* represent the average expression of A3G with different treatments and relative to the A3G-only reaction control (set to 100%). Data in **a–c** represent mean ± SD from three independent experiments. Statistical significance was determined using *t* test: *$p \leq 0.05$; **$p \leq 0.01$; ***$p \leq 0.001$. In each transfection, empty vector pcDNA3.1 was used to equalize DNA amounts. Values in **a–c** represent percentages of A3G-HA normalized against GAPDH or p24 and compared with control. Results are representative of at least three independent experiments

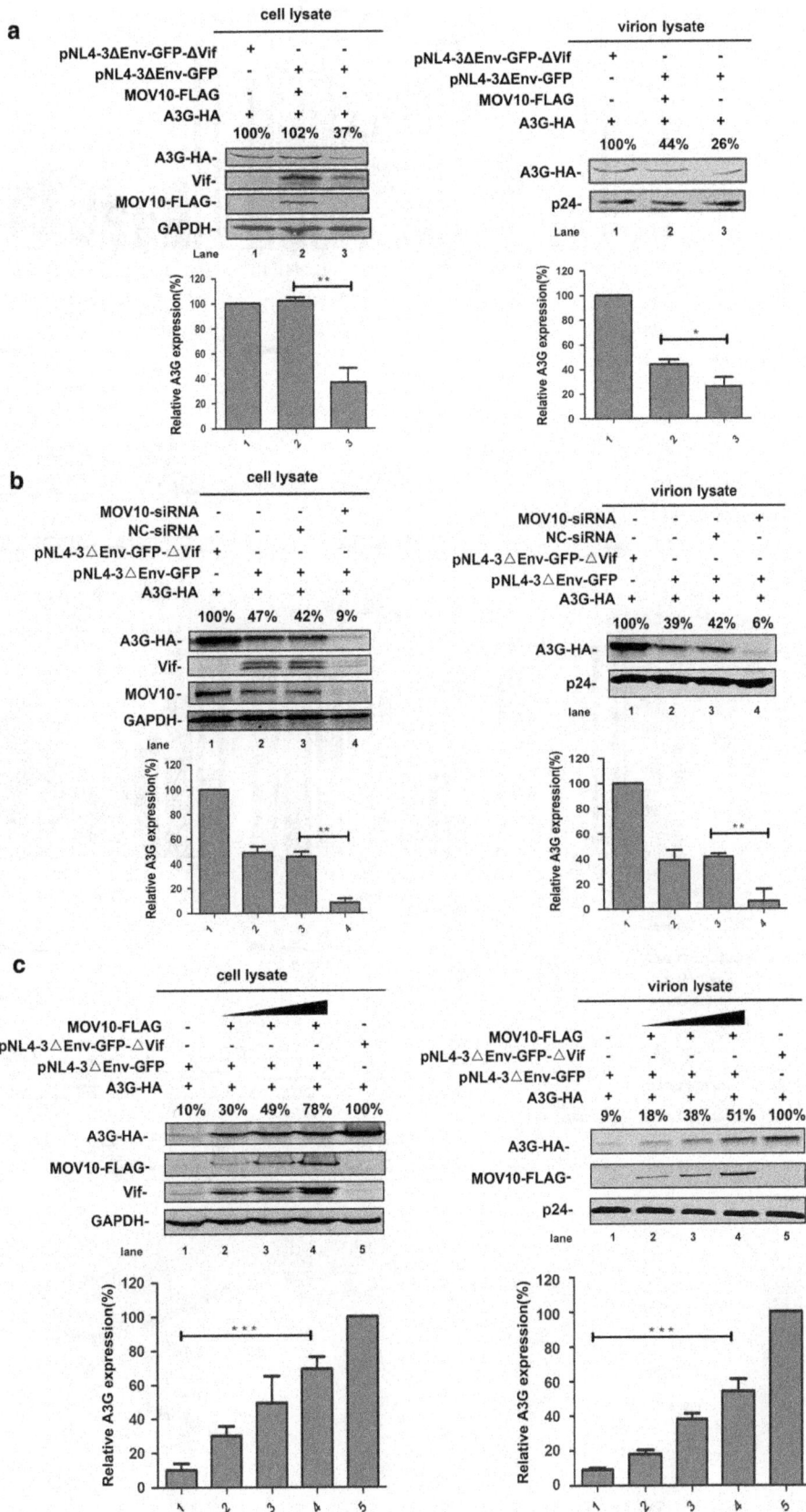

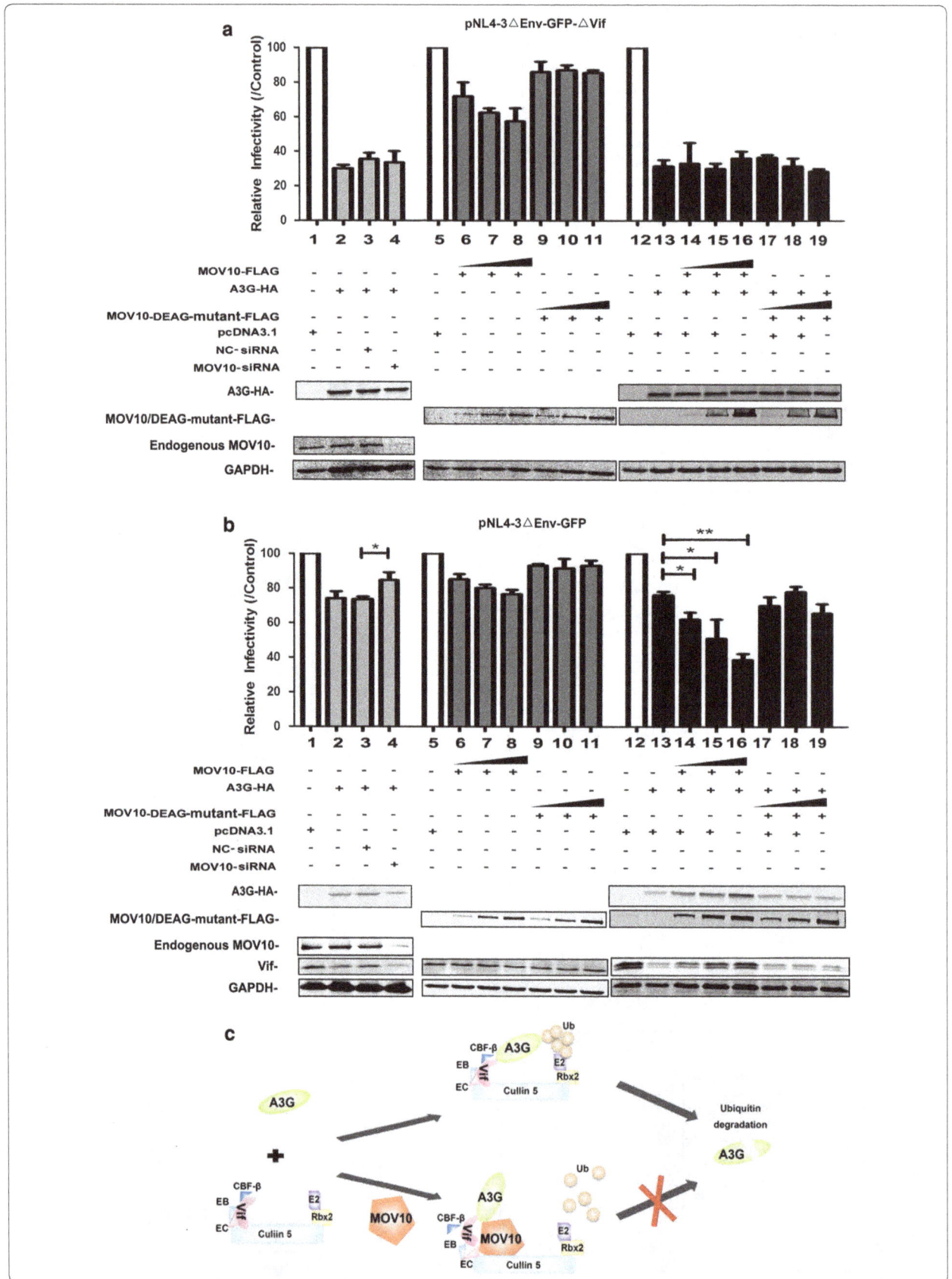

Fig. 10 MOV10 synergistically enhances the inhibitory effect of A3G on the infectivity of HIV-1. **a**, **b** *MOV10*-specific siRNA was transfected in 293T cells with pcDNA3.1-A3G-HA (0.8 μg), pCMV-VSV-G (2.5 μg), and pNL4-3ΔEnv-GFP-ΔVif (7.5 μg) or pNL4-3ΔEnv-GFP (7.5 μg). 293T cells were co-transfected with pCMV-VSV-G (2.5 μg), pNL4-3ΔEnv-GFP-ΔVif (7.5 μg) or pNL4-3ΔEnv-GFP (7.5 μg), and increasing amounts of pcDNA3.1-MOV10-FLAG (0.5–1.5 μg) or pcDNA3.1-MOV10-DEAG-mutant-FLAG (0.5–1.5 μg) in the presence or absence of pcDNA3.1-A3G-HA (0.8 μg). Culture supernatants containing 5 ng of p24 were used to infect TZM-bl cells and luciferase activity was determined at 72 h post infection. For viruses with different amounts of MOV10 but no A3G, and viruses with a fixed amount of A3G combined with different amounts of MOV10 or not, the data are plotted as relative infectivity, with the control virus (pcDNA3.1) set to 100%. Error bars represent standard errors from three independent experiments. Statistical significance was determined using t test: *$p \leq 0.05$; **$p \leq 0.01$. **c** A cartoon to show the interaction between MOV10, A3G, and Vif. In the absence of MOV10, the Vif-CBF-β-Cullin 5-ElonginB-ElonginC complex is stable and triggers the proteasomal degradation of A3G. In the presence of MOV10, the assembly of Vif-CBF-β-Cullin 5-ElonginB-ElonginC complex can be disturbed by MOV10, which leads to A3G escaping from Vif-induced proteasomal degradation

correlation between the helicase activity and anti-HIV-1 function of MOV10. Because the binding of MOV10-DEAG mutant with ElonginC or Cullin 5 decreased significantly, it almost lost the ability to protect A3G from Vif-mediated degradation, indicating that the helicase activity center of MOV10 is required for its inhibitory effect on Vif-mediated A3G degradation.

According to these data, we propose a model that, during the process of HIV-1 infection, MOV10 can interact with ElonginC and Cullin 5 to disturb the interaction of Vif with ElonginB, ElonginC, Cullin 5 or CBF-β and subsequently interfere with the assembly of Vif-CBF-β-Cullin 5-ElonginB-ElonginC complex which induces the ubiquitination of A3G. In this way, MOV10 prevents A3G from proteasomal degradation and subsequently enhances the level of A3G in virus-producing cells. It is well known that A3G can be packaged into HIV-1 virions and inhibit HIV-1 replication at multiple stages, the A3G level in newly-produced virions should be increased in the presence of MOV10 (Fig. 10c) [44]. Indeed, we found that the A3G level was significantly enhanced in virions by MOV10 overexpression and significantly reduced by MOV10 knockdown in the context of HIV-1 replication.

Moreover, the synergistic effects on the infectivity and replication of HIV-1 between MOV10 and A3G have been tested. Previous study has demonstrated that co-expression of MOV10 does not affect the inhibitory effect of A3G on the infectivity of ΔVif HIV-1 [29]. Our results also show the same phenomenon that the inhibitory effect of A3G plus MOV10 group on ΔVif HIV-1 is consistent with the effect of single A3G treatment group. As the anti-HIV-1 activity of A3G is more potent than that of MOV10, it will overspread the anti-HIV-1 effect of MOV10 when Vif deficiency. Nevertheless, consistent with our hypothesis, the infectivity of Vif-positive viral particles is synergistically inhibited by MOV10 and A3G. In 2010, Wang et al. [22] have shown that the replication of HIV-1 was enhanced by the depletion of endogenous MOV10 in permissive human T cell line (CEM-SS). Previous study also showed that MOV10

can be packaged into HIV-1 virions and inhibit viral replication at a postentry step [28]. However, little effect of MOV10 on HIV-1 replication in Hut78 T cells was reported by another group [58]. Considering that high concentration of the virus and short term infection will cover up the true effect of antiviral factors, we used low dose virus (5 ng of HIV-1 p24) to perform the experiment and extended the observation time. We found that the replication of wild-type HIV-1 was enhanced in MOV10-shRNA transduced non-permissive human T cells (H9), indicating that MOV10 and A3G can synergistically inhibit HIV-1 replication.

Conclusions
Therefore, our results reveal a novel anti-HIV-1 mechanism of MOV10: it prevents A3G from Vif-induced proteasomal degradation and then increases the levels of A3G both in cells and in newly-synthesized virions. In addition, because both MOV10 and A3G have anti-HIV-1 activity and belong to the interferon antiviral system, our findings suggested that these proteins are of synergistic anti-HIV-1 activities. These results will help us to get more comprehensive and profound understanding of MOV10 and A3G.

Methods
Plasmid construction and siRNAs synthesis
pcDNA3.1-A3G-HA, pcDNA3.1-GFP-HA, pcDNA3.1-MOV10-FLAG, pcDNA3.1-MOV10-HA, pcDNA3.1-rMOV10-FLAG, pcDNA3.1-MOV10-DEAG-mutant-HA, pcDNA3.1-MOV10-DEAG-mutant-FLAG and pcDNA3.1-Ub-FLAG were constructed as described previously [20, 32, 59]. pcDNA3.1-Vif-HA, pcDNA3.1-Vif-FLAG, pcDNA3.1-ElonginB-FLAG, pcDNA3.1-Cullin 5-FLAG, pcDNA3.1-CBF-β-FLAG, and were constructed by our lab [60]. HA or FLAG epitope tagged codon-optimized HIV-1 *vif* was constructed by chemically-synthesis of DNA fragment and subcloned into pcDNA3.1. Codon optimization was performed using the sequence of HIV-1$_{NL4-3}$ [61]. FLAG epitope tag sequence at 3'

terminus of ElonginB, Cullin 5, or CBF-β was amplified through reverse transcription-polymerase chain reaction (RT-PCR) with the mRNA of 293T cells as the template. ElonginC with FLAG tag sequence at its 3′ terminus was amplified via PCR from the pElonginC-HA plasmid, which was generously provided by Dr. Xianghui Yu in Jilin University [62]. Then, the tagged ElonginB, ElonginC, Cullin 5, or CBF-β was inserted into pcDNA3.1 vector. HIV-1 proviral construct pNL4-3-ΔEnv-GFP has been described in our previous reports [63, 64]. pNL4-3-ΔEnv-GFP-ΔVif, a *vif* defective construct, was generated from pNL4-3-ΔEnv-GFP. The *vif* gene in pNL4-3-ΔEnv-GFP-ΔVif was disrupted by PCR-mediated site-directed mutagenesis and introduced nonsense mutations at codon positions 26, 27 (AAA, CAC → TAA, TAG) and/or 33, 34 (ACT, AAA → TAA, TAG) [65]. The vector pLKO.1-TRC, which contains a U6 promoter and *puromycin* selection gene and was obtained from Addgene (plasmid # 10878), was used for expression of MOV10-shRNA or scrambled control (Scr)-shRNA. Forward oligo of MOV10-shRNA (TRCN0000425452): 5′-CCGGGGCCAGTGTTTCGAGAGTTTCCTCGAGG AAACTCTCGAAACACTGGCCTTTTTG-3′; reverse oligo of MOV10-shRNA: 5′-AATTCAAAAAGGCCAG TGTTTCGAGAGTTTCCTCGAGGAAACTCTCGAA ACACTGGCC-3′. Scr-shRNA forward oligo: 5′- CCGGA ACGTACGCGGAATACTTCGACTCGAGTCGAAGTA TTCCGCGTACGTTTTTTTG-3′; Scr-shRNA reverse oligo: 5′- AATTCAAAAAAACGTACGCGGAATACTT CGACTCGAGTCGAAGTATTCCGCGTACGTT-3′ [40]. All oligos were synthesized from Ribobio (Guangzhou, China).

The siGENOME SMART pool against MOV10 and siRNA for negative control were designed by Dharmacon and the target sequences for *MOV10*-specific siRNAs were chosen as described previously [20, 32]. *ElonginB*-specific siRNA, *ElonginC*-specific siRNA, and *Cullin 5*-specific siRNA were designed and synthesized by Ribobio (Guangzhou, China).

Cell culture and transfection
Human 293T cells were obtained from American Type Culture Collection (ATCC) and grown at 37 °C with 5% CO2 in Dulbecco's modified Eagle's medium (DMEM) (Invitrogen) supplemented with 10% fetal bovine serum (FBS) (Invitrogen) and 1% penicillin–streptomycin (Invitrogen). The cells were transfected with the indicated plasmids or siRNAs by lipofectamine 2000 (Invitrogen). The procedures described by the manufacturer were followed.

Co-immunoprecipitation and western blotting
Co-immunoprecipitation and western blotting assays were performed as previously described [20, 32]. In brief, human 293T cells were lysed with the lysis buffer (150 mM NaCl, 50 mM Tris–HCl [pH 7.5], 1 mM EDTA, 1% Triton X-100, 0.5% NP-40, plus PMSF and protease inhibitor cocktail [Sigma]) for 30 min at 4 °C. The cell lysates were clarified by centrifugation at 18,000g for 30 min at 4 °C, then mixed with anti-HA agarose beads (Sigma) and incubated at 4 °C for 4 h, followed by washing four times with cold lysis buffer and eluting in gel loading buffer. As indicated, the beads were treated with RNase mixture (DNase-free, Roche) (20 μg/ml) and incubated at 37 °C for 30 min. The immunoprecipitated samples were analyzed by SDS-PAGE and detected by western blotting. Anti-HA antibody (mouse monoclonal, Covance), anti-FLAG antibody (rabbit polyclonal, MBL), anti-GAPDH antibody (rabbit polyclonal, MBL), anti-MOV10 antibody (rabbit polyclonal, Abcam), anti-ElonginC antibody (rabbit polyclonal, Abcam), anti-Cullin 5 antibody (rabbit polyclonal, Abcam), anti-A3G antibody (rabbit polyclonal, Abcam), anti-Vif antibody (mouse monoclonal, Abcam), and anti-HIV-1 p24 antibody (rabbitpolyclonal antibodies made by our lab) were used as primary antibodies [64]. Quantity One program (Biorad) was used to quantify the western blotting results.

HIV-1 virus-like particle (VLP) purification
Human 293T cells were transfected with pNL4-3-ΔEnv-GFP or pNL4-3-ΔEnv-GFP-ΔVif and other indicated plasmids. After 48 h of transfection, cell supernatants were collected, centrifuged at 4 °C for 10 min at 8000 rpm (≈ 7000 g) and filtered through a 0.45 μm filter to remove cellular debris. And the cell-free supernatants were concentrated by ultracentrifugation through a 20% sucrose cushions at 4 °C for 2 h at 45,000 rpm (≈ 40,000 g) (HITACHI Preparative Ultracentrifuge, CP80WX). Then, the pellets were re-suspended in RIPA buffer containing protease inhibitor cocktail and subjected to immunoblotting.

Construction of MOV10-knockdown H9 cells
The pLKO.1-MOV10-shRNA or pLKO.1-Scr-shRNA was co-transfected with psPAX2 and pCMV-VSV-G into 293T cells. After 48 h, the supernatants were harvested and filtered with 0.45 μm filters (Millipore). Then, H9 cells were infected with MOV10-specific-shRNA-expressing or Scr-shRNA-expressing lentivirus respectively for 8 h and cultured with fresh medium. After 48 h, virus-infected H9 cells were selected by puromycin (1 μg/ml) for 2 weeks and subjected to the following experiments.

Wild-type HIV-1 infection

MOV10-knockdown H9 cells and negative control cells were infected with HIV-1$_{NL4-3}$ (p24 titer of 5 ng ml^{-1}) for 3 h and then cultured with fresh medium and detected p24 in culture supernatant at different days. After 12 days, cells were collected and treated with the transcription factor buffer set including fixation/permeabilization and fixation/wash buffers (BD Biosciences) according to the manufacturer supernatant at different days. After 12 days, cellFITC-conjugated anti-HIV-1 p24 antibody (Santa Cruz Biotechnology) for intracellular HIV-1 Gag (p24) expression. Then, p24 positive cells were sorted with BD Aria sorter for further analysis. Data was analyzed with FlowJo software (Tree Star, Ashland, OR).

Virus infectivity assay

Human 293T cells were co-transfected with pCMV-VSV-G, pNL4-3ΔEnv-GFP-ΔVif (or pNL4-3ΔEnv-GFP), and increasing amounts of pcDNA3.1-MOV10-FLAG or pcDNA31-MOV10-mutant-FLAG in the presence or absence of A3G-HA expressing plasmid. The virus-containing supernatant were collected at 48 h after transfection and filtered by a 0.45 μm filter. After normalization for HIV-1 p24 by enzyme-linked immunosorbent assay (ELISA, Clonetech), TZM-bl cells (2.5×10^5 cells per well in 24-well plates) were infected with virus which containing 5 ng of p24 capsid. And then, luciferase enzyme activity determinations at 72 h post infection were carried out.

Abbreviations

MOV10: Moloney leukemia virus 10; A3G: Apolipoprotein-B-mRNA-editing enzyme catalytic polypeptide-like 3G; USP: Ubiquitin–proteasome system.

Authors' contributions

CL and HZ designed this project. CC, XM, QH, and CL performed most of the experiments. CC, CL, and HZ analyzed the results and wrote the paper. XL, FH, JZ, and JX participated in some experiments. TP constructed ElonginB- and Cullin 5-expressing plasmids. All authors read and approved the final manuscript.

Author details

¹ Institute of Human Virology, Zhongshan School of Medicine, Sun Yat-sen University, Guangzhou 510080, China. ² Key Laboratory of Tropical Disease Control of Ministry of Education, Zhongshan School of Medicine, Sun Yat-sen University, Guangzhou 510080, China. ³ Department of Pathology, The First Affiliated Hospital, Sun Yat-sen University, Guangzhou 510080, China. ⁴ Department of Infectious Diseases, The Fifth Affiliated Hospital, Sun Yat-sen University, Zhuhai 519000, China.

Acknowledgements

We obtained pNL4-3ΔEnv-GFP from the National Institutes of Health AIDS Research and Reference Reagent Program. We thank Dr. Xianghui Yu (Jinli University, China) for the ElonginC-HA-expressing plasmid, pElonginC-HA.

Competing interests

The authors declare that they have no competing interests.

Funding

This work was supported by the National Natural Science Foundation of China (No. 81471935), the National Natural Science Foundation of China (NSFC-NIH project) (No. 81561128007), the Important Key Program of Natural Science Foundation of China (No. 81590765), the Introduction of Innovative R&D Team Program of Guangdong Province (No. 2009010058), and the Joint-innovation Program in Healthcare for Special Scientific Research Projects of Guangzhou, China (No. 201508020256).

References

1. Zhang H, Yang B, Pomerantz RJ, Zhang C, Arunachalam SC, Gao L. The cytidine deaminase CEM15 induces hypermutation in newly synthesized HIV-1 DNA. Nature. 2003;424:94–8.
2. Mariani R, Chen D, Schrofelbauer B, Navarro F, Konig R, Bollman B, Munk C, Nymark-McMahon H, Landau NR. Species-specific exclusion of APOBEC3G from HIV-1 virions by Vif. Cell. 2003;114:21–31.
3. Lecossier D, Bouchonnet F, Clavel F, Hance AJ. Hypermutation of HIV-1 DNA in the absence of the Vif protein. Science. 2003;300:1112.
4. Mangeat B, Turelli P, Caron G, Friedli M, Perrin L, Trono D. Broad antiretroviral defence by human APOBEC3G through lethal editing of nascent reverse transcripts. Nature. 2003;424:99–103.
5. Bourara K, Liegler TJ, Grant RM. Target cell APOBEC3C can induce limited G-to-A mutation in HIV-1. PLoS Pathog. 2007;3:1477–85.
6. Mehle A, Strack B, Ancuta P, Zhang C, McPike M, Gabuzda D. Vif overcomes the innate antiviral activity of APOBEC3G by promoting its degradation in the ubiquitin-proteasome pathway. J Biol Chem. 2004;279:7792–8.
7. Sheehy AM, Gaddis NC, Malim MH. The antiretroviral enzyme APOBEC3G is degraded by the proteasome in response to HIV-1 Vif. Nat Med. 2003;9:1404–7.
8. Conticello SG, Harris RS, Neuberger MS. The Vif protein of HIV triggers degradation of the human antiretroviral DNA deaminase APOBEC3G. Curr Biol. 2003;13:2009–13.
9. Stopak K, de Noronha C, Yonemoto W, Greene WC. HIV-1 Vif blocks the antiviral activity of APOBEC3G by impairing both its translation and intracellular stability. Mol Cell. 2003;12:591–601.
10. Marin M, Rose KM, Kozak SL, Kabat D. HIV-1 Vif protein binds the editing enzyme APOBEC3G and induces its degradation. Nat Med. 2003;9:1398–403.
11. Yu X, Yu Y, Liu B, Luo K, Kong W, Mao P, Yu XF. Induction of APOBEC3G ubiquitination and degradation by an HIV-1 Vif-Cul5-SCF complex. Science. 2003;302:1056–60.
12. Kobayashi M, Takaori-Kondo A, Miyauchi Y, Iwai K, Uchiyama T. Ubiquitination of APOBEC3G by an HIV-1 Vif-Cullin5-Elongin B-Elongin C complex is essential for Vif function. J Biol Chem. 2005;280:18573–8.
13. Jager S, Kim DY, Hultquist JF, Shindo K, LaRue RS, Kwon E, Li M, Anderson BD, Yen L, Stanley D, et al. Vif hijacks CBF-beta to degrade APOBEC3G and promote HIV-1 infection. Nature. 2012;481:371–5.
14. Yu Y, Xiao Z, Ehrlich ES, Yu X, Yu XF. Selective assembly of HIV-1 Vif-Cul5-ElonginB-ElonginC E3 ubiquitin ligase complex through a novel SOCS box and upstream cysteines. Genes Dev. 2004;18:2867–72.
15. Zhang W, Du J, Evans SL, Yu Y, Yu XF. T-cell differentiation factor CBF-beta regulates HIV-1 Vif-mediated evasion of host restriction. Nature. 2012;481:376–9.
16. Wang X, Wang X, Zhang H, Lv M, Zuo T, Wu H, Wang J, Liu D, Wang Z, Zhang J, et al. Interactions between HIV-1 Vif and human ElonginB-ElonginC are important for CBF-beta binding to Vif. Retrovirology. 2013;10:94.
17. Koonin EV. A new group of putative RNA helicases. Trends Biochem Sci. 1992;17:495–7.
18. Gregersen LH, Schueler M, Munschauer M, Mastrobuoni G, Chen W, Kempa S, Dieterich C, Landthaler M. MOV10 Is a 5′ to 3′ RNA helicase contributing to UPF1 mRNA target degradation by translocation along 3′ UTRs. Mol Cell. 2014;54:573–85.
19. Meister G, Landthaler M, Peters L, Chen PY, Urlaub H, Luhrmann R, Tuschl T. Identification of novel argonaute-associated proteins. Curr Biol. 2005;15:2149–55.
20. Liu C, Zhang X, Huang F, Yang B, Li J, Liu B, Luo H, Zhang P, Zhang H. APOBEC3G inhibits microRNA-mediated repression of translation by interfering with the interaction between Argonaute-2 and MOV10. J Biol Chem. 2012;287:29373–83.

21. El Messaoudi-Aubert S, Nicholls J, Maertens GN, Brookes S, Bernstein E, Peters G. Role for the MOV10 RNA helicase in polycomb-mediated repression of the INK4a tumor suppressor. Nat Struct Mol Biol. 2010;17:862–8.

22. Wang X, Han Y, Dang Y, Fu W, Zhou T, Ptak RG, Zheng YH. Moloney leukemia virus 10 (MOV10) protein inhibits retrovirus replication. J Biol Chem. 2010;285:14346–55.

23. Furtak V, Mulky A, Rawlings SA, Kozhaya L, Lee K, Kewalramani VN, Unutmaz D. Perturbation of the P-body component Mov10 inhibits HIV-1 infectivity. PLoS One. 2010;5:e9081.

24. Schoggins JW, Wilson SJ, Panis M, Murphy MY, Jones CT, Bieniasz P, Rice CM. A diverse array of gene products are effectors of the type I interferon antiviral response. Nature. 2011;472:481–5.

25. Schoggins JW, Rice CM. Interferon-stimulated genes and their antiviral effector functions. Curr Opin Virol. 2011;1:519–25.

26. Goodier JL, Cheung LE, Kazazian HH Jr. MOV10 RNA helicase is a potent inhibitor of retrotransposition in cells. PLoS Genet. 2012;8:e1002941.

27. Li X, Zhang J, Jia R, Cheng V, Xu X, Qiao W, Guo F, Liang C, Cen S. The MOV10 helicase inhibits LINE-1 mobility. J Biol Chem. 2013;288:21148–60.

28. Abudu A, Wang X, Dang Y, Zhou T, Xiang SH, Zheng YH. Identification of molecular determinants from Moloney leukemia virus 10 homolog (MOV10) protein for virion packaging and anti-HIV-1 activity. J Biol Chem. 2012;287:1220–8.

29. Burdick R, Smith JL, Chaipan C, Friew Y, Chen J, Venkatachari NJ, Delviks-Frankenberry KA, Hu WS, Pathak VK. P body-associated protein Mov10 inhibits HIV-1 replication at multiple stages. J Virol. 2010;84:10241–53.

30. Zheng YH, Jeang KT, Tokunaga K. Host restriction factors in retroviral infection: promises in virus-host interaction. Retrovirology. 2012;9:112.

31. Izumi T, Burdick R, Shigemi M, Plisov S, Hu WS, Pathak VK. Mov10 and APOBEC3G localization to processing bodies is not required for virion incorporation and antiviral activity. J Virol. 2013;87:11047–62.

32. Huang F, Zhang J, Zhang Y, Geng G, Liang J, Li Y, Chen J, Liu C, Zhang H. RNA helicase MOV10 functions as a co-factor of HIV-1 Rev to facilitate Rev/RRE-dependent nuclear export of viral mRNAs. Virology. 2015;486:15–26.

33. Donahue JP, Vetter ML, Mukhtar NA, D'Aquila RT. The HIV-1 Vif PPLP motif is necessary for human APOBEC3G binding and degradation. Virology. 2008;377:49–53.

34. Lu X, Zhang T, Xu Z, Liu S, Zhao B, Lan W, Wang C, Ding J, Cao C. Crystal structure of DNA cytidine deaminase ABOBEC3G catalytic deamination domain suggests a binding mode of full-length enzyme to single-stranded DNA. J Biol Chem. 2015;290:4010–21.

35. Feng Y, Baig TT, Love RP, Chelico L. Suppression of APOBEC3-mediated restriction of HIV-1 by Vif. Front Microbiol. 2014;5:450.

36. Kouno T, Luengas EM, Shigematsu M, Shandilya SM, Zhang J, Chen L, Hara M, Schiffer CA, Harris RS, Matsuo H. Structure of the Vif-binding domain of the antiviral enzyme APOBEC3G. Nat Struct Mol Biol. 2015;22:485–91.

37. Wang H, Liu B, Liu X, Li Z, Yu XF, Zhang W. Identification of HIV-1 Vif regions required for CBF-beta interaction and APOBEC3 suppression. PLoS One. 2014;9:e95738.

38. Wang H, Lv G, Zhou X, Li Z, Liu X, Yu XF, Zhang W. Requirement of HIV-1 Vif C-terminus for Vif-CBF-beta interaction and assembly of CUL5-containing E3 ligase. BMC Microbiol. 2014;14:290.

39. Kamura T, Burian D, Yan Q, Schmidt SL, Lane WS, Querido E, Branton PE, Shilatifard A, Conaway RC, Conaway JW. Muf1, a novel Elongin BC-interacting leucine-rich repeat protein that can assemble with Cul5 and Rbx1 to reconstitute a ubiquitin ligase. J Biol Chem. 2001;276:29748–53.

40. He Z, Zhang W, Chen G, Xu R, Yu XF. Characterization of conserved motifs in HIV-1 Vif required for APOBEC3G and APOBEC3F interaction. J Mol Biol. 2008;381:1000–11.

41. Schafer A, Bogerd HP, Cullen BR. Specific packaging of APOBEC3G into HIV-1 virions is mediated by the nucleocapsid domain of the gag polyprotein precursor. Virology. 2004;328:163–8.

42. Svarovskaia ES, Xu H, Mbisa JL, Barr R, Gorelick RJ, Ono A, Freed EO, Hu WS, Pathak VK. Human apolipoprotein B mRNA-editing enzyme-catalytic polypeptide-like 3G (APOBEC3G) is incorporated into HIV-1 virions through interactions with viral and nonviral RNAs. J Biol Chem. 2004;279:35822–8.

43. Zennou V, Perez-Caballero D, Gottlinger H, Bieniasz PD. APOBEC3G incorporation into human immunodeficiency virus type 1 particles. J Virol. 2004;78:12058–61.

44. Martin KL, Johnson M, D'Aquila RT. APOBEC3G complexes decrease human immunodeficiency virus type 1 production. J Virol. 2011;85:9314–26.

45. Shao Q, Wang Y, Hildreth JE, Liu B. Polyubiquitination of APOBEC3G is essential for its degradation by HIV-1 Vif. J Virol. 2010;84:4840–4.

46. Baig TT, Feng Y, Chelico L. Determinants of efficient degradation of APOBEC3 restriction factors by HIV-1 Vif. J Virol. 2014;88:14380–95.

47. Doerks T, Copley RR, Schultz J, Ponting CP, Bork P. Systematic identification of novel protein domain families associated with nuclear functions. Genome Res. 2002;12:47–56.

48. Dang Y, Siew LM, Zheng YH. APOBEC3G is degraded by the proteasomal pathway in a Vif-dependent manner without being polyubiquitylated. J Biol Chem. 2008;283:13124–31.

49. Bergeron JR, Huthoff H, Veselkov DA, Beavil RL, Simpson PJ, Matthews SJ, Malim MH, Sanderson MR. The SOCS-box of HIV-1 Vif interacts with ElonginBC by induced-folding to recruit its Cul5-containing ubiquitin ligase complex. PLoS Pathog. 2010;6:e1000925.

50. Wang J, Zhang W, Lv M, Zuo T, Kong W, Yu X. Identification of a Cullin5-ElonginB-ElonginC E3 complex in degradation of feline immunodeficiency virus Vif-mediated feline APOBEC3 proteins. J Virol. 2011;85:12482–91.

51. Guo Y, Dong L, Qiu X, Wang Y, Zhang B, Liu H, Yu Y, Zang Y, Yang M, Huang Z. Structural basis for hijacking CBF-beta and CUL5 E3 ligase complex by HIV-1 Vif. Nature. 2014;505:229–33.

52. Iwatani Y, Chan DS, Liu L, Yoshii H, Shibata J, Yamamoto N, Levin JG, Gronenborn AM, Sugiura W. HIV-1 Vif-mediated ubiquitination/degradation of APOBEC3G involves four critical lysine residues in its C-terminal domain. Proc Natl Acad Sci USA. 2009;106:19539–44.

53. Mehle A, Thomas ER, Rajendran KS, Gabuzda D. A zinc-binding region in Vif binds Cul5 and determines cullin selection. J Biol Chem. 2006;281:17259–65.

54. Skowyra D, Craig KL, Tyers M, Elledge SJ, Harper JW. F-box proteins are receptors that recruit phosphorylated substrates to the SCF ubiquitin-ligase complex. Cell. 1997;91:209–19.

55. Fribourgh JL, Nguyen HC, Wolfe LS, Dewitt DC, Zhang W, Yu XF, Rhoades E, Xiong Y. Core binding factor beta plays a critical role by facilitating the assembly of the Vif-cullin 5 E3 ubiquitin ligase. J Virol. 2014;88:3309–19.

56. Zhou X, Evans SL, Han X, Liu Y, Yu XF. Characterization of the interaction of full-length HIV-1 Vif protein with its key regulator CBFbeta and CRL5 E3 ubiquitin ligase components. PLoS One. 2012;7:e33495.

57. Kim DY, Kwon E, Hartley PD, Crosby DC, Mann S, Krogan NJ, Gross JD. CBF-beta stabilizes HIV Vif to counteract APOBEC3 at the expense of RUNX1 target gene expression. Mol Cell. 2013;49:632–44.

58. Arjan-Odedra S, Swanson CM, Sherer NM, Wolinsky SM, Malim MH. Endogenous MOV10 inhibits the retrotransposition of endogenous retroelements but not the replication of exogenous retroviruses. Retrovirology. 2012;9:53.

59. Li J, Chen C, Ma X, Geng G, Liu B, Zhang Y, Zhang S, Zhong F, Liu C, Yin Y, et al. Long noncoding RNA NRON contributes to HIV-1 latency by specifically inducing tat protein degradation. Nat Commun. 2016;7:11730.

60. Zhang S, Zhong L, Chen B, Pan T, Zhang X, Liang L, Li Q, Zhang Z, Chen H, Zhou J, et al. Identification of an HIV-1 replication inhibitor which rescues host restriction factor APOBEC3G in Vif-APOBEC3G complex. Antiviral Res. 2015;122:20–7.

61. Nguyen KL, Llano M, Akari H, Miyagi E, Poeschla EM, Strebel K, Bour S. Codon optimization of the HIV-1 vpu and vif genes stabilizes their mRNA and allows for highly efficient Rev-independent expression. Virology. 2004;319:163–75.

62. Zuo T, Liu D, Lv W, Wang X, Wang J, Lv M, Huang W, Wu J, Zhang H, Jin H, et al. Small-molecule inhibition of human immunodeficiency virus type 1 replication by targeting the interaction between Vif and ElonginC. J Virol. 2012;86:5497–507.

63. Huang J, Wang F, Argyris E, Chen K, Liang Z, Tian H, Huang W, Squires K, Verlinghieri G, Zhang H. Cellular microRNAs contribute to HIV-1 latency in resting primary CD4 + T lymphocytes. Nat Med. 2007;13:1241–7.

2

Global phosphoproteomics of CCR5-tropic HIV-1 signaling reveals reprogramming of cellular protein production pathways and identifies p70-S6K1 and MK2 as HIV-responsive kinases required for optimal infection of CD4+ T cells

Danica D. Wiredja[1], Caroline O. Tabler[1], Daniela M. Schlatzer[1], Ming Li[2], Mark R. Chance[1] and John C. Tilton[1]* ⬤

Abstract

Background: Viral reprogramming of host cells enhances replication and is initiated by viral interaction with the cell surface. Upon human immunodeficiency virus (HIV) binding to CD4+ T cells, a signal transduction cascade is initiated that reorganizes the actin cytoskeleton, activates transcription factors, and alters mRNA splicing pathways.

Methods: We used a quantitative mass spectrometry-based phosphoproteomic approach to investigate signal transduction cascades initiated by CCR5-tropic HIV, which accounts for virtually all transmitted viruses and the vast majority of viruses worldwide.

Results: CCR5-HIV signaling induced significant reprogramming of the actin cytoskeleton and mRNA splicing pathways, as previously described. In addition, CCR5-HIV signaling induced profound changes to the mRNA transcription, processing, translation, and post-translational modifications pathways, indicating that virtually every stage of protein production is affected. Furthermore, we identified two kinases regulated by CCR5-HIV signaling—p70-S6K1 (RPS6KB1) and MK2 (MAPKAPK2)—that were also required for optimal HIV infection of CD4+ T cells. These kinases regulate protein translation and cytoskeletal architecture, respectively, reinforcing the importance of these pathways in viral replication. Additionally, we found that blockade of CCR5 signaling by maraviroc had relatively modest effects on CCR5-HIV signaling, in agreement with reports that signaling by CCR5 is dispensable for HIV infection but in contrast to the critical effects of CXCR4 on cortical actin reorganization.

Conclusions: These results demonstrate that CCR5-tropic HIV induces significant reprogramming of host CD4+ T cell protein production pathways and identifies two novel kinases induced upon viral binding to the cell surface that are critical for HIV replication in host cells.

Keywords: HIV-1, CCR5, Signaling, Phosphoproteomics, Transcription, Splicing, Translation, Post-translational modifications

*Correspondence: jct63@case.edu
[1] Department of Nutrition, Center for Proteomics and Bioinformatics, School of Medicine, Case Western Reserve University, Cleveland, OH 44106, USA
Full list of author information is available at the end of the article

Background

HIV-1 enters cells via the interactions of gp120 with its primary receptor, CD4, and a coreceptor, typically CCR5 or CXCR4 for most clinical isolates. These events lead to conformational changes in gp120 that expose the fusion peptide of gp41 and lead to host and viral membrane fusion via the formation of an energetically favorable six-helix bundle conformation (reviewed in [1]). Transmission of HIV-1 is almost always associated with viruses that utilize CCR5 and these viruses predominate in the vast majority of infected individuals [2–7]. CXCR4-using viruses emerge in approximately 40% of patients infected with subtype B HIV [8, 9] and are associated with accelerated CD4+ T cell loss and progression to AIDS [2, 10, 11]. Emergence of CXCR4 is much less common in subtype C, which accounts for approximately half of infections worldwide [12–16].

CD4, CCR5, and CXCR4 are not only receptors and coreceptors for HIV-1 entry, but also have physiological roles in signal transduction in host immune cells. CD4 engagement results in the activation of the receptor tyrosine kinase p56^{Lck} while CCR5 and CXCR4 are G-protein coupled receptors (GPCRs) that link to Gα and Gβγ subunits, particularly Gα$_i$, Gα$_q$, and Gβγ (reviewed in [17]). HIV binding to the cell surface can induce signaling through CD4 and coreceptors and has been demonstrated to trigger calcium flux [18, 19] and to activate Pyk2 [20], phosphoinositol 3-kinase (PI3K) [19], Akt and Erk 1/2 [21], and the small GTPase Rac1 [22]. In addition, HIV can promote NF-κB, AP1, and NFAT translocation to the nucleus [23–25] and actin cytoskeleton rearrangement [21], including activation of cofilin, which reorganizes cortical actin barriers that restrict infection in primary CD4 T cells [26]. Rac1 and cofilin activation by HIV enhances viral entry into cells [22, 26], indicating that signaling through CD4 and coreceptor can induce rapid changes in cells that promote viral replication. However, signaling by HIV also can have longer-acting effects on the cellular environment: PI3 K activation by HIV was found to enhance infection via a post-entry step prior to integration [19] and, more recently, a phosphoproteomic screen demonstrated that CXCR4-tropic HIV causes extensive alterations to the cellular microenvironment including to the splicing factor SRm300 (SRRM2) that enhances viral production by regulating alternative splicing of HIV mRNAs [27].

Quantitative mass spectrometry-based phosphoproteomics is a powerful technique to broadly monitor phosphorylation changes in cells following exposure to a variety of stimuli. Here, we sought to build upon the study by Wojcechowskyj and colleagues [27] by performing a similar investigation but using CCR5-tropic HIV, which accounts for nearly all transmission events and the vast majority of infections. To gain additional insights, we examined phosphorylation changes at 1, 15, and 60 min after exposure to HIV and included conditions with the CCR5 antagonist maraviroc that blocks CCR5 signaling [28]. Together with an experimental setup closely related to that used by Wojchechowskyj, this design enabled comparisons between CCR5 and CXCR4-tropic HIV signaling, the transience or durability of phosphorylation changes, and how CCR5 signaling contributes to the overall reprogramming of host cells.

Here, we report that CCR5-tropic HIV signaling reprogrammed not only cellular mRNA splicing pathways, but also transcription, translation, and post-translational modification pathways. Signaling by HIV also induced rearrangement in phosphoproteins regulating cytoskeletal transport, endocytosis and movement of cargo along cytoskeletal networks. Surprisingly, many of these pathways were stimulated regardless of the presence of maraviroc, suggesting that the effects of HIV particles on cells are primarily due to CD4 signaling or from other host molecules incorporated into viruses rather than on the coreceptors themselves. These findings provide new insights into how HIV-1 actively manipulates the target cell environment to enhance its replication.

Results

Phosphoproteomics of CCR5-tropic HIV signaling in primary memory CD4+ T cells

HIV-1 binding to the cell surface induces signals within CD4+ T cells that have been characterized primarily using biochemical approaches [18–26]. More recently, Wojcechowskyj and colleagues used a mass spectrometry-based proteomics approach to identify proteins that were differentially phosphorylated in primary resting CD4+ T cells following a 1-min exposure to CXCR4-tropic HIV [27]. CXCR4 is expressed on the majority of CD4+ T cells [29]; however, CXCR4-tropic HIV-1 variants account for only a fraction of viruses worldwide and almost none that are involved in transmission and early infection [2–7]. To gain insight into phosphorylation changes induced by CCR5-tropic HIV-1 binding to cell surface receptors, we collected leukapheresis samples from several donors and removed naïve CD4+ T cells—which express little CCR5 and are not infected to an appreciable extent by R5-tropic HIV—by rosette depletion to yield pooled, unstimulated memory CD4+ T cells. 150×10^6 memory CD4+ T cells were exposed to 20 μg/ml p24 equivalent AT2-inactivated HIV-1 THRO or an equivalent protein concentration of non-viral extracellular vesicles. The high concentration of HIV was chosen to synchronize signaling events within CD4+ T cells as well as to maintain consistency with the CXCR4-tropic HIV phosphoproteomic study [27] to facilitate comparisons between R5- and X4-tropic HIV signaling. To further improve understanding of HIV-1 signaling events, we also exposed cells to R5-tropic HIV in the presence of 100 μM of the CCR5 antagonist maraviroc to block co-receptor signaling and included 1, 15, and 60 min stimulations for all experimental conditions to assess the durability of phosphorylation changes. A schematic of the experimental design is shown in Fig. 1a. Importantly, 100 μm maraviroc completely blocked entry of HIV-1 THRO into primary CD4+ T cells (Fig. 1b).

After applying filters to remove phosphopeptides demonstrating unreliable detection in three technical replicate controls (Fig. 1c), we removed peptides with non-phosphorylation post-translational modifications such as alkylation of cysteine residues. The final list contained 2816 phosphorylation sites from 1363 unique proteins using label-free proteomics. 1678 phosphorylation sites from 931 unique proteins were found to be HIV-responsive using an FDR cutoff of 0.001 (0.1%) compared to the respective extracellular vesicle control for at least one R5-tropic HIV-1 condition (Fig. 1d). The majority of peptides demonstrated modest fold-change variation (Fig. 1e); however a small number of peptides, particularly in the 1- and 15-min time points, showed much greater fold-change values Additional file 1: Table S1). We analyzed phosphopeptides with large fold-changes at both the 1- and 15-min time points and found nearly all were from proteins with roles in either (1) actin cytoskeletal architecture, endocytosis, and movement of vesicles along actin and tubulin networks, or (2) transcription, mRNA splicing and capping, translation, or acetylation of methionine residues on newly produced proteins. These data support previous studies demonstrating that these pathways are actively modulated by signaling upon HIV binding to the cell surface [22, 26, 27, 30].

Signaling by CCR5-tropic HIV results in phosphorylation patterns with both significant overlap and differences compared to CXCR4-tropic HIV

HIV-1 binding to the cell surface can signal through several different pathways. First, specific interactions between gp120 and the host receptors CD4 and CCR5/CXCR4 can trigger responses in their respective signal transduction cascades. CD4 activates the receptor tyrosine kinase p56^{Lck} while CCR5 and CXCR4 signal via Gα and Gβγ subunits, particularly Gα$_i$, Gα$_q$, and Gβγ (reviewed in [17]). Second, signaling from gp120 interacting with non-receptor molecules has also been reported, such as the induction of cdc42 in dendritic cells via engagement of DC-SIGN [31]. It is possible that Env proteins could signal through other, currently unidentified cellular receptors as well. Third, HIV-1 incorporates host proteins into virions including HLA-DR, LFA-1, and

ICAM-1 [32–34], which could also potentially induce signals in target cells. We reasoned that CCR5-tropic and CXCR4-tropic HIV would share considerable overlap in induced signaling pathways but could also vary due to potential signaling differences following CCR5 or CXCR4 engagement or due to the exclusion of naïve CD4+ T cells that are not readily infected by most HIV-1 isolates. Indeed, we found a considerable overlap between HIV-responsive proteins following CCR5- and CXCR4-HIV signaling (Fig. 2a), with 111 shared proteins between the two studies. Our study identified 63.4% (111/175, p < 1.0 × 10^{-15}) of the HIV-responsive proteins identified by Wojecechowskyj and colleagues and an additional 820 HIV-responsive proteins not identified by their study. The larger number of HIV-responsive proteins found here is likely due to a combination of factors, including a larger number of total phosphopeptides detected, indicating more robust coverage of the CD4+ T cell proteome and a larger number of experimental conditions including 1, 15, and 60 min time points and CCR5-signaling blockade with maraviroc.

To gain further insight into the proteins identified as HIV-responsive following CCR5-HIV signaling, we compared our results with a manually curated list of human proteins shown to interact with HIV—the HIV-1 human protein interaction database (HHPID). This comparison was of particular interest as signaling has previously been demonstrated to influence host proteins levels that subsequently affect viral replication within host cells [19, 22, 26, 27]. Again, we found a highly significant overlap (Fig. 2b), with 43.1% (401/931, p < 1.0 × 10^{-15}) of the HIV-responsive proteins identified here being part of the HHPID. The overlap between the HHPID, CCR5- and CXCR4-HIV signaling is shown in Fig. 2c. Shared proteins between the current study, CXCR4-HIV signaling, and the HHPID are listed in Additional file 1: Table S2.

CCR5-tropic HIV signaling extensively reprograms cellular pathways involved in protein production and cytoskeletal regulation

Following integration into the host chromosome, HIV is transcribed into mRNA by the cellular RNA polymerase II complex. HIV contains at least four splice donors (D1–D4) and eight splice acceptors (A1–A8) that result in over 40 varieties of spliced mRNA transcripts. Splicing is regulated in a temporal fashion, with fully spliced 1- to 2-kb transcripts appearing first, followed by intermediate 4- to 5-kb transcripts, and finally by full-length 9-kb mRNAs that encode the Gag-Pol proteins and comprise the genome of budding viruses. The phosphoproteomic analysis of CXCR4-tropic HIV signaling performed by Wojcechowskyj and colleagues revealed a reprogramming of the cellular mRNA splicing pathways and identified SRRM2 as an HIV responsive protein that was also required for optimal HIV replication. Five additional SR proteins involved in mRNA splicing were identified as HIV responsive, including SRRM1, ACIN1, PNN, PPIG, and TRA1.

Our results with CCR5-tropic signaling strongly support the finding that HIV actively modulates splicing pathways: 5 of 6 of the SR proteins identified as CXCR4-HIV responsive were also CCR5-HIV responsive, the lone exception being PPIG. In addition, we identified a large number of additional splicing regulators including serine/arginine-rich splicing factors (SRSF) 1, 2, 5, 6, 7, 9, 10 and 11 and the upstream SRSF kinase 1. In particular, the SRSF1, 2, 5, and 6 proteins have previously been implicated in binding to the splice-donor region of the major 5′ splice site of HIV [35]. HIV reprogramming of mRNA splicing is also apparent on a more global scale: there was a highly significant enrichment of HIV-responsive proteins that were members of mRNA splicing and major mRNA splicing pathways in the REACTOME database (Additional file 1: Table S3).

In addition to the splicing pathways, bioinformatic analysis of the REACTOME databases revealed significant enrichment of HIV-responsive proteins in several other pathways relating to mRNA and protein production pathways: transcriptional regulation, processing of capped intron-containing pre-mRNA, metabolism of proteins, and post-translational protein modifications. These results suggest that HIV signaling induces profound changes at multiple levels of protein production, from mRNA transcription to post-translational modifications. In particular, the eukaryotic translation initiation (EIF) proteins, S ribosomal proteins (RPS), secretory (SEC) proteins involved in ER to Golgi transport, and the ubiquitin specific peptidase (USP) families all demonstrated multiple members that were responsive to HIV signaling.

Signaling by Rho GTPases and Rho GTPase cycle pathways were also highly enriched for proteins responsive to HIV signaling. Rho GTPases regulate a variety of cellular processes including cytoskeletal dynamics, transcription, endosomal trafficking, cell cycle, cell adhesion and cytokinesis. The observation that HIV signaling influences Rho GTPase signaling pathways has been explored by our lab recently, in combination with a small molecule screen that implicated Rho GTPases in regulation of HIV infection [30]. Briefly, CCR5-tropic signaling was found to dramatically alter the cellular Rho GTPase landscape, regulating not only cdc42 and Rac1 GTPases but also at least 25 guanosine dissociation inhibitors (GDIs), guanosine exchange factors (GEFs) and GTPase activating proteins (GAPs) that influence GTPase signaling. Furthermore, inhibition of cdc42, RhoA or Rho-associated

protein kinase (ROCK) inhibited viral infection, demonstrating that the appropriate function of Rho family GTPases and their substrates is essential to optimal infection of CD4+ T cells. These results add to previous studies demonstrating that HIV-1 signaling actively regulates cytoskeletal dynamics and that inhibition of these pathways negatively affects viral replication [22, 26, 36].

Identification of kinases activated or inhibited by CCR5-tropic HIV

One of primary advantages of phosphoproteomics is that it enables collection of information on thousands of differentially regulated phosphorylation sites that are the result of changes in the activity of proximal kinases and phosphatases acting upon their substrates. Since different kinases have varying preferences for consensus substrate motifs, a variety of algorithms to infer and identify cellular kinase activity based on phosphoproteomic data have been developed, including Scansite [37], Group-base Prediction System (GPS) [38], and kinase-substrate enrichment analysis (KSEA) [39]. Using the kinase to phosphosite annotations from KSEA, we identified four kinases with significantly upregulated activity 15 min after exposure to CCR5-tropic HIV: MAPKAPK2 (MK2), RPS6KB1 (p70-S6K1), CHEK2 (checkpoint kinase 2, CHK2) and CSNK2A1 (casein kinase 2 subunit a1) (Fig. 3a). CSNK2A1 kinase was not significantly upregulated when phosphopeptides from cultures containing maraviroc were analyzed. None of the analyzed kinases were significant at the 1- and 60-min time points, suggesting that in this study signaling transduction induced by HIV was most pronounced 15 min after exposure.

To gain further insight into the role of CCR5 signaling, we performed KSEA analysis comparing the HIV plus maraviroc condition to HIV alone, focused on the 15-min time point where kinase analysis was most robust. The CSNK2A1 kinase was significantly down regulated in HIV plus MVC compared to HIV alone (Fig. 3b), consistent with the loss of significance in the overall KSEA analysis. In addition, BRCA1 signaling was significantly reduced and PRKCA (protein kinase C, isoform alpha) and CDK1 (cyclin dependent kinase 1) activity were significantly upregulated when CCR5 signaling was inhibited. However, most kinases were not affected by maraviroc-mediated blockade of CCR5 signaling. Finally, we also performed cluster-guided pathway enrichment analysis comparing cells treated with HIV plus MVC compared to HIV alone to identify global cellular pathways affected by MVC in the presence of HIV. Proteins in the unfolded protein response (UPR), metabolism of proteins, signaling, and immune system pathways demonstrated significantly decreased phosphorylation in the presence of MVC (Additional file 1: Table S4).

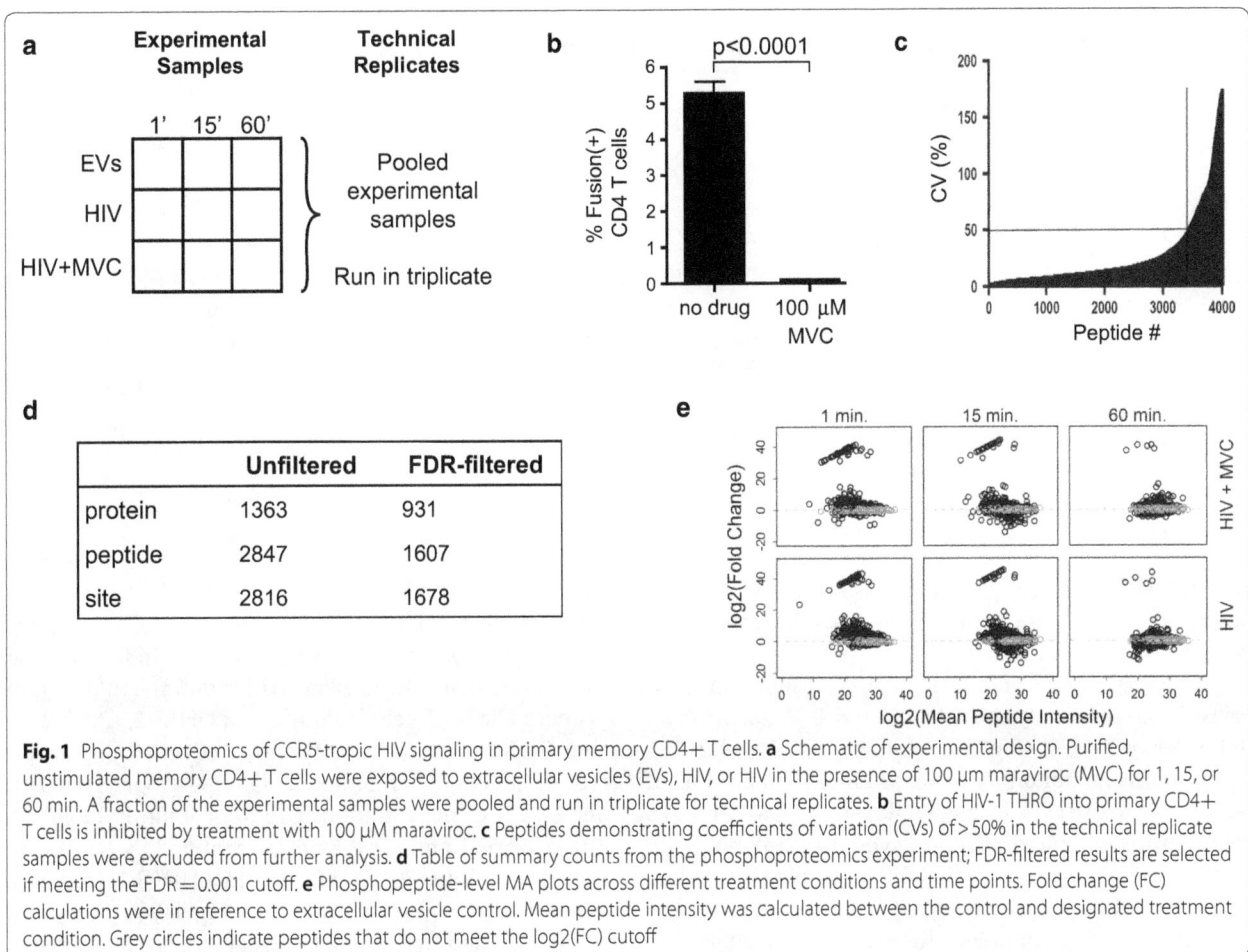

Fig. 1 Phosphoproteomics of CCR5-tropic HIV signaling in primary memory CD4+ T cells. **a** Schematic of experimental design. Purified, unstimulated memory CD4+ T cells were exposed to extracellular vesicles (EVs), HIV, or HIV in the presence of 100 μm maraviroc (MVC) for 1, 15, or 60 min. A fraction of the experimental samples were pooled and run in triplicate for technical replicates. **b** Entry of HIV-1 THRO into primary CD4+ T cells is inhibited by treatment with 100 μM maraviroc. **c** Peptides demonstrating coefficients of variation (CVs) of > 50% in the technical replicate samples were excluded from further analysis. **d** Table of summary counts from the phosphoproteomics experiment; FDR-filtered results are selected if meeting the FDR = 0.001 cutoff. **e** Phosphopeptide-level MA plots across different treatment conditions and time points. Fold change (FC) calculations were in reference to extracellular vesicle control. Mean peptide intensity was calculated between the control and designated treatment condition. Grey circles indicate peptides that do not meet the log2(FC) cutoff

Phosphorylation changes induced by CCR5-tropic HIV-1 signaling are transient, but induce long-lasting effects required for optimal infection of primary CD4+ T cells

Although KSEA analysis did not reveal annotated kinases with significantly altered phosphopeptide levels at the 1- or 60-min time points, a large number of phosphopeptides (typically lacking annotations in such databases) were differentially regulated in these conditions (Fig. 4). Interestingly, we observed that many phosphopeptides that were up-regulated at the 1- and 15-min time points appeared to be down-regulated 60 min after exposure, and vice versa, suggesting that the immediate phosphorylation events appear to be quite short-lived and do not simply return to baseline, but rather show a reversal of phosphorylation status.

To determine whether the effects of CCR5-HIV signaling are longer-lived, we examined the role of kinases identified by KSEA in further detail. Briefly, we generated combination reporter viruses that contain both a β-lactamase-Vpr fusion protein that can be used in conjunction with the fluorescent FRET substrate CCF2-AM

to monitor fusion with target cells [40, 41] as well as an *egfp* reporter gene that is expressed if fusion, uncoating, reverse transcription, nuclear import, integration into the host chromosome, Tat-dependent transcription and Rev-dependent mRNA export, and translation all occur successfully [42]. We purified primary resting CD4+ T cells from three healthy controls and infected with HIV-1 combination reporter viruses pseudotyped with patient-derived CCR5- or CXCR4-tropic Envs in the presence or absence of inhibitors targeting the differentially regulated kinases MK2 (PF 3644022), p70-S6K1 (PF 4708671), CHEK2 (Chk2 inhibitor) and CSNK2A1 (TBCA). In addition, we also included inhibitors of PKC (Go 6976) and its upstream regulator PDPK1 (GSK 2334470), ERK2 (TCS ERK11e), cyclin-dependent kinase 2 (CAS 222035-13-4), and calmodulin kinase (KN-62) as controls, as several of these have previously been demonstrated to affect HIV entry or replication [22, 43, 44]. Pharmacological inhibition of kinases was chosen over siRNA knockdown as the latter is still quite inefficient in primary CD4+ cells and certain barriers to infection in primary cells—such as

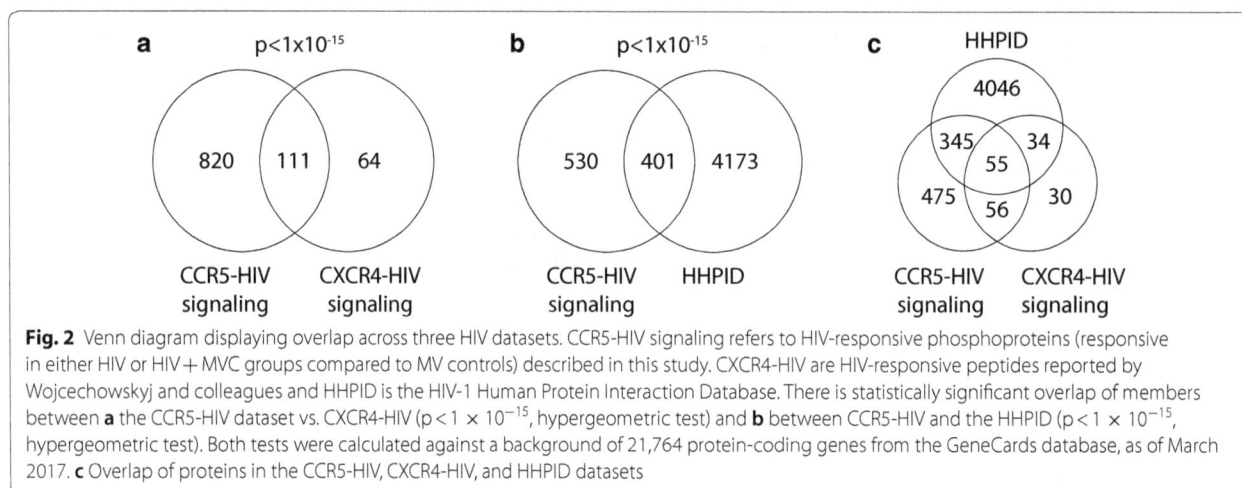

Fig. 2 Venn diagram displaying overlap across three HIV datasets. CCR5-HIV signaling refers to HIV-responsive phosphoproteins (responsive in either HIV or HIV + MVC groups compared to MV controls) described in this study. CXCR4-HIV are HIV-responsive peptides reported by Wojcechowskyj and colleagues and HHPID is the HIV-1 Human Protein Interaction Database. There is statistically significant overlap of members between **a** the CCR5-HIV dataset vs. CXCR4-HIV ($p < 1 \times 10^{-15}$, hypergeometric test) and **b** between CCR5-HIV and the HHPID ($p < 1 \times 10^{-15}$, hypergeometric test). Both tests were calculated against a background of 21,764 protein-coding genes from the GeneCards database, as of March 2017. **c** Overlap of proteins in the CCR5-HIV, CXCR4-HIV, and HHPID datasets

cortical actin—are not present in cell lines [26]. The gating strategy and representative fusion and infection plots are shown in Fig. 5a.

Two kinase inhibitors impacted HIV fusion with host cells: Go 6976, an inhibitor of PKC, and GSK 2334470, an inhibitor of PDPK1 (Fig. 5b, Additional file 1: Table S5). Both kinase inhibitors showed significant inhibition of CXCR4-tropic HIV-1 fusion, while only 10 μM Go 6976 significantly inhibited CCR5-tropic entry. Inhibition of PDPK1 did not appear to affect CCR5-tropic HIV fusion. Inhibitors of PKC have previously been shown to reduce HIV fusion by Harmon and Ratner [22], and PDPK1 is an upstream regulator of PKC activity [45, 46], supporting the importance of the PKC pathway in HIV infection. The difference in significance between CCR5- and CXCR4-tropic HIV may be due to the higher percentage of CD4+ T cells expressing CXCR4 [29], resulting in larger numbers of infected cells and reduced variability between conditions. Go 6976 and GSK 2334470 also reduced infection of CD4+ T cells by HIV as measured by EGFP accumulation (Fig. 5c). Finally, we determined the EGFP:fusion ratio, which represents the fraction of cells that progress to infection following fusion. Even after controlling for reduced fusion, infection was still significantly diminished by treatment with PKC and PDPK1 inhibitors (Additional file 1: Table S5, Fig. 5d), indicating that these kinases influence both fusion as well as post-entry stages of infection.

In addition to inhibitors of PKC and PDKP1, drugs targeting ERK2, calmodulin kinase, p70-S6K1, and MK2 all significantly reduced EGFP expression compared to no drug controls (Fig. 5c, Additional file 1: Table S5). Importantly, inhibition of HIV infection was not a result of cytotoxicity as only one condition reduced cellular viability below 90% of the control: 10 μM of the ERK2 inhibitor

TCS ERK11e. 1 μM of TCS ERK11e reduced infection significantly for both CCR5-tropic and CXCR4-tropic viruses while having no effect on viability, indicating that ERK2 activity is indeed required for optimal infection of primary CD4+ T cells. Inhibitors of CHEK2, CSNK2A1, and CDK2 did not significantly reduce CCR5-tropic HIV-1 infection but inhibited CXCR4-tropic HIV-1 at one or more concentrations (Additional file 1: Table S5). The p70-S6K1 and MK2 kinases identified by KSEA and shown here to be required for optimal HIV-1 infection of primary CD4+ T cells are known regulators of protein translation and cytoskeletal reorganization, respectively. These findings provide further evidence that these pathways are actively modulated by HIV-1 signaling and promote viral replication.

Discussion

It has long been recognized that viruses, including HIV, rely on manipulation of host cell machinery to complete their replication cycles. For instance, the accessory proteins Vif, Vpr, Vpu, and Nef facilitate viral replication by degrading or blocking the activity of cellular proteins including APOBEC3G [47], UNG2 [48], helicase-like transcription factor (HLTF) [49], tetherin [50], and serinc-3 and -5 [51, 52]. More recently, it has become apparent that HIV-1 manipulation of the host cell environment begins even earlier, with signals mediated through CD4 and coreceptor facilitating fusion by activating Rac1 [22] and cofilin [26] as well as promoting post-entry stages of replication via PI3 K [19] or the splicing factor SRm300 (SRRM2) [27]. The extent of remodeling of the host cell was impressively demonstrated through an unbiased phosphoproteomic approach by Wojcechowskyj and colleagues and revealed over 100 proteins differentially regulated by signaling of a CXCR4-tropic HIV.

Here, we sought to build upon these pioneering studies by examining cellular alterations due to CCR5-tropic HIV, which accounts for the vast majority of HIV infections worldwide and nearly all transmitted viruses [2–7]. We anticipated that substantial overlap would exist in cellular proteins regulated by CXCR4- and CCR5-tropic signaling, as both viruses can bind CD4 and incorporate similar host molecules, including HLA-DR, LFA-1, and ICAM-1, that can also initiate signaling events. Indeed, we found a highly significant overlap between phosphorylated peptides in this study using R5-tropic HIV and the report by Wojcechowskyj and colleagues using CXCR4-tropic HIV. In particular, our data confirm and extend the observation that HIV signaling strongly influences mRNA splicing pathways. In addition to identifying five of six SR proteins identified in the CXCR4-HIV phosphoproteomic study, we identified 29 additional proteins differentially regulated by CCR5-tropic HIV that are members of the major mRNA splicing pathway in the REACTOME database. These results reveal that the reprogramming of the mRNA splicing machinery induced by HIV signaling is considerably more extensive than previously appreciated.

mRNA splicing activity is highly coordinated with—and sometimes coupled to—transcription. Indeed, many proteins involved in mRNA splicing have also been implicated in transcription, RNA 3′-end formation, nuclear export, and translation (reviewed in [53]). These processes were also dramatically affected by CCR5-tropic HIV signaling and, along with splicing, accounted for six of the ten most overrepresented pathways in the REACTOME database. The importance of translational machinery was further supported by the kinase substrate enrichment analysis (KSEA), which revealed that p70-S6K1 activity was upregulated by HIV-1 signaling, and by the reporter virus assays that demonstrated that inhibition of p70-S6K1 reduced infection of in primary CD4+ T cells. The p70-S6K1 protein is activated by mTOR and subsequently phosphorylates the ribosomal S6 protein (RPS6), eukaryotic transcription initiation factor 4B (EIF4B), and eukaryotic elongation factor 2-kinase (eEF2 k) and is a positive regulator of protein translation (reviewed in [54]).

Many of the proteins identified as responsive to HIV signaling are involved in multiple processes and dissecting the exact mechanisms will require careful experimental work. For instance, a recent report demonstrated that the lens epithelium-derived growth factor (LEDGF/p75), encoded by the PSIP1 gene, interacts with splicing factors to target HIV integration to highly spliced genes [55]. LEDGF (PSIP1) and 33/60 of the LEDGF-interacting splicing proteins identified by Singh and colleagues [55] were identified here as CCR5-tropic HIV-responsive

phosphoproteins, suggesting that they may have effects at the level of integration site selection as well as at mRNA splicing. Similarly, the p70-S6K1 is not only a critical regulator of transcription but also an inhibitor of autophagy, which reduces HIV-1 infection by selectively degrading Tat in primary CD4+ T cells [56]. Therefore HIV-1 signaling through p70-S6K1 could enhance viral replication both via enhanced protein translation and reduced Tat degradation.

One surprising result from our study was that inhibition of CCR5 signaling by maraviroc had relatively modest effects on HIV-responsive phosphoproteins. In contrast, previous studies have reported that CXCR4-tropic HIV signaling is required for cofilin activation and rearrangement of cortical actin barriers [26]. There are several possibilities for these apparently contradictory results. First, maraviroc has been demonstrated to block RANTES signaling through CCR5 [28], but it is possible that HIV Env interacts with the receptor in a different manner that is not fully suppressed by maraviroc. Second, CCR5 and CXCR4 may induce different signaling pathways in CD4+ T cells; for instance CXCR4 is highly expressed on naïve CD4+ T cells [29] that were excluded from this study. However, our results are in agreement with reports demonstrating that signal transduction via CCR5 is not required for viral replication [57–60].

Conclusion

The results of this study confirm that HIV signaling has dramatic effects on cellular cytoskeletal regulation and on mRNA splicing pathways. We also demonstrate that CCR5-tropic HIV signaling induces significant reprogramming of virtually every stage of protein production: mRNA transcription, processing, translation, and post-translational protein modification. Furthermore, we identified two kinases not previously reported to have an effect on HIV replication—p70 S6K1 and MK2—that are induced by signaling and required for optimal infection of CD4+ T cells, providing new insights into how HIV manipulates host cells for viral replication.

Methods
Cells

This study was conducted according to the principles specified in the Declaration of Helsinki and under local ethical guidelines (Case Western Reserve University Institutional Review Board (IRB) #04-14-04). Normal donor samples were de-identified and obtained from leukapheresis from ALLCELLS, LLC. All donors were negative for HBV, HCV, and HIV. CD4+ T cells were isolated by adding additional autologous red blood cells to leukapheresis samples and RosetteSep CD4+ T cell enrichment kit antibodies (STEMCELL Technologies) prior to

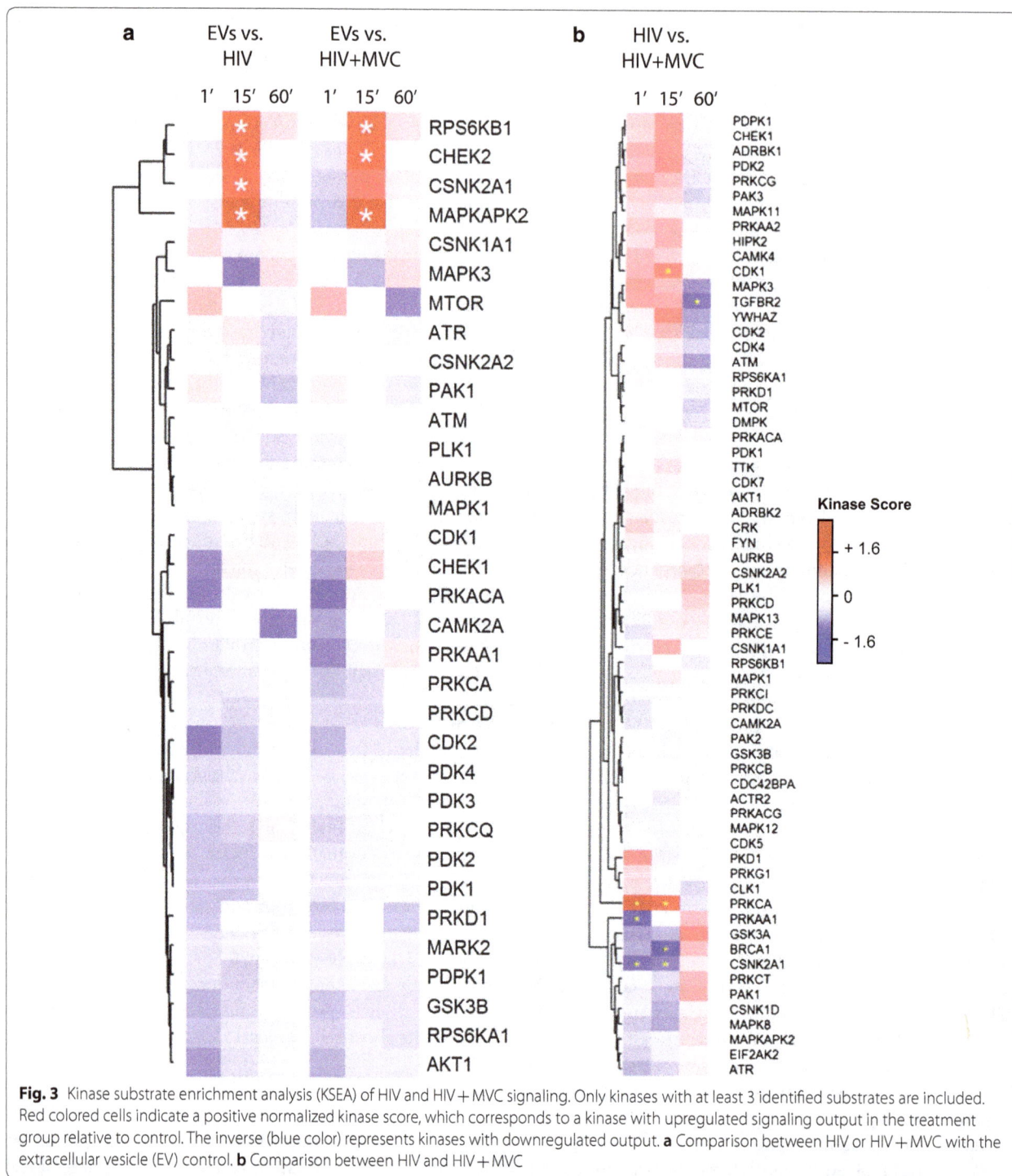

Fig. 3 Kinase substrate enrichment analysis (KSEA) of HIV and HIV + MVC signaling. Only kinases with at least 3 identified substrates are included. Red colored cells indicate a positive normalized kinase score, which corresponds to a kinase with upregulated signaling output in the treatment group relative to control. The inverse (blue color) represents kinases with downregulated output. **a** Comparison between HIV or HIV + MVC with the extracellular vesicle (EV) control. **b** Comparison between HIV and HIV + MVC

ficoll gradient separation. Cells were cryopreserved and treated with benzonase upon thawing, prior to infection.

Phosphoproteomic analysis of HIV-exposed CD4+ T cells
Memory CD4+ T cells were purified by negative selection from a leukapheresis pack using custom RosetteSep

kits (STEMCELL Technologies). Briefly, equal populations of 150×10^6 cells were exposed to: (1) 20 µg/ml p24 equivalent AT2-inactivated HIV-1 THRO, (2) AT-2 inactivated THRO in the presence of 100 µM maraviroc, or (3) equivalent protein concentrations of extracellular vesicles, for 1, 15, or 60 min. HIV-1 THRO is a

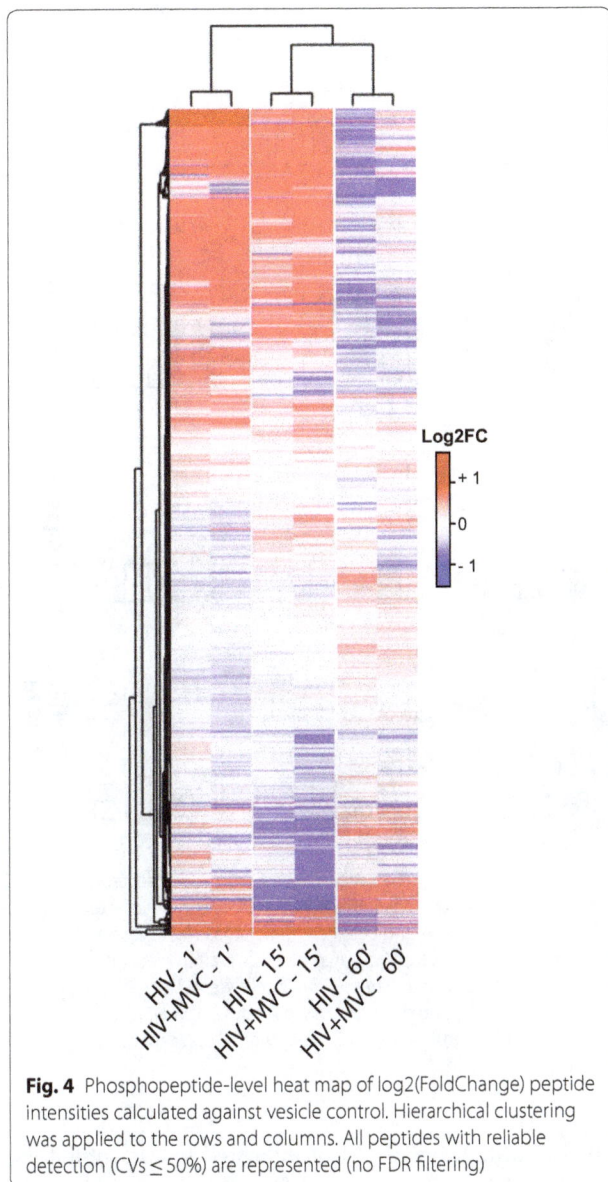

Fig. 4 Phosphopeptide-level heat map of log2(FoldChange) peptide intensities calculated against vesicle control. Hierarchical clustering was applied to the rows and columns. All peptides with reliable detection (CVs ≤ 50%) are represented (no FDR filtering)

were obtained as for the AT2-inactivated viruses with the exception that the HEK293T cells were not transfected with plasmids encoding THRO CL.29. Following exposure to virus or extracellular vesicles, cells were incubated with cold PBS containing protease and phosphatase inhibitors and washed and lysed with 2% SDS. Detergent removal was performed using the FASP cleaning procedure [62] and four hundred micrograms of each sample was digested enzymatically with a two step LysC/trypsin digestion. Phosphopeptides were enriched with titanium dioxide and enriched samples were analyzed by LC–MS/MS using a UPLC system (NanoAcquity, Waters) that was interfaced to Orbitrap ProVelos Elite mass spectrometer (Thermo Fisher). Technical replicates were performed by pooling equivalent protein amounts from each of the nine experimental samples following the titanium dioxide enrichment and analyzing them in triplicate by LC–MS/MS. Fold changes across time and treatment were determined for individual phosphopeptides compared to the corresponding extracellular vesicle controls. Unprocessed phosphoproteomic data is included in Additional file 1: Table S6.

Bioinformatic analyses
Statistics
Posterior probabilities for every peptide and subsequent false discovery rates (FDRs) were calculated per condition based on the mixture-model employed by Wojcechowskyj et al. Since each peptide has a total of 6 posterior probabilities (one per treatment condition), the max was chosen as the representative value for that peptide when filtering based on the 0.1% FDR cutoff. Details are provided in the supplemental R code, adapted from the one provided by Wojcechowskyj et al. The phosphoproteomic data filtered by coefficient of variation (CV) used for FDR calculations, along with the results of the FDR calculations, are included in Additional file 1: Table S7 and 8, respectively.

Pathway enrichment
Proteins containing at least one phosphopeptide meeting the FDR cutoff were analyzed for statistical overrepresentation of REACTOME pathways (version 58) using the PANTHER Gene List Analysis tool [63].

Kinase-substrate enrichment analysis (KSEA)
Kinase scoring was based on the method originally described by Casado et al. using the PhosphoSitePlus Kinase-Substrate dataset for substrate identification. In short, a kinase's output, reflected in its normalized score, is calculated from the collective phosphorylation changes

transmitted/founder virus isolated from a subject with early HIV infection that was found to be CCR5-tropic as evidenced by inhibition by TAK779 but not AMD3100 on TZM-bl cells and by its inability to replicate in PBMCs from a patient with the delta32-ccr5 mutation [61]. The AT2-inactivated viruses were derived from a cell clone of THRO (THRO CL.29) that was produced by co-culturing HEK293T cells transfected with the patient-derived THRO with A66-R5 cells and was identical in amino acid to the parental virus with the exception of Vif T68I, Vpu A8V, and Env R298K mutations. THRO CL.29 productively infected A66 cells expressing CCR5 but did not infect A66 cells that expressed CXCR4 (Julian Bess, personal communication). Extracellular vesicles

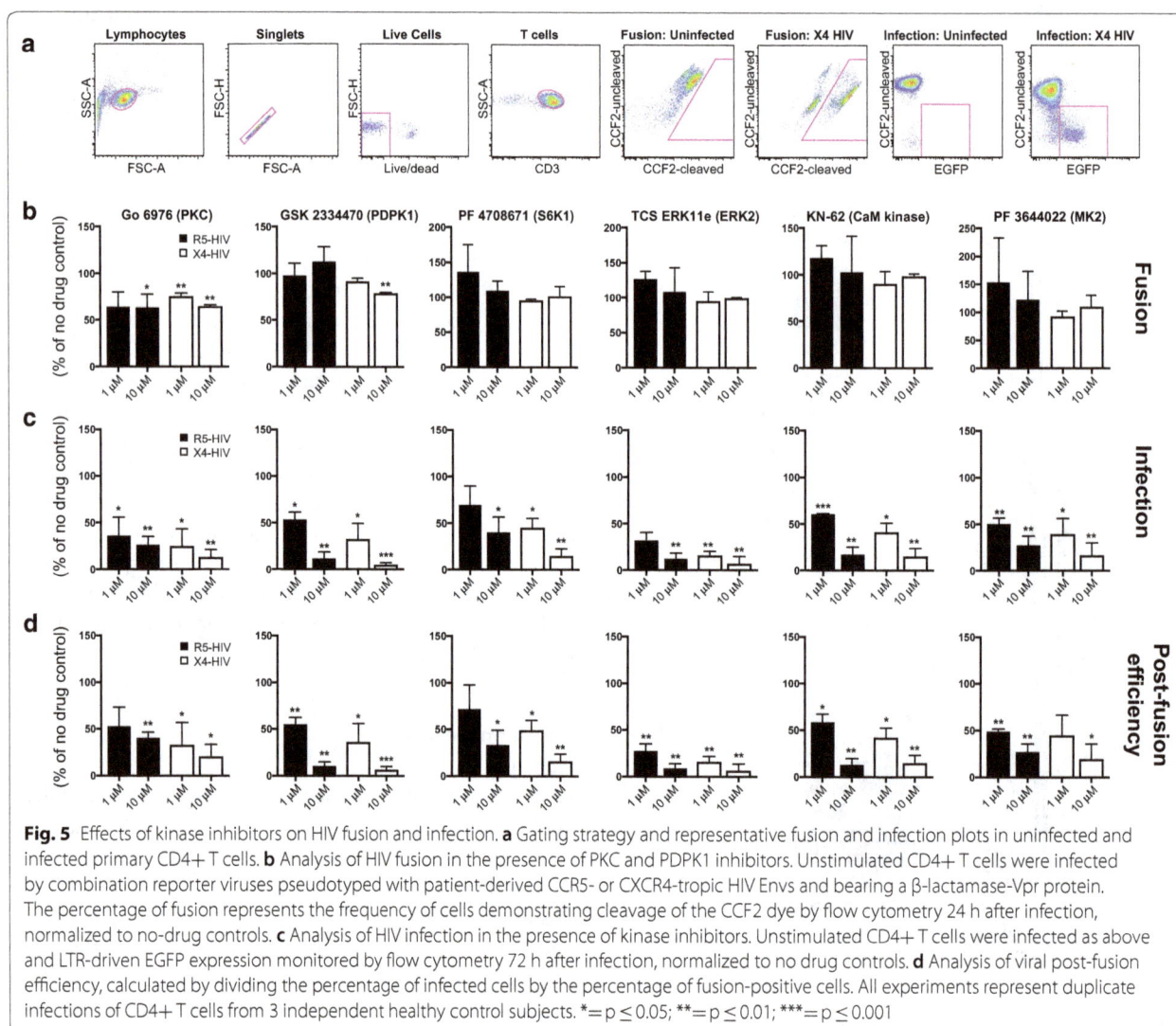

Fig. 5 Effects of kinase inhibitors on HIV fusion and infection. **a** Gating strategy and representative fusion and infection plots in uninfected and infected primary CD4+ T cells. **b** Analysis of HIV fusion in the presence of PKC and PDPK1 inhibitors. Unstimulated CD4+ T cells were infected by combination reporter viruses pseudotyped with patient-derived CCR5- or CXCR4-tropic HIV Envs and bearing a β-lactamase-Vpr protein. The percentage of fusion represents the frequency of cells demonstrating cleavage of the CCF2 dye by flow cytometry 24 h after infection, normalized to no-drug controls. **c** Analysis of HIV infection in the presence of kinase inhibitors. Unstimulated CD4+ T cells were infected as above and LTR-driven EGFP expression monitored by flow cytometry 72 h after infection, normalized to no drug controls. **d** Analysis of viral post-fusion efficiency, calculated by dividing the percentage of infected cells by the percentage of fusion-positive cells. All experiments represent duplicate infections of CD4+ T cells from 3 independent healthy control subjects. *=p ≤ 0.05; **=p ≤ 0.01; ***=p ≤ 0.001

of its identified substrates. A negative score (normalized by a weighted z-score) represents a kinase that has predominantly dephosphorylated substrates in the treatment condition relative to control. This, in turn, corresponds to downregulated signaling output with treatment. The inverse is true for a positive score. Statistical assessment was performed as originally described and utilized the z-test to assess the probability of achieving a more extreme score than the one observed. The KSEA scores and dataset used for KSEA analysis are included in Additional file 1: Table S9 and S10, respectively.

Infection experiments

1×10^6 unstimulated primary CD4+ T cells were plated per well in a 96-well format and incubated for 4 h at 37 °C with media alone or media supplemented with

10, 100 nM, 1, or 10 μM of indicated kinase inhibitors. Parallel plates were prepared for analysis of viral fusion and LTR-driven EGFP expression as previously described [42]. Following incubation with kinase inhibitors, cells were infected with 5 ng p24 equivalents of HIV-1 reporter virus strain NL4-3-deltaE-EGFP (obtained through the NIH AIDS Research and Reference Reagent Program, Division of AIDS, NIAID, NIH: pNL4-3-delta-E-EGFP (Cat #11100) from Drs. Haili Zhang, Yan Zhou, and Robert Siliciano) bearing the CCR5-tropic Env REJO. D12.1972 [64] or the CXCR4-tropic Env JOTO.TA1.2247 [65] and a β-lactamase-Vpr fusion protein [40, 41]. Plates were spinoculated for 2 h at 1200 rpm and 25 °C. Following centrifugation, cells were incubated for 1 h at 37° C. Cells for viral fusion analysis were treated with CCF2-AM, washed, and incubated overnight at room temperature in the presence of probenecid. For EGFP expression, cells were incubated at 37 °C for a total of 72 h prior to staining and processing. The following kinase inhibitors were added to cells 4 h prior to addition of virus and spinoculation: Go 6976 and PF3644022 (R&D Systems), PF 4708671, TBCA, TCS ERK11e, and GSK 2334470 (TOCRIS), KN-62 and CAS 222035-13-4 (Santa Cruz Biotechnology), and Chk2 inhibitor II hydrate (Sigma Aldrich) at the specified concentrations.

Flow cytometry

Cells were washed once with PBS containing 1% BSA and incubated with live/dead fixable yellow dead cell stain (Thermo Fisher), CD3 Brilliant Violet 650 (BioLegend), and CD4 Allophycocyanin (eBioscience) at 4 °C for 30 min. Cells were washed in PBS/BSA and fixed in PBS/BSA containing 1% paraformaldehyde prior to data acquisition. All samples were analyzed using an LSRII flow cytometer (Becton–Dickinson). A minimum of 50,000 events were collected per sample. FlowJo version 9.7.6 (TreeStar, Inc) was used for analysis. Flow cytometry plots were gated using fluorescence intensity. Summary data are presented as fusion (+) and infection (+) cells as a percentage of no drug controls. Post-infection efficiency represent the ratio of infection (+):fusion (+) cells, also expressed as a percentage of no drug controls. All summary data represent mean values with standard error of the mean unless stated otherwise. All differences with a p value of < 0.05 were considered statistically significant, correcting for multiple comparisons when appropriate. Statistical analyses were performed using student T-tests within GraphPad Prism v7.0.

Additional file

Additional file 1: Table S1. Phosphoproteomics data for peptides with large fold-changes at the 1- and 15- minute time points. **Table S2.** Shared proteins identified in the current study, CXCR4-HIV signaling, and the HIV-1 human protein interaction database. **Table S3.** Bioinformatic analysis of REACTOME pathways enriched for HIV-responsive phosphoproteins. **Table S4.** Cluster pathway enrichment analysis of HIV-responsive phosphoproteins. **Table S5.** Effects of kinase inhibitors on HIV-1 fusion, infection, and post-entry efficiency in primary CD4+ T cells.**Table S6.** Unprocessed proteomics data. **Table S7.** Phosphoproteomics data filtered by coefficient of variation (CV). **Table S8.** Phosphoproteomics data processed for false discovery rate (FDR) calculations. **Table S9.** Kinase-substrate enrichment analysis (KSEA) scores from phosphoproteomics data. **Table S10.** Dataset used for kinase-substrate enrichment analysis (KSEA) analysis.

Authors' contributions

DDW performed bioinformatics analysis and contributed to the manuscript. COT performed the phosphoproteomic setup and validation experiments. DMS digested samples, conducted the LC-MS/MS experiments, and contributed to the manuscript. ML provided biostatistics expertise. MRC supervised the statistical and bioinformatics analysis and edited the manuscript. JCT deigned the experiments, supervised the project, and wrote the manuscript. All authors read and approved the final manuscript.

Author details
[1] Department of Nutrition, Center for Proteomics and Bioinformatics, School of Medicine, Case Western Reserve University, Cleveland, OH 44106, USA. [2] Department of Population and Quantitative Health Sciences, School of Medicine, Case Western Reserve University, Cleveland, OH 44106, USA.

Acknowledgements
This work was supported by the Case Western Reserve University/University Hospitals Centers for AIDS Research: NIH Grant Number: P30 AI036219, NIH R21AI113148 (JCT), NIH R01GM117208 (MRC), and by the Clinical and Translation Science Collaborative of Cleveland, 4UL1TR000439. We would like to thank and acknowledge Terra Schaden-Ireland for generating the cell clone of THRO and Jeffery Lifson, Gregory Del Prete, and Julian Bess for preparing and sharing the AT2-inactivated CCR5-expressing HIV and control extracellular vesicles for phosphoproteomic experiments and analysis. We would also like to thank Jason Wojcechowskyj and Robert Doms for sharing insights and experimental details enabling comparisons with their phosphoproteomic analysis of HIV signaling via CD4 and CXCR4.

Competing interests
The authors declare that they have no competing interests.

References
1. Wilen CB, Tilton JC, Doms RW. Molecular mechanisms of HIV entry. Adv Exp Med Biol. 2012;726:223–42.
2. Schuitemaker H, Koot M, Kootstra NA, Dercksen MW, de Goede RE, van Steenwijk RP, et al. Biological phenotype of human immunodeficiency virus type 1 clones at different stages of infection: progression of disease is associated with a shift from monocytotropic to T-cell-tropic virus population. J Virol. 1992;66:1354–60.
3. van't Wout AB, Kootstra NA, Mulder-Kampinga GA, Albrecht-van Lent N, Scherpbier HJ, Veenstra J, et al. Macrophage-tropic variants initiate human immunodeficiency virus type 1 infection after sexual, parenteral, and vertical transmission. J Clin Invest. 1994;94:2060–7.
4. Cornelissen M, Mulder-Kampinga G, Veenstra J, Zorgdrager F, Kuiken C, Hartman S, et al. Syncytium-inducing (SI) phenotype suppression at seroconversion after intramuscular inoculation of a non-syncytium-inducing/SI phenotypically mixed human immunodeficiency virus population. J Virol Am Soc Microbiol. 1995;69:1810–8.
5. Spijkerman IJ, Koot M, Prins M, Keet IP, van den Hoek AJ, Miedema F, et al. Lower prevalence and incidence of HIV-1 syncytium-inducing phenotype among injecting drug users compared with homosexual men. AIDS. 1995;9:1085–92.
6. Huang Y, Paxton WA, Wolinsky SM, Neumann AU, Zhang L, He T, et al. The role of a mutant CCR5 allele in HIV-1 transmission and disease progression. Nat Med. 1996;2:1240–3.
7. de Roda Husman AM, Koot M, Cornelissen M, Keet IP, Brouwer M, Broersen SM, et al. Association between CCR5 genotype and the clinical course of HIV-1 infection. Ann Intern Med. 1997;127:882–90.
8. de Roda Husman AM, van Rij RP, Blaak H, Broersen S, Schuitemaker H. Adaptation to promiscuous usage of chemokine receptors is not a prerequisite for human immunodeficiency virus type 1 disease progression. J Infect Dis. 1999;180:1106–15.
9. Li S, Juarez J, Alali M, Dwyer D, Collman R, Cunningham A, et al. Persistent CCR5 utilization and enhanced macrophage tropism by primary blood human immunodeficiency virus type 1 isolates from advanced stages of disease and comparison to tissue-derived isolates. J Virol. 1999;73:9741–55.
10. Simmons G, Wilkinson D, Reeves JD, Dittmar MT, Beddows S, Weber J, et al. Primary, syncytium-inducing human immunodeficiency virus type 1 isolates are dual-tropic and most can use either Lestr or CCR5 as coreceptors for virus entry. J Virol. 1996;70:8355–60.
11. Connor RI, Sheridan KE, Ceradini D, Choe S, Landau NR. Change in coreceptor use correlates with disease progression in HIV-1-infected individuals. J Exp Med. 1997;185:621–8.

12. Abebe A, Demissie D, Goudsmit J, Brouwer M, Kuiken CL, Pollakis G, et al. HIV-1 subtype C syncytium- and non-syncytium-inducing phenotypes and coreceptor usage among Ethiopian patients with AIDS. AIDS. 1999;13:1305–11.

13. Peeters M, Vincent R, Perret JL, Lasky M, Patrel D, Liegeois F, et al. Evidence for differences in MT2 cell tropism according to genetic subtypes of HIV-1: syncytium-inducing variants seem rare among subtype C HIV-1 viruses. J Acquir Immune Defic Syndr Hum Retrovir. 1999;20:115–21.

14. Ping LH, Nelson JA, Hoffman IF, Schock J, Lamers SL, Goodman M, et al. Characterization of V3 sequence heterogeneity in subtype C human immunodeficiency virus type 1 isolates from Malawi: underrepresentation of X4 variants. J Virol. 1999;73:6271–81.

15. Cecilia D, Kulkarni SS, Tripathy SP, Gangakhedkar RR, Paranjape RS, Gadkari DA. Absence of coreceptor switch with disease progression in human immunodeficiency virus infections in India. Virology. 2000;271:253–8.

16. Jakobsen MR, Cashin K, Roche M, Sterjovski J, Ellett A, Borm K, et al. Longitudinal analysis of CCR5 and CXCR4 usage in a cohort of antiretroviral therapy-naïve subjects with progressive HIV-1 subtype C infection. PLoS ONE. 2013;8:e65950.

17. Wu Y, Yoder A. Chemokine coreceptor signaling in HIV-1 infection and pathogenesis. PLoS Pathog. 2009;5:e1000520.

18. Weissman D, Rabin RL, Arthos J, Rubbert A, Dybul M, Swofford R, et al. Macrophage-tropic HIV and SIV envelope proteins induce a signal through the CCR5 chemokine receptor. Nature. 1997;389:981–5.

19. François F, Klotman ME. Phosphatidylinositol 3-kinase regulates human immunodeficiency virus type 1 replication following viral entry in primary CD4+ T lymphocytes and macrophages. J Virol. 2003;77:2539–49.

20. Davis CB, Dikic I, Unutmaz D, Hill CM, Arthos J, Siani MA, et al. Signal transduction due to HIV-1 envelope interactions with chemokine receptors CXCR4 or CCR5. J Exp Med. 1997;186:1793–8.

21. Balabanian K, Harriague J, Décrion C, Lagane B, Shorte S, Baleux F, et al. CXCR4-tropic HIV-1 envelope glycoprotein functions as a viral chemokine in unstimulated primary CD4+ T lymphocytes. J Immunol. 2004;173:7150–60.

22. Harmon B, Ratner L. Induction of the Galpha(q) signaling cascade by the human immunodeficiency virus envelope is required for virus entry. J Virol. 2008;82:9191–205.

23. Briant L, Coudronnière N, Robert-Hebmann V, Benkirane M, Devaux C. Binding of HIV-1 virions or gp120-anti-gp120 immune complexes to HIV-1-infected quiescent peripheral blood mononuclear cells reveals latent infection. J Immunol. 1996;156:3994–4004.

24. Chirmule N, Goonewardena H, Pahwa S, Pasieka R, Kalyanaraman VS, Pahwa S. HIV-1 envelope glycoproteins induce activation of activated protein-1 in CD4+ T cells. J Biol Chem. 1995;270:19364–9.

25. Cicala C, Arthos J, Censoplano N, Cruz C, Chung E, Martinelli E, et al. HIV-1 gp120 induces NFAT nuclear translocation in resting CD4+ T-cells. Virology. 2006;345:105–14.

26. Yoder A, Yu D, Dong L, Iyer SR, Xu X, Kelly J, et al. HIV envelope-CXCR4 signaling activates cofilin to overcome cortical actin restriction in resting CD4 T cells. Cells. 2008;134:782–92.

27. Wojcechowskyj JA, Didigu CA, Lee JY, Parrish NF, Sinha R, Hahn BH, et al. Quantitative phosphoproteomics reveals extensive cellular reprogramming during HIV-1 entry. Cell Host Microbe. 2013;13:613–23.

28. Dorr P, Westby M, Dobbs S, Griffin P, Irvine B, Macartney M, et al. Maraviroc (UK-427,857), a potent, orally bioavailable, and selective small-molecule inhibitor of chemokine receptor CCR5 with broad-spectrum anti-human immunodeficiency virus type 1 activity. Antimicrob Agents Chemother. 2005;49:4721–32.

29. Bleul CC, Wu L, Hoxie JA, Springer TA, Mackay CR. The HIV coreceptors CXCR4 and CCR5 are differentially expressed and regulated on human T lymphocytes. Proc Natl Acad Sci USA. 1997;94:1925–30.

30. Lucera MB, Fleissner Z, Tabler CO, Schlatzer DM, Troyer Z, Tilton JC. HIV signaling through CD4 and CCR5 activates Rho family GTPases that are required for optimal infection of primary CD4+ T cells. Retrovirology. 2017;14:4.

31. Nikolic DS, Lehmann M, Felts R, Garcia E, Blanchet FP, Subramaniam S, et al. HIV-1 activates Cdc42 and induces membrane extensions in immature dendritic cells to facilitate cell-to-cell virus propagation. Blood. 2011;118:4841–52.

32. Orentas RJ, Hildreth JE. Association of host cell surface adhesion receptors and other membrane proteins with HIV and SIV. AIDS Res Hum Retroviruses. 1993;9:1157–65.

33. Capobianchi MR, Fais S, Castilletti C, Gentile M, Ameglio F, Dianzani F. A simple and reliable method to detect cell membrane proteins on infectious human immunodeficiency virus type 1 particles. J Infect Dis. 1994;169:886–9.

34. Meerloo T, Sheikh MA, Bloem AC, de Ronde A, Schutten M, van Els CA, et al. Host cell membrane proteins on human immunodeficiency virus type 1 after in vitro infection of H9 cells and blood mononuclear cells. An immuno-electron microscopic study. J Gen Virol. 1993;74(Pt 1):129–35.

35. Mueller N, Berkhout B, Das AT. HIV-1 splicing is controlled by local RNA structure and binding of splicing regulatory proteins at the major 5′ splice site. J Gen Virol. 2015;96:1906–17.

36. Sabo Y, Walsh D, Barry DS, Tinaztepe S, de Los SK, Goff SP, et al. HIV-1 induces the formation of stable microtubules to enhance early infection. Cell Host Microbe. 2013;14:535–46.

37. Yaffe MB, Leparc GG, Lai J, Obata T, Volinia S, Cantley LC. A motif-based profile scanning approach for genome-wide prediction of signaling pathways. Nat Biotechnol. 2001;19:348–53.

38. Xue Y, Ren J, Gao X, Jin C, Wen L, Yao X. GPS 2.0, a tool to predict kinase-specific phosphorylation sites in hierarchy. Mol Cell Proteom. 2008;7:1598–608.

39. Casado P, Rodriguez-Prados J-C, Cosulich SC, Guichard S, Vanhaesebroeck B, Joel S, et al. Kinase-substrate enrichment analysis provides insights into the heterogeneity of signaling pathway activation in leukemia cells. Sci Signal. 2013;6:rs6–rs6.

40. Cavrois M, De Noronha C, Greene WC. A sensitive and specific enzyme-based assay detecting HIV-1 virion fusion in primary T lymphocytes. Nat Biotechnol. 2002;20:1151–4.

41. Cavrois M, Neidleman J, Bigos M, Greene WC. Fluorescence resonance energy transfer-based HIV-1 virion fusion assay. Methods Mol Biol. 2004;263:333–44.

42. Tilton CA, Tabler CO, Lucera MB, Marek SL, Haqqani AA, Tilton JC. A combination HIV reporter virus system for measuring post-entry event efficiency and viral outcome in primary CD4+ T cell subsets. J Virol Methods. 2014;195:164–9.

43. Yang X, Gabuzda D. Regulation of human immunodeficiency virus type 1 infectivity by the ERK mitogen-activated protein kinase signaling pathway. J Virol. 1999;73:3460–6.

44. Ammosova T, Berro R, Jerebtsova M, Jackson A, Charles S, Klase Z, et al. Phosphorylation of HIV-1 Tat by CDK2 in HIV-1 transcription. Retrovirology. 2006;3:78.

45. Le Good JA, Ziegler WH, Parekh DB, Alessi DR, Cohen P, Parker PJ. Protein kinase C isotypes controlled by phosphoinositide 3-kinase through the protein kinase PDK1. Science. 1998;281:2042–5.

46. Park S-G, Schulze-Luehrman J, Hayden MS, Hashimoto N, Ogawa W, Kasuga M, et al. The kinase PDK1 integrates T cell antigen receptor and CD28 coreceptor signaling to induce NF-kappaB and activate T cells. Nat Immunol. 2009;10:158–66.

47. Sheehy AM, Gaddis NC, Choi JD, Malim MH. Isolation of a human gene that inhibits HIV-1 infection and is suppressed by the viral Vif protein. Nature. 2002;418:646–50.

48. Ahn J, Vu T, Novince Z, Guerrero-Santoro J, Rapic-Otrin V, Gronenborn AM. HIV-1 Vpr loads uracil DNA glycosylase-2 onto DCAF1, a substrate recognition subunit of a cullin 4A-ring E3 ubiquitin ligase for proteasome-dependent degradation. J Biol Chem. 2010;285:37333–41.

49. Hrecka K, Hao C, Shun M-C, Kaur S, Swanson SK, Florens L, et al. HIV-1 and HIV-2 exhibit divergent interactions with HLTF and UNG2 DNA repair proteins. Proc Natl Acad Sci USA. 2016;113:E3921–30.

50. Neil SJD, Zang T, Bieniasz PD. Tetherin inhibits retrovirus release and is antagonized by HIV-1 Vpu. Nature. 2008;451:425–30.

51. Usami Y, Wu Y, Göttlinger HG. SERINC3 and SERINC5 restrict HIV-1 infectivity and are counteracted by Nef. Nature. 2015;526:218–23.

52. Rosa A, Chande A, Ziglio S, De Sanctis V, Bertorelli R, Goh SL, et al. HIV-1 Nef promotes infection by excluding SERINC5 from virion incorporation. Nature. 2015;526:212–7.

53. Mahiet C, Swanson CM. Control of HIV-1 gene expression by SR proteins. Biochem Soc Trans. 2016;44:1417–25.

54. Magnuson B, Ekim B, Fingar DC. Regulation and function of ribosomal protein S6 kinase (S6K) within mTOR signalling networks. Biochem J. 2012;441:1–21.

55. Singh PK, Plumb MR, Ferris AL, Iben JR, Wu X, Fadel HJ, et al. LEDGF/p75 interacts with mRNA splicing factors and targets HIV-1 integration to highly spliced genes. Genes Dev. 2015;29:2287–97.

56. Sagnier S, Daussy CF, Borel S, Robert-Hebmann V, Faure M, Blanchet FP, et al. Autophagy restricts HIV-1 infection by selectively degrading Tat in CD4+ T lymphocytes. J Virol. 2015;89:615–25.

57. Alkhatib G, Locati M, Kennedy PE, Murphy PM, Berger EA. HIV-1 coreceptor activity of CCR5 and its inhibition by chemokines: independence from G protein signaling and importance of coreceptor downmodulation. Virology. 1997;234:340–8.

58. Aramori I, Ferguson SS, Bieniasz PD, Zhang J, Cullen B, Cullen MG. Molecular mechanism of desensitization of the chemokine receptor CCR-5: receptor signaling and internalization are dissociable from its role as an HIV-1 co-receptor. EMBO J. 1997;16:4606–16.

59. Gosling J, Monteclaro FS, Atchison RE, Arai H, Tsou CL, Goldsmith MA, et al. Molecular uncoupling of C–C chemokine receptor 5-induced chemotaxis and signal transduction from HIV-1 coreceptor activity. Proc Natl Acad Sci USA. 1997;94:5061–6.

60. Amara A, Vidy A, Boulla G, Mollier K, Garcia-Perez J, Alcamí J, et al. G protein-dependent CCR5 signaling is not required for efficient infection of primary T lymphocytes and macrophages by R5 human immunodeficiency virus type 1 isolates. J Virol. 2003;77:2550–8.

61. Ochsenbauer C, Edmonds TG, Ding H, Keele BF, Decker J, Salazar MG, et al. Generation of transmitted/founder HIV-1 infectious molecular clones and characterization of their replication capacity in CD4 T lymphocytes and monocyte-derived macrophages. J Virol. 2012;86:2715–28.

62. Wiśniewski JR, Zougman A, Nagaraj N, Mann M. Universal sample preparation method for proteome analysis. Nat Methods. 2009;6:359–62.

63. Mi H, Muruganujan A, Casagrande JT, Thomas PD. Large-scale gene function analysis with the PANTHER classification system. Nat Protoc. 2013;8:1551–66.

64. Keele BF, Giorgi EE, Salazar-Gonzalez JF, Decker JM, Pham KT, Salazar MG, et al. Identification and characterization of transmitted and early founder virus envelopes in primary HIV-1 infection. Proc Natl Acad Sci USA. 2008;105:7552–7.

65. Wilen CB, Parrish NF, Pfaff JM, Decker JM, Henning EA, Haim H, et al. Phenotypic and immunologic comparison of clade B transmitted/founder and chronic HIV-1 envelope glycoproteins. J Virol. 2011;85:8514–27.

3

Prediction of HIV-associated neurocognitive disorder (HAND) from three genetic features of envelope gp120 glycoprotein

Masato Ogishi[1,2]* 🔾 and Hiroshi Yotsuyanagi[1]

Abstract

Background: HIV-associated neurocognitive disorder (HAND) remains an important and yet potentially underdiagnosed manifestation despite the fact that the modern combination antiretroviral therapy (cART) has achieved effective viral suppression and greatly reduced the incidence of life-threatening events. Although HIV neurotoxicity is thought to play a central role, the potential of viral genetic signature as diagnostic and/or prognostic biomarker has yet to be fully explored.

Results: Using a manually curated sequence metadataset (80 specimens, 2349 sequences), we demonstrated that only three genetic features are sufficient to predict HAND status regardless of sampling tissues; the accuracy reached 100 and 94% in the hold-out testing subdataset and the entire dataset, respectively. The three genetic features stratified HAND into four distinct clusters. Extrapolating the classification to the 1619 specimens registered in the Los Alamos HIV Sequence Database, the global HAND prevalence was estimated to be 46%, with significant regional variations (30–71%). The R package *HANDPrediction* was implemented to ensure public availability of key codes.

Conclusions: Our analysis revealed three amino acid positions in gp120 glycoprotein, providing the basis of the development of novel cART regimens specifically optimized for HAND-associated quasispecies. Moreover, the classifier can readily be translated into a diagnostic biomarker, warranting prospective validation.

Keywords: HIV-associated neurocognitive disorder (HAND), HIV envelope gp120 glycoprotein, Machine learning, Biomarker

Background

Neurocognitive impairments during the course of chronic HIV infection, called HIV-associated neurocognitive disorder (HAND), remain as an unconquered clinical entity despite the improvement of combination antiretroviral therapy (cART) over the last 20 years [1, 2]. HAND is a comprehensive concept encompassing the broad spectrum of motor, cognitive, and neuropsychiatric impairment, in which persistent HIV infection in the central nervous system (CNS) plays a fundamental role.

According to the criteria proposed by the HIV Neurobehavioral Research Center (HNRC), HAND is stratified into three conditions, namely, asymptomatic neurocognitive impairment (ANI), mild neurocognitive disorder (MND), and HIV-associated dementia (HAD) [3]. In a large cohort study from the U.S., prevalence estimates of ANI, MND and HAD were inferred at 33, 12 and 2%, respectively [4]. Other cohort studies yielded similar estimates [5–7]. Despite its wide prevalence, diagnostic and therapeutic strategies are quite limited; currently, there is no molecularly defined biomarkers, and prompt initiation of cART is the only clinically available treatment, though its effectiveness on preventing the progression of neurocognitive impairment is still in hot controversy

*Correspondence: oogishi-tky@umin.ac.jp
[2] National Center for Global Health and Medicine, Tokyo, Japan
Full list of author information is available at the end of the article

[8, 9]. Indeed, as cART has become more accessible in resource-limited settings worldwide, thereby extending the expected lifespan of HIV-infected patients, the global burden of HAND is expected to be steadily on the rise. Recently, accumulating evidence suggests that persistent viral replication and ongoing diversification in the CNS compartment even in patients with undetectably suppressed viremia could lead to the emergence of neurotoxic quasispecies and thereby contribute to the progression of HAND [10, 11]. In this context, defining etiologically relevant diagnostic and/or prognostic biomarkers and optimal regimens based on those biomarkers in the era of modern cART is an inevitable step forward to improve current clinical practice.

Neurotoxic HIV viral quasispecies have been hypothesized to play an indispensable role in HAND pathogenesis. Although the mechanisms of HIV neurotoxicity has yet to be thoroughly clarified, several studies have suggested that there is a link between HAND and the neurotoxicity exerted by the orchestrated actions of several HIV proteins including trans-activating protein (*Tat*) and envelope glycoprotein (*Env*) [12]. Particularly, gp120, a fragment proteolytically cleaved from the *Env* protein, may mediate neuronal damage via direct induction of apoptosis both in rodents and primary human brain tissue culture [13–15]. On the other hand, hypervariable region 3 (V3) located at the middle of gp120 is primarily responsible for the genotypic and phenotypic diversity of HIV. A loop structure formed by V3 (V3 loop) interacts with chemokine coreceptors CCR5 and/or CXCR4, thereby determining multifaceted viral phenotypes including cell tropism [16]. Studies of CNS-derived viral isolates have indicated the links between CCR5 tropism, macrophage/microglia tropism, and the compartmentalization and persistent replication of viruses in the CNS [17–19]. Considering these insights, it is plausible to hypothesize that the gp120 glycoprotein serves as a primary, if not exclusive, determinant of both neurotropism, i.e., the ability to cross the blood–brain barrier and maintain replicative capacity in the CNS compartment, and neurotoxicity, i.e., the capability of igniting and/or fueling neurocognitive impairments. In this context, Pillai et al. [20] studied the C2V3 *env* subregion, and reported that the fifth residue of the V3 loop significantly correlated with neurocognitive deficit, although they did not explore the predictive significance of this signature. Indeed, a single amino acid signature is unlikely to be adequate to explain HIV adaptation during the course of HAND progression; thus, the combination of various signatures should be explored.

Machine learning (ML) is a highly promising technique for exploring a vastly large set of parameters to yield a potent classifier without prespecifying mathematical models. To gain optimized predictive accuracy, ML algorithms iteratively evaluate three types of error: training errors, validation errors (i.e., in-sample errors), and generalization errors (i.e., out-of-sample errors). The ultimate goal of ML-based prediction is to construct a classifier which has minimal generalization errors to unobserved real-world data. When a training dataset is provided, ML algorithms internally evaluate training errors to find the best set of parameters specific to the algorithm, and validation errors are evaluated by methods such as cross-validation (CV). When multiple algorithms with different sets of parameters are compared, the classifier with the smallest validation errors is selected. Then, the generalization errors should be evaluated with a testing dataset independent from model construction and selection.

Holman and Gabuzda applied ML-based approach to a manually collected metadataset of *env* C2V3C3 sequences derived from patients with or without HIV-associated dementia (HAD), reporting 75% accuracy for predicting HAD-associated *env* sequences [21]. Although their work provided intriguing insights into HIV neuropathogenesis, its generalizability is limited by several caveats. First, they reported the predictive accuracy via leave-one-out cross-validation. However, this corresponds to the validation error and may be a too optimistic estimation of the generalization error because of overfitting of the model against the training dataset. Rather, hold-out validation with no classifier retraining is necessary to correctly evaluate the generalization error. Second, although they only tested a simple rule-based classification algorithm, this could be outperformed by several recently implemented machine learning algorithms and an ensemble of those classifiers. Lastly, they attempted to construct a sequence-level classifier, and they empirically set a threshold at 95% of the patient's sequences for classifying the patient as having HAD. However, such empirical criteria should be carefully interpreted for potential overfitting. Moreover, since it is plausible to assume that even patients with HAD harbor non-neurotoxic quasispecies, and vice versa for patients without clinically apparent neurocognitive impairments, a patient-level set of features capturing the diversity of intrapatient quasispecies could be more predictive rather than a sequence-level set of features.

The purpose of this retrospective analysis is to propose a potential biomarker for HAND. To this end, the most predictive genetic signatures were explored by generating an ML-based HAND prediction model. A thorough literature search led to the construction of the most comprehensive metadataset to date, comprised of 2494 *env* C2V3C3 sequences from 9 studies involving 85 specimens from 43 patients. Iterative ML and stepwise feature reduction yielded three genetic features. A final ensemble classifier achieved accuracy of 100 and 94% in the hold-out testing subdataset and as a whole, respectively. Specimens from various sampling sources were classifiable using the same genetic features. Clustering analysis stratified HAND into four distinct clusters. The datasets, the main analysis workflow, and the in-house functions were made publicly available so as to maximize the reproducibility of the entire work.

Results

Construction of annotated HIV *env* sequence metadataset
A large, curated sequence dataset annotated with relevant clinical information is indispensable for ML-based prediction of the HAND status. Initially, we considered using The HIVBrainSeqDB [22] (http://hivbrainseqdb.dfci.harvard.edu/HIVSeqDB/) or The HAND Database [23] (http://www.handdatabase.org/). However, because these databases did not seem comprehensive, we decided to conduct a manual literature review. A thorough literature search resulted in the construction of a manually curated metadataset derived from 9 studies involving 40 patients, and consisting of 2494 HIV *env* C2V3C3 sequences (see "Methods" section for details), among which 2358 were unique (Additional file 1: Table 1). Sequences isolated from HAND and NonHAND cases formed several phylogenetically distinct clusters (Additional file 1: Fig. 1). Supported by this observation, we decided to further explore ML-based approach to construct a classifier predicting the HAND status from the C2V3C3 sequences.

Machine learning for predicting HAND status
The 2349 C2V3C3 sequences derived from HAND or NonHAND patients were converted into a numerical matrix using the 76 AAIndex schemes relevant to the physicochemical properties of amino acids. Patients diagnosed as either HIV-associated encephalitis (HIVE) or non-specific neuropsychiatric disorder (NPD) were excluded. Next, sequences were grouped by patient and sampling source, and representative statistics (e.g. mean and standard deviation) were calculated for each alignment position. Features with little variance, and a set of highly correlated features were excluded. In this manner, a total of 3169 patient-level predictive features were generated for 80 specimens. We performed ML with five distinct algorithms with ten different random seeds for hold-out data splitting. Stacking of the five classifiers was also attempted.

The mean and the best accuracy of the stacked classifiers trained using all features were 63 and 78%, respectively, in the hold-out validation subdataset (Fig. 1a and Additional file 1: Table 2). However, since this is extremely over-parametrized analysis, we attempted to reduce the number of features. First, algorithm-specific feature importance was calculated for each classifier, and the 20 most important ones were screened (Additional file 1: Table 3). Next, features selected by two or more distinct algorithms were selected. Finally, distributions between HAND and NonHAND cases were compared. P values were calculated by Welch's t test, and adjustment for multiple comparisons was done according to the method controlling the false discovery rate (FDR)

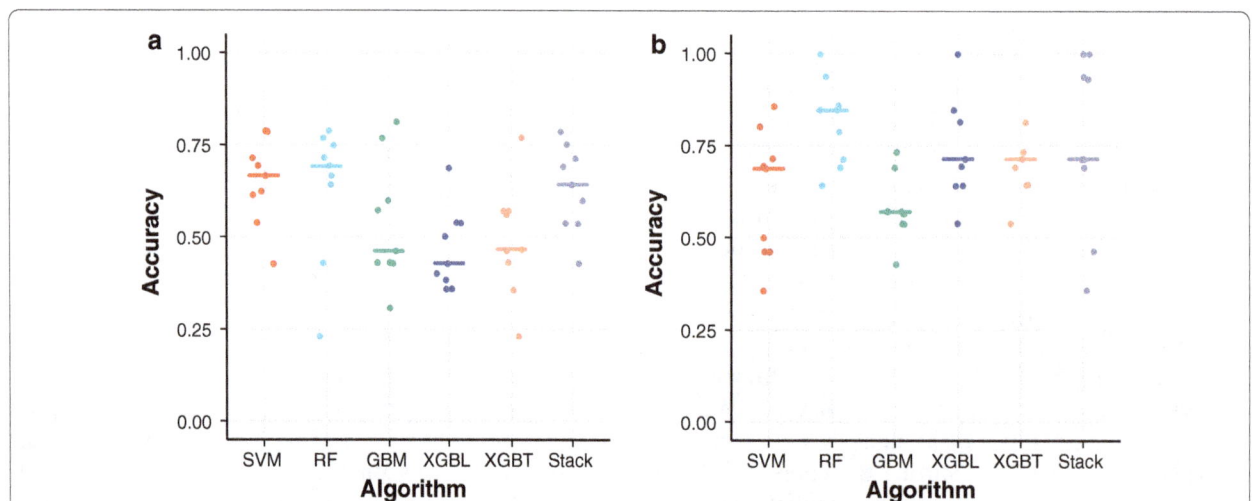

Fig. 1 Performance of ML-based classifiers predicting HAND. The in-house metadataset constructed from an extensive literature search was divided into the training and testing subdatasets. Five ML classifiers and their stacked classifier were trained using the training subdataset, and their accuracies were evaluated using the testing subdataset. Stacking algorithm was XGBT. **a** Classifiers trained using all features. **b** Classifiers trained with three minimal features. Dots represent ML attempts with different random seeds. SVM, support vector machine; RF, random forest; GBM, gradient boosting machine; XGBL, extreme gradient boosting with linear booster; XGBT, extreme gradient boosting with tree booster; Stack, the stacked classifier

originally reported by Benjamini and Hochberg [24]. Features with adjusted P values of lower than 0.05 were retained. In this manner, seven important features were uncovered (Additional file 1: Fig. 2). Encouraged by the observation that feature reduction did improve the predictive accuracy, we further deciphered the best set of features by means of stepwise feature reduction (Table 1 and Additional file 1: Table 4). Surprisingly, we observed the highest accuracy being 100% in the testing subdataset in two different algorithms (Fig. 1b). These classifiers used only three features. The mean and the best accuracy of the stacked classifiers were 76 and 100%, respectively (Fig. 1b and Additional file 1: Table 5). The accuracy of the best stacked classifier for the whole dataset was 94%, where the HAND status was predicted correctly in 75 out of 80 specimens. The distributions of Bayesian posterior probabilities showed that this classifier is expected to work well when the prior probability of HAND lies within the range from ~ 25% to ~ 50% (Additional file 1: Figure 3). Finally, as an external validation, all of the three specimens obtained from two patients with NPD were classified as HAND. One specimen was obtained from Patient 196, who was not diagnosed as HAD due to lack of information in the original paper despite the evidence of neuropsychiatric impairment [25]. The other two specimens were obtained from Subject 7115 at July 8th, 2002 [26]. Although the diagnosis of HAD could not be made due to confounding conditions at that moment, the same patient was diagnosed as moderate to severe HAD 2 years later. These two cases highlight the potential utility of our sequence-based HAND classifier as a diagnostic aid.

The distributions of the most important features were significantly different between the HAND and NonHAND cases (Fig. 2a). At position 291 (Pos291), the maximum value of the AAIndex DIGM050101, which represents a hydrostatic pressure asymmetry index, was shown to be the most predictive. The difference between the HAND and NonHAND cases was explained by the decrease of the frequency of 291S in the HAND group (Fig. 2b). Meanwhile, the other two important AAIndices, namely, KARP850102 and BHAR880101, are related to the flexibility of the

residue. Variants enriched in the HAND cases such as 315 K/S and 340D/K/S contributed to the different feature distributions (Fig. 2).

Molecular stratification of HAND through the minimal set of genetic features

HAND is a diagnosis of exclusion, thus inherently harboring some heterogeneity. We noticed that, although the stacked classifier predicts the HAND status with high confidence, the subordinate classifiers returned considerably varied probabilities to the same cases, indicating that each of the classifiers captures distinct aspects of the triad of the genetic features. Indeed, clustering analysis revealed four distinct HAND-rich clusters (H1-H4) with characteristic genetic landscapes (Fig. 3a). Clusters enriched with NonHAND cases were combined as N. Random forest algorithm successfully constructed a classifier for these five categories, with the estimated accuracy from internal CV being 94%. A representative decision tree with the median number of nodes was shown in Fig. 3b. The tree understandably reflects the similarities between H2 and H4, and those between H1 and H3. When each amino acid variants were considered to be features, no apparent cluster-specific enrichment occurred, underscoring the effectiveness of our AAIndex-based feature generation framework (Additional file 1: Fig. 3).

To unveil the characteristics of each of the HAND clusters, we next applied the random forest classifier to the entire dataset obtained from The HAND Database (http://www.handdatabase.org/), which is a recently published, manually curated database of HIV sequences with clinical metadata [16] (Fig. 4). Collectively, 26 out of 33 (79%) HAD cases were classified into one of the HAND clusters, whereas all of the twenty cases originally annotated as not neurocognitively impaired were predicted as such (100%). Interestingly, nine out of eleven (82%) HIVE cases were predicted as N. Moreover, remaining two HIVE cases and the 6 cases with HAD and overlapping HIVE were classified as H2. These observations highlight the uniqueness of H2, potentially bridging the two distinct disease entities, namely, HAND and HIVE.

Table 1 Important AAIndices identified in this study

AAIndex ID	Description	Reference
DIGM050101	Hydrostatic pressure asymmetry index	Di Giulio [47]
KARP850102	Flexibility parameter for one rigid neighbor	Karplus and Schulz [48]
BHAR880101	Average flexibility indices	Bhaskaran and Ponnuswamy [49]

For further information regarding each AAIndex, visit the AAIndex website (http://www.genome.jp/aaindex/) [42]

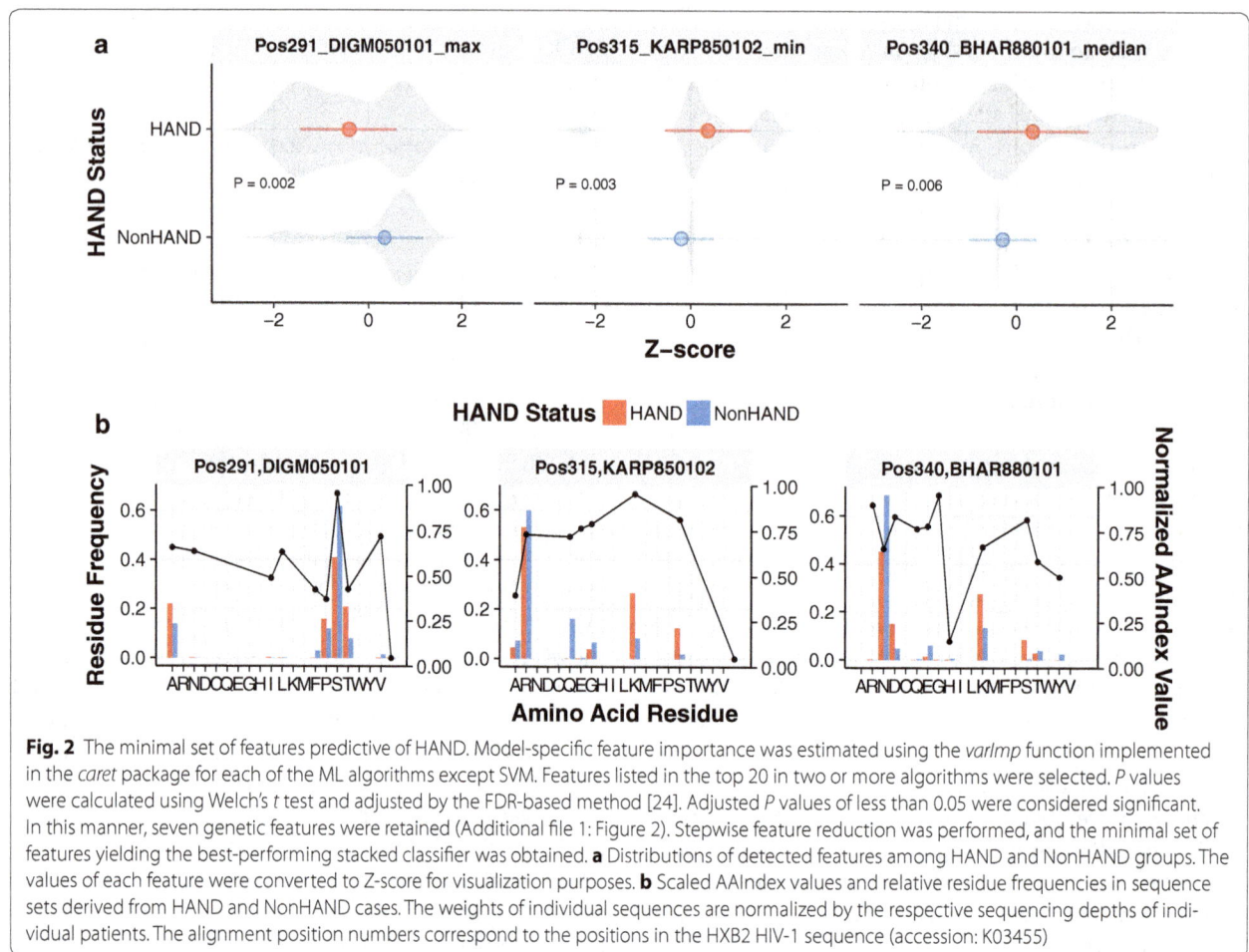

Fig. 2 The minimal set of features predictive of HAND. Model-specific feature importance was estimated using the *varImp* function implemented in the *caret* package for each of the ML algorithms except SVM. Features listed in the top 20 in two or more algorithms were selected. *P* values were calculated using Welch's *t* test and adjusted by the FDR-based method [24]. Adjusted *P* values of less than 0.05 were considered significant. In this manner, seven genetic features were retained (Additional file 1: Figure 2). Stepwise feature reduction was performed, and the minimal set of features yielding the best-performing stacked classifier was obtained. **a** Distributions of detected features among HAND and NonHAND groups. The values of each feature were converted to Z-score for visualization purposes. **b** Scaled AAIndex values and relative residue frequencies in sequence sets derived from HAND and NonHAND cases. The weights of individual sequences are normalized by the respective sequencing depths of individual patients. The alignment position numbers correspond to the positions in the HXB2 HIV-1 sequence (accession: K03455)

Estimation of the global burden of HAND

One major obstacle against the epidemiological study regarding HAND is the dearth of molecularly defined biomarkers. Currently, a careful neuropsychiatric examination is the only solid basis; in addition to this, various tests including brain CT/MRI and the cerebrospinal fluid (CSF) analysis are frequently required to exclude various mimicking diseases such as meningoencephalitis, toxoplasmosis, and primary CNS lymphoma. Biomarkers measurable from peripheral plasma could greatly reduce the burden for diagnostic procedures, and thereby facilitate epidemiological and other clinical studies particularly in resource-limited settings.

In view of this application, we retrospectively estimated the global burden of HAND from the entire sequence dataset deposited in the Los Alamos HIV Sequence Database (https://www.hiv.lanl.gov/content/sequence/HIV/mainpage.html), the largest database to date. Collectively, 46% of the cases were predicted as HAND, which was slightly higher than estimates from historical cohorts [4–7] (Fig. 5a). Among the predicted

HAND cases, H1 was the most common cluster, followed by H2, H3, and H4 (Fig. 5a). Geographically dissecting, Caribbean region was the region with the largest predicted HAND burden (71%), whereas Sub-Saharan Africa was the lowest prevalence (30%). Among HAND clusters, H1 was dominant in Sub-Saharan Africa and Asia/Middle-East/Oceania (97 and 85%, respectively). In other regions, no single dominant cluster was noted. Caribbean region was characterized by the high prevalence of H3 (59%). Europe and North America regions had relatively high prevalence of H2 (54 and 38%, respectively). These regional differences in viral genetic landscape might be associated with various factors such as ethnicity and human leucocyte antigen (HLA) allele frequencies. Among the HAND clusters, H1 had a moderately higher viral load and lower CD4$^+$ T-cell count compared to H2. Meanwhile, H3 had a statistically higher CD4$^+$ T-cell count compared to H1 (Additional file 1: Figure 5). These trends were unchanged even when the *P* values were adjusted according to the FDR-based method [24].

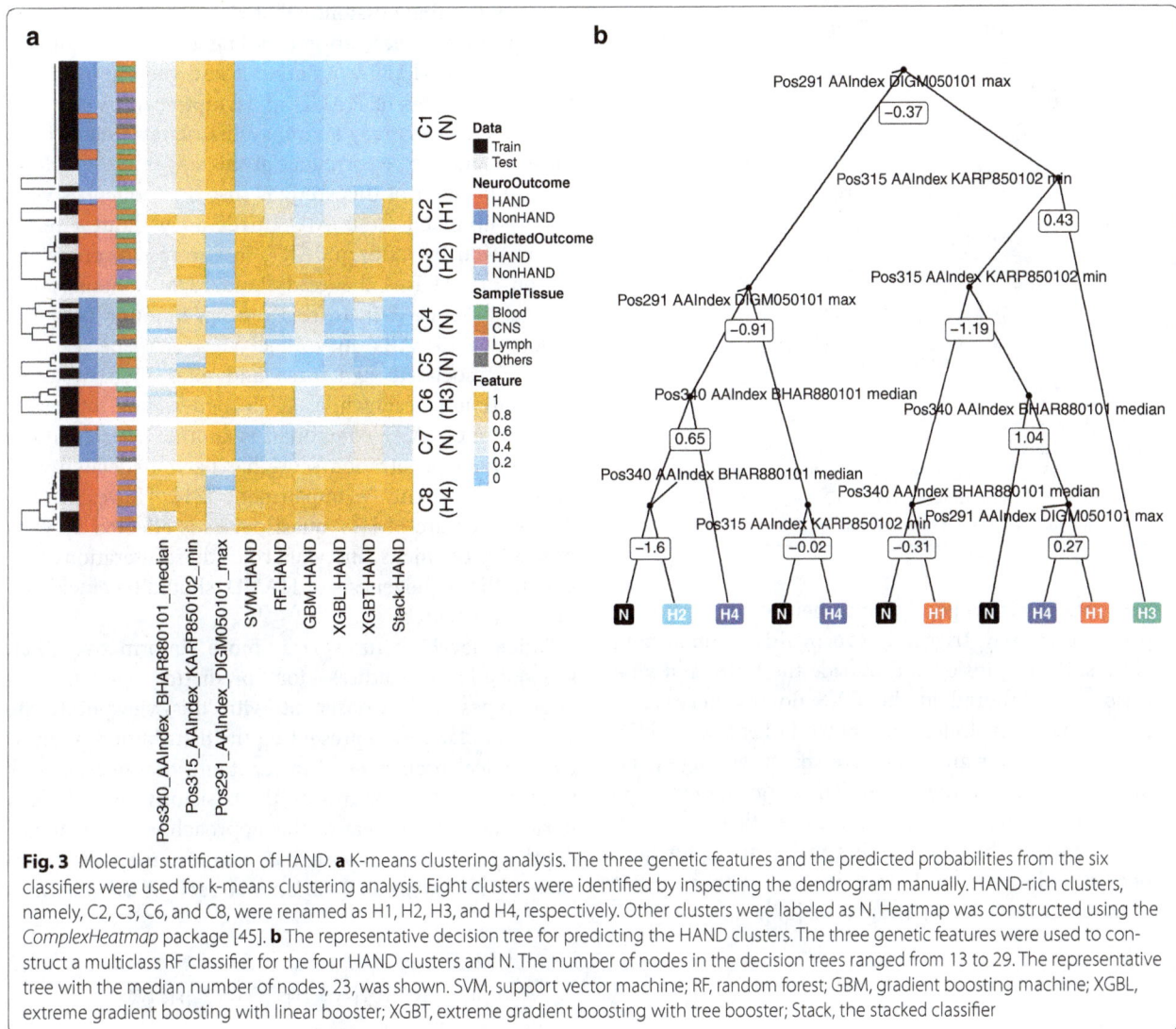

Fig. 3 Molecular stratification of HAND. **a** K-means clustering analysis. The three genetic features and the predicted probabilities from the six classifiers were used for k-means clustering analysis. Eight clusters were identified by inspecting the dendrogram manually. HAND-rich clusters, namely, C2, C3, C6, and C8, were renamed as H1, H2, H3, and H4, respectively. Other clusters were labeled as N. Heatmap was constructed using the *ComplexHeatmap* package [45]. **b** The representative decision tree for predicting the HAND clusters. The three genetic features were used to construct a multiclass RF classifier for the four HAND clusters and N. The number of nodes in the decision trees ranged from 13 to 29. The representative tree with the median number of nodes, 23, was shown. SVM, support vector machine; RF, random forest; GBM, gradient boosting machine; XGBL, extreme gradient boosting with linear booster; XGBT, extreme gradient boosting with tree booster; Stack, the stacked classifier

Data and code availability for future research

Both the datasets and the in-house functions created in this study were bundled as the R package *HAND-Prediction*, and distributed on GitHub (https://github.com/masato-ogishi/HANDPrediction). To facilitate future research, the entire analysis workflow was also publicly distributed as an HTML document (Additional file 2).

Discussion

In this work, the three genetic features of the HIV *env* gene most predictive of the HAND status were identified through the construction of a highly accurate classifier via machine learning (ML). The surprisingly small number of features, three, strongly counter-argues the possibility of overfitting and supports the generalizability of

the model to external datasets. The set of features stratified the 37 specimens derived from HAND cases into four clusters. The stratification process was successfully recapitulated by random forest algorithm, which enabled extrapolation of the genetic feature-based classification of HAND status. Estimation of global burden of HAND was demonstrated using the Loa Alamos HIV sequence database. The regional differences in the relative frequencies of HAND clusters probed by this retrospective analysis underscore the potential usefulness of our framework as an aid for epidemiological research, thereby warranting prospective validation.

In contrast to previous studies, neurotoxicity was stringently distinguished from neurotropism during the construction of the metadataset in this study. This is because it is inappropriate to discuss those two distinct

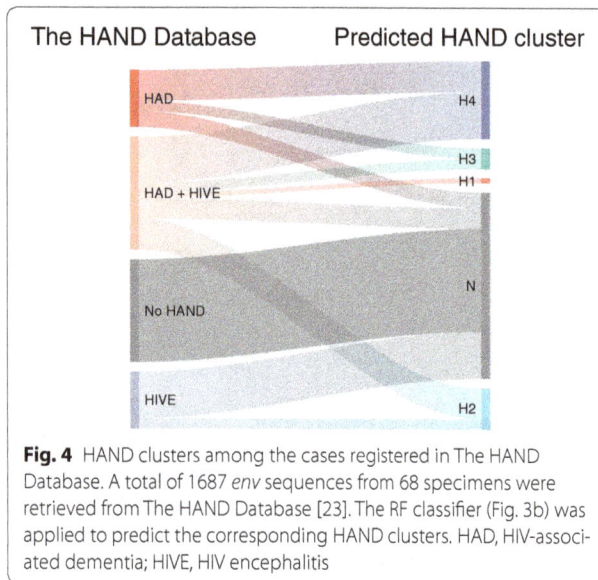

Fig. 4 HAND clusters among the cases registered in The HAND Database. A total of 1687 *env* sequences from 68 specimens were retrieved from The HAND Database [23]. The RF classifier (Fig. 3b) was applied to predict the corresponding HAND clusters. HAD, HIV-associated dementia; HIVE, HIV encephalitis

It is an exciting possibility that viral sequences obtained from peripheral circulation could be used as a diagnostic biomarker of HAND. Whether these genetic biomarkers provide clues to HAND at asymptomatic stage is of great interest, as many neuropsychiatric tests suffer from lower diagnostic performance at this stage [28, 29]. However, one caveat of this study is that the sequences were mainly obtained from AIDS patients without viremia suppression by modern cART. In contrast, prompt initiation of cART is the gold standard of contemporary clinical practice [30]. In this setting, immune reconstitution due to cART may affect viral quasispecies with HAND-associated signatures and alter their systemic distributions. Meanwhile, CNS penetration effectiveness score of cART compound is another consideration, since higher penetration score has been associated with lower neurocognitive impairment [31]. However, how the architecture of HIV quasispecies is affected by various cART regimens, and what roles these alterations may play in the pathogenesis of HAND, should be elucidated in future research.

Patient-level features are more informative than sequence-level features for predicting patient-level phenotypes [32]. Consistent with this viewpoint, the summary statistics representing the distribution of physicochemical properties of intrapatient viral quasispecies were used as the features on the basis of which ML was performed. One caveat of this approach is the sequence depth per patient; observed relative frequencies of each of the amino acid variants at each of the positions

phenotypes interchangeably, since neurotoxic viral quasispecies that may trigger neurocognitive impairment could reside both inside and outside the CNS, and viral quasispecies harbored in the CNS do not necessarily exert neurotoxicity. Indeed, as shown in Fig. 3a, HAND-associated genetic signatures were shared among specimens derived from the CNS, lymphatic system, and peripheral circulation. This indicates that selection pressure outside the CNS is not a major driver for quasispecies evolution, which is consistent with a recent observational study led by Stefic et al. [27].

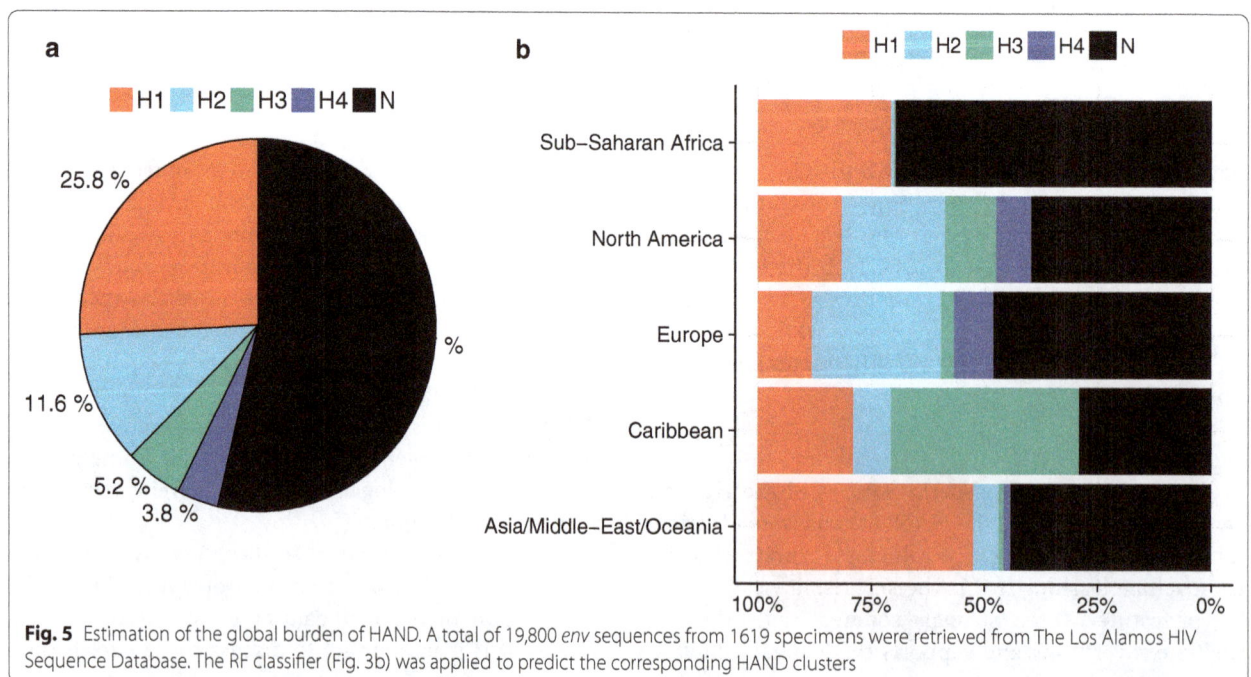

Fig. 5 Estimation of the global burden of HAND. A total of 19,800 *env* sequences from 1619 specimens were retrieved from The Los Alamos HIV Sequence Database. The RF classifier (Fig. 3b) was applied to predict the corresponding HAND clusters

may not reflect true intrapatient abundance with limited sequencing depth. Alternatively, next-generation sequencing platform could allow researchers to estimate relative abundance of variants with remarkably improved accuracy. We have previously shown that intrapatient abundances of viral quasispecies could be reliably estimated bioinformatically from short-read sequence datasets generated by the Illumina MiSeq platform [33]. This process is known as "quasispecies reconstruction". Integration of high-throughput sequencing technology and quasispecies reconstruction could enable more accurate estimations of intrapatient quasispecies abundance with augmented scalability. Such large-scale datasets could bolster the precision and accuracy of the HAND prediction framework presented in this work.

A number of gp120 variants have been associated with neurotropism and/or neurotoxicity. For example, Dunfee et al. [34] reported T283N as a neurotoxic variant causing enhanced macrophage infectivity and neuronal degeneration. Duenas-Decamp et al. [27] showed that the otherwise non-macrophage-tropic strain LN40 can be transformed into a macrophage-tropic strain by introducing 283 N substitution. However, in an already macrophage-tropic strain (B33), substitution of 283 N into 283T did not alter tropism, indicating the existence of other determinants [27]. In our analysis, three positions, namely, Pos291, Pos315, and, Pos340, were identified to be the most predictive for HAND status (Fig. 2b). Holman and Gabuzda also reported the involvement of Pos315 in HAND-predicting signature [21]. Pos315 resides in the tip of the V3-loop, and various variants such as R315K, R315T, and R315Q have been associated with reduced efficacy of neutralizing antibodies (NAbs) [35–38]. In our analysis, R315K and R315Q were enriched in the HAND and NonHAND cases, respectively (Fig. 2b). Although the other two positions, Pos291 and Pos340, were less intensively studied, S291 (enriched in NonHAND) has been associated with decreased infectivity to macrophages in R5 virus [27]. Meanwhile, compartmentalization of N340, a variant enriched in NonHAND in our analysis, to the CNS was observed in some cases [39]. Both S291 and N340 were also identified in this study (Additional file 1: Figure 4).

The current concept of HAND is heterogeneous due to its nature of being diagnosed on the basis of symptomatic criteria and by exclusion of other confounding conditions. To our knowledge, there is no attempt to date to molecularly stratify the disease entity. In this work, four HAND clusters were identified based on a clustering analysis. Particularly, H2 is interesting because it was associated with HIVE (Fig. 4). Since H2 and the closest cluster H4 were distinguished by the Pos340 feature (Fig. 3), and H4 was associated with both HAD

and HAD + HIVE (Fig. 4), Pos340 might be important in separating HAND and HIVE. Moreover, geographically speaking, both H2 and H4 seemed to be enriched in Europe and North America (Fig. 5). Such geographical difference, if is the case, should be taken into consideration when interpreting various research on HAND from various nations. The biological and epidemiological relevance of those variants and clusters has yet to be elucidated, thus warranting further research.

This study has some limitations, similarly to prior studies. First, since this is a retrospective observational study, no causative link can be definitively established. Amino acid signatures detected could be relevant to the neurotoxicity of HIV, but should not be interpreted as causative of HAND. Second, although unprecedented size, the numbers of unique specimens and patients were fairly small. Although we successfully reduced the number of required genetic features down to three, the risk of overfitting to the entire dataset should not be negated. Prospective collection of the adequate size of specimens would be the only strategy to effectively resolve this concern. Third, since most of the currently available *env* sequences were derived from HAD cases, the most severe form of HAND, the utility of our analysis in predicting early-stage HAND has yet to be fully verified. Similarly to this point, the effect of cART regimens on the evolutionary trajectory of viral quasispecies should also be taken into consideration in future research. We do not argue that our analysis provides all answers; rather, we hope this work could be a starting point. Therefore, we made publicly available the datasets, the custom codes, and the entire analysis workflow for the community.

Conclusions

In this study, robust prediction of HAND status from three genetic features derived from the HIV *env* sequences was demonstrated. Furthermore, based on the combination of these three genetic features, we stratified HAND into four clusters with unique characteristics. These results could be utilized as a diagnostic aid after prospectively validation. Finally, the biological and epidemiological significance of newly discovered genetic features, potentially providing the basis of the development of novel cART regimens specifically optimized for HAND-associated quasispecies, are to be elucidated in future research.

Methods

Computational analysis

All computational analyses were conducted using R ver. 3.4.1 (https://www.r-project.org/) [40]. The latest versions of R packages were consistently used. The dataset and the scripts generated in this study are available as the

R package *HANDPrediction* on GitHub (https://github.com/masato-ogishi/HANDPrediction). The entire analysis workflow is also available as an HTML document (Additional file 2).

Assembly of the HIV *env* sequence metadataset

A thorough literature search was conducted to collect previously published studies on HIV neurotoxicity and/or neurotropism. Sequences and accompanying metadata were retrieved from the Los Alamos HIV Sequence Database (http://www.hiv.lanl.gov/content/sequence/HIV/mainpage.html/) and manually curated. Diagnoses of HIV-associated neurological conditions were retrieved from original publications for all of the cases. The subcategories of HAND (AMI, MND, and HAD) were combined as 'HAND', and the AIDS-dementia complex (ADC) was also considered 'HAND' in this study. HIVE and other NPDs were labeled as such. Cases with no neurocognitive impairments were labeled as 'NonHAND' regardless of other CNS diseases including bacterial meningitis, toxoplasmosis, and CNS lymphoma. The sample sources were categorized into one of the following categories: 'CNS', 'Blood', 'Lymph', and 'Others'.

Alignment of HIV *env* sequences

The HXB2 HIV-1 sequence (accession: K03455) was used as a reference. The *env* region was identified by mapping sequences to the reference sequence using Geneious ver 8.1.8 (www.geneious.com). The built-in Geneious mapper was used with the "Medium Sensitivity" option selected. Default parameters were used. Sequences not mapped to the reference were discarded from the metadataset. The *env* C2V3C3 regions were manually determined, clipped, and re-aligned with MAFFT [41]. The alignment was refined and translated using the HIVAlign tool with the HMM-align option selected (https://www.hiv.lanl.gov/content/sequence/VIRALIGN/viralign.html). Alignment gaps shared by the reference sequence and more than 75% of the aligned sequences were manually removed. Sequences containing stop codons inside the C2V3C3 region were discarded.

Machine learning

AAIndex matrix

AAIndex metrics (http://www.genome.jp/aaindex/) [42] were adopted as quantitative measures of biophysicochemical properties of each amino acid. A total of 531 AAIndices were retrieved from the *BioSeqClass* package available in *Bioconductor* [43]. The 76 AAIndices whose names matched with one of the following phrases were selected for machine learning: 'Hydro', 'Charge', 'Polar', 'Distribution', and 'Flexi'. A C2V3C3 sequence was converted to a numerical vector comprising a set of AAIndex values corresponding to each amino acid residue at each alignment position. For all gaps and ambiguities (i.e., two or more amino acid residues indicated), values for all AAIndices were set to zero. In this manner, all sequences were converted to a numerical matrix, which had 76×189 (188 alignment positions plus one gap) columns.

Hold-out validation

The metadataset was split into the training and testing subdatasets at a ratio of 4:1. Note that the metadataset was split at the patient level, not at the sequence level. Sequence-level data splitting is inappropriate because the HAND vs NonHAND status is assigned to patients, not to individual sequences, and the genetic relatedness of the sequences derived from the same patient will likely lead to biased classification.

Preprocessing

In the training subdataset, columns with zero variance and near-zero variance were removed using the *preProcess* function with the 'zv' and 'nzv' method implemented in the *caret* package [44]. Then, highly correlating columns were filtered using *preProcess* with the 'corr' method. After these filtration steps, 3169 unique features were retained. Finally, the features were centered and scaled using *preProcess* with the 'center' and 'scale' methods. All preprocessing steps were carried out with default parameter settings. In the testing phase, the same preprocessing conditions prepared in the training phase were applied.

Machine learning with different algorithms

For simplicity, binary classification was attempted, i.e., HAND vs NonHAND. The following algorithms were compared for performance: support vector machine (SVM), random forest (RF), gradient boosting machine (GBM), extreme gradient boosting with linear booster (XGBL), and extreme gradient boosting with tree booster (XGBT), all of which are implemented in the *caret* package. "Stacking" of the classifiers was done using XGBT as a supervised learning algorithm. Ten-fold repeated three-fold CV was conducted in the training phase to improve the generalizability of the classifiers. Their predictive performances, i.e., sensitivity, specificity, and overall accuracy, were estimated using the testing subdataset.

Feature importance analysis

Model-specific feature importance was estimated using the *varImp* function implemented in the *caret* package. All models except SVM tested in this study have their own feature importance measures. The 20 most important features from each of the models were combined, and features detected in two or more different models were selected. Next, the distribution of the feature values among the HAND and NonHAND groups were compared by Welch's t test, and P values were adjusted by the FDR-based method by Benjamini and Hochberg [24]. Features whose adjusted P values were less than 0.05 were selected. Finally, stepwise feature reduction was iteratively performed. ML was performed on the training subdataset with one of the features removed, and the accuracy in the testing subdataset. The removed feature giving the highest accuracy of the stacked classifier was removed for the next iteration.

Clustering analysis

K-means clustering was performed on the minimal set of the most important features, and the predicted probabilities by each of the classifiers. Visualization of the heatmap and dendrograms were performed using the *ComplexHeatmap* package [45]. Clusters enriched with the HAND cases were identified by manual inspection of the dendrogram. Clusters enriched with the NonHAND cases were combined and labeled as 'N'. The minimal set of the most important features was used to construct a multiclass random forest classifier classifying the HAND clusters and N using the entire dataset.

Characterization of HAND clusters using The HAND Database

The HAND Database [23] (http://database.handdatabase.org/) was used to characterize each of the HAND clusters. The entire dataset was downloaded as is. A total of 1687 *env* sequences from 68 specimens were obtained. Sequences were aligned to the HXB2 reference sequence, converted to a numerical matrix, preprocessed using the preprocessing models prepared in the training phase. For each specimen, the corresponding HAND cluster was assigned by the multiclass random forest classifier trained during the clustering analysis. The original labels of neuropathological conditions and the prediction results were linked and visualized as a Sankey plot using the *googleVis* package [46].

Estimation of the global burden of HAND using the Los Alamos HIV Sequence Database

The Los Alamos HIV Sequence Database (https://www.hiv.lanl.gov/content/sequence/HIV/mainpage.html) was used to demonstrate a retrospective estimation of the global burden of HAND. The sequences whose "culture method" were either "primary" or "uncultured" were downloaded. A total of 19800 *env* sequences from 1619 specimens were obtained. HAND status was predicted as described above.

Abbreviations

HIV: human immunodeficiency virus type 1; HAND: HIV-associated neurocognitive disorder; cART: combination antiretroviral therapy; CNS: the central nervous system; HNRC: HIV Neurobehavioral Research Center; ANI: asymptomatic neurocognitive impairment; MND: mild neurocognitive disorder; HAD: HIV-associated dementia; ML: machine learning; CV: cross-validation; HIVE: HIV-associated encephalitis; NPD: non-specific neuropsychiatric disorder; FDR: false discovery rate; CSF: cerebrospinal fluid; AIDS: acquired immunodeficiency syndrome; NAb: neutralizing antibody; ADC: AIDS-dementia complex; SVM: support vector machine; RF: random forest; GBM: gradient boosting machine; XGBL: extreme gradient boosting with linear booster; XGBT: extreme gradient boosting with tree booster; CI: confidential interval.

Authors' contributions

MO and HY designed the study; MO performed data analyses, prepared figures and tables, and drafted the manuscript; MO and HY, wrote the manuscript. Both authors read and approved the final manuscript.

Author details

[1] Division of Infectious Diseases and Applied Immunology, Research Hospital, The Institute of Medical Science, The University of Tokyo, Tokyo, Japan. [2] National Center for Global Health and Medicine, Tokyo, Japan.

Acknowledgements

We thank Dr. Couture-Cossette for thoughtful comments.

Competing interests

The authors declare that they have no competing interests.

Funding

This research received no specific grant from any funding agency in the public, commercial, or not-for-profit sectors.

References

1. Saylor D, Dickens AM, Sacktor N, Haughey N, Slusher B, Pletnikov M, et al. HIV-associated neurocognitive disorder—pathogenesis and prospects for treatment. Nat Rev Neurol. 2016;12:234–48.
2. Clifford DB, Ances BM. HIV-associated neurocognitive disorder. Lancet Infect Dis. 2013;13:976–86.
3. Antinori A, Arendt G, Becker JT, Brew BJ, Byrd DA, Cherner M, et al. Updated research nosology for HIV-associated neurocognitive disorders. Neurology. 2007;69:1789–99.
4. Heaton RK, Clifford DB, Franklin DR, Woods SP, Ake C, Vaida F, et al. HIV-associated neurocognitive disorders persist in the era of potent antiretroviral therapy: Charter Study. Neurology. 2010;75:2087–96.
5. Chan LG, Kandiah N, Chua A. HIV-associated neurocognitive disorders (HAND) in a South Asian population—contextual application of the 2007 criteria. BMJ Open. 2012;2:e000662.
6. Yusuf AJ, Hassan A, Mamman AI, Muktar HM, Suleiman AM, Baiyewu O. Prevalence of HIV-associated neurocognitive disorder (HAND) among patients attending a tertiary health facility in Northern Nigeria. J Int Assoc Provid AIDS Care. 2014;116:1477–90.
7. Sacktor N, Skolasky RL, Seaberg E, Munro C, Becker JT, Martin E, et al. Prevalence of HIV-associated neurocognitive disorders in the Multicenter AIDS Cohort Study. Neurology. 2015;86:334–40.
8. Crum-Cianflone NF, Moore DJ, Letendre S, Roediger MP, Eberly L, Weintrob A, et al. Low prevalence of neurocognitive impairment in early diagnosed and managed HIV-infected persons. Neurology. 2013;80:371–9.
9. Oliveira MF, Chaillon A, Nakazawa M, Vargas M, Letendre SL, Strain MC, et al. Early antiretroviral therapy is associated with lower HIV DNA molecular diversity and lower inflammation in cerebrospinal fluid but does not prevent the establishment of compartmentalized HIV DNA populations. PLoS Pathog. 2017;13:e1006112.
10. Simioni S, Cavassini M, Annoni J-M, Rimbault Abraham A, Bourquin I, Schiffer V, et al. Cognitive dysfunction in HIV patients despite long-standing suppression of viremia. AIDS. 2010;24:1243–50.
11. Peluso MJ, Ferretti F, Peterson J, Lee E, Fuchs D, Boschini A, et al. Cerebrospinal fluid HIV escape associated with progressive neurologic dysfunction in patients on antiretroviral therapy with well controlled plasma viral load. AIDS. 2012;26:1765–74.

12. Toggas SM, Masliah E, Rockenstein EM, Rall GF, Abraham CR, Mucke L. Central nervous system damage produced by expression of the HIV-1 coat protein gp120 in transgenic mice. Nature. 1994;367:188–93.

13. Jana A, Pahan K. Human immunodeficiency virus type 1 gp120 induces apoptosis in human primary neurons through redox-regulated activation of neutral sphingomyelinase. Neuroscience. 2004;24:9531–40.

14. Zhang K, Rana F, Silva C, Ethier J, Wehrly K, Chesebro B, et al. Human immunodeficiency virus type 1 envelope-mediated neuronal death: uncoupling of viral replication and neurotoxicity. J Virol. 2003;77:6899–912.

15. Bachis A, Cruz MI, Mocchetti I. M-tropic HIV envelope protein gp120 exhibits a different neuropathological profile than T-tropic gp120 in rat striatum. Eur J Neurosci. 2010;32:570–8.

16. Hartley O, Klasse PJ, Sattentau QJ, Moore JP. V3: HIV's switch-hitter. AIDS Res Hum Retroviruses. 2005;21:171–89.

17. Rossi F, Querido B, Nimmagadda M, Cocklin S, Navas-Martín S, Martín-García J. The V1-V3 region of a brain-derived HIV-1 envelope glycoprotein determines macrophage tropism, low CD4 dependence, increased fusogenicity and altered sensitivity to entry inhibitors. Retrovirology. 2008;5:89.

18. Albright AV, Shieh JT, Itoh T, Lee B, Pleasure D, O'Connor MJ, et al. Micro-glia express CCR5, CXCR4, and CCR3, but of these, CCR5 is the principal coreceptor for human immunodeficiency virus type 1 dementia isolates. J Virol. 1999;73:205–13.

19. Gorry PR, Taylor J, Holm GH, Mehle A, Morgan T, Cayabyab M, et al. Increased CCR5 affinity and reduced CCR5/CD4 dependence of a neurovirulent primary human immunodeficiency virus type 1 isolate. J Virol. 2002;76:6277–92.

20. Pillai SK, Pond SLK, Liu Y, Good BM, Strain MC, Ellis RJ, et al. Genetic attributes of cerebrospinal fluid-derived HIV-1 env. Brain. 2006;129:1872–83.

21. Holman AG, Gabuzda D. A machine learning approach for identifying amino acid signatures in the HIV env gene predictive of dementia. PLoS ONE. 2012;7:e49538.

22. Holman AG, Mefford ME, O'Connor N, Gabuzda D. HIVBrainSeqDB: a database of annotated HIV envelope sequences from brain and other anatomical sites. AIDS Res Ther. 2010;7:43.

23. Griffin TZ, Kang W, Ma Y, Zhang M. The HAND Database: a gateway to understanding the role of HIV in HIV-associated neurocognitive disorders. BMC Med Genomics. 2015;8:70.

24. Benjamini Y, Hochberg Y. Controlling the false discovery rate: a practical and powerful approach to multiple testing. J R Stat Soc Ser B. 1995;57:289–300.

25. Shapshak P, Segal DM, Crandall KA, Fujimura RK, Zhang BT, Xin KQ, et al. Independent evolution of HIV type 1 in different brain regions. AIDS Res Hum Retroviruses. 1999;15:811–20.

26. Schnell G, Joseph S, Spudich S, Price RW, Swanstrom R. HIV-1 replication in the central nervous system occurs in two distinct cell types. PLoS Pathog. 2011;7:e1002286.

27. Duenas-Decamp MJ, Peters PJ, Burton D, Clapham PR. Determinants flanking the CD4 binding loop modulate macrophage tropism of human immunodeficiency virus type 1 R5 envelopes. J Virol. 2009;83:2575–83.

28. Bloch M, Kamminga J, Jayewardene A, Bailey M, Carberry A, Vincent T, et al. A screening strategy for HIV-associated neurocognitive disorders that accurately identifies patients requiring neurological review. Clin Infect Dis. 2016;63:687–93.

29. Krista J, Siefried BJB, Brew BJ, Siefried KJ, Draper B, Cysique LA. Is the HIV dementia scale a reliable tool for assessing HIV-related neurocognitive decline? J AIDS Clin Res. 2014;5:1–7.

30. INSIGHT START Study Group, Lundgren JD, Babiker AG, Gordin F, Emery S, Grund B, et al. Initiation of antiretroviral therapy in early asymptomatic HIV infection. N Engl J Med. 2015;373:795–807.

31. Smurzynski M, Wu K, Letendre S, Robertson K, Bosch RJ, Clifford DB, et al. Effects of central nervous system antiretroviral penetration on cognitive functioning in the ALLRT cohort. AIDS. 2011;25:357–65.

32. Vignuzzi M, Stone JK, Arnold JJ, Cameron CE, Andino R. Quasispecies diversity determines pathogenesis through cooperative interactions in a viral population. Nature. 2006;439:344–8.

33. Ogishi M, Yotsuyanagi H, Tsutsumi T, Gatanaga H, Ode H, Sugiura W, et al. Deconvoluting the composition of low-frequency hepatitis C viral quasispecies: comparison of genotypes and NS3 resistance-associated variants between HCV/HIV coinfected hemophiliacs and HCV monoinfected patients in Japan. PLoS ONE. 2015;10:e0119145.

34. Dunfee RL, Thomas ER, Gorry PR, Wang J, Taylor J, Kunstman K, et al. The HIV Env variant N283 enhances macrophage tropism and is associated with brain infection and dementia. Proc Natl Acad Sci USA. 2006;103:15160–5.

35. Pantophlet R, Wilson IA, Burton DR. Improved design of an antigen with enhanced specificity for the broadly HIV-neutralizing antibody b12. Protein Eng Des Sel. 2004;17:749–58.

36. Pantophlet R, Wrin T, Cavacini LA, Robinson JE, Burton DR. Neutralizing activity of antibodies to the V3 loop region of HIV-1 gp120 relative to their epitope fine specificity. Virology. 2008;381:251–60.

37. Pantophlet R, Aguilar-Sino RO, Wrin T, Cavacini LA, Burton DR. Analysis of the neutralization breadth of the anti-V3 antibody F425-B4e8 and re-assessment of its epitope fine specificity by scanning mutagenesis. Virology. 2007;364:441–53.

38. Kuwata T, Enomoto I, Baba M, Matsushita S. Incompatible natures of the HIV-1 envelope in resistance to the CCR5 antagonist cenicriviroc and to neutralizing antibodies. Antimicrob Agents Chemother. 2015;60:437–50.

39. Strain MC, Letendre S, Pillai SK, Russell T, Ignacio CC, Günthard HF, et al. Genetic composition of human immunodeficiency virus type 1 in cerebrospinal fluid and blood without treatment and during failing antiretroviral therapy. J Virol. 2005;79:1772–88.

40. R Core Team. R: a language and environment for statistical computing. Vienna: R Foundation for Statistical Computing; 2016.

41. Katoh K, Misawa K, Kuma K, Miyata T. MAFFT: a novel method for rapid multiple sequence alignment based on fast Fourier transform. Nucleic Acids Res. 2002;30:3059–66.

42. Kawashima S, Pokarowski P, Pokarowska M, Kolinski A, Katayama T, Kanehisa M. AAindex: amino acid index database, progress report 2008. Nucleic Acids Res. 2008;36:202–5.

43. Gentleman RC, Carey VJ, Bates DM, Bolstad B, Dettling M, Dudoit S, et al. Bioconductor: open software development for computational biology and bioinformatics. Genome Biol. 2004;5:R80.

44. Kuhn M. Building predictive models in R using the caret package. J Stat Softw. 2008;28:1–26.

45. Gu Z, Eils R, Schlesner M. Complex heatmaps reveal patterns and correlations in multidimensional genomic data. Bioinformatics. 2016;32:2847–9.

46. Gesmann M, de Castillo D. Using the google visualisation API with R. R J. 2011;3:40–4.

47. Di Giulio M. A comparison of proteins from *Pyrococcus furiosus* and *Pyrococcus abyssi*: barophily in the physicochemical properties of amino acids and in the genetic code. Gene. 2005;346:1–6.

48. Karplus PA, Schulz GE. Prediction of chain flexibility in proteins. Naturwissenschaften. 1985;72:212–3.

49. Bhaskaran R, Ponnuswamy PK. Positional flexibilities of amino acid residues in globular proteins. Int J Pept Protein Res. 2009;32:241–55.

4

New World feline APOBEC3 potently controls inter-genus lentiviral transmission

Yoriyuki Konno[1,2], Shumpei Nagaoka[1,2], Izumi Kimura[1,3], Keisuke Yamamoto[1,4], Yumiko Kagawa[1,5], Ryuichi Kumata[1,6], Hirofumi Aso[1,3,7], Mahoko Takahashi Ueda[8], So Nakagawa[8,9], Tomoko Kobayashi[10], Yoshio Koyanagi[1] and Kei Sato[1,11,12*]

Abstract

Background: The apolipoprotein B mRNA-editing enzyme catalytic polypeptide-like 3 (APOBEC3; A3) gene family appears only in mammalian genomes. Some A3 proteins can be incorporated into progeny virions and inhibit lentiviral replication. In turn, the lentiviral viral infectivity factor (Vif) counteracts the A3-mediated antiviral effect by degrading A3 proteins. Recent investigations have suggested that lentiviral *vif* genes evolved to combat mammalian APOBEC3 proteins, and have further proposed that the Vif-A3 interaction may help determine the co-evolutionary history of cross-species lentiviral transmission in mammals.

Results: Here we address the co-evolutionary relationship between two New World felids, the puma (*Puma concolor*) and the bobcat (*Lynx rufus*), and their lentiviruses, which are designated puma lentiviruses (PLVs). We demonstrate that PLV-A Vif counteracts the antiviral action of APOBEC3Z3 (A3Z3) of both puma and bobcat, whereas PLV-B Vif counteracts only puma A3Z3. The species specificity of PLV-B Vif is irrespective of the phylogenic relationships of feline species in the genera *Puma, Lynx* and *Acinonyx*. We reveal that the amino acid at position 178 in the puma and bobcat A3Z3 is exposed on the protein surface and determines the sensitivity to PLV-B Vif-mediated degradation. Moreover, although both the puma and bobcat *A3Z3* genes are polymorphic, their sensitivity/resistance to PLV Vif-mediated degradation is conserved.

Conclusions: To the best of our knowledge, this is the first study suggesting that the host A3 protein potently controls inter-genus lentiviral transmission. Our findings provide the first evidence suggesting that the co-evolutionary arms race between lentiviruses and mammals has occurred in the New World.

Keywords: Lentivirus, FIV, APOBEC3, Vif, Evolutionary arms race, Puma, Bobcat, PLV, New World

Background

The apolipoprotein B mRNA editing enzyme catalytic polypeptide-like 3 (APOBEC3; A3) proteins are cellular cytidine deaminases that are specifically encoded in mammals but not in other vertebrates [1, 2]. Mammalian A3 proteins, particularly primate A3 proteins, are considered cellular intrinsic immune factors that potently restrict lentiviral replication. To exhibit antiviral activity, some A3 proteins are incorporated into the released progeny virions and enzymatically insert guanine-to-adenine hypermutations into the viral genome, thereby halting viral replication. In turn, the lentiviral protein, viral infectivity factor (Vif), antagonizes the A3-mediated antiviral action by degrading A3 proteins via the ubiquitin/proteasome-dependent pathway (reviewed in [3]).

Elucidating co-evolutionary relationships between hosts and their viruses is an intriguing topic in virology and is crucial to understanding how viruses influence their hosts' evolution and vice versa. Cell-based virological experiments are essential for a better understanding of the evolutionary conflict between mammals and their viruses, including lentiviruses. For instance, since the

*Correspondence: ksato@ims.u-tokyo.ac.jp
[12] Division of Systems Virology, Department of Infectious Disease Control, International Research Center for Infectious Diseases, Institute of Medical Science, The University of Tokyo, 4-6-1 Shirokanedai, Minato-ku, Tokyo 1088639, Japan
Full list of author information is available at the end of the article

interaction between host A3 and lentiviral Vif is species specific, various investigations focusing on the functional relationship between A3 and Vif have recently been conducted in combination with molecular phylogenetic approaches (reviewed in [4]). This strategy stems from the "Red Queen hypothesis [5]", which proposes that host and viral proteins have competed with one another for survival over time [6–8]. However, since most previous observations are based the Old World evolutionary events [4], whether the evolutionary arms race between mammals and lentiviruses has occurred in the New World is unclear.

Feline immunodeficiency virus (FIV) is a lentivirus that was first isolated in 1987 from domestic cats (*Felis catus*) with chronic AIDS-like disorders [9]. Domestic cats encode multiple *A3* genes, and the feline A3 protein (designated A3Z3) potently impairs FIV replication by incorporating into nascent virions [10–15]. In response, FIV Vif antagonizes the antiviral activity of feline A3Z3 by degrading this protein [11–15]. To elucidate the evolutionary relationship between FIV and felids, we have recently reported that the domestic cat *A3Z3* is polymorphic and that a haplotype of the domestic cat A3Z3 is resistant to Vif-mediated degradation by FIVfca, which is the FIV that infects domestic cats [12]. Our findings suggest that the domestic cat *A3Z3* is under positive selection due to evolutionary selective pressure caused by FIVfca or related ancestral viruses [12, 14].

In addition to FIVfca in domestic cats, various FIV types have been identified in other felids, such as FIVple in lions (*Panthera leo*), FIVpco in pumas (*Puma concolor*), and FIVlru in bobcats (*Lynx rufus*) (reviewed in [16]). Interestingly, although these felids become infected with a specific FIV species, Lee et al. [17] recently reported that a subcluster of FIVpco co-circulated in both pumas and bobcats in North America. The authors designated these viruses (FIVpco and FIVlru) puma lentiviruses (PLVs) and re-classified them as follows: PLV-A includes the FIVpco and FIVlru strains co-circulating in both pumas and bobcats, and PLV-B includes FIVpco strains circulating only in pumas (Fig. 1a) [17–19]. This scenario is the first known case indicating cross-species transmission (CST) of a lentivirus between hosts of different genera (*Puma* and *Lynx*) at present. Since *A3* genes are under positive selection [12, 20–22], the A3 sequences are highly variable among hosts of different genera. Furthermore, we can reasonably hypothesize that the specificity in which Vif counteracts the host A3 also differs in each host genus. These findings and insights raise the hypothesis that Vif-A3 interplay between FIV and the two New World felids (puma and bobcat) is closely associated with the mode of CST among lentiviruses, which may illustrate the history

of the co-evolutionary arms race between lentiviruses and felids in the New World.

In this study, we perform cell-based virological experiments and demonstrate that the species specificity of the Vif proteins of PLV-A and PLV-B is different between each other. Through the combinational investigations of experimental virology and molecular phylogenetics, we also provide evidence suggesting that bobcat A3Z3 plays a role as the species barrier specifically against PLV-B. Moreover, we determine the amino acid residue responsible for the sensitivity to PLV-B Vif-dependent degradation. This is the first report addressing the co-evolutionary interplay between antiviral A3 of the two New World felids and feline lentiviral Vif.

Results

Bobcat A3Z3 is resistant to PLV-B Vif-mediated degradation

To elucidate the co-evolutionary relationship between PLVs and their host felids, particularly between viral Vif and host A3Z3, first we constructed a phylogenetic tree of FIV *vif* gene. As shown in Fig. 1a, FIVfca and FIVple formed clusters based on their hosts. In sharp contrast, the FIVlru sequences were co-mingled with some FIVpco sequences, whereas the other FIVpco sequences formed a cluster (Fig. 1a). These results are consistent with the phylogeny of the full-length FIV sequences shown in a previous study [17]. According to this previous report, here we designated the FIVlru and co-mingled FIVpco sequences PLV-A and the other FIVpco sequences PLV-B. The sequence identities of PLV-A Vif and PLV-B Vif were 90.1 ± 4.8 and $85.7 \pm 7.1\%$, respectively, whereas the Vif sequence identity between PLV-A and PLV-B was $40.6 \pm 1.1\%$. Thus, the PLV-A Vif and PLV-B Vif sequences clearly differed.

Next, we focused on the host felid evolutionary relationships. Based on comprehensive genetic information, a previous study [23] described the evolutionary history of the felids of interest in this study (Fig. 1b). The common ancestor of the puma (*Puma concolor*) and the bobcat (*Lynx rufus*) is estimated to have crossed the Bering Isthmus from Eurasia to the New World approximately 8.0–8.5 million years ago (Mya) and to have diverged approximately 7.2 Mya [23]. The puma diverged from the cheetah (*Acinonyx jubatus*) approximately 4.9 Mya, whereas the bobcat was branched from the lynx (*Lynx lynx*) approximately 3.2 Mya (Fig. 1b) [23]. Puma and bobcat resided in the New World, whereas lynx and cheetah returned to Eurasia approximately 1.2–1.6 Mya (Fig. 1b) [23]. To assess the phylogenetic relationships of the *A3Z3* genes of these felids, we collected body hairs from a bobcat and a cheetah from Japanese zoos and determined their *A3Z3* sequences (see Additional file 1: Fig. S1 and Additional file 2: Table S1). As shown in

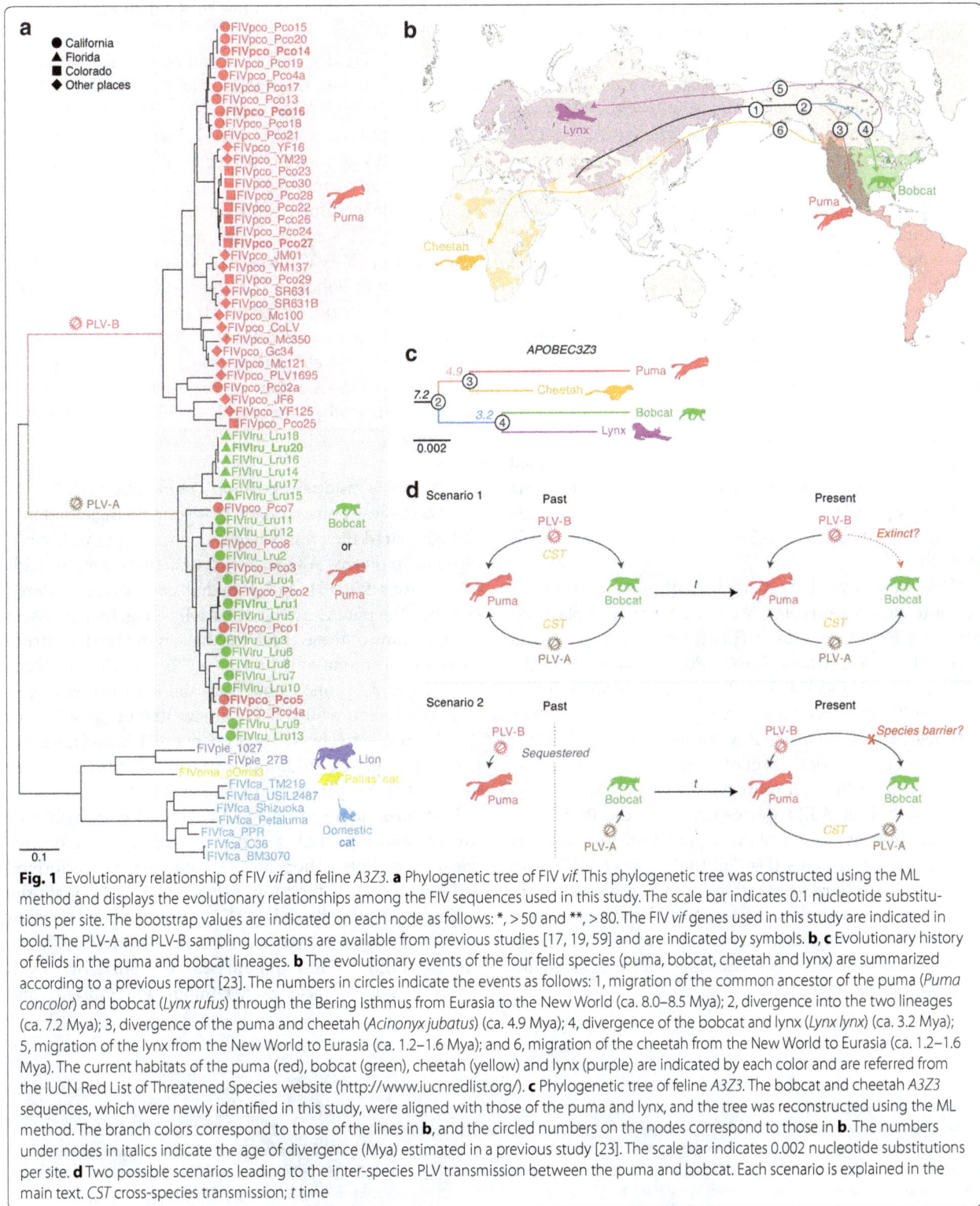

Fig. 1 Evolutionary relationship of FIV *vif* and feline *A3Z3*. **a** Phylogenetic tree of FIV *vif*. This phylogenetic tree was constructed using the ML method and displays the evolutionary relationships among the FIV sequences used in this study. The scale bar indicates 0.1 nucleotide substitutions per site. The bootstrap values are indicated on each node as follows: *, > 50 and **, > 80. The FIV *vif* genes used in this study are indicated in bold. The PLV-A and PLV-B sampling locations are available from previous studies [17, 19, 59] and are indicated by symbols. **b, c** Evolutionary history of felids in the puma and bobcat lineages. **b** The evolutionary events of the four felid species (puma, bobcat, cheetah and lynx) are summarized according to a previous report [23]. The numbers in circles indicate the events as follows: 1, migration of the common ancestor of the puma (*Puma concolor*) and bobcat (*Lynx rufus*) through the Bering Isthmus from Eurasia to the New World (ca. 8.0–8.5 Mya); 2, divergence into the two lineages (ca. 7.2 Mya); 3, divergence of the puma and cheetah (*Acinonyx jubatus*) (ca. 4.9 Mya); 4, divergence of the bobcat and lynx (*Lynx lynx*) (ca. 3.2 Mya); 5, migration of the lynx from the New World to Eurasia (ca. 1.2–1.6 Mya); and 6, migration of the cheetah from the New World to Eurasia (ca. 1.2–1.6 Mya). The current habitats of the puma (red), bobcat (green), cheetah (yellow) and lynx (purple) are indicated by each color and are referred from the IUCN Red List of Threatened Species website (http://www.iucnredlist.org/). **c** Phylogenetic tree of feline *A3Z3*. The bobcat and cheetah *A3Z3* sequences, which were newly identified in this study, were aligned with those of the puma and lynx, and the tree was reconstructed using the ML method. The branch colors correspond to those of the lines in **b**, and the circled numbers on the nodes correspond to those in **b**. The numbers under nodes in italics indicate the age of divergence (Mya) estimated in a previous study [23]. The scale bar indicates 0.002 nucleotide substitutions per site. **d** Two possible scenarios leading to the inter-species PLV transmission between the puma and bobcat. Each scenario is explained in the main text. *CST* cross-species transmission; *t* time

Fig. 1c, the topology of the phylogenetic tree of the *A3Z3* genes form these four felids corresponded to their evolutionary relationships.

Based on these observations, two scenarios are assumed. The first scenario was that both PLV-A and PLV-B co-circulated in pumas and bobcats in the New

World but PLV-B became extinct only in the bobcat population ("scenario 1" in Fig. 1d). The other possibility was that PLV-A and PLV-B were specific viruses in bobcats and pumas, respectively, in the past. After co-habitation of these two feline species in the New World, PLV-A was transferred from bobcats to pumas, whereas PLV-B CST from pumas to bobcats was hampered for unknown reasons ("scenario 2" in Fig. 1d).

To experimentally investigate the interplay between PLVs and their hosts, we analyzed the antiviral activity of the puma and bobcat A3Z3 proteins. In the absence of PLV Vif, both puma and bobcat A3Z3 were expressed at comparable levels and are incorporated into the released particles of *vif*-deficient FIV (strain Petaluma) in a dose-dependent manner (Fig. 2a). In addition, the infectivity of *vif*-deficient FIV was suppressed by both puma and bobcat A3Z3 proteins in a dose-dependent manner (Fig. 2b). Interestingly, although the protein expression (Fig. 2a, top) and incorporation levels in the released virions (Fig. 2a, bottom) were similar between the puma and bobcat A3Z3 s, the antiviral effect was significantly higher for the puma A3Z3 than for the bobcat A3Z3 (Fig. 2b).

Next, we analyzed the sensitivity of puma and bobcat A3Z3 to PLV Vif proteins. We used expression plasmids for three PLV-A Vif strains (Lru1, Lru20 and Pco5) and three PLV-B Vif strains (Pco14, Pco16 and Pco27). The sampling years and locations for each virus are summarized in Table 1. As shown in Fig. 2c, the puma A3Z3 was degraded by all of the PLV Vif proteins tested in this study, and the antiviral effect of puma A3Z3 was counteracted by these PLV Vif proteins (Fig. 2d). In sharp contrast, the bobcat A3Z3 was degraded by the PLV-A Vif proteins but was resistant to degradation mediated by the PLV-B Vif proteins (Fig. 2e, top). Bobcat A3Z3 was incorporated into nascent virions even in the presence of PLV-B Vif (Fig. 2e, bottom), which significantly decreased viral infectivity (Fig. 2f). Taken together, these findings suggest that bobcat A3Z3 is resistant to PLV-B Vif-mediated degradation.

Puma A3Z3 is uniquely sensitive to PLV-B Vif-mediated degradation

As shown in Fig. 1b, the puma and bobcat are evolutionarily similar to the cheetah (*Acinonyx jubatus*) and the lynx (*Lynx lynx*), respectively. To address whether the sensitivity of host A3Z3 to PLV-B Vif is associated with the host phylogeny, we constructed expression plasmids for cheetah and lynx A3Z3 proteins and performed similar experiments. Our results revealed that both cheetah and lynx A3Z3 were degraded by PLV-A Vif but were resistant to PLV-B Vif-mediated degradation (Fig. 3a, b, top). Similar to bobcat A3Z3, the cheetah and lynx A3Z3 proteins were incorporated into the released virions even in the presence of PLV-B Vif (Fig. 3a, b, bottom) resulting in an antiviral effect (Fig. 3c, d). These findings suggest that the PLV-A Vif antagonizes all four feline A3Z3 tested in this study, whereas PLV-B Vif antagonizes only the puma A3Z3.

The threonine residue at position 178 of bobcat A3Z3 confers the resistance to PLV-B Vif-mediated degradation

We compared the amino acid sequence of puma, bobcat, cheetah and lynx A3Z3s and found three amino acids at positions 90, 131 and 178 that consistently differed between the puma and the other felids (Fig. 4a). To assess the positions of these three residues in the tertiary structures of the puma and bobcat A3Z3 proteins, we constructed A3Z3 protein homology models for these felids (Fig. 4b). Residues 90 and 178 are located in alpha-helices 3 and 6, respectively, whereas residue 131 is positioned in the loop (Fig. 4c). Additionally, residues 90 and 178 are localized on the protein surface (Fig. 4d).

To determine the amino acid residue(s) responsible for the resistance to PLV-B Vif-mediated degradation, we constructed lines of bobcat A3Z3 mutants and performed cell-based loss-of-function experiments. Although the bobcat A3Z3 E90K and I131T mutants were resistant to PLV-B Vif-mediated degradation (strain Pco27), the bobcat A3Z3 T178M mutant was degraded by PLV-B Vif (Fig. 5a). We also used combination mutants and

(See figure on next page.)
Fig. 2 Resistance of bobcat A3Z3 to PLV-B Vif-dependent degradation. **a, b** Antiviral effects of the puma and bobcat A3Z3 proteins. Different amounts of HA-tagged expression plasmids for puma or bobcat A3Z3 (0, 50, 100, 200 and 400 ng) and the three plasmids used to produce the *vif*-deficient FIV-based reporter virus (FIV plasmids; pFP93 [200 ng], pTiger-luc [150 ng] and pMD.G [50 ng]) were co-transfected into HEK293T cells. **a** Western blotting. Representative results are shown. **b** FIV reporter assay. FIV infectivity is shown as the percentage of the value of "no A3Z3". **c–f** Puma and bobcat A3Z3 sensitivity to PLV Vif. HA-tagged expression plasmids for puma (**c, d**) and bobcat (**e, f**) A3Z3 (200 ng) and the three plasmids used to produce the *vif*-deficient FIV-based reporter virus (FIV plasmids; pFP93 [200 ng], pTiger-luc [150 ng] and pMD.G [50 ng]) were co-transfected with or without His-tagged PLV Vif expression plasmids (400 ng) into HEK293T cells. **c, e** Western blotting. Representative results are shown. **d, f** FIV reporter assay. FIV infectivity is shown as the percentage of the value of "no A3Z3". In **b**, asterisks indicate significant differences (P < 0.05 by Student's t test) between puma A3Z3 and bobcat A3Z3. In **d** and **f**, asterisks indicate significant differences (P < 0.05 by Student's t test) versus "no Vif". The assays were independently performed in triplicate. Data represent averages with SDs

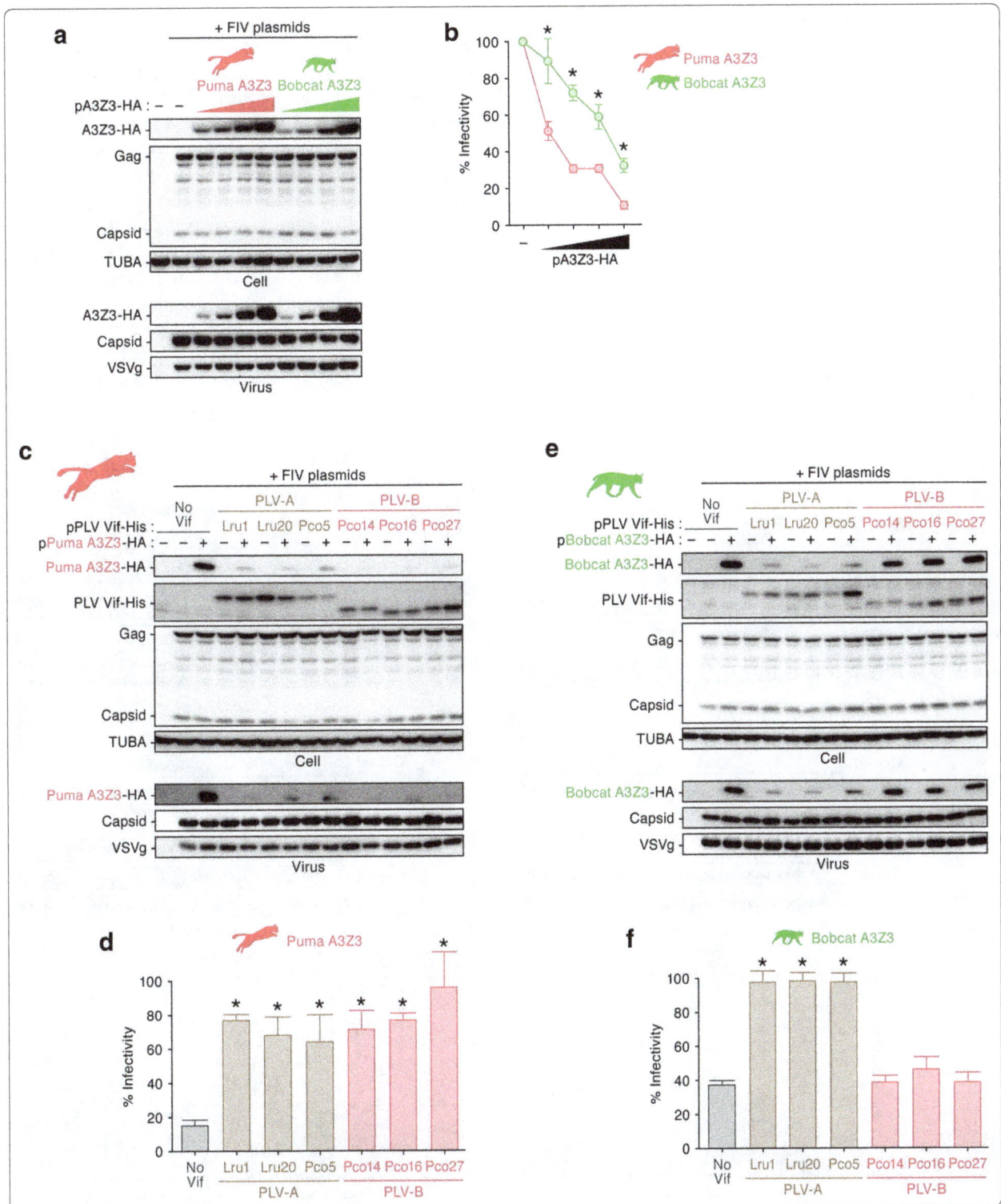

Table 1 PLV Vif used in this study

Group	Strain	Sampling location	Sampling year	Accession nos.
PLV-A	Lru1	California	1996	KF906143
PLV-A	Lru20	Florida	2010	KF906162
PLV-A	Pco5	California	2004	KF906167
PLV-B	Pco14	California	2002	KF906182
PLV-B	Pco16	California	2011	KF906193
PLV-B	Pco27	Colorado	2008	KF906194

found those harboring the T178M substitution lost the ability to resist PLV-B Vif-mediated degradation (strain Pco27) (Fig. 5a). In the presence of PLV-B Vif, incorporation of bobcat A3Z3 derivatives possessing the T178M

mutation into the released viruses was impaired (Fig. 5a, bottom), and the derivatives' antiviral effects were abrogated (Fig. 5b). To determine whether this observation was strain-specific, we performed similar experiments using the other PLV-B strains (Pco14 and Pco16). Similar to strain Pco27 (Fig. 5a, b), the Vif proteins of the other PLV-B strains degraded the bobcat A3Z3 T178M mutant (Fig. 5c) and significantly recovered viral infectivity (Fig. 5d). These findings suggest that the resistance of bobcat A3Z3 to PLV-B Vif-mediated degradation is determined by the amino acid residue at position 178.

To validate the importance of the amino acid at position 178 to sensitivity to PLV-B Vif-mediated degradation, we performed gain-of-function experiments based on the puma A3Z3. By substituting the methionine

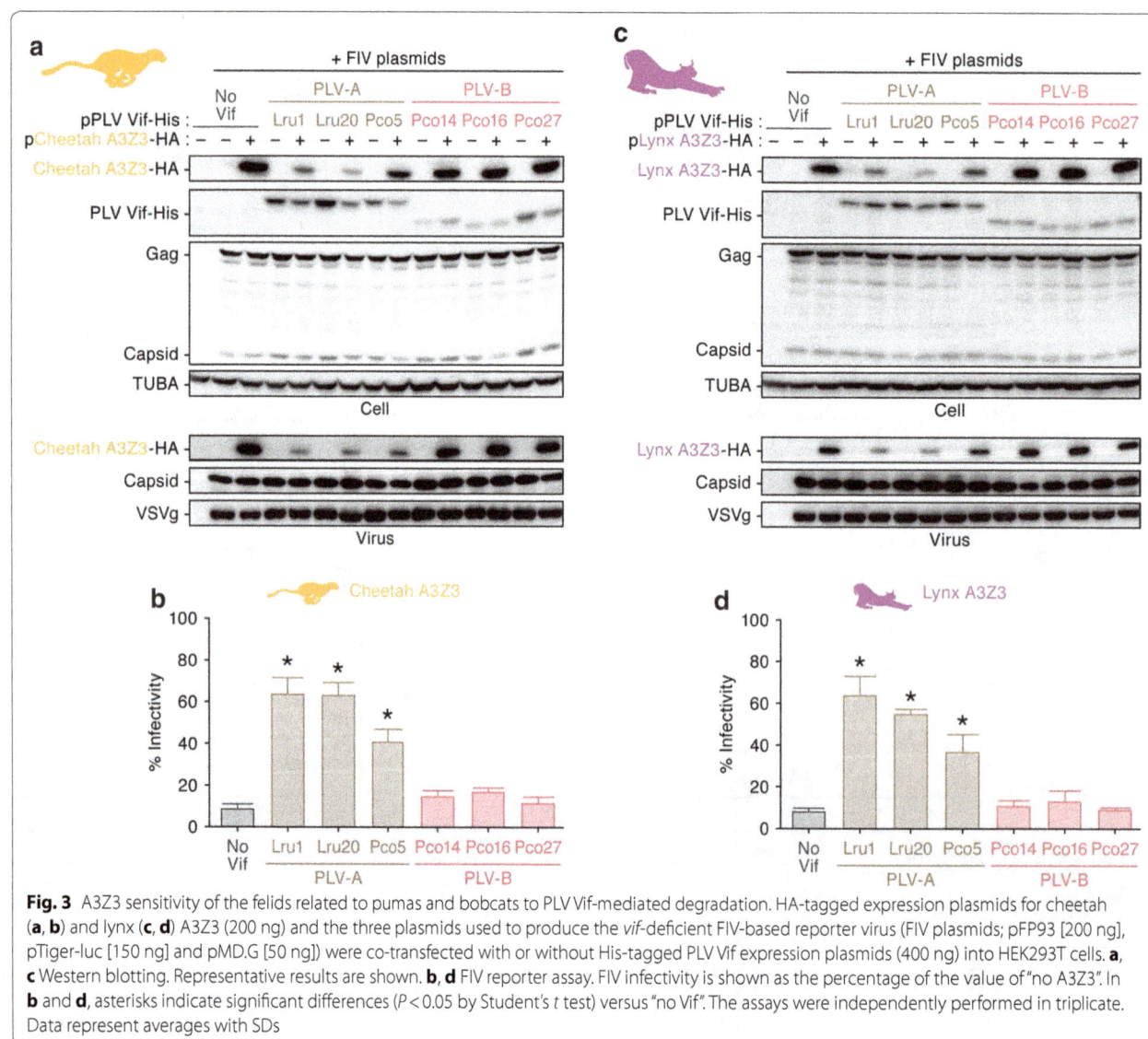

Fig. 3 A3Z3 sensitivity of the felids related to pumas and bobcats to PLV Vif-mediated degradation. HA-tagged expression plasmids for cheetah (**a**, **b**) and lynx (**c**, **d**) A3Z3 (200 ng) and the three plasmids used to produce the *vif*-deficient FIV-based reporter virus (FIV plasmids; pFP93 [200 ng], pTiger-luc [150 ng] and pMD.G [50 ng]) were co-transfected with or without His-tagged PLV Vif expression plasmids (400 ng) into HEK293T cells. **a**, **c** Western blotting. Representative results are shown. **b**, **d** FIV reporter assay. FIV infectivity is shown as the percentage of the value of "no A3Z3". In **b** and **d**, asterisks indicate significant differences ($P < 0.05$ by Student's *t* test) versus "no Vif". The assays were independently performed in triplicate. Data represent averages with SDs

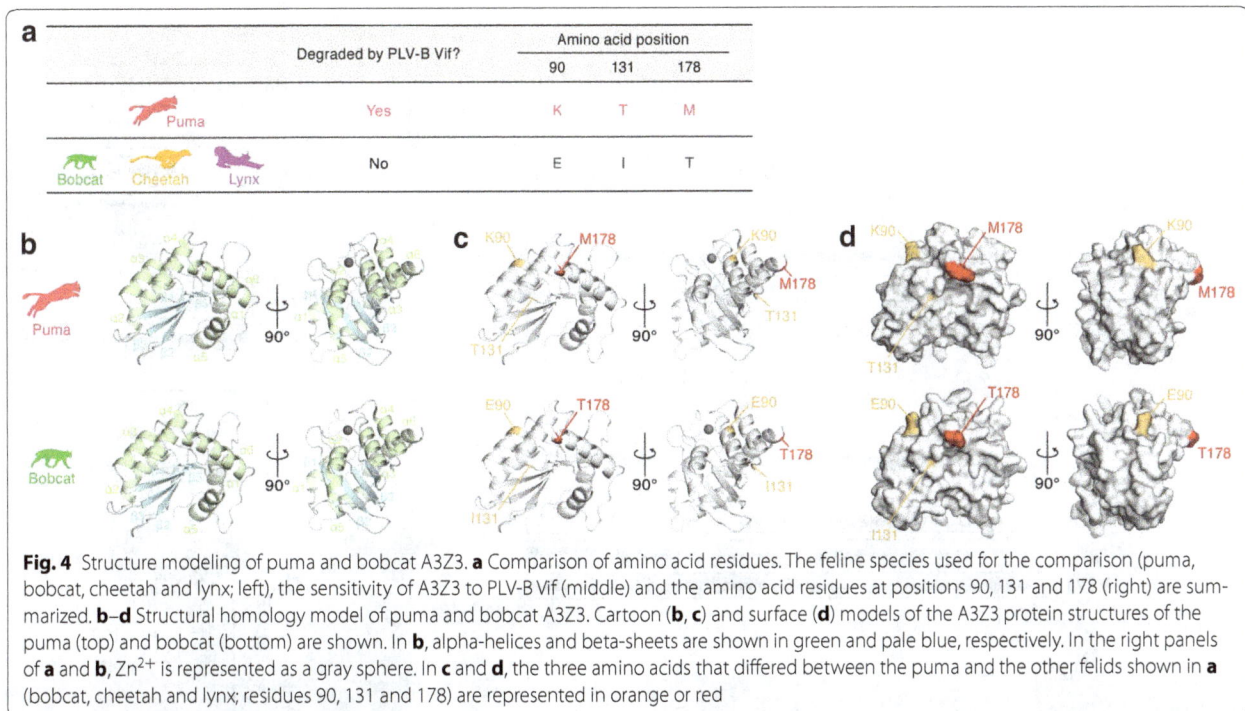

Fig. 4 Structure modeling of puma and bobcat A3Z3. **a** Comparison of amino acid residues. The feline species used for the comparison (puma, bobcat, cheetah and lynx; left), the sensitivity of A3Z3 to PLV-B Vif (middle) and the amino acid residues at positions 90, 131 and 178 (right) are summarized. **b**–**d** Structural homology model of puma and bobcat A3Z3. Cartoon (**b**, **c**) and surface (**d**) models of the A3Z3 protein structures of the puma (top) and bobcat (bottom) are shown. In **b**, alpha-helices and beta-sheets are shown in green and pale blue, respectively. In the right panels of **a** and **b**, Zn^{2+} is represented as a gray sphere. In **c** and **d**, the three amino acids that differed between the puma and the other felids shown in **a** (bobcat, cheetah and lynx; residues 90, 131 and 178) are represented in orange or red

residue at position 178 of the puma A3Z3 to threonine, the puma A3Z3 mutant became resistant to PLV-B Vif-mediated degradation (Fig. 6a, top). The puma A3Z3 M178T mutant was efficiently incorporated into the released virions (Fig. 6a, bottom) and exhibited significant antiviral activity (Fig. 6b). Taken together, these findings suggest that the amino acid at position 178 in the bobcat/puma A3Z3 plays a pivotal role in conferring resistance to PLV-B Vif-mediated degradation.

Puma and bobcat A3Z3 are polymorphic

Previous studies have revealed that mammalian *A3* genes, including feline *A3Z3* genes, are under positive selection and are highly diversified due to evolutionary selective pressures presumably caused by the ancestral FIV Vif [23]. For instance, the domestic cat *A3Z3* is polymorphic [24], and a haplotype of the domestic cat A3Z3 renders resistance to FIVfca Vif-mediated degradation [12]. These previous findings raise the possibility that the puma and bobcat *A3Z3* genes are also polymorphic and that the PLV Vif sensitivity may differ among haplotypes. To address this possibility, we additionally determined the *A3Z3* sequences of five pumas, one bobcat as well as one cheetah. As shown in Fig. 7a, we detected additional puma and bobcat *A3Z3* haplotypes and designated them haplotype II (hap II). One nonsynonymous mutation was detected in the puma A3Z3 hap II (a c392t mutation resulting in T131I amino acid substitution), and a heterozygous sequence was detected in the bobcat A3Z3 hap

II (g347r; a g347a mutation resulting in a R116H amino acid substitution) (Fig. 7a). Next, we mapped these residues on the protein homology model. Both residue 131 of the puma A3Z3 (Fig. 4b) and residue 116 of the bobcat A3Z3 (Additional file 3: Fig. S2) are positioned in the loop structure. Then, we prepared expression plasmids for these haplotypes and assessed their antiviral activity and sensitivity to PLV Vif. As shown in Fig. 7b, puma and bobcat A3Z3 hap II were expressed at similar levels to their hap I derivatives. Notably, in the absence of PLV Vif, the antiviral effects of the puma and bobcat A3Z3 hap II were significantly higher than those of the hap I derivatives (Fig. 7c). In particular, the bobcat A3Z3 hap II exhibited stronger antiviral activity in a dose-dependent manner (Fig. 7c). Moreover, puma A3Z3 hap II was sensitive to both the PLV-A and PLV-B Vifs (Fig. 7d, e), whereas the bobcat A3Z3 hap II was sensitive to PLV-A Vif but was resistant to PLV-B Vif-mediated degradation (Fig. 7e, f). Taken together, these findings suggest that the puma and bobcat *A3Z3* genes are polymorphic and that the bobcat A3Z3 hap II exhibits a higher antiviral effect than the hap I derivative, whereas the PLV Vif sensitivity phenotype is conserved within each species.

Discussion

In this study, we identified the *A3Z3* sequences of two felids, the bobcat and cheetah, and demonstrated that PLV-A Vif counteracted the A3Z3 proteins of both the puma and bobcat lineages, whereas PLV-B Vif

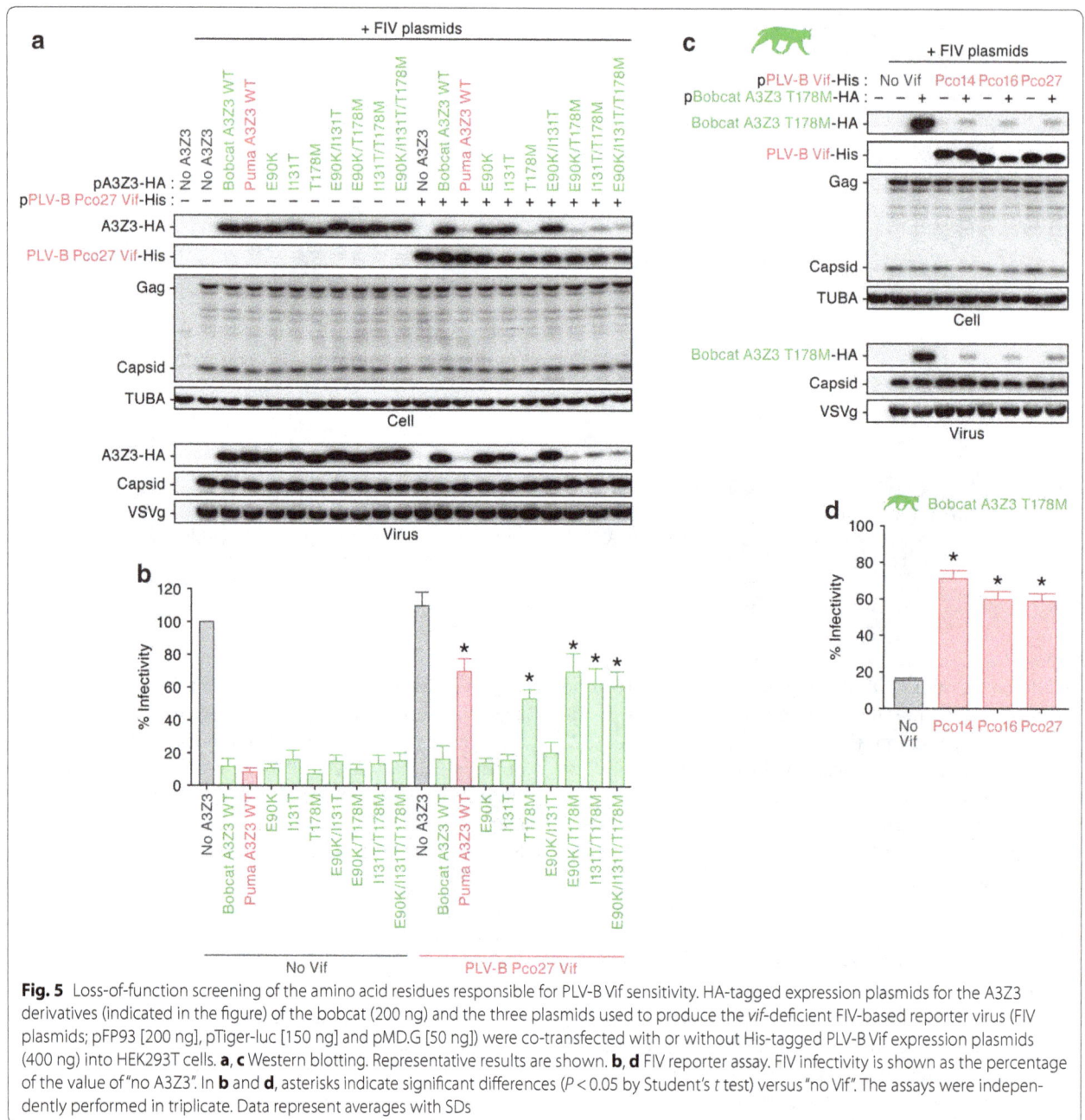

Fig. 5 Loss-of-function screening of the amino acid residues responsible for PLV-B Vif sensitivity. HA-tagged expression plasmids for the A3Z3 derivatives (indicated in the figure) of the bobcat (200 ng) and the three plasmids used to produce the *vif*-deficient FIV-based reporter virus (FIV plasmids; pFP93 [200 ng], pTiger-luc [150 ng] and pMD.G [50 ng]) were co-transfected with or without His-tagged PLV-B Vif expression plasmids (400 ng) into HEK293T cells. **a**, **c** Western blotting. Representative results are shown. **b**, **d** FIV reporter assay. FIV infectivity is shown as the percentage of the value of "no A3Z3". In **b** and **d**, asterisks indicate significant differences ($P < 0.05$ by Student's t test) versus "no Vif". The assays were independently performed in triplicate. Data represent averages with SDs

counteracted only the puma A3Z3 (Figs. 1, 2, 3). Through loss-of-function (Fig. 5) and gain-of-function (Fig. 6) experiments, we also determined that the amino acid at position 178 of the puma and bobcat A3Z3 was responsible for the sensitivity to PLV-B Vif. In addition, structural modeling suggested that this residue was exposed to the protein surface (Fig. 4). Furthermore, although the puma and bobcat *A3Z3* genes were polymorphic, the sensitivity to PLV-B Vif was conserved in each species (Fig. 7). Some previous studies have addressed the potential of

OWM A3G to restrict HIV-1 infection [25, 26]. However, OWMs do not infect with HIV-1 in nature. Therefore, to the best of our knowledge, this study is the first to suggest that inter-species lentiviral transmission in nature is controlled by a host A3 protein.

As summarized in Fig. 1a, d, PLV-A is shared by both pumas and bobcats in North America, whereas PLV-B is detected only in pumas. Through cell-based virological experiments, here we demonstrated that PLV-A Vif degraded the A3Z3 protein of feline lineages including

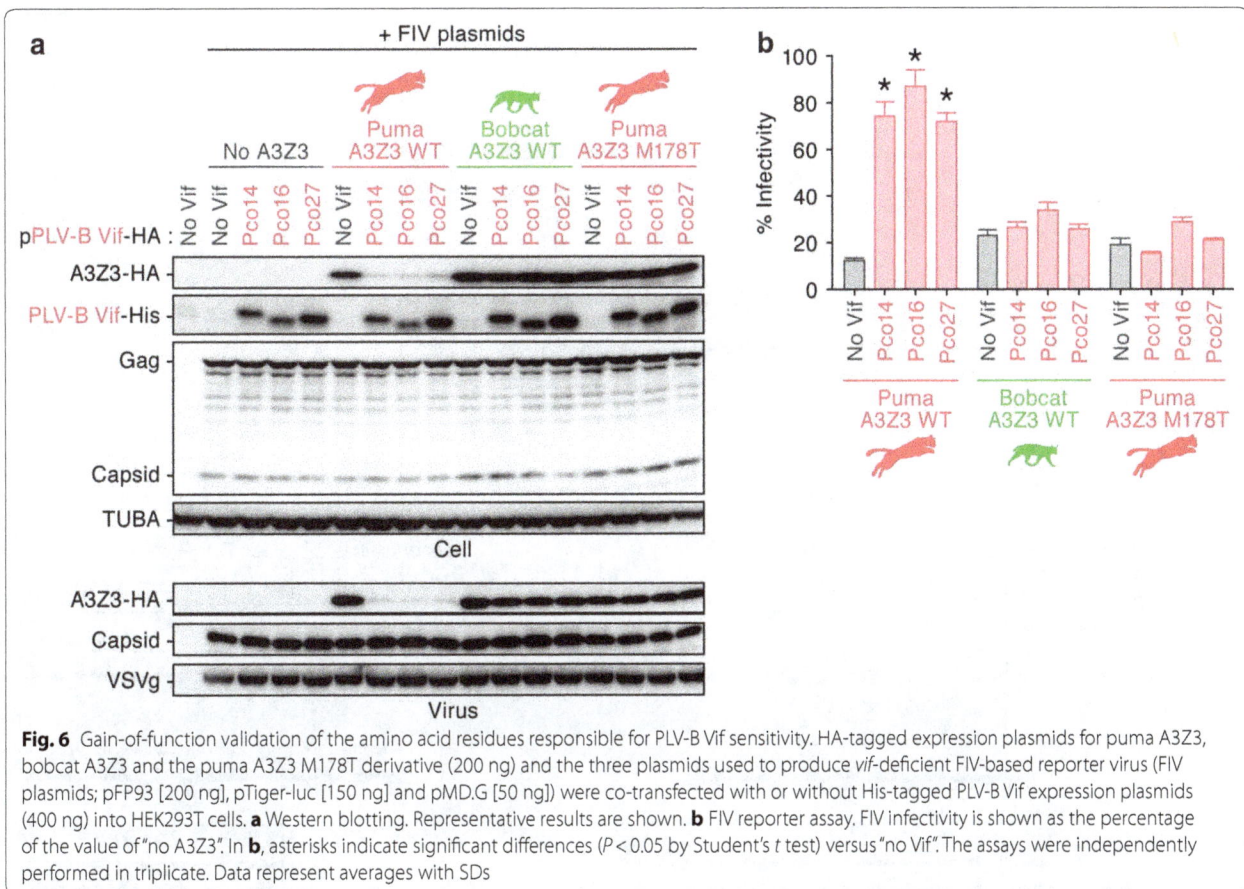

Fig. 6 Gain-of-function validation of the amino acid residues responsible for PLV-B Vif sensitivity. HA-tagged expression plasmids for puma A3Z3, bobcat A3Z3 and the puma A3Z3 M178T derivative (200 ng) and the three plasmids used to produce *vif*-deficient FIV-based reporter virus (FIV plasmids; pFP93 [200 ng], pTiger-luc [150 ng] and pMD.G [50 ng]) were co-transfected with or without His-tagged PLV-B Vif expression plasmids (400 ng) into HEK293T cells. **a** Western blotting. Representative results are shown. **b** FIV reporter assay. FIV infectivity is shown as the percentage of the value of "no A3Z3". In **b**, asterisks indicate significant differences (*P* < 0.05 by Student's *t* test) versus "no Vif". The assays were independently performed in triplicate. Data represent averages with SDs

puma and bobcat, whereas PLV-B Vif counteracted only the puma A3Z3. Additionally, the bobcat A3Z3 exhibited a significant antiviral effect even in the presence of PLV-B Vif. Because the functionality of PLV Vif is independent of the sampling location and year (Fig. 2 and Table 1), our results suggest that the functional relationship between PLV Vif and feline A3Z3 is conserved. Moreover, we found a polymorphism in the puma *A3Z3*, but the sensitivity of the puma A3Z3 variants to PLV-B Vif-mediated degradation was also conserved (Fig. 6). These findings suggest that "scenario 2" reasonably explains the difference in species tropism between PLV-A and PLV-B and that bobcat A3Z3 acts as a species barrier to restrict PLV-B CST of PLV-B from pumas (Fig. 1d). To the best of our knowledge, this is the first report demonstrating that the host A3 protein is the factor that restricts non-primate lentiviral CST.

Consistent with our results, PLV-A and PLV-B form clusters by sampling location [17–19]. Moreover, the PLV-As detected in pumas (FIVpco) and bobcats (FIV-lru), particularly those isolated in California, were highly co-mingled in a cluster (Fig. 1a). These observations suggest that PLV-As have been transmitted relatively

recently from bobcats to pumas after geological sequestration, and we can assume that this bobcat-to-puma CST event occurs frequently at least in California.

Our findings in New World felids were reminiscent of the fact that simian immunodeficiency viruses (SIVs) in Old World monkeys (OWMs) were transferred to chimpanzees, which originated in the emergence of a novel SIV in chimpanzees (SIVcpz) (reviewed in [27, 28]). SIV CST from OWMs to chimpanzees in Africa is explained phylogenetically and is assumed to be due to the prey-predator relationship between OWMs and chimpanzees. Small OWMs are the prey of chimpanzees in the wild; thus, chimpanzees are frequently exposed to various SIVs that infect their OWM prey species [29, 30]. Similarly, pumas are a top carnivore in the New World [31] and bobcats are their prey [32, 33]. Therefore, pumas may be frequently exposed to PLV-A in bobcats via prey-predator interactions, leading to bobcat-to-puma CST; this possibility is consistent with a previous assumption based on phylogenetic analyses [17].

Although PLV-A Vif degraded all of the feline A3Z3 proteins tested in this study, PLV-B Vif counteracted only the puma A3Z3, suggesting the evolutionary convergence

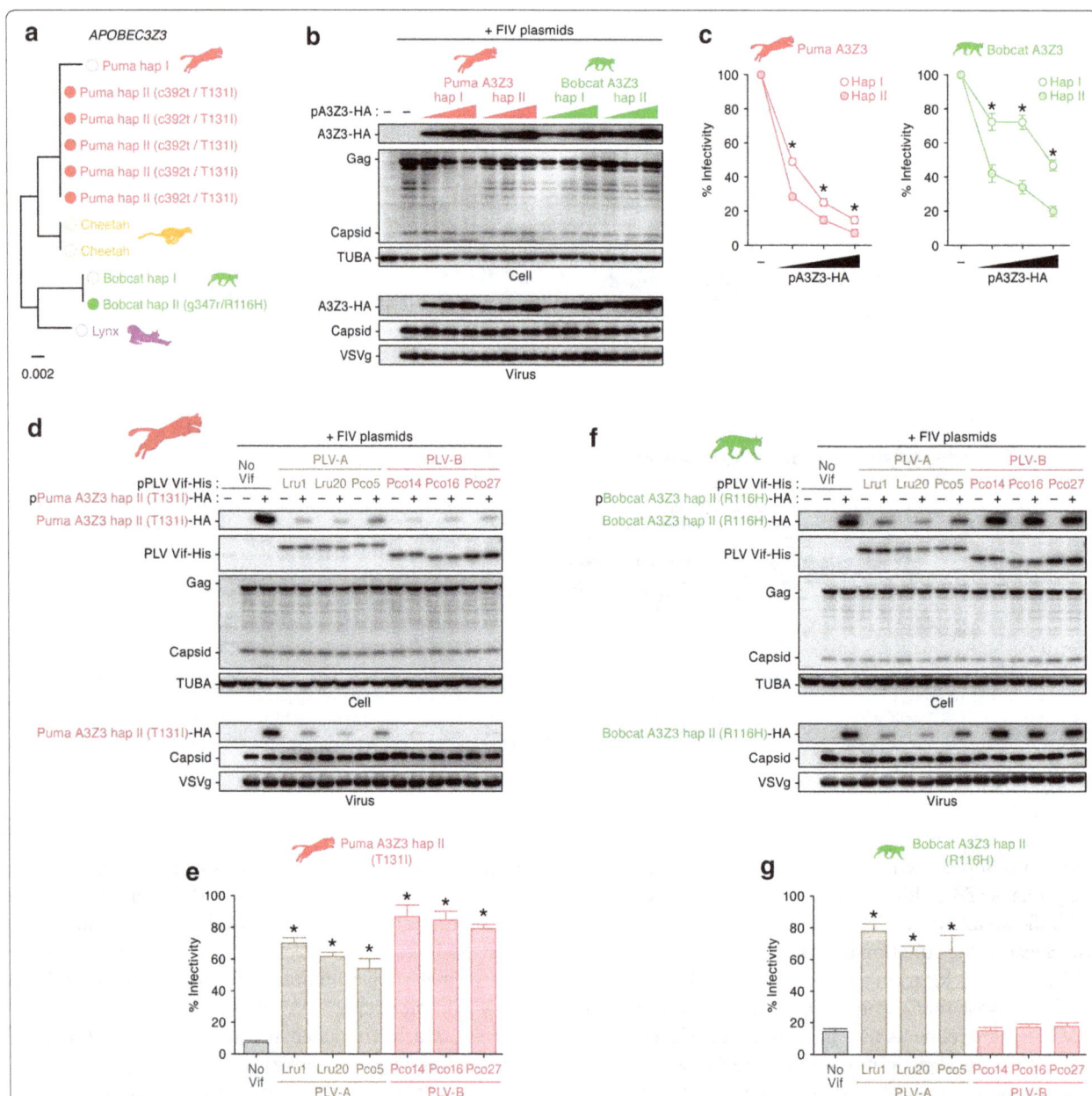

Fig. 7 Polymorphisms of puma and bobcat *A3Z3* and their association with PLV Vif sensitivity. **a** Feline *A3Z3* polymorphisms. Additional *A3Z3* sequences from five pumas, one cheetah and one bobcat were determined and the phylogenetic tree was reconstructed using the ML method. The *A3Z3* sequences used in the experiments above (summarized in Fig. 1c) are indicated with open circles and designated hap I. Additional *A3Z3* haplotypes detected in the puma and bobcat are indicated with filled circles and designated hap II. The nucleotide/amino acid substitutions detected in puma and bobcat A3Z3 hap II are indicated in parentheses. Note that the new cheetah *A3Z3* sequence was identical to the previously determined sequence (Fig. 1c). The scale bar indicates 0.002 nucleotide substitutions per site. **b–f** Antiviral activity of the puma and bobcat A3Z3 hap II proteins and their sensitivity to PLV Vif. **b, c** Different amounts of HA-tagged expression plasmids for A3Z3 hap I and II of puma or bobcat (0, 100, 200 and 400 ng) and the three plasmids used to produce the *vif*-deficient FIV-based reporter virus (FIV plasmids; pFP93 [200 ng], pTiger-luc [150 ng] and pMD.G [50 ng]) were co-transfected into HEK293T cells. **b** Western blotting. Representative results are shown. **c** FIV reporter assay. FIV infectivity is shown as the percentage of the value of "no A3Z3". Note that "hap I" is identical to those used in the other experiments shown in Figs. 1, 2, 4, 5 and 6. **d–g** HA-tagged expression plasmids for puma A3Z3 hap II (**d, e**) or bobcat A3Z3 hap II (**f, g**) (200 ng) and the three plasmids used to produce the *vif*-deficient FIV-based reporter virus (FIV plasmids; pFP93 [200 ng], pTiger-luc [150 ng] and pMD.G [50 ng]) were co-transfected with or without His-tagged PLV Vif expression plasmids (400 ng) into HEK293T cells. **d, f** Western blotting. Representative results are shown. **e, g** FIV reporter assay. FIV infectivity is shown as the percentage of the value of "no A3Z3". In **b**, asterisks indicate significant differences ($P < 0.05$ by Student's t test) between hap I and hap II. In **e** and **g**, asterisks indicate significant differences ($P < 0.05$ by Student's t test) versus "no Vif". The assays were independently performed in triplicate. Data represent averages with SDs

of the puma and PLV-B. Compton and Emerman reported that the Vif protein of an SIV infecting colobus monkey (*Colobus guereza*), which is an OWM in Africa, counteracted only colobus A3G [34]. Based on findings for the A3G-Vif interaction in colobus monkeys, the authors proposed convergent evolution of colobus monkeys and SIVcor and further suggested that the convergent co-evolution of these monkeys and viruses occurred at least 12 Mya [34]. Similarly, the puma diversified from the cheetah approximately 4.9 Mya (Fig. 1c) [23]. Puma and cheetah habitats were separated approximately 1.2–1.6 Mya after cheetahs immigrated from the New World to Eurasia (Fig. 1b) [23]. Since the cheetah A3Z3 was not counteracted by the PLV-B Vif (Fig. 3), our findings suggested that the co-evolutionary convergence of the puma and PLV-B arose at least 1.2–1.6 Mya. Moreover, OWMs exhibit higher viral RNA loads without any disorders [35]. Since SIVs circumvent the immune pressure from host monkeys because they are naturally infected, SIVs are less diversified in African OWMs, which is assumed to be due to the co-existence of SIVs in OWMs over a long period [35]. Lee et al. [17] recently showed that the PLV-B plasma viral RNA load in pumas was significantly higher than PLV-A loads in both pumas and bobcats, whereas PLV-B was less diversified than PLV-A. This is the first study suggesting the convergent co-evolution of a mammal (puma) and a lentivirus (PLV-B) in the New World, and PLV-B can be concluded to have co-evolved with pumas over a long period, similar to apathogenic SIV infections in OWMs.

Through mutagenesis experiments, we demonstrated that the amino acid at position 178 determined the sensitivity to PLV-B Vif-dependent degradation (Fig. 5). Since both the gain- and loss-of-function experiments indicated the importance of this residue, the species specificity of PLV-B Vif against puma and bobcat A3Z3 was determined by this single amino acid. In addition, the structural biology investigation revealed that this amino acid residue was exposed on the A3Z3 protein surface (Fig. 4). In our previous study [12], we revealed that there are at least seven haplotypes in the domestic cat *A3Z3* and that a domestic cat A3Z3 haplotype (designated haplotype V in our previous study) was resistant to FIVfca Vif-mediated degradation. Furthermore, we demonstrated that amino acid residue 65 of the domestic cat A3Z3 determines the sensitivity to FIVfca Vif [12]. Similar to this study, residue 65 in the domestic cat A3Z3 was also exposed on the protein surface, which suggested that this residue was associated with the interaction with FIV Vif [12]. However, the amino acid residue at position 65 was positioned at alpha-helix 2 in the domestic cat A3Z3 [12], whereas the residue 178 was located at alpha-helix 6 in the puma and bobcat A3Z3 (Fig. 5). Therefore, our

findings suggest that these residues render resistance to FIV Vif in a different manner.

In addition to A3, other cellular proteins such as tripartite motif containing protein 5 (TRIM5) [36] and tetherin [37, 38] are known as restriction factors that inhibit lentiviral replication in primates. Therefore, it might be possible that these restriction factors in pumas and/or bobcats may also play roles in preventing FIV CST. However, feline TRIM5 is not functional because of the insertion of premature stop codon [39], and feline tetherin is unable to restrict spreading FIV infection [40]. Furthermore, although FIV Vif is a functional antagonist against feline A3, FIV lacks functional proteins that potently counteract TRIM5 and tetherin [39, 40]. Primates encode several restriction factors against lentiviruses; however, only A3 is convincing to be a restriction factor in felids. Therefore, feline A3 may play a pivotal role in controlling CST in felids.

In summary, we demonstrated that bobcat A3Z3 was resistant to PLV-B Vif-dependent degradation, whereas PLV-A Vif overcame the antiviral action mediated by both the puma and bobcat A3Z3. The co-evolutionary relationship between primate A3 proteins and their lentiviral Vifs has been rigorously investigated [20, 22, 34, 41–44]; however, few studies, including ours, have addressed the evolutionary dynamics of non-primate A3 and non-primate lentiviruses [4, 12, 14]. Here, we provided evidence suggesting that lentiviral CST between different genera (*Puma* and *Lynx*) was controlled by the Vif-A3 interaction. To the best of our knowledge, this is the first report providing evidence of the co-evolutionary arms race between mammals and lentiviruses in the New World.

Methods

Ethics statement

To determine the feline *A3Z3* sequences, blood, body hair or cryopreserved muscle tissue of pumas, bobcats and cheetahs were kindly provided by the following facilities: Tennoji zoo, Osaka, Japan; Kobe City Oji zoo, Hyogo, Japan; Omoriyama zoo, Akita, Japan; Tama Zoological Park, Tokyo, Japan; Izu Animal Kingdom, Shizuoka, Japan; and Shizuoka Municipal Nihondaira zoo, Shizuoka, Japan. Sampling was performed in accordance with the guideline of Tokyo University of Agriculture, Japan. All experimental protocols were approved by a committee at Tokyo University of Agriculture, Japan.

Sequencing PCR of the feline *A3Z3* genes

Sequencing PCR of feline *A3Z3* was performed as previously described [45, 46]. Briefly, genomic DNA was extracted from the samples described above using the DNA Extractor FM kit (Wako) or the DNeasy Blood &

Tissue it (Qiagen). PCR was performed using the Prime-STAR GXL DNA polymerase (Takara) and the primers are listed in Additional file 2: Table S1. The obtained PCR products were purified by gel extraction using the QIAquick gel extraction kit (Qiagen). The nucleotide sequences were determined by a DNA sequencing service (Fasmac, Kanagawa, Japan) and the data were analyzed using Sequencher v5.1 software (Gene Codes Corporation).

Molecular phylogenetic analysis of the FIV *vif* and feline *A3Z3* genes

Molecular phylogenetic analyses were performed as previously described [12, 14, 45–47]. Briefly, the sequences of PLV Vif and feline *A3Z3*, some of which were newly identified in this study (Figs. 1a, c, 7a), were aligned using ClustalW implemented in MEGA7 [48]. The alignments were verified manually at the amino acid level. Phylogenetic trees (Figs. 1a, c, 7a) were reconstructed using the maximum likelihood (ML) method with PhyML [49]. To calculate the amino acid sequence diversity of PLV Vif, 26 and 34 amino acid sequences from PLV-A and PLV-B Vif (summarized in Fig. 1a) are used, respectively. A multiple alignment was generated using L-INS-i in MAFFT [50]. The gapped regions were removed using trimAl with the nogaps option [51], and 227 amino acid sites were used for the analysis. Then, we performed pairwise comparisons of 60 amino acid sequences to calculate the amino acid sequence identity using MEGA7 [48].

Plasmid construction

The expressing plasmids for HA-tagged puma and lynx A3Z3 were kindly provided by Dr. Carsten Münk [15]. The expressing plasmids for HA-tagged bobcat and cheetah A3Z3 were constructed by using the genomic DNA fragments and the primers listed in Additional file 2: Table S1. The point mutants of HA-tagged puma and bobcat A3Z3 were constructed by using a GeneArt site-directed mutagenesis system (Thermo Fisher Scientific). Each wild-type plasmid was used as the template, and the primers used are listed in Additional file 2: Table S1. The His-tagged PLV-A Vif (strains Lru1, Lru20 and Pco5) and PLV-B (strains Pco14, Pco16 and Pco27) were obtained from GeneArt gene synthesis service (Thermo Fisher Scientific). The obtained DNA fragments were digested with BamHI and SalI and inserted into the BamHI-SalI site of pDON-AI plasmid (Takara). The nucleotide sequences were determined by a DNA sequencing service (Fasmac, Kanagawa, Japan) and the data were analyzed by Sequencher v5.1 software (Gene Codes Corporation).

Cell culture and transfection

HEK293T cells (CRL-11268; ATCC) were cultured in Dulbecco's modified Eagle medium (Sigma-Aldrich) supplemented with 10% heat-inactivated fetal calf serum and antibiotics (Thermo Fisher Scientific). Transfection was performed by using PEI Max (GE Healthcare) in accordance with the manufacturers procedures and described previously [12, 14, 45–47, 52]. To analyze the dose-dependent anti-FIV activity of feline A3Z3, pFP93 (pFIVgagpolΔvif; a replication incompetent *vif*-deficient FIV packaging construct derived from clone FIV-34TF10 [GenBank accession number M25381]; kindly provided by Dr. Eric M. Poeschla) (200 ng), pTiger-luc (pFIVΨ-luc) (150 ng), and pMD.G (pVSVg; a vesicular stomatitis virus G [VSVg] expression plasmid) (50 ng) were co-transfected into HEK293T cells (1×10^5 cells) with feline A3Z3 expression plasmid (50, 100, 200, or 400 ng). To analyze the functional relationship between feline A3Z3 and PLV-Vif, feline A3Z3 expression plasmid (200 ng), pFP93 (200 ng), pTiger-luc (150 ng), and pMD.G (50 ng) were co-transfected into HEK293T cells with or without His-tagged PLV Vif expression plasmid (400 ng). After 48 h post-transfection, the transfected cells and culture supernatants were harvested as previously described [12–14, 45–47, 52].

Western blotting and virus reporter assay

Western blotting and reporter assay were performed as previously described [12–14, 45–47, 52]. For the Western blotting of virus particles, 340 μl of the culture supernatant was ultracentrifuged at $100,000 \times g$ for 1 h at 4 °C using a TL-100 instrument (Beckman), and the pellet was lysed with $1 \times$ SDS buffer. For the Western blotting of transfected cells, the cells were lysed with RIPA buffer (50 mM Tris–HCl buffer [pH 7.6], 150 mM NaCl, 1% Nonidet P-40, 0.5% sodium deoxycholate, 0.1% SDS) with protease inhibitor cocktail (Roche). The following antibodies for Western blotting: anti-His polyclonal antibody (OGHis; Medical and Biological Laboratories), anti-HA antibody (3F10; Roche), anti-FIV p24 Capsid antibody (PAK3-2C1; Santa Cruz Biotechnology); anti-alpha-tubulin (TUBA) antibody (DM1A; Sigma), and anti-VSVg antibody (P5DA; Roche). For FIV reporter assays, HEK293T cells were used for the target of infection. Ten microliter of the culture supernatant of transfected cells was inoculated into HEK293T cells in a 96-well plate (Nunc), and the firefly luciferase activity was measured by using the BrillianStar-LT assay system (Toyo-b-net) and the 2030 ARVO X multilabel counter instrument (PerkinElmer) according to the manufacturers' procedures.

Protein homology modeling

Homology modeling was performed using the SWISS-MODEL server [53–56]. After BLAST searches [57] of the bobcat and puma A3Z3 amino acid sequences against protein data bank sequence entries (http://www.rcsb.org/pdb/), the crystal structure of human APOBEC3A (PDB: 5KEG) [58] was selected as the best template for homology modeling per the Global Model Quality Estimations, QMEAN statistical parameters, and modeled sequence length. Each generated model was minimized and refined using Discovery Studio (Dassault Systèmes BIOVIA, Discovery Studio Modeling Environment, Release 4.1, San Diego: Dassault Systèmes, 2007). Mutant models and 3D images were generated with PyMOL (The PyMOL Molecular Graphics System, version 1.8 Schrödinger, LLC).

Statistical analyses

The data are expressed as averages with the standard deviations (SDs), and statistically significant differences were determined using Student's *t* test.

Accession numbers

The *A3Z3* sequences of five pumas, two bobcats and two cheetahs were submitted to DDBJ (accession numbers LC376039-LC376042).

Additional files

Additional file 1: Figure S1. Scheme of the feline genome encoding *APOBEC3Z3* and the position of the primers used in this study. The scheme used for *Felis catus* chromosome B4, including the exons of feline *APOBEC3Z3*, is shown. The primers used for PCR/sequencing are shown as red arrowheads, and the names are identical to those in Table S1.

Additional file 2: Table S1. Primers used in this study. A full list of the primers used in this study.

Additional file 3: Figure S2. Structure homology model of bobcat A3Z3 hap II. Cartoon (top and middle) and surface (bottom) models of the A3Z3 protein structures of bobcat hap I (A) and hap II (B) are shown. In the top panel, alpha-helices and beta-sheets are shown in green and pale blue, respectively. Zn^{2+} is represented as a gray sphere. In the middle and bottom panels, the amino acid that differed between hap I (R116) and hap II (H116) is represented in orange.

Abbreviations

A3: apolipoprotein B mRNA-editing enzyme catalytic polypeptide-like 3 (APOBEC3); A3Z3: APOBEC3Z3; CST: cross-species transmission; FIV: feline immunodeficiency virus; ML: maximum likelihood; Mya: million years ago; OWM: Old World monkey; PLV: puma lentivirus; SIV: simian immunodeficiency virus; SD: standard deviation; TRIM5: tripartite motif containing protein 5; TUBA: alpha-tubulin; Vif: viral infectivity factor; VSVg: vesicular stomatitis virus G.

Authors' contributions

KS conceived the study and designed experiments; Y.Konno, S.Nagaoka, IK, KY, Y.Kagawa, RK, HA and TK performed experiments; Y.Konno, S.Nagaoka, IK, KY and HA analyzed data; MTU and S.Nakagawa constructed protein homology models; S.Nakagawa and KS performed phylogenetic analyses; KS wrote the

paper; and Y.Konno, S.Nagaoka, IK, MTU, S.Nakagawa, Y.Koyanagi and KS edited the manuscript. All authors read and approved the final manuscript.

Author details

[1] Laboratory of Systems Virology, Institute for Frontier Life and Medical Sciences, Kyoto University, Kyoto, Japan. [2] Graduate School of Biostudies, Kyoto University, Kyoto, Japan. [3] Graduate School of Pharmaceutical Sciences, Kyoto University, Kyoto, Japan. [4] Graduate School of Medicine, Kyoto University, Kyoto, Japan. [5] Faculty of Medicine, Kyoto University, Kyoto, Japan. [6] Faculty of Science, Kyoto University, Kyoto, Japan. [7] Faculty of Pharmaceutical Sciences, Kyoto University, Kyoto, Japan. [8] Micro/Nano Technology Center, Tokai University, Kanagawa, Japan. [9] Department of Molecular Life Science, Tokai University School of Medicine, Tokai University, Kanagawa, Japan. [10] Department of Animal Science, Faculty of Agriculture, Tokyo University of Agriculture, Kanagawa, Japan. [11] CREST, Japan Science and Technology Agency, Saitama, Japan. [12] Division of Systems Virology, Department of Infectious Disease Control, International Research Center for Infectious Diseases, Institute of Medical Science, The University of Tokyo, 4-6-1 Shirokanedai, Minato-ku, Tokyo 1088639, Japan.

Acknowledgements

We thank Carsten Münk (Heinrich-Heine-Universität, Düsseldorf, Germany) and Eric M. Poeschla (University of Colorado, USA) for providing experimental materials and Tennoji zoo (Osaka, Japan), Kobe City Oji zoo (Hyogo, Japan), Omoriyama zoo (Akita, Japan), Tama Zoological Park (Tokyo, Japan), Izu Animal Kingdom (Shizuoka, Japan), and Shizuoka Municipal Nihondaira zoo (Shizuoka, Japan) for kindly providing feline samples.

Competing interests

The authors declare that no competing interests exist.

Funding

This study was supported in part by AMED J-PRIDE 17fm0208006h0001 (to KS); JST CREST (to KS); JSPS KAKENHI Grants-in-Aid for Scientific Research C 15K07166 (to KS), Scientific Research B (Generative Research Fields) 16KT0111 (to KS), and Scientific Research on Innovative Areas 16H06429 (to S. Nakagawa and KS), 16K21723 (to S.Nakagawa and KS), 17H05823 (to S. Nakagawa) and 17H05813 (to KS); Takeda Science Foundation (to KS); Salt Science Research Foundation (to KS); Smoking Research Foundation (to KS); Chube Ito Foundation (to KS); Fordays Self-Reliance Support in Japan (to KS); Mishima Kaiun Memorial Foundation (to KS); Tobemaki Foundation (to KS); ONO Medical Research Foundation (to KS); MEXT-Supported Program for the Strategic Research Foundation at Private Universities (to S.Nakagawa and MTU); Joint Usage/Research Center program of Institute for Frontier Life and Medical Sciences Kyoto University (to S.Nakagawa); JSPS Core-to-Core program, A. Advanced Research Networks (to Y.Koyanagi); and AMED Research on HIV/AIDS 16fk0410203h002 (to Y.Koyanagi).

References

1. Koito A, Ikeda T. Intrinsic restriction activity by AID/APOBEC family of enzymes against the mobility of retroelements. Mob Genet Elem. 2011;1:197–202.

2.   LaRue RS, Andresdottir V, Blanchard Y, Conticello SG, Derse D, Emerman M, et al. Guidelines for naming nonprimate APOBEC3 genes and proteins. J Virol. 2009;83:494–7.

3.   Harris RS, Dudley JP. APOBECs and virus restriction. Virology. 2015;479–480:131–45.

4.   Nakano Y, Aso H, Soper A, Yamada E, Moriwaki M, Juarez-Fernandez G, et al. A conflict of interest: the evolutionary arms race between mammalian APOBEC3 and lentiviral Vif. Retrovirology. 2017;14:31.

5.   Dawkins R, Krebs JR. Arms races between and within species. Proc R Soc Lond B Biol Sci. 1979;205:489–511.

6.   Duggal NK, Emerman M. Evolutionary conflicts between viruses and restriction factors shape immunity. Nat Rev Immunol. 2012;12:687–95.

7.   Gifford RJ. Viral evolution in deep time: lentiviruses and mammals. Trends Genet. 2012;28:89–100.

8.   Kirchhoff F. Immune evasion and counteraction of restriction factors by HIV-1 and other primate lentiviruses. Cell Host Microbe. 2010;8:55–67.

9.   Pedersen NC, Ho EW, Brown ML, Yamamoto JK. Isolation of a T-lymphotropic virus from domestic cats with an immunodeficiency-like syndrome. Science. 1987;235:790–3.

10. Münk C, Beck T, Zielonka J, Hotz-Wagenblatt A, Chareza S, Battenberg M, et al. Functions, structure, and read-through alternative splicing of feline APOBEC3 genes. Genome Biol. 2008;9:R48.

11. Wang J, Zhang W, Lv M, Zuo T, Kong W, Yu X. Identification of a Cullin5-ElonginB-ElonginC E3 complex in degradation of feline immunodeficiency virus Vif-mediated feline APOBEC3 proteins. J Virol. 2011;85:12482–91.

12. Yoshikawa R, Izumi T, Yamada E, Nakano Y, Misawa N, Ren F, et al. A naturally occurring domestic cat APOBEC3 variant confers resistance to FIV infection. J Virol. 2015;90:474–85.

13. Yoshikawa R, Nakano Y, Yamada E, Izumi T, Misawa N, Koyanagi Y, et al. Species-specific differences in the ability of feline lentiviral Vif to degrade feline APOBEC3 proteins. Microbiol Immunol. 2016;60:272–9.

14. Yoshikawa R, Takeuchi JS, Yamada E, Nakano Y, Misawa N, Kimura Y, et al. Feline immunodeficiency virus evolutionarily acquires two proteins, vif and protease, capable of antagonizing Feline APOBEC3. J Virol. 2017;91:e00250-17.

15. Zielonka J, Marino D, Hofmann H, Yuhki N, Löchelt M, Münk C. Vif of feline immunodeficiency virus from domestic cats protects against APOBEC3 restriction factors from many felids. J Virol. 2010;84:7312–24.

16. Pecon-Slattery J, Troyer JL, Johnson WE, O'Brien SJ. Evolution of feline immunodeficiency virus in Felidae: implications for human health and wildlife ecology. Vet Immunol Immunopathol. 2008;123:32–44.

17. Lee J, Malmberg JL, Wood BA, Hladky S, Troyer R, Roelke M, et al. Feline immunodeficiency virus cross-species transmission: implications for emergence of new lentiviral infections. J Virol. 2017;91:e02134-16.

18. Franklin SP, Troyer JL, Terwee JA, Lyren LM, Boyce WM, Riley SP, et al. Frequent transmission of immunodeficiency viruses among bobcats and pumas. J Virol. 2007;81:10961–9.

19. Lee JS, Bevins SN, Serieys LE, Vickers W, Logan KA, Aldredge M, et al. Evolution of puma lentivirus in bobcats (Lynx rufus) and mountain lions (Puma concolor) in North America. J Virol. 2014;88:7727–37.

20. Sawyer SL, Emerman M, Malik HS. Ancient adaptive evolution of the primate antiviral DNA-editing enzyme APOBEC3G. PLoS Biol. 2004;2:E275.

21. Vallender EJ, Lahn BT. Positive selection on the human genome. Hum Mol Genet. 2004;13(2):R245–54.

22. Krupp A, McCarthy KR, Ooms M, Letko M, Morgan JS, Simon V, et al. APOBEC3G polymorphism as a selective barrier to cross-species transmission and emergence of pathogenic SIV and AIDS in a primate host. PLoS Pathog. 2013;9:e1003641.

23. Johnson WE, Eizirik E, Pecon-Slattery J, Murphy WJ, Antunes A, Teeling E, et al. The late Miocene radiation of modern Felidae: a genetic assessment. Science. 2006;311:73–7.

24. de Castro FL, Junqueira DM, de Medeiros RM, da Silva TR, Costenaro JG, Knak MB, et al. Analysis of single-nucleotide polymorphisms in the APOBEC3H gene of domestic cats (Felis catus) and their association with the susceptibility to feline immunodeficiency virus and feline leukemia virus infections. Infect Genet Evol. 2014;27:389–94.

25. Hatziioannou T, Princiotta M, Piatak M Jr, Yuan F, Zhang F, Lifson JD, et al. Generation of simian-tropic HIV-1 by restriction factor evasion. Science. 2006;314:95.

26. Schrofelbauer B, Senger T, Manning G, Landau NR. Mutational alteration of human immunodeficiency virus type 1 Vif allows for functional interaction with nonhuman primate APOBEC3G. J Virol. 2006;80:5984–91.

27. Hahn BH, Shaw GM, De Cock KM, Sharp PM. AIDS as a zoonosis: scientific and public health implications. Science. 2000;287:607–14.

28. Sharp PM, Hahn BH. The evolution of HIV-1 and the origin of AIDS. Philos Trans R Soc Lond B Biol Sci. 2010;365:2487–94.

29. Gogarten JF, Akoua-Koffi C, Calvignac-Spencer S, Leendertz SA, Weiss S, Couacy-Hymann E, et al. The ecology of primate retroviruses: an assessment of 12 years of retroviral studies in the Tai national park area, Cote d Ivoire. Virology. 2014;460–461:147–53.

30. Leendertz SA, Locatelli S, Boesch C, Kucherer C, Formenty P, Liegeois F, et al. No evidence for transmission of SIVwrc from western red colobus monkeys (Piliocolobus badius badius) to wild West African chimpanzees (Pan troglodytes verus) despite high exposure through hunting. BMC Microbiol. 2011;11:24.

31. Lomolino MV, Riddle BR, Whittaker RJ, Brown JH: Distributions of Communities. In: Biogeography. 4th ed. Sunderland: Oxford University Press; 2010. pp. 121–164.

32. Wynne EM, Mathew WA, Jonathan NP. Quantifying risk and resource use for a large carnivore in an expanding urban-wildland interface. J Appl Ecol. 2015;53:371–8.

33. Smith JA, Wang Y, Wilmers CC. Top carnivores increase their kill rates on prey as a response to human-induced fear. Proc Biol Sci. 2015;282(1802):20142711.

34. Compton AA, Emerman M. Convergence and divergence in the evolution of the APOBEC3G-Vif interaction reveal ancient origins of simian immunodeficiency viruses. PLoS Pathog. 2013;9:e1003135.

35. Coffin JM. HIV population dynamics in vivo: implications for genetic variation, pathogenesis, and therapy. Science. 1995;267:483–9.

36. Stremlau M, Owens CM, Perron MJ, Kiessling M, Autissier P, Sodroski J. The cytoplasmic body component TRIM5alpha restricts HIV-1 infection in Old World monkeys. Nature. 2004;427:848–53.

37. Neil SJ, Zang T, Bieniasz PD. Tetherin inhibits retrovirus release and is antagonized by HIV-1 Vpu. Nature. 2008;451:425–30.

38. Van Damme N, Goff D, Katsura C, Jorgenson RL, Mitchell R, Johnson MC, et al. The interferon-induced protein BST-2 restricts HIV-1 release and is downregulated from the cell surface by the viral Vpu protein. Cell Host Microbe. 2008;3:245–52.

39. McEwan WA, Schaller T, Ylinen LM, Hosie MJ, Towers GJ, Willett BJ. Truncation of TRIM5 in the Feliformia explains the absence of retroviral restriction in cells of the domestic cat. J Virol. 2009;83:8270–5.

40. Dietrich I, McMonagle EL, Petit SJ, Vijayakrishnan S, Logan N, Chan CN, et al. Feline tetherin efficiently restricts release of feline immunodeficiency virus but not spreading of infection. J Virol. 2011;85:5840–52.

41. Compton AA, Hirsch VM, Emerman M. The host restriction factor APOBEC3G and retroviral Vif protein coevolve due to ongoing genetic conflict. Cell Host Microbe. 2012;11:91–8.

42. Compton AA, Malik HS, Emerman M. Host gene evolution traces the evolutionary history of ancient primate lentiviruses. Philos Trans R Soc Lond B Biol Sci. 2013;368:20120496.

43. Jern P, Coffin JM. Host-retrovirus arms race: trimming the budget. Cell Host Microbe. 2008;4:196–7.

44. OhAinle M, Kerns JA, Li MM, Malik HS, Emerman M. Antiretroelement activity of APOBEC3H was lost twice in recent human evolution. Cell Host Microbe. 2008;4:249–59.

45. Kobayashi T, Takeuchi JS, Ren F, Matsuda K, Sato K, Kimura Y, et al. Characterization of red-capped mangabey tetherin: implication for the co-evolution of primates and their lentiviruses. Sci Rep. 2014;4:5529.

46. Yamada E, Yoshikawa R, Nakano Y, Misawa N, Kobayashi T, Ren F, et al. A naturally occurring bovine APOBEC3 confers resistance to bovine lentiviruses: implication for the co-evolution of bovids and their lentiviruses. Sci Rep. 2016;6:33988.

47. Takeuchi JS, Ren F, Yoshikawa R, Yamada E, Nakano Y, Kobayashi T, et al. Coevolutionary dynamics between tribe Cercopithecini tetherins and their lentiviruses. Sci Rep. 2015;5:16021.

48. Kumar S, Stecher G, Tamura K. MEGA7: molecular evolutionary genetics analysis version 7.0 for bigger datasets. Mol Biol Evol. 2016;33:1870–4.

49. Guindon S, Dufayard JF, Lefort V, Anisimova M, Hordijk W, Gascuel O. New algorithms and methods to estimate maximum-likelihood phylogenies: assessing the performance of PhyML 3.0. Syst Biol. 2010;59:307–21.

50. Katoh K, Standley DM. MAFFT multiple sequence alignment software version 7: improvements in performance and usability. Mol Biol Evol. 2013;30:772–80.

51. Capella-Gutierrez S, Silla-Martinez JM, Gabaldon T. trimAl: a tool for automated alignment trimming in large-scale phylogenetic analyses. Bioinformatics. 2009;25:1972–3.

52. Nakano Y, Misawa N, Juarez-Fernandez G, Moriwaki M, Nakaoka S, Funo T, et al. HIV-1 competition experiments in humanized mice show that APOBEC3H imposes selective pressure and promotes virus adaptation. PLoS Pathog. 2017;13:e1006348.

53. Biasini M, Bienert S, Waterhouse A, Arnold K, Studer G, Schmidt T, et al. SWISS-MODEL: modelling protein tertiary and quaternary structure using evolutionary information. Nucleic Acids Res. 2014;42:W252–8.

54. Guex N, Peitsch MC, Schwede T. Automated comparative protein structure modeling with SWISS-MODEL and Swiss-PdbViewer: a historical perspective. Electrophoresis. 2009;30(Suppl 1):S162–73.

55. Bordoli L, Kiefer F, Arnold K, Benkert P, Battey J, Schwede T. Protein structure homology modeling using SWISS-MODEL workspace. Nat Protoc. 2009;4:1–13.

56. Altschul SF, Madden TL, Schaffer AA, Zhang J, Zhang Z, Miller W, et al. Gapped BLAST and PSI-BLAST: a new generation of protein database search programs. Nucleic Acids Res. 1997;25:3389–402.

57. Arnold K, Bordoli L, Kopp J, Schwede T. The SWISS-MODEL workspace: a web-based environment for protein structure homology modelling. Bioinformatics. 2006;22:195–201.

58. Kouno T, Silvas TV, Hilbert BJ, Shandilya SMD, Bohn MF, Kelch BA, et al. Crystal structure of APOBEC3A bound to single-stranded DNA reveals structural basis for cytidine deamination and specificity. Nat Commun. 2017;8:15024.

59. Bruen TC, Poss M. Recombination in feline immunodeficiency virus genomes from naturally infected cougars. Virology. 2007;364:362–70.

5

CLIP-related methodologies and their application to retrovirology

Paul D. Bieniasz[1] and Sebla B. Kutluay[2]* ⓘ

Abstract

Virtually every step of HIV-1 replication and numerous cellular antiviral defense mechanisms are regulated by the binding of a viral or cellular RNA-binding protein (RBP) to distinct sequence or structural elements on HIV-1 RNAs. Until recently, these protein–RNA interactions were studied largely by in vitro binding assays complemented with genetics approaches. However, these methods are highly limited in the identification of the relevant targets of RBPs in physiologically relevant settings. Development of crosslinking-immunoprecipitation sequencing (CLIP) methodology has revolutionized the analysis of protein–nucleic acid complexes. CLIP combines immunoprecipitation of covalently crosslinked protein–RNA complexes with high-throughput sequencing, providing a global account of RNA sequences bound by a RBP of interest in cells (or virions) at near-nucleotide resolution. Numerous variants of the CLIP protocol have recently been developed, some with major improvements over the original. Herein, we briefly review these methodologies and give examples of how CLIP has been successfully applied to retrovirology research.

Background

Following the integration of proviral DNA into the host cell chromosome, genesis of new HIV-1 particles is initiated by the host RNA Polymerase II-mediated synthesis of a single poly-cistronic viral RNA species [1]. This transcript undergoes varying levels of alternative splicing generating over 40 different RNA species, an event orchestrated by the host cellular splicing machinery and cis-acting elements on viral RNAs [1, 2]. Like cellular mRNAs, all viral RNAs contain 5′ 7-methylguanosine (m7G) caps and 3′ polyA tails [1, 3]. While fully spliced viral RNAs can exit the nucleus via canonical nuclear export pathways, the partially spliced and unspliced viral RNAs depend on the viral Rev and cellular Crm1 proteins for nuclear export [4]. All viral mRNAs are subsequently translated in the cytosol, but the unspliced full-length viral RNAs also serve as the viral genome and are packaged into virions by the viral major structural protein Gag. Following their release from the plasma membrane, particles undergo a maturation step triggered by the viral protease enzyme. During this process, Gag and Gag-Pol proteins are cleaved into their constituent domains, the CA domain of Gag forms a conical lattice and the viral RNA genome condenses with the cleaved NC domain of Gag and viral enzymes inside this conical core [5, 6]. Thus, virtually every step in HIV-1 replication depends on a complex and changing set of interactions between viral RNAs and the multitude of trans-acting viral and cellular RNA-binding proteins. Historically, the interactions between these proteins and their RNA targets have largely been mapped by genetic studies, complemented by limited in vitro approaches. Comprehensive analysis of these interactions in physiologically relevant settings was effectively impossible prior to the recent development of cutting-edge next-generation sequencing-based methodologies. These methods, collectively referred to as CLIP (crosslinking-immunoprecipitation coupled with next-generation sequencing), allow the global identification of RNA targets of RNA-binding proteins (RBPs) in physiological settings in unprecedented detail. In this review, we provide a detailed outline of the existing CLIP methodologies, discuss their advantages and shortcomings (based partly on our own experience) and give examples of how CLIP has been successfully applied to retrovirology research.

*Correspondence: kutluay@wustl.edu
[2] Department of Molecular Microbiology, Washington University School of Medicine, Saint Louis, MO 63110, USA
Full list of author information is available at the end of the article

(See figure on next page.)
Fig. 1 Outline of CLIP

Principles of CLIP and variant methodologies

In simple terms, CLIP is a powerful methodology with which one can identify the RNA targets of RNA-binding proteins in physiological settings, ranging from live cells to virus particles and even animal tissues. The inception of the original CLIP protocol [7, 8] and its subsequent coupling to next-generation sequencing [9] has revolutionized the study of protein–RNA interactions. Since then, several other versions of CLIP have been developed. The salient steps of the existing CLIP methodologies are (Fig. 1): (1) protein–RNA complexes are covalently crosslinked in live cells/tissues/virions; (2) Cells/tissues/virions are lysed and treated with limited amounts of RNases leaving small fragments of RNA molecules (~ 20 to 50 nucleotides) protected by the protein of interest; (3) Protein–RNA complexes are immunoprecipitated, and non-specific RNAs and proteins are removed by stringent washes. Because the protein–RNA complexes are covalently crosslinked, these stringent conditions, in principle, do not affect purification of target protein–RNA adducts. (4) The purified protein–RNA complexes are radioactively labeled and separated by SDS-PAGE. (5) Bound RNA is isolated either directly from SDS-PAGE gels or from nitrocellulose membranes following transfer by Proteinase K treatment. (6) Eluted RNA is ligated to adapters, reverse transcribed, the resulting cDNA is PCR amplified and subjected to sequencing. (7) Sequencing reads are processed and mapped to reference genomes. Depending on the method used, the resulting library contains nucleotide substitutions or deletions at the site of crosslinking, which allows mapping of the site of protein–RNA interactions at near-nucleotide resolution. Subsequent analyses include determination of the significantly enriched binding sites, identification of the binding motifs within them as well as other custom analyses. In the remainder of this section we will review the currently existing CLIP methods and give an overview of the widely used CLIP data analysis tools and pipelines.

HITS-CLIP

Historically, protein–RNA interactions were studied largely using in vitro binding assays with pure proteins and RNAs. Alternatively, GST-pulldown and immunoprecipitation-based assays were conducted on cell lysates followed by downstream quantitative analysis of RNA by Q-RT-PCR or microarrays. A major drawback of these cell lysate-based approaches was their limited ability to identify direct interactions between a RBP and its target RNA molecules. Their limited power was due at least in

part to the presence of contaminating protein and RNA molecules in the isolated RBP-RNA complexes. Development of the original CLIP protocol [7, 8], in which the protein–RNA complexes were UV-crosslinked in vivo and immunoprecipitated under stringent conditions to remove the contaminating proteins and RNA molecules marked the first advancement over these traditional methods. While the initial CLIP methodology relied on cloning and subsequent sequencing of the RNA targets, the coupling of CLIP to high-throughput sequencing, HITS-CLIP, allowed global transcriptome-wide analysis of RBP-RNA crosslinks [9]. HITS-CLIP relies on UV crosslinking of protein–RNA complexes at UV254 nm. As such, HITS-CLIP can be applied to animal tissues due to its high level of penetration. Following crosslinking and immunoprecipitation of protein–RNA complexes, ligation to the radioactively labeled 5′ adapter is performed while the protein–RNA adducts are attached to beads. This allows the removal of unligated 5′ adapter by further rounds of bead washing, which substantially reduces the appearance of adapter–adapter ligation products following downstream processing. The isolated protein–RNA adducts are separated by SDS-PAGE and transferred to nitrocellulose membranes. As naked RNA molecules are not retained on the nitrocellulose membranes, protein–RNA complexes are purified further during this step. Transfer to nitrocellulose membranes has been utilized in other CLIP approaches and in our experience confers a major advantage over the originally described PAR-CLIP approach described below. Protein-crosslinked RNA is further purified from nitrocellulose membranes by proteinase K treatment, ligated to the 3′ adapters and PCR-amplified prior to sequencing. Detailed bioinformatics analyses of HITS-CLIP datasets revealed that reverse transcriptase (RT) introduces deletions at the site of crosslinking [10], albeit at a fairly low frequency, allowing HITS-CLIP to reach to near nucleotide-resolution identification of binding sites.

PAR-CLIP

A major advantage of PAR-CLIP [11] over HITS-CLIP is the use of ribonucleoside analogs, including 4-thiouridine (4SU) and 6-thioguanosine (6SG), that significantly enhance the efficiency of protein–RNA crosslinking. In PAR-CLIP experiments, cells are typically grown in the presence of ribonucleoside analogs for up to 16 h and UV-crosslinked at a longer wavelength (365 nm). As such, in contrast to HITS-CLIP, application of PAR-CLIP is largely limited to cell culture systems (an exception

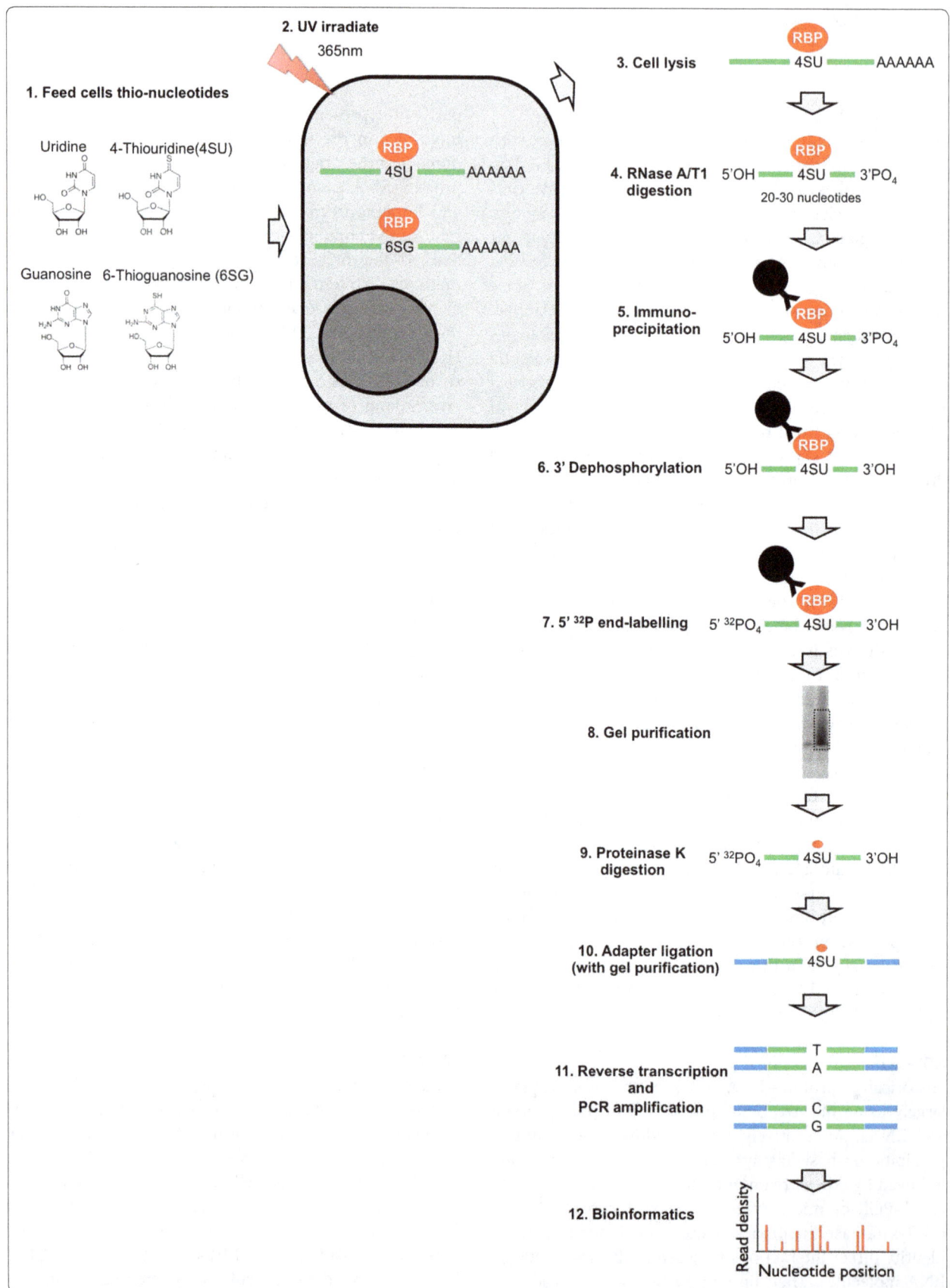

being *C. elegans* which can be grown in 4SU containing media and efficiently UV-crosslinked due to its transparency [12]). Although the original PAR-CLIP description utilized an inducible tagged RNA-binding protein [11], we and many other groups have successfully adapted PAR-CLIP to study endogenous proteins, including HIV-1 NC and IN [13, 14], Argonaute [15–18], as well as other proteins involved in RNA biogenesis and metabolism [19–24]. A potential disadvantage of the PAR-CLIP protocol is the cellular toxicity that may be induced by 4SU treatment depending on the cell type, the dose and incubation time [25]. Thus, optimal conditions that allow efficient protein–RNA crosslinking without major toxicity should be determined on a case-by-case basis. Nevertheless, PAR-CLIP allows accurate nucleotide resolution mapping of target RNA sites due to mutations introduced by RT (T-to-C for 4SU and G-to-A for 6SG) precisely at the site of crosslinking during cDNA synthesis. While allowing nucleotide resolution mapping, use of ribonucleoside analogs may inadvertently enrich RNA elements with distinct nucleotide composition or alter RNA structure [26], which may subsequently affect protein binding. Careful validation of PAR-CLIP experiments with different ribonucleoside analogs and RNases should, in principle, address these potential problems.

iCLIP

Identification of the precise crosslinking site in the HITS-CLIP and PAR-CLIP approaches relies respectively on deletions and substitutions introduced by RT during cDNA synthesis. However, read-through at crosslinking sites appears to be a relatively rare event as compared to truncations that occur as a result of RT stalling at these sites [27, 28]. Thus, a major shortcoming of HITS-CLIP and PAR-CLIP approaches is the loss of a large fraction (estimated to be > 80%) of the starting material due to the inability to recover truncated reverse transcription products. iCLIP [29] has been designed to address this problem by ligation of a 3′ adapter while protein–RNA complexes are still on beads followed by introduction of a two-part cleavable adaptor into cDNA during reverse transcription. The resulting cDNA is circularized and subsequently linearized with a restriction enzyme, which allows the recovery of a larger fraction of truncated cDNAs. In addition, as circularization is done at high temperatures, structured cDNA molecules are recovered at a much higher efficiency. As a result of this enrichment, iCLIP can yield higher complexity libraries and has been proposed to perform better than previous approaches in identification of the precise site of crosslinking [28–30]. Application of iCLIP on a large scale by the ENCODE consortium indicated that the success rate in generating libraries was low for many RBPs, which was ascribed to

the low efficiency of the circularization step [31]. However, several studies that utilized iCLIP have generated libraries with sufficiently high complexity and sensitivity, and these parameters were not carefully assessed by the ENCODE consortium. The remainder of the iCLIP protocol is similar to HITS-CLIP and PAR-CLIP approaches. BrdU-CLIP [32] and FAST-iCLIP [33] are iterations of the iCLIP protocol, which provide alternative cDNA and RNA purification methods, respectively. For example, by exchanging the 3′ ddC blocker from the standard iCLIP 3′ adaptor with a 3′ biotin moiety and subsequent purification of ligation products on streptavidin beads, FAST-iCLIP is reported to reduce the time required to perform iCLIP by 50%.

eCLIP

The eCLIP protocol [31] proposes to address some of the shortcomings of previous CLIP approaches by including two separate adapter ligation steps (i.e. in the HITS-CLIP and PAR-CLIP protocols). In eCLIP, the immunoprecipitated RNA is first ligated to an indexed 3′ RNA adapter while complexes are still on the immunoprecipitation beads, and to a 3′ single-stranded (ss) DNA adapter after reverse transcription. As reverse transcription frequently terminates at the RBP-RNA crosslinking site, the ligation of the 3′ ssDNA adapter to the terminated cDNA fragments allows higher recovery rates of the starting material and helps in identification of the binding sites as in iCLIP. In addition, as the first 3′ RNA adapter already contains the indeces, samples can be combined at an earlier stage than in other protocols saving processing time. While adapter ligations conducted on beads has been inefficient in our hands (see below), the authors suggest that increased T4 RNA ligase concentration and the addition of high concentrations of polyethylene glycol (PEG8000) and DMSO in ligation reactions enable ligation efficiencies of up to > 90% [31]. In addition, RNA radiolabeling and autoradiographic visualization steps can be omitted allowing even faster library preparation times. However, these steps in our experience are highly important to purify the target protein–RNA complexes away from other proteins and RNA molecules that have non-specifically immunoprecipitated. Thus, the specificity of eCLIP libraries should be carefully evaluated, as also reviewed by a recent study [34]. Finally, inclusion of a size-matched input control (SMInput) in eCLIP enables efficient background normalization and controls for any inherent biases in library generation. The remainder of the eCLIP protocol shares many of the same steps as other CLIP approaches, in particular iCLIP.

irCLIP

Similar to eCLIP, irCLIP has been developed to overcome some of the shortcomings of previous CLIP methodologies by simplifying the library generation steps, increasing the yield and complexity of the CLIP library, and allowing faster processing times. One of the major differences of this approach is the utilization of a 3′ adapter conjugated to an infrared fluorescent dye [35], which provides a more sensitive and faster way of tracking the target RNA molecules compared to radioactive labeling. Similar to FAST-iCLIP, the adapter ligated RNA library is purified by streptavidin beads. CLIP has an inherent bias against identification of protein binding events on structured RNA elements due to stalling of RT at these sites. Although not proven, irCLIP may mitigate this problem by utilizing thermostable enzymes for circularization and reverse transcription steps to take place at 60 °C, which helps to resolve potential RNA secondary structures [35]. Other aspects of the irCLIP protocol, such as on-bead nuclease digestions and Proteinase K digestion in SDS have previously been utilized within the context of PAR-CLIP experiments [11, 14]. As in iCLIP and eCLIP, the irCLIP procedure achieves single-nucleotide resolution by recovery of truncated cDNAs after the reverse transcription stage.

Customizing CLIP

The major shortcomings of all of the above CLIP approaches include technically challenging and labor-intensive protocols, and loss of the starting material at several inefficient steps in the procedure. This problem is further exacerbated if the initial protein–RNA complexes are not abundant due to low levels of expression in cells (virions), low crosslinking or immunoprecipitation efficiencies. These problems can often lead to a final library with insufficient complexity and enrichment of environmental contaminating sequences. When we adapted the CLIP protocol to study HIV-1 Gag-RNA interactions [36], we took advantage of both HITS-CLIP and PAR-CLIP protocols as detailed in [14]. In our experience, 4-SU-mediated crosslinking yielded more abundant Gag-, MA- and NC-RNA complexes, that was critical for generating libraries with sufficient sequence diversity for successful sequencing. While the original PAR-CLIP protocol relied on electroelution of protein–RNA complexes from SDS-PAGE gels, we opted for transfer of protein–RNA complexes to nitrocellulose membranes following SDS-PAGE (as in HITS-CLIP). As naked RNA oligonucleotides are not immobilized on nitrocellulose membranes, this step provides an added level of protein–RNA complex purification. While the HITS-CLIP and many other protocols call for ligation of adapters while the protein–RNA complexes are on beads, the PAR-CLIP library

generation protocol in solution was significantly more efficient in our hands with 3′ and 5′ adapter ligations routinely working at > 90 and 50% efficiency. Although seemingly more cumbersome, sequential ligation of adapters provides more control over monitoring the ligation efficiency and substantially decreases contaminating adapter–adapter ligation products. Additionally, we have utilized barcoded and degenerate sequence containing adapters, which enabled us to combine multiple samples (typically up to eight) and distinguish between independent ligation versus PCR overamplification events, respectively. Finally, due to some of the potential inherent biases of the PAR-CLIP approach discussed above, we typically validate our findings using different ribonucleosides (4SU vs. 6SG) and RNases (RNase A vs. RNase T1).

CLIP data analyses

CLIP data analyses can be summarized in four major steps: (1) pre-processing of sequencing reads. (2) mapping of reads to reference genomes, (3) subjecting mapped reads to cluster finding algorithms to define binding sites, (4) analysis of binding sites for enrichment of certain features including where within a gene body the binding site is located, presence of distinct motifs or nucleotide composition. Recently a few pipelines that can perform the majority of these steps have been developed and include the PARCLIPsuite [37], CLIPZ [38], CIMS [39] and CLIP-seq tools [40]. Below, we will go through some of the publicly available and most frequently used standalone tools that can be utilized for analyses of CLIP data sets. For a more detailed review of these tools and algorithms we refer the readers to detailed recent reviews [41–44]. Implementing many of these analysis pipelines requires some level of coding knowledge and familiarity with shell scripting.

1. Pre-processing of sequencing reads: The resulting CLIP libraries in all of the above protocols will contain some form of 3′ and 5′ adaptors. In the majority of cases, these adaptors contain barcodes and degenerate sequences (N_{3-10}), which allow multiplexing and differentiating between independent ligation versus PCR overamplification events, respectively. In these circumstances, a typical pipeline will involve removing low quality reads, collapsing of raw reads into unique reads, demultiplexing samples, discarding short reads (typically less than 15 nucleotides) and trimming the adaptors prior to mapping. One of the most commonly used tools is the FASTX_toolkit (http://hannonlab.cshl.edu/fastx_toolkit/), which provides a number of functions to accomplish all of these steps. Other alternatives, with more limited

functions include Cutadapt [45], Trimmomatic [46], PRINSEQ [47] as well as custom scripts.

2. Mapping to reference genomes: The reads that pass the above filtering steps are mapped onto reference genomes or transcriptomes. The most commonly used mapping algorithms used for this task include Bowtie [48], Bowtie2 [49], STAR [50], Novoalign (http://www.novocraft.com/products/novoalign/), RMAP [51], TopHat [52], GSnap [53], SOAP [54] and BWA [55], some with unique advantages over others depending on whether mapping is done on a genome versus transcriptome. The choice of algorithm and the parameters for mapping will need to be finely tuned depending on which CLIP methodology is employed and the properties of the RBP of interest. For example, PAR-CLIP reads are expected to contain a number of T-to-C substitutions, and thus mismatches (typically ≤ 2 for reads between 15 and 40 nucleotides) should be allowed during mapping. While all algorithms allow mapping with mismatches, not all can handle deletions, which arise as a result of UV_{254} nm crosslinking in HITS-CLIP and related methods. For example while the original Bowtie algorithm did not allow gaps during alignment, Bowtie2 was developed to enable alignments with indels. Similarly, if mapping is done on transcriptomes, alignment algorithms such as STAR, which allow higher accuracy and speed for mapping spliced transcripts should be preferred. However, mapping to the transcriptome will clearly lead to the exclusion of reads derived from introns, which may constitute the primary binding sites for various splicing regulatory proteins. Thus, a general strategy whereby CLIP reads are mapped first to the transcriptome and the remaining reads are mapped to the genome may work the best for proteins for which there is no information on the types of targeted RNA molecules.

3. Peak calling: The next essential step in CLIP analysis is identification of the true binding sites by what is often referred to as *peak calling*. In simple terms, peak calling is the process by which clusters of reads that map to distinct locations are separated from background reads that may stem from unspecific binding events or contaminants during the CLIP procedure. Peaks are typically defined based on a number of variables such as read depth relative to surrounding regions, presence of expected and absence of unwanted mutations (as in the case of PAR-CLIP-based approaches) and peak shape. While peak calling can be based solely on CLIP data, additional controls such as data derived from replicates and negative controls (i.e. immunoprecipitations done with isotype controls and/or conducted

in lysates lacking the RBP of interest) can further increase specificity of peak calling. Comparison of the CLIP peaks with transcript abundance derived from matching RNA-seq experiments allows the discrimination of whether a binding event is merely a result of transcript abundance or a more specific interaction between the RBP and its target RNA. Several peak calling programs have been developed and include Piranha [56], CLIPper [57], PIPE-CLIP [58], Pyicos [59] that work with all CLIP variants, and PARalyzer [60] and wavClusteR that are specifically developed for PAR-CLIP analysis. For more details on the statistical models underlying these programs, we refer the readers to detailed reviews on this topic [41, 42].

4. Post-processing analyses: Following the identification of peaks, further analyses are typically conducted to identify the specific rules that may determine protein binding. For example, many studies generally assess what classes of RNAs and where within those transcripts binding sites are located and whether there are distinct motifs within the binding sites. While the former analyses are done usually by custom scripts, programs such as MEME [61], HOMER [62] and cERMIT [63] are commonly used for motif discovery. Finally, binding sites derived from CLIP experiments can further be analyzed by programs that are commonly used in gene expression profiling experiments for gene ontology and pathway analyses.

Application of CLIP techniques in retrovirology
Novel insights into selective HIV-1 genome packaging
All major steps of HIV-1 particle assembly are orchestrated by the major structural protein, Gag [6]. Gag undergoes major changes in its subcellular localization, structure and oligomeric state during this process. Immediately following its synthesis, Gag exists as a diffuse pool of monomers and low-order multimers in the cytosol, where it initially binds to the viral RNA genome [64, 65]. Concurrent with binding to the plasma membrane Gag undergoes a major structural change and oligomerizes around the viral genome [65]. Following the release of immature particles from the host cell's plasma membrane, particles undergo maturation—Gag is subjected to several proteolytic cleavages, which liberates NC and other constituent domains. NC remains bound to the viral genome and condenses with it inside the remodeled conical capsid lattice. Thus, a crucial property of Gag is its ability to select two copies of the viral genome for packaging in the cytosol and remain bound to them through various subcellular settings and configurations.

The mechanism by which HIV-1 selectively packages a dimeric unspliced viral genome is based largely on prior observations with simple retroviruses, as well as genetic studies and limited in vitro data. Selective packaging of the HIV-1 genome is governed in part by binding of the nucleocapsid (NC) domain of Gag to a highly structured *cis*-acting packaging element, psi (Ψ), within the 5' leader of the viral genome, composed of sequences in the unique 5' region (U5) and between the tRNA primer binding site (PBS) and the 5' portion of the Gag open reading frame (ORF). However, disruption of Ψ only modestly decreases HIV-1 RNA encapsidation [66–68], and sequences outside Ψ can increase virion RNA levels and viral vector titers [69–73]. In addition, viral RNA is not necessary for particle assembly and cellular RNAs can be packaged in its absence [74, 75]. Thus, although several lines of evidence have long indicated that sequences other than Ψ can contribute to genome packaging, determining the identities and features of these elements remained a challenge, due largely to lack of proper assays to study this process in cells.

Application of the CLIP methodology to the study of Gag-RNA interactions during different stages of particle assembly in cells revealed previously unanticipated rules of selective genome packaging [14]. First, nucleotide-resolution mapping of Gag binding to the HIV-1 genome in the cytosol revealed selective binding to sequences that coincide nearly precisely with a minimal element that can drive genome packaging. This minimal psi (Ψ) element adopts alternative structures, one of which favors genome packaging [76–78]. Second, in addition to Ψ, cytoplasmic Gag was bound to additional discrete elements on the viral RNA, including Rev Responsive Element (RRE), another highly structured region that mediates the export of HIV-1 RNAs from the nucleus. Although Gag-RRE interactions appeared to be dispensable for genome packaging, a more recent study has implied a role for it in preventing Gag from moving away from the viral RNA genome in the cytosol [79]. Third, mapping of Gag binding sites within the cellular mRNAs revealed a striking contrast between the binding preference of cytosolic versus membrane-bound Gag; while cytosolic Gag preferentially bound to GU-rich motifs, A-rich mRNA sequences were found to be enriched in plasma membrane-bound mRNA molecules. Remarkably, the nucleotide composition of the cellular mRNA targets of Gag at the plasma membrane mirrored the unusual A-rich nucleotide composition of the HIV-1 genome [14]. Finally, upon proteolytic cleavage of Gag in mature virions, the NC binding preference reverted back to GU-rich mRNA sequences and discrete viral RNA elements including Ψ. Together, these findings suggest that upon binding of monomeric Gag to the viral genome through Ψ, multimerization-dependent changes in the RNA binding specificity of Gag may drive the selective packaging of the A-rich viral genome. In line with this

model, a recent study has shown that longer segments of the Gag ORF, but not Ψ alone, can gradually increase the packaging of heterologous RNAs into virions [80]. Thus as part of the selective RNA packaging process, the role of Gag-Ψ interaction may be to nucleate further assembly of Gag oligomers on the viral genome [81].

HIV-1 MA-tRNA interactions

In addition to the NC domain, the matrix (MA) domain of Gag had long been suspected to bind RNA, based largely on in vitro assays [82–87]. The N-terminal basic amino acids of MA that are thought to bind RNA also mediate binding to cellular membranes [83, 88–92]. However, MA-RNA interaction has been thought to be fairly non-specific, and whether it actually occurs in cells could not be addressed until the application of the CLIP methodology. By releasing MA from Gag by Factor Xa protease-mediated cleavage as part of the CLIP procedure, following UV-crosslinking of Gag-expressing cells, MA was bound to a specific set of tRNAs in the cytosol [36]. In fact, MA-tRNA interactions constituted the most frequent binding event between cytosolic Gag and RNA. Notably, MA-tRNA interaction was lost upon binding of Gag to the plasma membrane and RNase treatment of cell lysates expressing Gag led to significantly higher levels of membrane associated Gag [36]. Together, these findings suggested that occlusion of MA basic residues by specific tRNAs may target HIV-1 assembly to the plasma membrane and prevent nonproductive assembly on intracellular membranes. Alternatively, tRNA binding by MA may temporally regulate membrane binding and assembly [93]. Recent in vitro liposome binding assays also revealed that a specific set of RNAs, including Ψ, total yeast tRNA and tRNA^{Pro} can inhibit Gag binding to negatively charged lipid membranes lacking PI(4, 5)P$_2$ [94]. Interestingly, tRNA^{Lys}, which was one of the most frequently bound to tRNAs by MA in cells [36], did not prevent Gag binding to liposomes [94]. As this study only tested the ability of in vitro transcribed tRNAs in regulating Gag membrane binding, it remains to be seen whether tRNAs containing the complete set of post-transcriptional modifications exhibit differences in MA binding in vitro.

In addition to regulation of Gag membrane binding, MA-tRNA interactions could have other functions. An obvious possibility is regulation of viral and/or host translation. As a result of the unusually A-rich nature of the HIV-1 genome [95–97], Ile, Lys, Glu and Val codons are overrepresented in the Gag and Pol ORFs [98]. Notably, tRNA^{Lys}, tRNA^{Glu} and tRNA^{Val} were found to be amongst the most frequently bound by MA, suggesting the possibility of MA enhancing the translation of Gag and Pol by sequestering these specific set of tRNAs. Alternatively, it is conceivable that by sequestering tRNAs, MA could inhibit translation of host mRNAs whose products may block viral replication. Indeed, one report has suggested that interaction of MA with host translation elongation factors via a tRNA bridge could inhibit in vitro translation [84]. It remains to be determined whether MA-tRNA interactions in a relevant infection setting can influence viral or host translation. Finally, it is possible that if not bound by tRNAs, the basic patch on MA may nonspecifically bind to the viral genome and even prevent the proper interaction of NC with the genome, which may inhibit subsequent steps of infection. In a similar scenario, MA binding to small RNAs might be a mechanism to avoid aggregation by a protein that has two distinct RNA binding domains and an intrinsic tendency to multimerize.

Role of IN-RNA interactions in particle maturation

The morphological changes that occur during HIV-1 particle maturation are often thought to be dependent only on proteolytic cleavage of Gag. The cleaved CA domain of Gag forms the conical lattice within which the viral genome condenses, along with the cleaved NC domain of Gag as well as viral enzymes integrase (IN) and reverse transcriptase (RT), cleavage products of the Pol polyprotein. However, more than two decades ago, mutational studies of the HIV-1 IN indicated that it may also play an active role in proper particle maturation [99–110]. In particular, a set of mutations referred to as Class II IN mutations, were shown to lead to the formation of morphologically aberrant "eccentric" particles, in which the viral ribonucleoproteins complexes (vRNPs) are mislocalized outside the conical CA lattice [101, 103, 111]. Although IN is known to bind DNA through several charged residues scattered throughout the protein (reviewed in [112]) and can bind to RNA in vitro with some specificity [113], why and how mutations within IN would specifically lead to mislocalization of vRNPs in virions remained enigmatic.

The recent development of allosteric integrase inhibitors (ALLINIs) reignited research in this area. While ALLINIs were initially developed to target IN binding to the cellular cofactor LEDGF, it was later shown that these compounds primarily act during particle maturation and lead to morphological aberrations in particles similar to those induced by the aforementioned Class II IN mutations [114–119]. Biochemical analysis of IN in vitro and in virions revealed that ALLINIs induce aberrant IN multimerization [103, 111, 120–123] through catalytic core domain–C-terminal domain interactions at the dimer–dimer interface [116]. By employing CLIP and complementary in vitro approaches, recent studies have shown that low-order multimers of IN binds to distinct structured elements on the viral genome, including TAR, with high affinity [13]. Notably, while ALLINIs indirectly block these interactions by inducing IN oligomerization, mutations of basic amino acids within the C-terminal domain of IN can abolish IN-RNA binding directly without altering the multimeric state of IN. Inhibition of IN-RNA interactions leads to mislocalization vRNPs and IN outside the conical capsid core [124]. Surprisingly, CLIP experiments reveal that the pattern of NC binding on the vRNA genome seems to be unaffected by IN mutations or ALLINIs, despite the mislocalization of vRNPs in eccentric particles [124]. Together, these aberrations in virion morphology are accompanied by premature degradation of vRNPs and IN, and spatial separation of RT from vRNPs, explaining the early reverse transcription block of these particles in target cells [124]. Thus, CLIP has been key in unveiling the key role of IN-RNA interactions during virion morphogenesis that ensure the correct localization of core components inside the CA lattice during particle maturation.

Incorporation of APOBEC3 proteins into virions

While viral RNAs contain sequence and structural elements that regulate key steps in HIV-1 replication, they can also be recognized by host defense mechanisms. Infiltration of the host APOBEC3 (A3) proteins into virus particles by binding viral RNAs is a prime example of this process. A3 proteins are a family of cytidine deaminases that inhibit the replication of a broad range of viruses and retroelements (reviewed in [125, 126]). A3s inhibit replication in two ways. One mechanism involves the deamination of cytidines to uridines in (–) strand DNA during reverse transcription, resulting in the accumulation dG-to-dA mutations on the coding strand [127–130] and lethal hypermutation. Additionally, A3 proteins have been shown to induce a deamination-independent block, by binding to reverse transcriptase and inhibiting reverse transcription [131–135]. Packaging of A3 proteins into HIV-1 virions is required for their antiviral activity and depends on the NC domain of Gag and its associated RNA [136–141]. A3 proteins appear to be promiscuous RNA binding proteins and it has been difficult to determine whether they selectively target viral or cellular RNAs to infiltrate into particles. For example, there is evidence to indicate that viral genome [142], 7SL RNA, a cellular RNA that is normally part of the signal recognition particle and is enriched in retroviral particles [143], or both cellular and viral RNAs [140, 141] can mediate packaging of A3G into particles. As many of these studies largely relied only on genetic assays, whether A3 proteins exhibit any preference towards a specific set of RNAs, or sequence features within them in a relevant setting remained unknown. Nevertheless, the presence of a discrete RNA binding domain in A3G implies some level of selectivity in RNA binding, much like other RBPs [144, 145].

Three recent studies employing CLIP have provided insight into the RNA-binding properties of several A3 proteins in infected cells and in virions [146, 147]. The earlier iCLIP-based study indicated that although the viral genome is enriched amongst A3F and A3G-bound RNAs, a diverse set of RNAs could drive the incorporation of A3F and A3G into virions [146]. A subsequent PAR-CLIP-based study confirmed some of these findings in that A3 proteins were shown to bind similar classes of cellular RNAs and HIV-1 RNA was bound preferentially over cellular RNAs in infected cells. However, the PAR-CLIP approach provided a higher resolution assessment of A3-RNA interactions in cells, likely due to the ability to more accurately identify the site of crosslinking. Most importantly, detailed analysis of A3 binding sites revealed that the A3 proteins partly mimic the RNA-binding specificity of NC, in that they target RNA sequences that are G-rich and A-rich [147]. This model provides some explanation of how A3 proteins are incorporated efficiently into virions in the presence of a vast excess of cellular RNA molecules. This model invokes a bias in the binding of A3 proteins to RNA molecules of a given sequence composition, as a way of maintaining broad RNA binding specificity, while removing the need to occupy all mRNA sequences present in an infected cell. One recent study, the first to reveal a crystal structure of an A3 protein in complex with an RNA showed that the A3H protein has a particular propensity to bind to seven-nucleotide duplexes, in a manner that was independent of the nucleotide sequences forming the duplexes [148]. Accompanying CLIP experiments showed that the sites in the HIV-1 genome to which A3H was most frequently bound were invariably predicted to contain 7nt duplexes.

Role of zinc finger antiviral protein (ZAP) in imposing compositional bias on viral genomes

The genomes of vertebrates are marked with a paucity of CG dinucleotides [149], a feature that is well understood to have been caused by the action of CG-specific DNA methyl transferases and methyl-cytosine deamination, over hundreds of millions of years. More mysteriously, inspection of the composition of the genomes of RNA viruses in vertebrates, reveal that they mimic this CG-poor state, even though they are not substrates for DNA methyl transferases [150–152]. Recent work, in the context of HIV-1 has shown that the paucity of CG dinucleotides is essential for viral replication, and that the appearance of too many CG dinucleotides in the viral genome causes cytoplasmic depletion of viral RNA [153]. The apparently destabilizing effect of CG dinucleotides

was cumulative, and found to be induced by CG dinucleotides in both translated portions of an mRNA and also in untranslated exons. Further experiments showed that zinc finger antiviral protein (ZAP) [154] a protein that encodes four CCCH zinc fingers in is N-terminal domain is essential the for mediating the deleterious effects of CG dinucleotides. Indeed, HIV-1 mutants containing segments whose CG-content mimicked a random nucleotide sequence could not replicate in unmanipulated cells containing an intact ZAP gene, but could replicate with wild-type kinetics in cells rendered ZAP-deficient by CRISPR-Cas9 editing [153].

While previous studies had shown that ZAP had antiviral activity against a number of RNA viruses, several conventional techniques could not identify a common sequence motif or RNA feature that could explain how ZAP was able to specifically target viral RNA sequences [154, 155]. RNA elements that could confer sensitivity to ZAP when inserted into a reporter RNA were large, leading to the proposal that a specific tertiary structure constituted a ZAP recognition site. However, RNA elements that conferred sensitivity to ZAP did so in both orientations [156], effectively refuting these models. CLIP experiments showed unambiguously that ZAP binds directly and selectively to RNA elements that contain CG dinucleotides, but exhibits no preferential binding to RNA elements containing GC or any other dinucleotide [153]. Interestingly, these results suggest that ZAP arose to exploit a compositional difference between host mRNAs and RNAs from viruses have high CG content. However, the dinucleotide composition of HIV-1, appears to have adapted to evade ZAP and it is possible that ZAP has driven the purging of CG dinucleotides from a range of RNA viruses.

Identification of m⁶A marks on HIV-1 RNAs

Like proteins and DNA, RNA can undergo a number of chemical modifications that subsequently affect its metabolism, function and localization. While tRNAs and rRNAs are subjected to the most diverse set of modifications, recent transcriptome-wide studies revealed the presence of numerous mRNAs modifications [157–162]. Methylation of adenosine at the N6 position (m^6A) is the most prevalent of these and has been proposed to regulate several aspects of RNA metabolism, including splicing, nuclear export, localization, stability and translation [163]. m^6A modification is catalyzed by a nuclear "writer" protein complex, composed of two methyltransferase-like enzymes, METTL3 and MTTL4, and their cofactor Wilms tumor 1-associated protein (WTAP). This modification can be reversed by two RNA demethylases, or "erasers", ALKBH5 (a-ketoglutamarate-dependent dioxygenase homolog 5) and FTO (fat mass and obesity associated). m^{6}A-modifications on mRNAs can be bound by three related cytosolic "reader" proteins called YTH-domain containing family 1 (YTHDF1), YTHDF2, and YTHDF3. Exactly how binding of these proteins on modified nucleotides regulate mRNA metabolism is currently unknown. Nonetheless, m^{6}A modifications can be found on mRNAs of diverse viruses that replicate in the nucleus, including SV40 [164], adenovirus [165, 166], influenza A virus [167] as well as retroviruses such as avian sarcoma virus [168] and Rous sarcoma virus [169, 170]. Until recently, whether HIV-1 mRNAs contained m^{6}A modifications and how this affected virus replication was not known.

Three recent studies have addressed this question by immunoprecipitating methylated HIV-1 RNAs from infected cells using a m^{6}A-specific antibody followed by high throughput sequencing of the immunoprecipitated mRNAs [171–173]. Strikingly, there was virtually no overlap in the m^{6}A sites identified in these independent studies. This lack of consistency can in part be explained by the different approaches taken. The first published study that has utilized a RIP-seq approach, in which m^{6}A-modified RNAs were immunoprecipitated from cell lysates and sequenced, found m^{6}A modifications throughout the viral genome [172]. In contrast, a later study, which included a PAR-CLIP-based crosslinking step following immunoprecipitation of m^{6}A-modified RNAs, found that the m^{6}A modifications were exclusively localized within the viral 3′ UTRs [171]. Importantly, parallel YTHDF PAR-CLIP experiments conducted in this latter study revealed binding sites at or near the modified nucleotides, reinforcing the findings from m^{6}A-specific immunoprecipitations [171]. A third study similarly coupled YTHDF HITS-CLIP with m^{6}A-seq [173] and identified putative modification sites within 3′ and 5′ UTRs of HIV-1 mRNAs. Notably, none of these sites overlapped with those identified in the former studies. Thus, while CLIP methodologies have been highly instrumental in identification of m^{6}A sites on HIV-1 RNAs, cross-validation of reagents (i.e. cell lines, viruses, m^{6}A antibodies) and methods (i.e. m^{6}A-seq, PAR- vs. HITS-CLIP) will be necessary to reach to a consensus in future studies.

Conclusions

Application of the CLIP methods to questions in retrovirology will undoubtedly continue to increase, given the large number of RBPs that are known and continuing to emerge as key regulators of retroviral replication. Several poorly explored areas in retrovirology will benefit from these approaches. One of the immediate applications of this methodology will be in determining how the alternative splicing of HIV-1 transcripts is regulated by cellular hnRNP and SR splicing-regulatory proteins. Although

the families of hnRNP and SR proteins constitute more than 50 proteins, only a few have been shown to play roles in HIV-1 RNA splicing. In addition, none of the studies performed to date determined where on viral RNAs these proteins bind. Instead, in vitro splicing reporters and genetic assays were used, which are prone to artefacts. Another exciting area of research where CLIP and related methodologies may make a major impact is the sensing of viral nucleic acids in infected cells. HIV-1 infection induces high levels of interferon and other cytokines during the acute phase of infection, suggesting that viral nucleic acids are sensed in infected cells. While a few isolated studies indicated that viral reverse transcription products or RNA elements can be sensed in certain settings, it remains to be determined what features of viral nucleic acids are sensed and whether viral RNA or DNA elicits an inflammatory response. While A3 proteins provide a good example of how viral RNAs can be targeted by antiviral host proteins, it is plausible that many other cellular proteins that can recognize and target viral RNAs. CLIP will be a key tool in unveiling novel cellular proteins that participate at the HIV-1-host interface. Finally, although CLIP has so far only been applied to HIV-1 biology, it will certainly find broad applications in retrovirology and virology more generally as the methods and next-generation sequencing becomes more accessible.

Authors' contributions
Both authors read and approved the final manuscript.

Author details
[1] Howard Hughes Medical Institute and Laboratory of Retrovirology, The Rockefeller University, New York, NY 10065, USA. [2] Department of Molecular Microbiology, Washington University School of Medicine, Saint Louis, MO 63110, USA.

Acknowledgements
Not applicable.

Competing interests
The authors declare they have no competing interests.

Funding
Funding was provided by National Institute of General Medical Sciences (Grant Nos. U54 GM-103297, GM-122458) and National Institute of Allergy and Infectious Diseases (Grant No. AI-50111).

References
1. Karn J, Stoltzfus CM. Transcriptional and posttranscriptional regulation of HIV-1 gene expression. Cold Spring Harb Perspect Med. 2012;2:a006916.
2. Stoltzfus CM. Chapter 1. Regulation of HIV-1 alternative RNA splicing and its role in virus replication. Adv Virus Res. 2009;74:1–40.
3. Leblanc J, Weil J, Beemon K. Posttranscriptional regulation of retroviral gene expression: primary RNA transcripts play three roles as pre-mRNA, mRNA, and genomic RNA. Wiley Interdiscip Rev RNA. 2013;4:567–80.

4. Cullen BR. Nuclear mRNA export: insights from virology. Trends Biochem Sci. 2003;28:419–24.

5. Briggs JA, Krausslich HG. The molecular architecture of HIV. J Mol Biol. 2011;410:491–500.

6. Sundquist WI, Krausslich HG. HIV-1 assembly, budding, and maturation. Cold Spring Harb Perspect Med. 2012;2:a006924.

7. Ule J, Jensen KB, Ruggiu M, Mele A, Ule A, Darnell RB. CLIP identifies Nova-regulated RNA networks in the brain. Science. 2003;302:1212–5.

8. Ule J, Jensen K, Mele A, Darnell RB. CLIP: a method for identifying protein-RNA interaction sites in living cells. Methods. 2005;37:376–86.

9. Licatalosi DD, Mele A, Fak JJ, Ule J, Kayikci M, Chi SW, Clark TA, Schweitzer AC, Blume JE, Wang X, Darnell JC, Darnell RB. HITS-CLIP yields genome-wide insights into brain alternative RNA processing. Nature. 2008;456:464–9.

10. Zhang C, Darnell RB. Mapping in vivo protein-RNA interactions at single-nucleotide resolution from HITS-CLIP data. Nat Biotechnol. 2011;29:607–14.

11. Hafner M, Landthaler M, Burger L, Khorshid M, Hausser J, Berninger P, Rothballer A, Ascano M Jr, Jungkamp AC, Munschauer M, Ulrich A, Wardle GS, Dewell S, Zavolan M, Tuschl T. Transcriptome-wide identification of RNA-binding protein and microRNA target sites by PAR-CLIP. Cell. 2010;141:129–41.

12. Jungkamp AC, Stoeckius M, Mecenas D, Grun D, Mastrobuoni G, Kempa S, Rajewsky N. In vivo and transcriptome-wide identification of RNA binding protein target sites. Mol Cell. 2011;44:828–40.

13. Kessl JJ, Kutluay SB, Townsend D, Rebensburg S, Slaughter A, Larue RC, Shkriabai N, Bakouche N, Fuchs JR, Bieniasz PD, Kvaratskhelia M. HIV-1 integrase binds the viral RNA genome and is essential during virion morphogenesis. Cell. 2016;166:1257–68.

14. Kutluay SB, Bieniasz PD. Analysis of HIV-1 Gag-RNA interactions in cells and virions by CLIP-seq. Methods Mol Biol. 2016;1354:119–31.

15. Gottwein E, Corcoran DL, Mukherjee N, Skalsky RL, Hafner M, Nusbaum JD, Shamulailatpam P, Love CL, Dave SS, Tuschl T, Ohler U, Cullen BR. Viral microRNA targetome of KSHV-infected primary effusion lymphoma cell lines. Cell Host Microbe. 2011;10:515–26.

16. Hafner M, Lianoglou S, Tuschl T, Betel D. Genome-wide identification of miRNA targets by PAR-CLIP. Methods. 2012;58:94–105.

17. Jaskiewicz L, Bilen B, Hausser J, Zavolan M. Argonaute CLIP—a method to identify in vivo targets of miRNAs. Methods. 2012;58:106–12.

18. Kishore S, Jaskiewicz L, Burger L, Hausser J, Khorshid M, Zavolan M. A quantitative analysis of CLIP methods for identifying binding sites of RNA-binding proteins. Nat Methods. 2011;8:559–64.

19. Chang X, Li B, Rao A. RNA-binding protein hnRNPLL regulates mRNA splicing and stability during B-cell to plasma-cell differentiation. Proc Natl Acad Sci USA. 2015;112:E1888–97.

20. Degrauwe N, Schlumpf TB, Janiszewska M, Martin P, Cauderay A, Provero P, Riggi N, Suva ML, Paro R, Stamenkovic I. The RNA binding protein IMP2 preserves glioblastoma stem cells by preventing let-7 target gene silencing. Cell Rep. 2016;15:1634–47.

21. Kim KK, Yang Y, Zhu J, Adelstein RS, Kawamoto S. Rbfox3 controls the biogenesis of a subset of microRNAs. Nat Struct Mol Biol. 2014;21:901–10.

22. Schonemann L, Kuhn U, Martin G, Schafer P, Gruber AR, Keller W, Zavolan M, Wahle E. Reconstitution of CPSF active in polyadenylation: recognition of the polyadenylation signal by WDR33. Genes Dev. 2014;28:2381–93.

23. Uemura Y, Oshima T, Yamamoto M, Reyes CJ, Costa Cruz PH, Shibuya T, Kawahara Y. Matrin3 binds directly to intronic pyrimidine-rich sequences and controls alternative splicing. Genes Cells. 2017. https://doi.org/10.1111/gtc.12512.

24. Lee AS, Kranzusch PJ, Cate JH. eIF3 targets cell-proliferation messenger RNAs for translational activation or repression. Nature. 2015;522:111–4.

25. Burger K, Muhl B, Kellner M, Rohrmoser M, Gruber-Eber A, Windhager L, Friedel CC, Dolken L, Eick D. 4-thiouridine inhibits rRNA synthesis and causes a nucleolar stress response. RNA Biol. 2013;10:1623–30.

26. Testa SM, Disney MD, Turner DH, Kierzek R. Thermodynamics of RNA-RNA duplexes with 2- or 4-thiouridines: implications for antisense design and targeting a group I intron. Biochemistry. 1999;38:16655–62.

27. Urlaub H, Hartmuth K, Luhrmann R. A two-tracked approach to analyze RNA-protein crosslinking sites in native, nonlabeled small nuclear ribonucleoprotein particles. Methods. 2002;26:170–81.

28. Sugimoto Y, Konig J, Hussain S, Zupan B, Curk T, Frye M, Ule J. Analysis of CLIP and iCLIP methods for nucleotide-resolution studies of protein-RNA interactions. Genome Biol. 2012;13:R67.

29. Konig J, Zarnack K, Rot G, Curk T, Kayikci M, Zupan B, Turner DJ, Luscombe NM, Ule J. iCLIP reveals the function of hnRNP particles in splicing at individual nucleotide resolution. Nat Struct Mol Biol. 2010;17:909–15.

30. Haberman N, Huppertz I, Attig J, Konig J, Wang Z, Hauer C, Hentze MW, Kulozik AE, Le Hir H, Curk T, Sibley CR, Zarnack K, Ule J. Insights into the design and interpretation of iCLIP experiments. Genome Biol. 2017;18:7.

31. Van Nostrand EL, Pratt GA, Shishkin AA, Gelboin-Burkhart C, Fang MY, Sundararaman B, Blue SM, Nguyen TB, Surka C, Elkins K, Stanton R, Rigo F, Guttman M, Yeo GW. Robust transcriptome-wide discovery of RNA-binding protein binding sites with enhanced CLIP (eCLIP). Nat Methods. 2016;13:508–14.

32. Weyn-Vanhentenryck SM, Mele A, Yan Q, Sun S, Farny N, Zhang Z, Xue C, Herre M, Silver PA, Zhang MQ, Krainer AR, Darnell RB, Zhang C. HITS-CLIP and integrative modeling define the Rbfox splicing-regulatory network linked to brain development and autism. Cell Rep. 2014;6:1139–52.

33. Flynn RA, Martin L, Spitale RC, Do BT, Sagan SM, Zarnegar B, Qu K, Khavari PA, Quake SR, Sarnow P, Chang HY. Dissecting noncoding and pathogen RNA-protein interactomes. RNA. 2015;21:135–43.

34. Lee FCY, Ule J. Advances in CLIP technologies for studies of protein–RNA interactions. Mol Cell. 2018;69:354–69.

35. Zarnegar BJ, Flynn RA, Shen Y, Do BT, Chang HY, Khavari PA. irCLIP platform for efficient characterization of protein–RNA interactions. Nat Methods. 2016;13:489–92.

36. Kutluay SB, Zang T, Blanco-Melo D, Powell C, Jannain D, Errando M, Bieniasz PD. Global changes in the RNA binding specificity of HIV-1 gag regulate virion genesis. Cell. 2014;159:1096–109.

37. Garzia A, Meyer C, Morozov P, Sajek M, Tuschl T. Optimization of PAR-CLIP for transcriptome-wide identification of binding sites of RNA-binding proteins. Methods. 2017;118–119:24–40.

38. Khorshid M, Rodak C, Zavolan M. CLIPZ: a database and analysis environment for experimentally determined binding sites of RNA-binding proteins. Nucleic Acids Res. 2011;39:D245–52.

39. Moore MJ, Zhang C, Gantman EC, Mele A, Darnell JC, Darnell RB. Mapping Argonaute and conventional RNA-binding protein interactions with RNA at single-nucleotide resolution using HITS-CLIP and CIMS analysis. Nat Protoc. 2014;9:263–93.

40. Maragkakis M, Alexiou P, Nakaya T, Mourelatos Z. CLIPSeqTools–a novel bioinformatics CLIP-seq analysis suite. RNA. 2016;22:1–9.

41. Bottini S, Pratella D, Grandjean V, Repetto E, Trabucchi M. Recent computational developments on CLIP-seq data analysis and microRNA targeting implications. Brief Bioinform. 2017. https://doi.org/10.1093/bib/bbx063.

42. Uhl M, Houwaart T, Corrado G, Wright PR, Backofen R. Computational analysis of CLIP-seq data. Methods. 2017;118–119:60–72.

43. Liu Q, Zhong X, Madison BB, Rustgi AK, Shyr Y. Assessing computational steps for CLIP-Seq data analysis. Biomed Res Int. 2015;2015:196082.

44. Reyes-Herrera PH, Ficarra E. Computational methods for CLIP-seq data processing. Bioinform Biol Insights. 2014;8:199–207.

45. Chen C, Khaleel SS, Huang H, Wu CH. Software for pre-processing Illumina next-generation sequencing short read sequences. Source Code Biol Med. 2014;9:8.

46. Bolger AM, Lohse M, Usadel B. Trimmomatic: a flexible trimmer for Illumina sequence data. Bioinformatics. 2014;30:2114–20.

47. Schmieder R, Edwards R. Quality control and preprocessing of metagenomic datasets. Bioinformatics. 2011;27:863–4.

48. Langmead B, Trapnell C, Pop M, Salzberg SL. Ultrafast and memory-efficient alignment of short DNA sequences to the human genome. Genome Biol. 2009;10:R25.

49. Langmead B, Salzberg SL. Fast gapped-read alignment with Bowtie 2. Nat Methods. 2012;9:357–9.

50. Dobin A, Davis CA, Schlesinger F, Drenkow J, Zaleski C, Jha S, Batut P, Chaisson M, Gingeras TR. STAR: ultrafast universal RNA-seq aligner. Bioinformatics. 2013;29:15–21.

51. Smith AD, Chung WY, Hodges E, Kendall J, Hannon G, Hicks J, Xuan Z, Zhang MQ. Updates to the RMAP short-read mapping software. Bioinformatics. 2009;25:2841–2.

52. Trapnell C, Pachter L, Salzberg SL. TopHat: discovering splice junctions with RNA-Seq. Bioinformatics. 2009;25:1105–11.

53. Wu TD, Nacu S. Fast and SNP-tolerant detection of complex variants and splicing in short reads. Bioinformatics. 2010;26:873–81.

54. Li R, Li Y, Kristiansen K, Wang J. SOAP: short oligonucleotide alignment program. Bioinformatics. 2008;24:713–4.

55. Li H, Durbin R. Fast and accurate short read alignment with Burrows–Wheeler transform. Bioinformatics. 2009;25:1754–60.

56. Uren PJ, Bahrami-Samani E, Burns SC, Qiao M, Karginov FV, Hodges E, Hannon GJ, Sanford JR, Penalva LO, Smith AD. Site identification in high-throughput RNA-protein interaction data. Bioinformatics. 2012;28:3013–20.

57. Lovci MT, Ghanem D, Marr H, Arnold J, Gee S, Parra M, Liang TY, Stark TJ, Gehman LT, Hoon S, Massirer KB, Pratt GA, Black DL, Gray JW, Conboy JG, Yeo GW. Rbfox proteins regulate alternative mRNA splicing through evolutionarily conserved RNA bridges. Nat Struct Mol Biol. 2013;20:1434–42.

58. Chen B, Yun J, Kim MS, Mendell JT, Xie Y. PIPE-CLIP: a comprehensive online tool for CLIP-seq data analysis. Genome Biol. 2014;15:R18.

59. Althammer S, Gonzalez-Vallinas J, Ballare C, Beato M, Eyras E. Pyicos: a versatile toolkit for the analysis of high-throughput sequencing data. Bioinformatics. 2011;27:3333–40.

60. Corcoran DL, Georgiev S, Mukherjee N, Gottwein E, Skalsky RL, Keene JD, Ohler U. PARalyzer: definition of RNA binding sites from PAR-CLIP short-read sequence data. Genome Biol. 2011;12:R79.

61. Bailey TL, Boden M, Buske FA, Frith M, Grant CE, Clementi L, Ren J, Li WW, Noble WS. MEME SUITE: tools for motif discovery and searching. Nucleic Acids Res. 2009;37:W202–8.

62. Heinz S, Benner C, Spann N, Bertolino E, Lin YC, Laslo P, Cheng JX, Murre C, Singh H, Glass CK. Simple combinations of lineage-determining transcription factors prime cis-regulatory elements required for macrophage and B cell identities. Mol Cell. 2010;38:576–89.

63. Georgiev S, Boyle AP, Jayasurya K, Ding X, Mukherjee S, Ohler U. Evidence-ranked motif identification. Genome Biol. 2010;11:R19.

64. Jouvenet N, Simon SM, Bieniasz PD. Imaging the interaction of HIV-1 genomes and Gag during assembly of individual viral particles. Proc Natl Acad Sci USA. 2009;106:19114–9.

65. Kutluay SB, Bieniasz PD. Analysis of the initiating events in HIV-1 particle assembly and genome packaging. PLoS Pathog. 2010;6:e1001200.

66. Clever JL, Parslow TG. Mutant human immunodeficiency virus type 1 genomes with defects in RNA dimerization or encapsidation. J Virol. 1997;71:3407–14.

67. Laham-Karam N, Bacharach E. Transduction of human immunodeficiency virus type 1 vectors lacking encapsidation and dimerization signals. J Virol. 2007;81:10687–98.

68. McBride MS, Panganiban AT. Position dependence of functional hairpins important for human immunodeficiency virus type 1 RNA encapsidation in vivo. J Virol. 1997;71:2050–8.

69. Berkowitz RD, Hammarskjold ML, Helga-Maria C, Rekosh D, Goff SP. 5′ regions of HIV-1 RNAs are not sufficient for encapsidation: implications for the HIV-1 packaging signal. Virology. 1995;212:718–23.

70. Chamanian M, Purzycka KJ, Wille PT, Ha JS, McDonald D, Gao Y, Le Grice SF, Arts EJ. A cis-acting element in retroviral genomic RNA links Gag-Pol ribosomal frameshifting to selective viral RNA encapsidation. Cell Host Microbe. 2013;13:181–92.

71. Das AT, Klaver B, Klasens BI, van Wamel JL, Berkhout B. A conserved hairpin motif in the R-U5 region of the human immunodeficiency virus type 1 RNA genome is essential for replication. J Virol. 1997;71:2346–56.

72. McBride MS, Schwartz MD, Panganiban AT. Efficient encapsidation of human immunodeficiency virus type 1 vectors and further characterization of cis elements required for encapsidation. J Virol. 1997;71:4544–54.

73. Richardson JH, Child LA, Lever AM. Packaging of human immunodeficiency virus type 1 RNA requires cis-acting sequences outside the 5′ leader region. J Virol. 1993;67:3997–4005.

74. Muriaux D, Mirro J, Harvin D, Rein A. RNA is a structural element in retrovirus particles. Proc Natl Acad Sci USA. 2001;98:5246–51.

75. Rulli SJ Jr, Hibbert CS, Mirro J, Pederson T, Biswal S, Rein A. Selective and nonselective packaging of cellular RNAs in retrovirus particles. J Virol. 2007;81:6623–31.

76. Keane SC, Heng X, Lu K, Kharytonchyk S, Ramakrishnan V, Carter G, Barton S, Hosic A, Florwick A, Santos J, Bolden NC, McCowin S, Case DA, Johnson BA, Salemi M, Telesnitsky A, Summers MF. RNA structure. Structure of the HIV-1 RNA packaging signal. Science. 2015;348:917–21.

77. Keane SC, Van V, Frank HM, Sciandra CA, McCowin S, Santos J, Heng X, Summers MF. NMR detection of intermolecular interaction sites in the dimeric 5′-leader of the HIV-1 genome. Proc Natl Acad Sci USA. 2016;113:13033–8.

78. Lu K, Heng X, Garyu L, Monti S, Garcia EL, Kharytonchyk S, Dorjsuren B, Kulandaivel G, Jones S, Hiremath A, Divakaruni SS, LaCotti C, Barton S, Tummillo D, Hosic A, Edme K, Albrecht S, Telesnitsky A, Summers MF. NMR detection of structures in the HIV-1 5′-leader RNA that regulate genome packaging. Science. 2011;334:242–5.

79. Becker JT, Sherer NM. Subcellular localization of HIV-1 gag-pol mRNAs regulates sites of virion assembly. J Virol. 2017;91:e02315–6.

80. Liu Y, Nikolaitchik OA, Rahman SA, Chen J, Pathak VK, Hu WS. HIV-1 sequence necessary and sufficient to package non-viral RNAs into HIV-1 particles. J Mol Biol. 2017. https://doi.org/10.1016/j.jmb.2017.06.018.

81. Comas-Garcia M, Datta SA, Baker L, Varma R, Gudla PR, Rein A. Dissection of specific binding of HIV-1 Gag to the 'packaging signal' in viral RNA. Elife. 2017. https://doi.org/10.7554/eLife.27055.

82. Alfadhli A, Still A, Barklis E. Analysis of human immunodeficiency virus type 1 matrix binding to membranes and nucleic acids. J Virol. 2009;83:12196–203.

83. Chukkapalli V, Oh SJ, Ono A. Opposing mechanisms involving RNA and lipids regulate HIV-1 Gag membrane binding through the highly basic region of the matrix domain. Proc Natl Acad Sci USA. 2010;107:1600–5.

84. Cimarelli A, Luban J. Translation elongation factor 1-alpha interacts specifically with the human immunodeficiency virus type 1 Gag polyprotein. J Virol. 1999;73:5388–401.

85. Levin JG, Mitra M, Mascarenhas A, Musier-Forsyth K. Role of HIV-1 nucleocapsid protein in HIV-1 reverse transcription. RNA Biol. 2010;7:754–74.

86. Ramalingam D, Duclair S, Datta SA, Ellington A, Rein A, Prasad VR. RNA aptamers directed to human immunodeficiency virus type 1 Gag polyprotein bind to the matrix and nucleocapsid domains and inhibit virus production. J Virol. 2011;85:305–14.

87. Ott DE, Coren LV, Gagliardi TD. Redundant roles for nucleocapsid and matrix RNA-binding sequences in human immunodeficiency virus type 1 assembly. J Virol. 2005;79:13839–47.

88. Chukkapalli V, Inlora J, Todd GC, Ono A. Evidence in support of RNA-mediated inhibition of phosphatidylserine-dependent HIV-1 Gag membrane binding in cells. J Virol. 2013;87:7155–9.

89. Hill CP, Worthylake D, Bancroft DP, Christensen AM, Sundquist WI. Crystal structures of the trimeric human immunodeficiency virus type 1 matrix protein: implications for membrane association and assembly. Proc Natl Acad Sci USA. 1996;93:3099–104.

90. Saad JS, Miller J, Tai J, Kim A, Ghanam RH, Summers MF. Structural basis for targeting HIV-1 Gag proteins to the plasma membrane for virus assembly. Proc Natl Acad Sci USA. 2006;103:11364–9.

91. Shkriabai N, Datta SA, Zhao Z, Hess S, Rein A, Kvaratskhelia M. Interactions of HIV-1 Gag with assembly cofactors. Biochemistry. 2006;45:4077–83.

92. Zhou W, Parent LJ, Wills JW, Resh MD. Identification of a membrane-binding domain within the amino-terminal region of human immunodeficiency virus type 1 Gag protein which interacts with acidic phospholipids. J Virol. 1994;68:2556–69.

93. Holmes M, Zhang F, Bieniasz PD. Single-cell and single-cycle analysis of HIV-1 Replication. PLoS Pathog. 2015;11:e1004961.

94. Todd GC, Duchon A, Inlora J, Olson ED, Musier-Forsyth K, Ono A. Inhibition of HIV-1 Gag-membrane interactions by specific RNAs. RNA. 2017;23:395–405.

95. Kypr J, Mrazek J. Unusual codon usage of HIV. Nature. 1987;327:20.

96. Grantham P, Perrin P. AIDS virus and HTLV-I differ in codon choices. Nature. 1986;319:727–8.

97. Sharp PM. What can AIDS virus codon usage tell us? Nature. 1986;324:114.

98. Berkhout B, van Hemert FJ. The unusual nucleotide content of the HIV RNA genome results in a biased amino acid composition of HIV proteins. Nucleic Acids Res. 1994;22:1705–11.

99. Bukovsky A, Gottlinger H. Lack of integrase can markedly affect human immunodeficiency virus type 1 particle production in the presence of an active viral protease. J Virol. 1996;70:6820–5.

100. Engelman A. In vivo analysis of retroviral integrase structure and function. Adv Virus Res. 1999;52:411–26.

101. Engelman A, Englund G, Orenstein JM, Martin MA, Craigie R. Multiple effects of mutations in human immunodeficiency virus type 1 integrase on viral replication. J Virol. 1995;69:2729–36.

102. Johnson BC, Metifiot M, Ferris A, Pommier Y, Hughes SH. A homology model of HIV-1 integrase and analysis of mutations designed to test the model. J Mol Biol. 2013;425:2133–46.

103. Jurado KA, Wang H, Slaughter A, Feng L, Kessl JJ, Koh Y, Wang W, Ballandras-Colas A, Patel PA, Fuchs JR, Kvaratskhelia M, Engelman A. Allosteric integrase inhibitor potency is determined through the inhibition of HIV-1 particle maturation. Proc Natl Acad Sci USA. 2013;110:8690–5.

104. Mohammed KD, Topper MB, Muesing MA. Sequential deletion of the integrase (Gag-Pol) carboxyl terminus reveals distinct phenotypic classes of defective HIV-1. J Virol. 2011;85:4654–66.

105. Lu R, Limon A, Devroe E, Silver PA, Cherepanov P, Engelman A. Class II integrase mutants with changes in putative nuclear localization signals are primarily blocked at a postnuclear entry step of human immunodeficiency virus type 1 replication. J Virol. 2004;78:12735–46.

106. Lu R, Ghory HZ, Engelman A. Genetic analyses of conserved residues in the carboxyl-terminal domain of human immunodeficiency virus type 1 integrase. J Virol. 2005;79:10356–68.

107. Limon A, Devroe E, Lu R, Ghory HZ, Silver PA, Engelman A. Nuclear localization of human immunodeficiency virus type 1 preintegration complexes (PICs): V165A and R166A are pleiotropic integrase mutants primarily defective for integration, not PIC nuclear import. J Virol. 2002;76:10598–607.

108. Leavitt AD, Robles G, Alesandro N, Varmus HE. Human immunodeficiency virus type 1 integrase mutants retain in vitro integrase activity yet fail to integrate viral DNA efficiently during infection. J Virol. 1996;70:721–8.

109. Jenkins TM, Engelman A, Ghirlando R, Craigie R. A soluble active mutant of HIV-1 integrase: involvement of both the core and carboxyl-terminal domains in multimerization. J Biol Chem. 1996;271:7712–8.

110. Shehu-Xhilaga M, Hill M, Marshall JA, Kappes J, Crowe SM, Mak J. The conformation of the mature dimeric human immunodeficiency virus type 1 RNA genome requires packaging of pol protein. J Virol. 2002;76:4331–40.

111. Fontana J, Jurado KA, Cheng N, Ly NL, Fuchs JR, Gorelick RJ, Engelman AN, Steven AC. Distribution and redistribution of HIV-1 nucleocapsid protein in immature, mature, and integrase-inhibited virions: a role for integrase in maturation. J Virol. 2015. https://doi.org/10.1128/JVI.01522-15.

112. Engelman A, Cherepanov P. Retroviral integrase structure and DNA recombination mechanism. Microbiol Spectr. 2014;2:1–22.

113. Allen P, Worland S, Gold L. Isolation of high-affinity RNA ligands to HIV-1 integrase from a random pool. Virology. 1995;209:327–36.

114. Christ F, Voet A, Marchand A, Nicolet S, Desimmie BA, Marchand D, Bardiot D, Van der Veken NJ, Van Remoortel B, Strelkov SV, De Maeyer M, Chaltin P, Debyser Z. Rational design of small-molecule inhibitors of the LEDGF/p75-integrase interaction and HIV replication. Nat Chem Biol. 2010;6:442–8.

115. Fader LD, Malenfant E, Parisien M, Carson R, Bilodeau F, Landry S, Pesant M, Brochu C, Morin S, Chabot C, Halmos T, Bousquet Y, Bailey MD, Kawai SH, Coulombe R, LaPlante S, Jakalian A, Bhardwaj PK, Wernic

D, Schroeder P, Amad M, Edwards P, Garneau M, Duan J, Cordingley M, Bethell R, Mason SW, Bos M, Bonneau P, Poupart MA, Faucher AM, Simoneau B, Fenwick C, Yoakim C, Tsantrizos Y. Discovery of BI 224436, a noncatalytic site integrase inhibitor (NCINI) of HIV-1. ACS Med Chem Lett. 2014;5:422–7.

116. Gupta K, Brady T, Dyer BM, Malani N, Hwang Y, Male F, Nolte RT, Wang L, Velthuisen E, Jeffrey J, Van Duyne GD, Bushman FD. Allosteric inhibition of human immunodeficiency virus integrase: late block during viral replication and abnormal multimerization involving specific protein domains. J Biol Chem. 2014;289:20477–88.

117. Kessl JJ, Jena N, Koh Y, Taskent-Sezgin H, Slaughter A, Feng L, de Silva S, Wu L, Le Grice SF, Engelman A, Fuchs JR, Kvaratskhelia M. Multimode, cooperative mechanism of action of allosteric HIV-1 integrase inhibitors. J Biol Chem. 2012;287:16801–11.

118. Le Rouzic E, Bonnard D, Chasset S, Bruneau JM, Chevreuil F, Le Strat F, Nguyen J, Beauvoir R, Amadori C, Brias J, Vomscheid S, Eiler S, Levy N, Delelis O, Deprez E, Saib A, Zamborlini A, Emiliani S, Ruff M, Ledoussal B, Moreau F, Benarous R. Dual inhibition of HIV-1 replication by integrase-LEDGF allosteric inhibitors is predominant at the post-integration stage. Retrovirology. 2013;10:144.

119. van Bel N, van der Velden Y, Bonnard D, Le Rouzic E, Das AT, Benarous R, Berkhout B. The allosteric HIV-1 integrase inhibitor BI-D affects virion maturation but does not influence packaging of a functional RNA genome. PLoS ONE. 2014;9:e103552.

120. Balakrishnan M, Yant SR, Tsai L, O'Sullivan C, Bam RA, Tsai A, Niedziela-Majka A, Stray KM, Sakowicz R, Cihlar T. Non-catalytic site HIV-1 integrase inhibitors disrupt core maturation and induce a reverse transcription block in target cells. PLoS ONE. 2013;8:e74163.

121. Desimmie BA, Schrijvers R, Demeulemeester J, Borrenberghs D, Weydert C, Thys W, Vets S, Van Remoortel B, Hofkens J, De Rijck J, Hendrix J, Bannert N, Gijsbers R, Christ F, Debyser Z. LEDGINs inhibit late stage HIV-1 replication by modulating integrase multimerization in the virions. Retrovirology. 2013;10:57.

122. Sharma A, Slaughter A, Jena N, Feng L, Kessl JJ, Fadel HJ, Malani N, Male F, Wu L, Poeschla E, Bushman FD, Fuchs JR, Kvaratskhelia M. A new class of multimerization selective inhibitors of HIV-1 integrase. PLoS Pathog. 2014;10:e1004171.

123. Gupta K, Turkki V, Sherrill-Mix S, Hwang Y, Eilers G, Taylor L, McDanal C, Wang P, Temelkoff D, Nolte RT, Velthuisen E, Jeffrey J, Van Duyne GD, Bushman FD. Structural basis for inhibitor-induced aggregation of HIV integrase. PLoS Biol. 2016;14:e1002584.

124. Madison MK, Lawson DQ, Elliott J, Ozanturk AN, Koneru PC, Townsend D, Errando M, Kvaratskhelia M, Kutluay SB. Allosteric HIV-1 integrase inhibitors lead to premature degradation of the viral RNA genome and integrase in target cells. J Virol. 2017. https://doi.org/10.1128/JVI.00821-17.

125. Harris RS, Dudley JP. APOBECs and virus restriction. Virology. 2015;479–480:131–45.

126. Stavrou S, Ross SR. APOBEC3 proteins in viral immunity. J Immunol. 2015;195:4565–70.

127. Harris RS, Bishop KN, Sheehy AM, Craig HM, Petersen-Mahrt SK, Watt IN, Neuberger MS, Malim MH. DNA deamination mediates innate immunity to retroviral infection. Cell. 2003;113:803–9.

128. Mangeat B, Turelli P, Caron G, Friedli M, Perrin L, Trono D. Broad antiretroviral defence by human APOBEC3G through lethal editing of nascent reverse transcripts. Nature. 2003;424:99–103.

129. Zhang H, Yang B, Pomerantz RJ, Zhang C, Arunachalam SC, Gao L. The cytidine deaminase CEM15 induces hypermutation in newly synthesized HIV-1 DNA. Nature. 2003;424:94–8.

130. Lecossier D, Bouchonnet F, Clavel F, Hance AJ. Hypermutation of HIV-1 DNA in the absence of the Vif protein. Science. 2003;300:1112.

131. Holmes RK, Koning FA, Bishop KN, Malim MH. APOBEC3F can inhibit the accumulation of HIV-1 reverse transcription products in the absence of hypermutation. Comparisons with APOBEC3G. J Biol Chem. 2007;282:2587–95.

132. Iwatani Y, Chan DS, Wang F, Maynard KS, Sugiura W, Gronenborn AM, Rouzina I, Williams MC, Musier-Forsyth K, Levin JG. Deaminase-independent inhibition of HIV-1 reverse transcription by APOBEC3G. Nucleic Acids Res. 2007;35:7096–108.

133. Newman EN, Holmes RK, Craig HM, Klein KC, Lingappa JR, Malim MH, Sheehy AM. Antiviral function of APOBEC3G can be dissociated from cytidine deaminase activity. Curr Biol. 2005;15:166–70.

134. Gillick K, Pollpeter D, Phalora P, Kim EY, Wolinsky SM, Malim MH. Suppression of HIV-1 infection by APOBEC3 proteins in primary human CD4(+) T cells is associated with inhibition of processive reverse transcription as well as excessive cytidine deamination. J Virol. 2013;87:1508–17.

135. Pollpeter D, Parsons M, Sobala AE, Coxhead S, Lang RD, Bruns AM, Papaioannou S, McDonnell JM, Apolonia L, Chowdhury JA, Horvath CM, Malim MH. Deep sequencing of HIV-1 reverse transcripts reveals the multifaceted antiviral functions of APOBEC3G. Nat Microbiol. 2018;3:220–33.

136. Alce TM, Popik W. APOBEC3G is incorporated into virus-like particles by a direct interaction with HIV-1 Gag nucleocapsid protein. J Biol Chem. 2004;279:34083–6.

137. Cen S, Guo F, Niu M, Saadatmand J, Deflassieux J, Kleiman L. The interaction between HIV-1 Gag and APOBEC3G. J Biol Chem. 2004;279:33177–84.

138. Luo K, Liu B, Xiao Z, Yu Y, Yu X, Gorelick R, Yu XF. Amino-terminal region of the human immunodeficiency virus type 1 nucleocapsid is required for human APOBEC3G packaging. J Virol. 2004;78:11841–52.

139. Schafer A, Bogerd HP, Cullen BR. Specific packaging of APOBEC3G into HIV-1 virions is mediated by the nucleocapsid domain of the gag polyprotein precursor. Virology. 2004;328:163–8.

140. Svarovskaia ES, Xu H, Mbisa JL, Barr R, Gorelick RJ, Ono A, Freed EO, Hu WS, Pathak VK. Human apolipoprotein B mRNA-editing enzyme-catalytic polypeptide-like 3G (APOBEC3G) is incorporated into HIV-1 virions through interactions with viral and nonviral RNAs. J Biol Chem. 2004;279:35822–8.

141. Zennou V, Perez-Caballero D, Gottlinger H, Bieniasz PD. APOBEC3G incorporation into human immunodeficiency virus type 1 particles. J Virol. 2004;78:12058–61.

142. Khan MA, Kao S, Miyagi E, Takeuchi H, Goila-Gaur R, Opi S, Gipson CL, Parslow TG, Ly H, Strebel K. Viral RNA is required for the association of APOBEC3G with human immunodeficiency virus type 1 nucleoprotein complexes. J Virol. 2005;79:5870–4.

143. Wang T, Tian C, Zhang W, Luo K, Sarkis PT, Yu L, Liu B, Yu Y, Yu XF. 7SL RNA mediates virion packaging of the antiviral cytidine deaminase APOBEC3G. J Virol. 2007;81:13112–24.

144. Auweter SD, Oberstrass FC, Allain FH. Sequence-specific binding of single-stranded RNA: is there a code for recognition? Nucleic Acids Res. 2006;34:4943–59.

145. Lunde BM, Moore C, Varani G. RNA-binding proteins: modular design for efficient function. Nat Rev Mol Cell Biol. 2007;8:479–90.

146. Apolonia L, Schulz R, Curk T, Rocha P, Swanson CM, Schaller T, Ule J, Malim MH. Promiscuous RNA binding ensures effective encapsidation of APOBEC3 proteins by HIV-1. PLoS Pathog. 2015;11:e1004609.

147. York A, Kutluay SB, Errando M, Bieniasz PD. The RNA binding specificity of human APOBEC3 proteins resembles that of HIV-1 nucleocapsid. PLoS Pathog. 2016;12:e1005833.

148. Bohn JA, Thummar K, York A, Raymond A, Brown WC, Bieniasz PD, Hatziioannou T, Smith JL. APOBEC3H structure reveals an unusual mechanism of interaction with duplex RNA. Nat Commun. 2017;8:1021.

149. Karlin S, Mrazek J. Compositional differences within and between eukaryotic genomes. Proc Natl Acad Sci. 1997;94(19):10227–32.

150. Karlin S, Doerfler W, Cardon LR. Why is CpG suppressed in the genomes of virtually all small eukaryotic viruses but not in those of large eukaryotic viruses? J Virol. 1994;68:2889–97.

151. Rima BK, McFerran NV. Dinucleotide and stop codon frequencies in single-stranded RNA viruses. J Gen Virol. 1997;78(Pt 11):2859–70.

152. Greenbaum BD, Levine AJ, Bhanot G, Rabadan R. Patterns of evolution and host gene mimicry in influenza and other RNA viruses. PLoS Pathog. 2008;4:e1000079.

153. Takata MA, Goncalves-Carneiro D, Zang TM, Soll SJ, York A, Blanco-Melo D, Bieniasz PD. CG dinucleotide suppression enables antiviral defence targeting non-self RNA. Nature. 2017;550:124–7.

154. Gao G, Guo X, Goff SP. Inhibition of retroviral RNA production by ZAP, a CCCH-type zinc finger protein. Science. 2002;297:1703–6.

155. Muller S, Moller P, Bick MJ, Wurr S, Becker S, Gunther S, Kummerer BM. Inhibition of filovirus replication by the zinc finger antiviral protein. J Virol. 2007;81:2391–400.

156. Guo X, Carroll JW, Macdonald MR, Goff SP, Gao G. The zinc finger antiviral protein directly binds to specific viral mRNAs through the CCCH zinc finger motifs. J Virol. 2004;78:12781–7.

157. Carlile TM, Rojas-Duran MF, Zinshteyn B, Shin H, Bartoli KM, Gilbert WV. Pseudouridine profiling reveals regulated mRNA pseudouridylation in yeast and human cells. Nature. 2014;515:143–6.

158. Dominissini D, Moshitch-Moshkovitz S, Schwartz S, Salmon-Divon M, Ungar L, Osenberg S, Cesarkas K, Jacob-Hirsch J, Amariglio N, Kupiec M, Sorek R, Rechavi G. Topology of the human and mouse m6A RNA methylomes revealed by m6A-seq. Nature. 2012;485:201–6.

159. Dominissini D, Nachtergaele S, Moshitch-Moshkovitz S, Peer E, Kol N, Ben-Haim MS, Dai Q, Di Segni A, Salmon-Divon M, Clark WC, Zheng G, Pan T, Solomon O, Eyal E, Hershkovitz V, Han D, Dore LC, Amariglio N, Rechavi G, He C. The dynamic N(1)-methyladenosine methylome in eukaryotic messenger RNA. Nature. 2016;530:441–6.

160. Meyer KD, Saletore Y, Zumbo P, Elemento O, Mason CE, Jaffrey SR. Comprehensive analysis of mRNA methylation reveals enrichment in 3' UTRs and near stop codons. Cell. 2012;149:1635–46.

161. Schwartz S, Bernstein DA, Mumbach MR, Jovanovic M, Herbst RH, Leon-Ricardo BX, Engreitz JM, Guttman M, Satija R, Lander ES, Fink G, Regev A. Transcriptome-wide mapping reveals widespread dynamic-regulated pseudouridylation of ncRNA and mRNA. Cell. 2014;159:148–62.

162. Squires JE, Patel HR, Nousch M, Sibbritt T, Humphreys DT, Parker BJ, Suter CM, Preiss T. Widespread occurrence of 5-methylcytosine in human coding and non-coding RNA. Nucleic Acids Res. 2012;40:5023–33.

163. Yue Y, Liu J, He C. RNA N6-methyladenosine methylation in post-transcriptional gene expression regulation. Genes Dev. 2015;29:1343–55.

164. Canaani D, Kahana C, Lavi S, Groner Y. Identification and mapping of N6-methyladenosine containing sequences in simian virus 40 RNA. Nucleic Acids Res. 1979;6:2879–99.

165. Hashimoto SI, Green M. Multiple methylated cap sequences in adenovirus type 2 early mRNA. J Virol. 1976;20:425–35.

166. Sommer S, Salditt-Georgieff M, Bachenheimer S, Darnell JE, Furuichi Y, Morgan M, Shatkin AJ. The methylation of adenovirus-specific nuclear and cytoplasmic RNA. Nucleic Acids Res. 1976;3:749–65.

167. Krug RM, Morgan MA, Shatkin AJ. Influenza viral mRNA contains internal N6-methyladenosine and 5'-terminal 7-methylguanosine in cap structures. J Virol. 1976;20:45–53.

168. Dimock K, Stoltzfus CM. Sequence specificity of internal methylation in B77 avian sarcoma virus RNA subunits. Biochemistry. 1977;16:471–8.

169. Beemon K, Keith J. Localization of N6-methyladenosine in the Rous sarcoma virus genome. J Mol Biol. 1977;113:165–79.

170. Kane SE, Beemon K. Precise localization of m6A in Rous sarcoma virus RNA reveals clustering of methylation sites: implications for RNA processing. Mol Cell Biol. 1985;5:2298–306.

171. Kennedy EM, Bogerd HP, Kornepati AV, Kang D, Ghoshal D, Marshall JB, Poling BC, Tsai K, Gokhale NS, Horner SM, Cullen BR. Posttranscriptional m(6)A editing of HIV-1 mRNAs enhances viral gene expression. Cell Host Microbe. 2016;19:675–85.

172. Lichinchi G, Gao S, Saletore Y, Gonzalez GM, Bansal V, Wang Y, Mason CE, Rana TM. Dynamics of the human and viral m(6)A RNA methylomes during HIV-1 infection of T cells. Nat Microbiol. 2016;1:16011.

173. Tirumuru N, Zhao BS, Lu W, Lu Z, He C, Wu L. N(6)-methyladenosine of HIV-1 RNA regulates viral infection and HIV-1 Gag protein expression. Elife. 2016. https://doi.org/10.7554/eLife.15528.

6

Structural alteration of DNA induced by viral protein R of HIV-1 triggers the DNA damage response

Kenta Iijima[1], Junya Kobayashi[2] and Yukihito Ishizaka[1*]

Abstract

Background: Viral protein R (Vpr) is an accessory protein of HIV-1, which is potentially involved in the infection of macrophages and the induction of the ataxia-telangiectasia and Rad3-related protein (ATR)-mediated DNA damage response (DDR). It was recently proposed that the SLX4 complex of structure-specific endonuclease is involved in Vpr-induced DDR, which implies that aberrant DNA structures are responsible for this phenomenon. However, the mechanism by which Vpr alters the DNA structures remains unclear.

Results: We found that Vpr unwinds double-stranded DNA (dsDNA) and invokes the loading of RPA70, which is a single-stranded DNA-binding subunit of RPA that activates the ATR-dependent DDR. We demonstrated that Vpr influenced RPA70 to accumulate in the corresponding region utilizing the LacO/LacR system, in which Vpr can be tethered to the LacO locus. Interestingly, RPA70 recruitment required chromatin remodelling via Vpr-mediated ubiquitination of histone H2B. On the contrary, Q65R mutant of Vpr, which lacks ubiquitination activity, was deficient in both chromatin remodelling and RPA70 loading on to the chromatin. Moreover, Vpr-induced unwinding of dsDNA coincidently resulted in the accumulation of negatively supercoiled DNA and covalent complexes of topoisomerase 1 and DNA, which caused DNA double-strand breaks (DSBs) and DSB-directed integration of proviral DNA. Lastly, we noted the dependence of Vpr-promoted HIV-1 infection in resting macrophages on topoisomerase 1.

Conclusions: The findings of this study indicate that Vpr-induced structural alteration of DNA is a primary event that triggers both DDR and DSB, which ultimately contributes to HIV-1 infection.

Background

Combined antiretroviral therapy (cART) for human immunodeficiency virus-1 (HIV-1)-positive patients suppresses viral replication to a non-detectable level, thereby preventing immunodeficiency caused by T cell depletion. Unfortunately, the interruption of the cART regimen allows the expansion of viral replication from long-lived reservoir cells [1]. Because macrophages comprise the major cell population involved in the formation of viral reservoirs [2, 3], understanding the mode of viral infection in resting macrophages is crucial.

*Correspondence: zakay@ri.ncgm.go.jp
[1] Department of Intractable Diseases, National Center for Global Health and Medicine, 1-21-1 Toyama, Shinjuku-ku, Tokyo 162-8655, Japan
Full list of author information is available at the end of the article

Viral protein R (Vpr) is an accessory gene of HIV-1, which encodes a virion-associated nuclear protein that is made up of 96 amino acids (aa) [4] and can facilitate viral infection in resting macrophages [5–8]. The induction of cell-cycle abnormality at the G_2/M phase is a well-investigated function of Vpr among its pleiotropic activities [9]. Notably, Vpr induces a DNA damage response (DDR) involving ATR/ATRIP-Chk1 activation, the phosphorylation of histone H2AX (γH2AX) and the formation of BRCA1, 53BP1, RAD51 and FANCD2 foci [10–14]. Structural analyses revealed that Vpr contains three alpha helices with self-dimerisation properties along with a flexible carboxy (C)-terminal region with a basic stretch that is involved in DNA binding [15, 16], both of which were attributable to the cell-cycle abnormalities at the G_2/M phase [17]. Originally, Vpr-induced G_2/M arrest was proposed to contribute to viral infection by delaying cell death, thereby providing longer periods for viral replication [18]; however, its biological significance in resting macrophages remains largely unclear.

Regarding the upstream events that potentially trigger Vpr-induced DDR, several lines of evidence suggest that Vpr expression provokes replication stress, thereby inducing chromatin loading of the replication protein A 70-kDa subunit (RPA70), which is a DNA-binding subunit of the single-strand DNA (ssDNA) binding heterotrimeric protein [12, 19]). Considering that DNA binding of RPA70 triggers the ATR/ATRIP-Chk1 pathway responsible for G_2/M cell-cycle arrest [20], it is imperative to determine the mechanism of RPA70 loading onto the chromatin. Furthermore, cellular ubiquitination by Vpr is also required for DDR activation: the Q65R mutant of Vpr, which cannot bind DDB1/VprBP, an adaptor protein for Cul4 E3-ligase, is defective for the G_2/M checkpoint activation and cellular ubiquitination [21–24]. Although these findings imply that Vpr modulates RPA70 loading onto the chromatin in close functional association with the DDB1/VprBP-Cul4-dependent ubiquitination pathway, no cellular targets of Vpr-dependent ubiquitination have yet been identified.

For determining whether Vpr influences the structural alteration of DNA, Kichler et al. [25] performed an electron microscopic study and proposed that the C-terminal moiety of Vpr can aggregate plasmid DNA. Moreover, Lyonnais et al. [26] found that Vpr mediates the bridging and stretching of DNA helices. These observations strongly suggest that Vpr is capable of altering DNA structures. Generally, aberrant DNA structures interfere with DNA replication and transcription and may cause DNA damage. Such molecular consequences have been well-characterised in the context of DNA topological stress induced by camptothecin (CPT) and etoposide [27], which inhibit topoisomerase 1 (Topo1) and Topo2, respectively. Topo1 is involved in the relaxation of excess supercoils on dsDNA, whereas Topo2 is involved in the disentangling of dsDNA strands through cycles of cleavage and re-ligation. Chemical inhibition of re-ligation after relief of DNA distortions results in the formation of covalent complexes between Topo1 or Topo2 and cleaved DNA ends, which potentially induce DNA double-strand breaks (DSBs) due to subsequent collision of replication or transcription [27, 28].

Because Vpr itself does not possess DNA cleavage activity, Vpr must induce the DDR with the aid of host factor(s) [16]. Several cellular proteins, including UNG2, HTLF and SLX4 have been suggested as candidates for participation in Vpr-induced DDR [14, 29, 30]. UNG2 and HTLF are DNA repair proteins, and suppression of their functions leads to aggravation of DNA damage [29, 30]. On the other hand, Laguette et al. [14] suggested that

Vpr causes the premature activation of the SLX4-Mus81/Eme1 complex, which is a structure-specific nuclease complex, and promotes the cleavage of its target DNA structures, including DNA replication and recombination intermediates [14]. These observations suggest that cellular proteins involved in replication stress or its repair contribute to Vpr-induced DDR induction.

The findings of this study revealed that Vpr-induced structural alteration of DNA lead to RPA70 loading and negative supercoil formations. We demonstrated lines of evidence supporting that such Vpr-induced structural alteration of DNA is an upstream event that leads to DDR induction as well as DSB formation. Similar activity was observed at the cellular level; when Vpr was artificially recruited onto a specific chromosomal locus, it induced RPA70 loading, accumulation of negative supercoils, formation of a Topo1-DNA covalent complex (Topo1-cc) and DSBs in the corresponding region. Notably, Vpr also induced the ubiquitination of histone H2B, thereby increasing histone mobility and promoting RPA70 loading onto the chromatin. Together with the data regarding the Vpr-induced promotion of viral DNA integration in resting macrophages in a Topo1-dependent manner, we proposed that the structural alteration of DNA by Vpr acts as a trigger event for DDR and DSBs induction, which ultimately contributes to HIV-1 infection.

Results

Vpr unwinds supercoiled DNA and alters its topological configuration

To elucidate the activity of Vpr on dsDNA, we first performed atomic force microscopy (AFM) to analyse the structural alteration of dsDNA. In these experiments, supercoiled dsDNA was incubated in a buffer solution with recombinant Vpr protein (rVpr), attached onto a freshly cleaved mica surface through a gentle Ni^{2+}-mediated interaction, and then subjected to analysis [31]. AFM under liquid conditions can avoid potential artefacts resulting from the fixation or staining of DNA. Typical morphological changes and height profiles are shown in Fig. 1a. Markedly, treatment with chloroquine (Chlq), which is a DNA intercalator, resulted in the conversion of dsDNA into a highly expanded and de-condensed form (Fig. 1a, compare upper and middle panel and Additional file 1: Figure S1a). Interestingly, rVpr induced similar morphological changes in DNA (bottom panel). Each height profile was measured, and the root-mean-square (RMS) of the roughness (Rq) was calculated on the basis of the integrated data; Rq indicates the status and bulkiness of condensed dsDNA. As shown in Fig. 1b, the Rq value was significantly reduced by treatment with Chlq and rVpr (see also Additional file 1: Figure S1b). In contrast, ΔC12, which is a Vpr mutant that lacked the

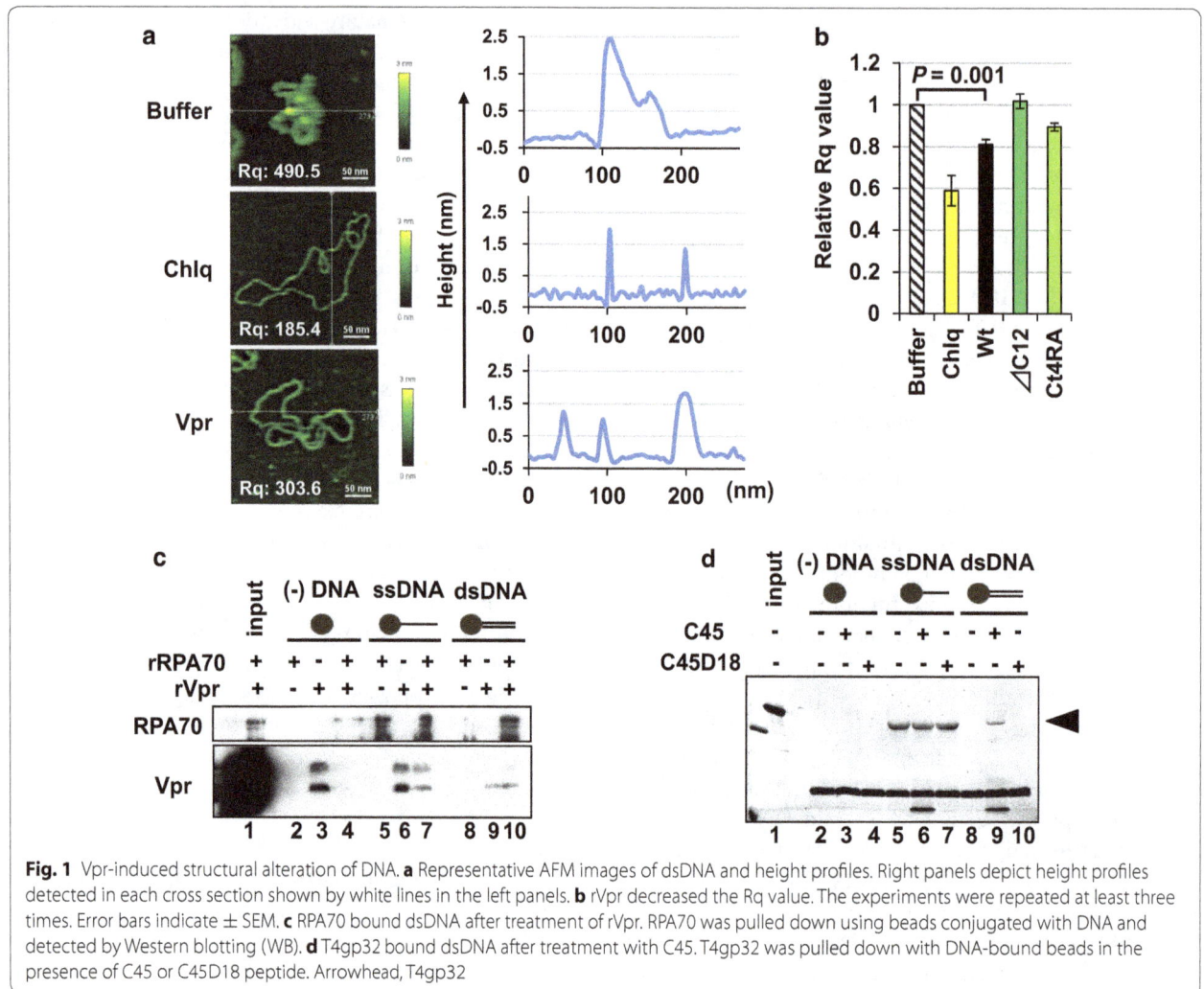

Fig. 1 Vpr-induced structural alteration of DNA. **a** Representative AFM images of dsDNA and height profiles. Right panels depict height profiles detected in each cross section shown by white lines in the left panels. **b** rVpr decreased the Rq value. The experiments were repeated at least three times. Error bars indicate ± SEM. **c** RPA70 bound dsDNA after treatment of rVpr. RPA70 was pulled down using beads conjugated with DNA and detected by Western blotting (WB). **d** T4gp32 bound dsDNA after treatment with C45. T4gp32 was pulled down with DNA-bound beads in the presence of C45 or C45D18 peptide. Arrowhead, T4gp32

C-terminal 12 aa [16], did not affect the Rq value (Fig. 1b and Additional file 1: Figure S1b). Similarly, the Ct4RA mutant, in which all four arginines (R) of the RxRRxR motif of the C-terminal region were replaced with alanines (A), showed lower activity than Vpr-Wt (Fig. 1b and Additional file 1: Figure S1b, c). These data suggest that Vpr influences the structural alteration of dsDNA by interacting via positively charged residues in its C-terminal stretch. Notably, other Vpr mutants, including Q65R, R77Q and R80A, showed similar activity with Vpr-Wt (Additional file 1: Figure S1c).

Our initial experiment using AFM suggested that Vpr generates an ssDNA stretch in the dsDNA molecule. To confirm this, we tested whether RPA70 formed an association with dsDNA when treated with rVpr. As shown in Fig. 1c, Western blotting (WB) after a pull-down procedure detected RPA70 when dsDNA and RPA70 were incubated with rVpr (compare lanes 8–10). To further confirm the dependence of RPA70 loading on the

C-terminal stretch of Vpr, we performed experiments using C45, which is a peptide made up of 45 aa of the C-terminal Vpr [32]. In this experiment, we used T4gp32 (T4 gene 32 protein), a well-established ssDNA-binding protein of the T4 phage [33, 34]. Consistent with the first experiment, we observed that T4gp32 bound dsDNA in the presence of C45 (Fig. 1d, lane 9). In contrast, no association was detected between dsDNA and T4gp32 when C45D18, which is a truncated form of C45 lacking the C-terminal 18 aa, was incubated (lane 10). Because Vpr did not interact with RPA70 or T4gp32 (Additional file 2: Figure S2a for RPA70 and Figure S2b for T4gp32), the data suggest that Vpr-induced unwinding of dsDNA occurred through its positively charged C-terminal region.

When circular-dsDNA is relaxed in one part of a dsDNA, topological changes are aroused in the other (Fig. 2a, step-1). Such dsDNA with differential topologies can be detected using a DNA supercoiling assay [35], in which dsDNA is treated with *Escherichia coli* Topo1, followed by deproteinisation with proteinase K (ProK). On treatment with *E. coli* Topo1, negative supercoiling was removed through a nicking and re-ligation cycle (Fig. 2a, step-2), whereas treatment with ProK removed Vpr and Topo1, and generated relaxed forms of dsDNA (RFs) (Fig. 2a, step-3). Since agarose electrophoresis can separate each topoisomer, rVpr induced the formation of a slower-migrating species of DNA, representing RFs (Fig. 2b, lanes 6–8). Similar experiments were performed using various mutants of Vpr (Fig. 2c), indicating that Vpr-Wt increased the RFs of dsDNA (lane 5), whereas ΔC12 or Ct4RA did not (lanes 17 and 20). In contrast, Vpr mutants (Q65R, R77Q and R80A) showed activities comparable with that of Vpr-Wt (Fig. 2c, lanes 8, 11 and 14, respectively).

Expression of Vpr induces the Topo1-cc formation

Topo1-cc formation induces SSBs (DNA single-strand breaks) and DDR [27], while collision of a replication fork or transcription with the complex triggers DSB [27, 28]. To maintain genomic stability, Topo1-cc is removed by tyrosyl-DNA phosphodiesterase 1 (TDP1) and degraded by the SUMO/ubiquitin-mediated proteasomal degradation pathway [27, 36, 37]. For characterising the functional link between Vpr and Topo1 at the cellular level, we examined the Topo1 protein using Mit-23 cells, in which the tetracycline promoter tightly regulates Vpr expression [17]. When doxycycline (Dox) is added to these cells, Vpr is expressed at a level comparable with that in HIV-1 infected cells [38]. As observed in Fig. 3a, Vpr expression led to reduction in the level of Topo1 (relative level decreased to 0.71); an immunohistochemical analysis revealed that the nuclear

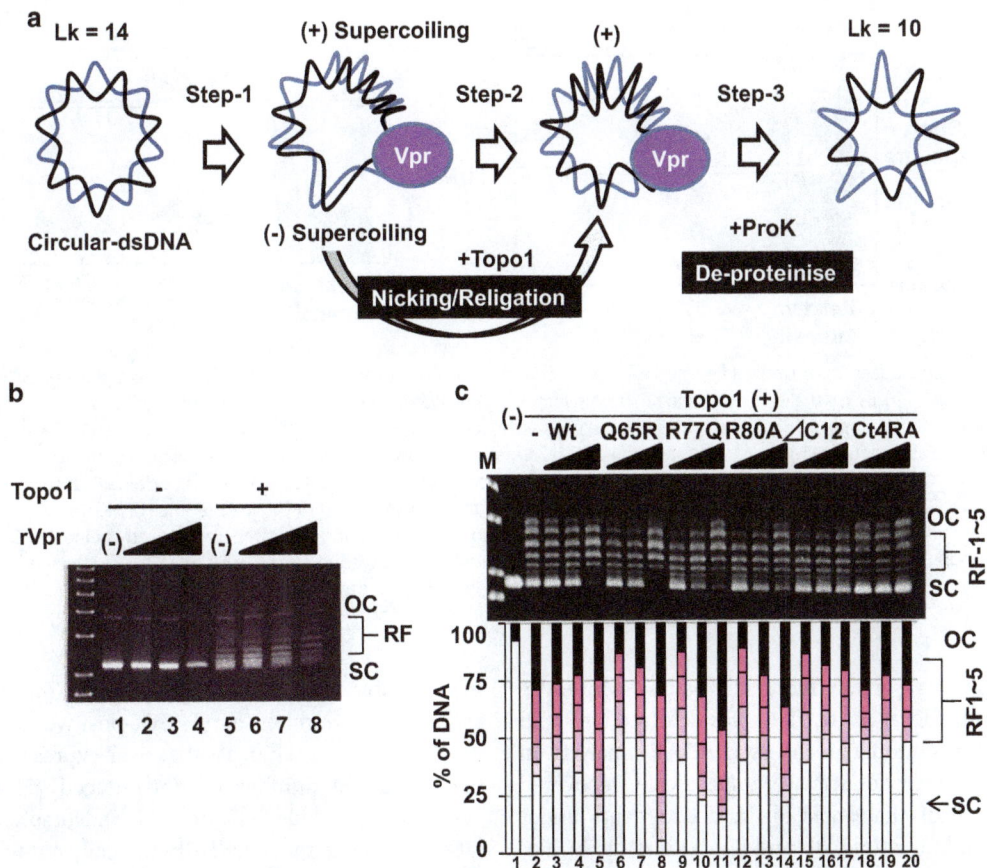

Fig. 2 Vpr induced topological changes on DNA. a Schematic representation of experimental procedure for DNA supercoiling assay. Possible induction of partial unwinding of dsDNA by Vpr induces negative and positive supercoiling (Step-1). In the presence of *E. coli* Topo1, negative supercoiling (lower side) is relieved by nicking/relegation activity (Step-2). After the de-proteinisation, net amounts of linking number (Lk) are decreased (Step-3). b DNA supercoiling assay with rVpr-Wt. The effects of various amounts of rVpr were tested using *E. coli* Topo1. *OC* open circular, *RF* relaxed form, *SC* supercoiled. c DNA supercoiling assay with mutants of Vpr. Intensities of each topoisomer were quantified, and their relative amounts are shown in the bottom graph

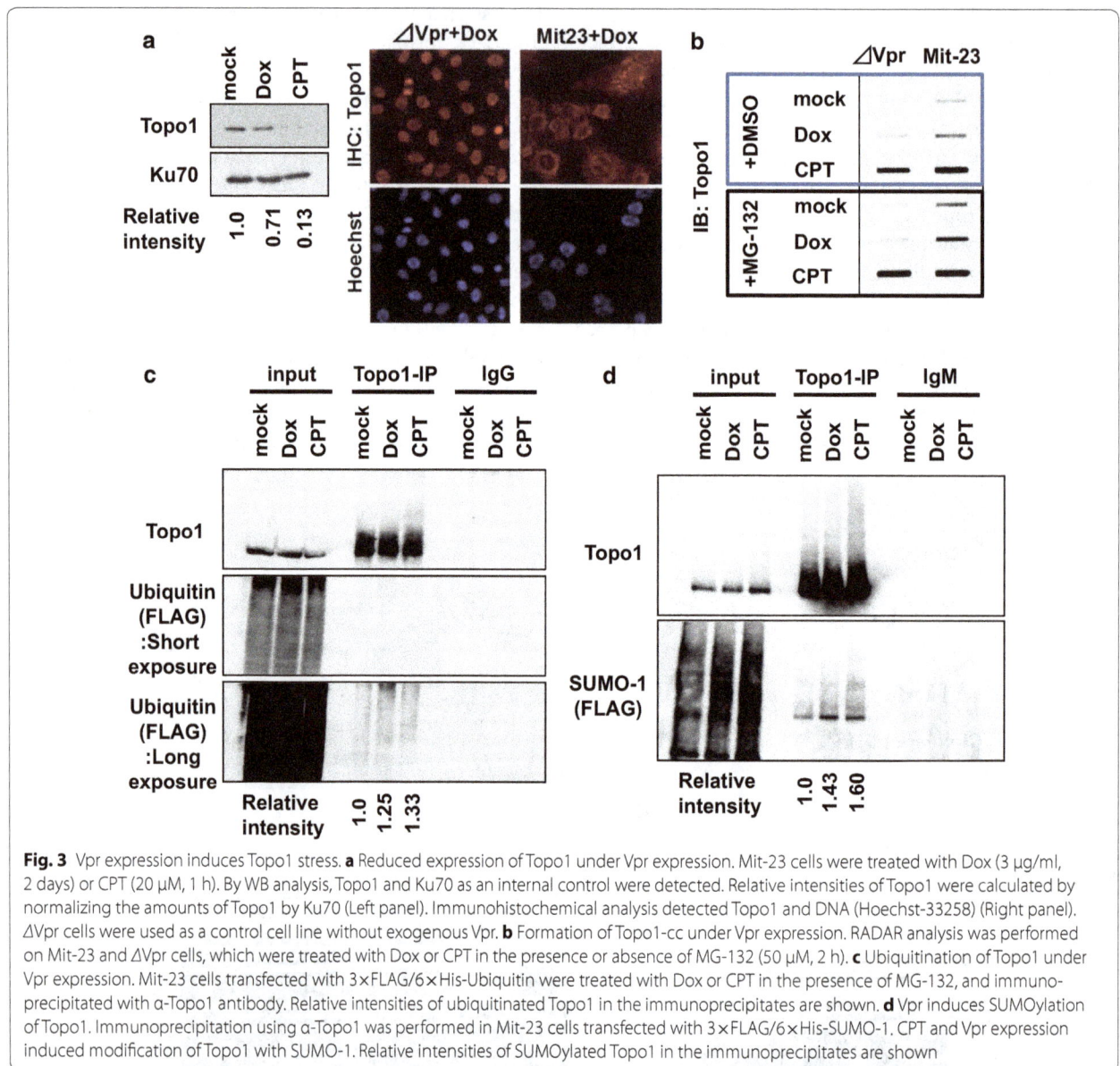

Fig. 3 Vpr expression induces Topo1 stress. **a** Reduced expression of Topo1 under Vpr expression. Mit-23 cells were treated with Dox (3 µg/ml, 2 days) or CPT (20 µM, 1 h). By WB analysis, Topo1 and Ku70 as an internal control were detected. Relative intensities of Topo1 were calculated by normalizing the amounts of Topo1 by Ku70 (Left panel). Immunohistochemical analysis detected Topo1 and DNA (Hoechst-33258) (Right panel). ΔVpr cells were used as a control cell line without exogenous Vpr. **b** Formation of Topo1-cc under Vpr expression. RADAR analysis was performed on Mit-23 and ΔVpr cells, which were treated with Dox or CPT in the presence or absence of MG-132 (50 µM, 2 h). **c** Ubiquitination of Topo1 under Vpr expression. Mit-23 cells transfected with 3×FLAG/6×His-Ubiquitin were treated with Dox or CPT in the presence of MG-132, and immunoprecipitated with α-Topo1 antibody. Relative intensities of ubiquitinated Topo1 in the immunoprecipitates are shown. **d** Vpr induces SUMOylation of Topo1. Immunoprecipitation using α-Topo1 was performed in Mit-23 cells transfected with 3×FLAG/6×His-SUMO-1. CPT and Vpr expression induced modification of Topo1 with SUMO-1. Relative intensities of SUMOylated Topo1 in the immunoprecipitates are shown

signal of Topo1 was greatly reduced (Fig. 3a). Moreover, an increase in the level of Topo1-cc was detected by Rapid approach to DNA adducts recovery (RADAR) analysis, in which DNA–protein adducts were specifically recovered in the presence of chaotropic ion and detergents under denaturing conditions (Fig. 3b and Additional file 3: Figure S3a, b) [39]. Vpr-induced accumulation of Topo1-cc was enhanced by treatment with MG-132, which is a proteasomal inhibitor (Fig. 3b). Moreover, the Vpr expression increased the susceptibility of Topo1 to ubiquitination (Fig. 3c) and SUMOylation (Fig. 3d).

To demonstrate the involvement of Topo1 in Vpr-induced DDR, we performed RNA interference (RNAi) experiment (knockdown efficiency is shown in Additional

file 4: Table S1). Down-regulation of *Topo1* by siRNA reduced the number of γH2AX-positive cells (Figs. 4a, b, $P = 0.007$), whereas the over-expression of TDP1 decreased the number of Vpr-induced γH2AX-positive cells (Additional file 5: Figure S4a, b). Notably, down-regulation of *DDB1* and *VprBP* dramatically reduced cell-cycle arrest (Fig. 4c, d), whereas that of *Topo1* partially attenuated the Vpr-induced G_2/M arrest. Because accumulation of Topo1-cc can lead to DSB formation [27, 28], we examined whether DSBs were induced in cells under Vpr expression. As shown in Fig. 4e, f, a neutral comet assay, which is a highly sensitive method to detect DSBs, revealed that Vpr induced DSB. In this case, the down-regulation of *Topo1* significantly attenuated Vpr-induced DSB (Fig. 4f).

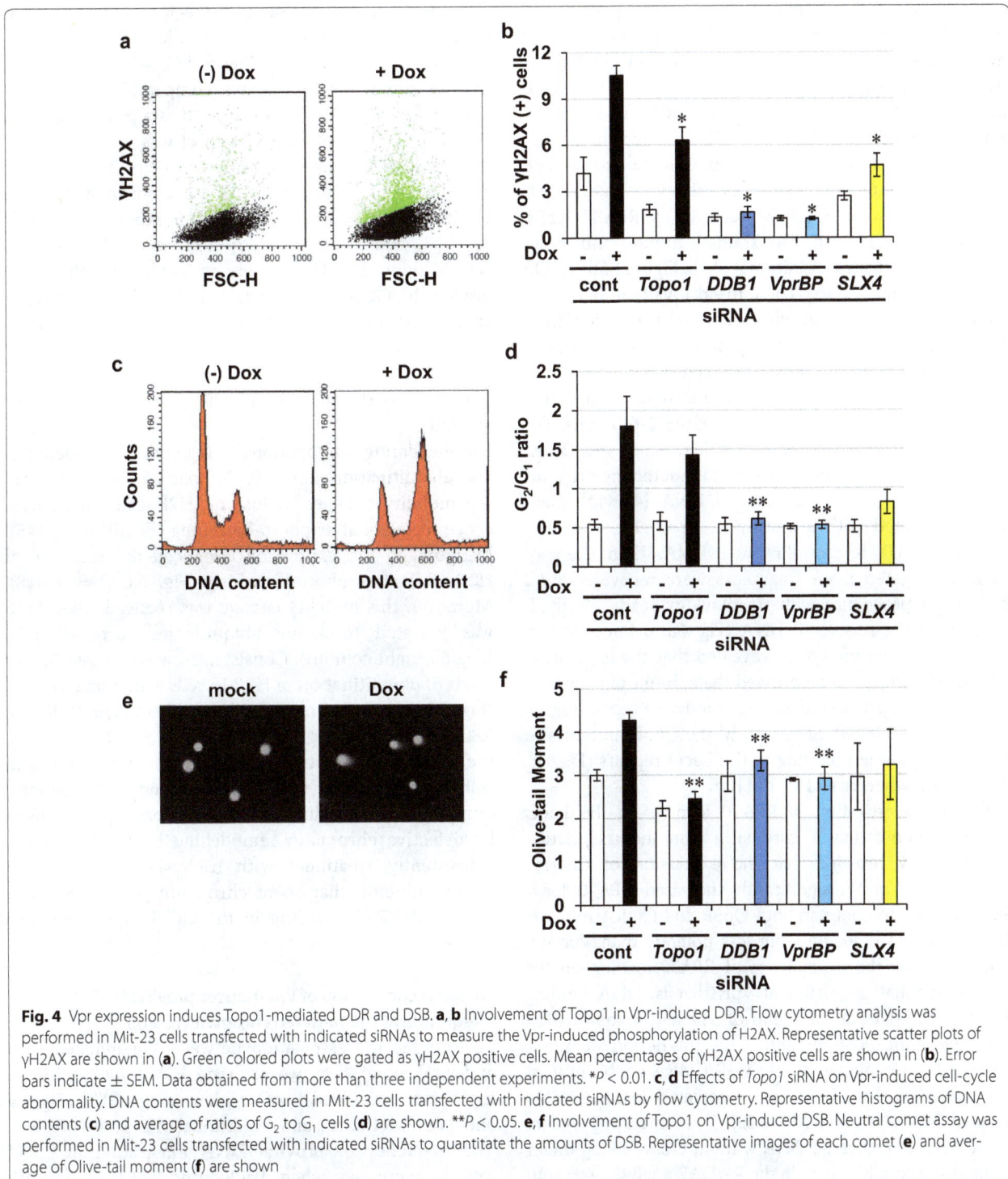

Fig. 4 Vpr expression induces Topo1-mediated DDR and DSB. **a**, **b** Involvement of Topo1 in Vpr-induced DDR. Flow cytometry analysis was performed in Mit-23 cells transfected with indicated siRNAs to measure the Vpr-induced phosphorylation of H2AX. Representative scatter plots of γH2AX are shown in (**a**). Green colored plots were gated as γH2AX positive cells. Mean percentages of γH2AX positive cells are shown in (**b**). Error bars indicate ± SEM. Data obtained from more than three independent experiments. *$P < 0.01$. **c**, **d** Effects of *Topo1* siRNA on Vpr-induced cell-cycle abnormality. DNA contents were measured in Mit-23 cells transfected with indicated siRNAs by flow cytometry. Representative histograms of DNA contents (**c**) and average of ratios of G_2 to G_1 cells (**d**) are shown. **$P < 0.05$. **e**, **f** Involvement of Topo1 on Vpr-induced DSB. Neutral comet assay was performed in Mit-23 cells transfected with indicated siRNAs to quantitate the amounts of DSB. Representative images of each comet (**e**) and average of Olive-tail moment (**f**) are shown

Forced accumulation of Vpr on a targeted DNA locus induces structural alteration of DNA and DDR

To investigate Vpr-induced structural alteration of DNA in the cell, we used U2OS/2-6-3, a human osteosarcoma cell line containing 200 copies of a construct composed of 256 *lac operator* (LacO) repeats at a single locus on 1p36 [40]. This cell line can be used to analyse the molecular events in a specific region of chromosomal DNA. When a fused protein of Vpr and Lac repressor (LacR) was expressed, Vpr was recruited to the LacO repeats (Fig. 5a)

[40–42], which was confirmed by detecting mCherry-focus accumulated on a single distinct region in the nucleus (Fig. 5b, left panel). In these cells, mCherry-positive focus was precisely co-localised with all DDR-related molecules when a fused molecule of Cherry-LacR-Vpr was expressed: the following DDR-related molecules were examined: γH2AX (Fig. 5b, middle panels and Additional file 6: Figure S5a), phosphorylated ataxia telangiectasia mutated (ppATM-Ser1981), ppRPA32-Ser33, ppRAD17-Ser645 and FK2-stained mono- and poly-ubiquitin conjugates (Additional file 6: Figure S5b–e). On the other hand, Cherry-LacR fused Ovalbumin (OVA), which is a control molecule, generated no DDR signals overlapping with the mCherry-positive focus (Fig. 5b, upper panels and Additional file 6: Figure S5).

We next attempted to detect the structural alteration of DNA in the LacO repeats of U2OS/2-6-3 cells. For this purpose, we first used a psoralen, which is a DNA-intercalating cross-linker used for detecting regions containing negatively supercoiled DNA [43, 44]. Cells were incubated with a biotinylated psoralen and irradiated with UV to cross-link with DNA. Then, the psoralen-conjugated DNA fragments were recovered by a pull-down procedure with streptavidin beads. A qPCR analysis of the recovered DNA (Fig. 5a, primers shown as arrows below the boxes) revealed that the expression of LacR-fused Vpr-Wt increased the amount of psoralen-bound DNA corresponding with the LacO repeat region (Fig. 5c, $P = 0.0058$). Surprisingly, the Q65R mutant also increased psoralen binding to the LacO repeats (Fig. 5c, $P = 0.034$), whereas Ct4RA did not.

Further investigation of RPA70 loading on the LacO repeat region using a chromatin immunoprecipitation (ChIP) assay revealed that the expression of Cherry-LacR fused Vpr-Wt significantly increased RPA70 loading (Fig. 5d). In contrast, both Q65R and Ct4RA mutants increased RPA70 loading, but less potently than Vpr-Wt, which implies the dependence of RPA70 loading on the dual functional properties of Vpr; that is, DNA binding through the C-terminal region of Vpr and ubiquitination defective in the Q65R mutant. To test this notion, we monitored RPA70 loading with the Q65R/Ct4RA double mutant and observed that this mutant completely lost the ability to load RPA70 (Fig. 5d, $P = 0.22$). To evaluate the level of Topo1-cc, we recovered DNA without cross-linking under denaturing conditions, as in the RADAR analysis, and subjected the samples to ChIP assay done with the α-Topo1 antibody. Vpr-Wt significantly induced Topo1-cc accumulation on the LacO repeat region, whereas the Q65R and Ct4RA mutants did not (Fig. 5e, $P = 0.049$ for Vpr-Wt). As both Q65R and Ct4RA were severely defective in Topo1-cc accumulation, the coordinated functions of Vpr were required for provoking such downstream events.

We next quantified DSBs at the region where Vpr accumulated using a ligation-mediated (LM)-PCR (see Methods and Additional file 7: Figure S6) [41]. Surprisingly, Vpr-Wt induced DSBs at a level comparable with that by Fok1 endonuclease, which was used as a positive control (Fig. 5f). In contrast, the DSB level was not elevated in the Q65R and C-terminal mutants of Vpr. Requirement of Topo1 for Vpr-induced DSBs was confirmed also by a Cre/loxP-mediated Cherry-LacR-Vpr expression system, in which expression of Cherry-LacR-Vpr in U2OS/2-6-3 cells is induced by Cre expression (Additional file 8: Figure S7a, b). Obtained data again showed that down-regulation of *Topo1* suppressed Topo1-cc and DSB formation (Additional file 8: Figure S7c, d).

Vpr-mediated chromatin remodelling is required for RPA70 loading

For elucidating the functional link between Vpr-dependent ubiquitination and RPA70 loading, we measured the mobility changes of histone H2B using a fluorescence recovery after photo-bleaching (FRAP) assay [45]. Intriguingly, Vpr expression enhanced the recovery of H2B-GFP after photo-bleaching (Fig. 6a, $P = 0.018$). Moreover, this mobility change was reduced when H2B was mutated to a non-ubiquitinated form (K120R) (Fig. 6b, right column). Consistently, we observed higher levels of ubiquitination of H2B in cells expressing Vpr-Wt (Fig. 6c, lane 4), but not in cells expressing Q65R, R77Q, R80A and Ct4RA (Fig. 6c, lanes 6, 8, 10 and 12). Notably, the enhanced mobility of H2B-GFP was not detected in cells expressing the Q65R mutant (Fig. 6d, right column), implying that the reduction of RPA70 loading was caused by defective chromatin remodelling by Q65R mutant. Consistently, treatment with trichostatin A (TSA), a HDAC inhibitor that opens chromatin [46], successfully recovered RPA70 loading in the Q65R-expressing cells (Fig. 6e).

Forced accumulation of Vpr induces proviral DNA integration at the targeted chromatin region

To examine the association between Vpr-induced DSB and viral integration, we analysed HIV-1 integration in the Vpr-accumulated LacO region using qPCR (Fig. 7a and see "Methods" and Additional file 9: Figure S8). The frequency of proviral DNA integration in LacO repeats increased when LacR-fused Fok1 or Vpr-Wt was co-expressed at the time of HIV-1 infection (Additional file 10: Figure S9, Additional file 11: Figure S10). For demonstrating the direct effects of virion-associated Vpr, we prepared lentiviral particles composed of defective integrase (IN-D64A) and Cherry-LacR-fused Vpr (CLV) or Cherry-Vpr (CV) (Fig. 7b), infected them into U2OS/2-6-3 cells and performed qPCR. When CLV

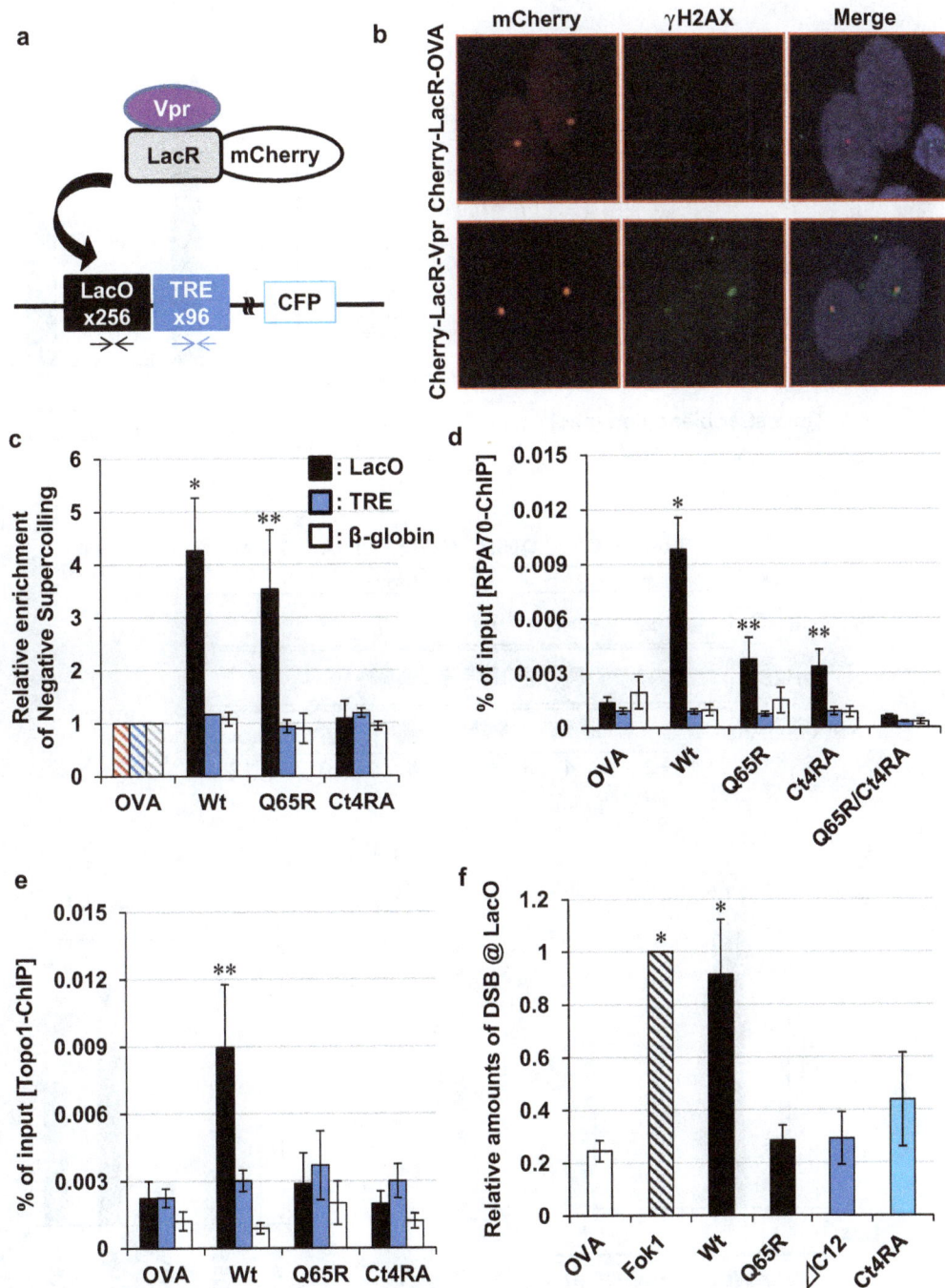

Fig. 5 Forced accumulation of Vpr induces DDR in the targeted region. **a** Schematic of experiments using the LacO/LacR system. In U2OS/2-6-3 cells, 200 copies of p3216PECMS2β, which contains 256 copies of the LacO sequence and 96 copies of the tetracycline response element (TRE) upstream of the CFP coding region are integrated into a single site. In this cell lines, the LacR-Vpr fusion is forcibly recruited to the LacO repeat region (curved arrow). Arrows indicate PCR primers used for amplification of the LacO (red) and TRE (blue) regions (nucleotide sequence is shown in Additional file 20: Table S3). **b** Co-localised signals of Cherry-LacR-Vpr and DDR marker. Phosphorylated H2AX (γH2AX) was detected as a representative DDR marker after 2 days of transfection with indicated construct. **c** Formation of negatively supercoiled DNA in the Vpr-accumulated region. Two days after transfection, a psoralen-bound DNA was recovered and subjected to qPCR analysis with the primers shown in Fig. 5a. The relative copy numbers of LacO (red column), TRE (blue column), and β-globin (as a negative control; blank column) are shown. Error bars indicate ± SEM. *P < 0.01; **P < 0.05. **d** Enhanced loading of RPA70 by Vpr. Loading of RPA70 was quantitated by ChIP assay. **e** Formation of Topo1-cc by Vpr. ChIP assay was performed without cross-linking. MG-132 was treated for 2 h at 50 μM. **f** DSB induction by Vpr. LM-PCR was performed to measure the amounts of DSB-ends in the LacO repeat region. Each column indicates the amount of DSBs relative to LacR-fused Fok1 (positive control)

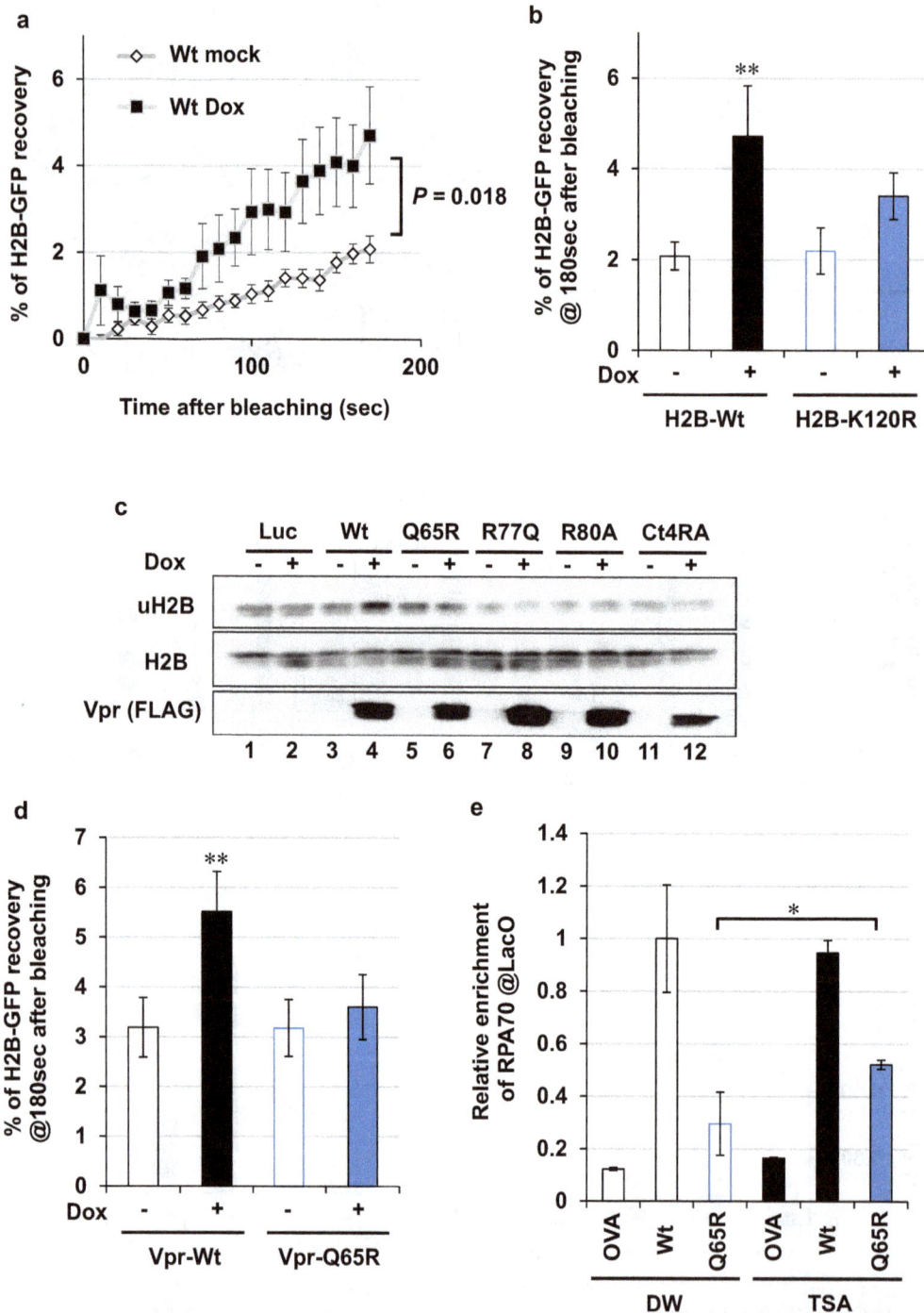

Fig. 6 Vpr induces chromatin remodelling through histone H2B ubiquitination. **a** Increased mobility of H2B under Vpr expression. The FRAP assay was performed using Mit-23 cells with H2B-GFP. The collected values for the recovery rate of each GFP signal were subjected to statistical analysis. Error bars indicate ± SEM. **b** Vpr-induced mobilization of H2B depends on ubiquitination. Mean percentages of H2B-GFP recovery after 180 s of photo-bleaching were compared. $**P < 0.05$. **c** H2B was ubiquitinated by Vpr-Wt expression. For this experiment, we newly established cell lines (HT1080vRxt-Vpr), in which expression of Vpr-Wt (lanes 3 and 4), Vpr-Q65R (lanes 5 and 6), Vpr-R77Q (lanes 7 and 8), Vpr-R80A (lanes 9 and 10) and Vpr-Ct4RA (lanes 11 and 12) can be controlled by the tetracycline promoter, and ubiquitination of H2B on K120 was examined after Dox treatment (5 µg/ml, 2 days). As a negative control, a clone expressing Luciferase (Luc) was also included (lanes 1 and 2). Total H2B and Dox-induced expression of Vpr were detected. **d** Mobility of H2B was not increased by the Q65R mutant of Vpr. Graph shows mean percentages of H2B-GFP recovery after 180 s of photo-bleaching. **e** Defect of the Q65R mutant for RPA70 loading was rescued by TSA. After treatment with TSA (50 nM, 16 h), RPA70 loading onto the LacO repeats was quantitated by ChIP assay. $*P < 0.01$

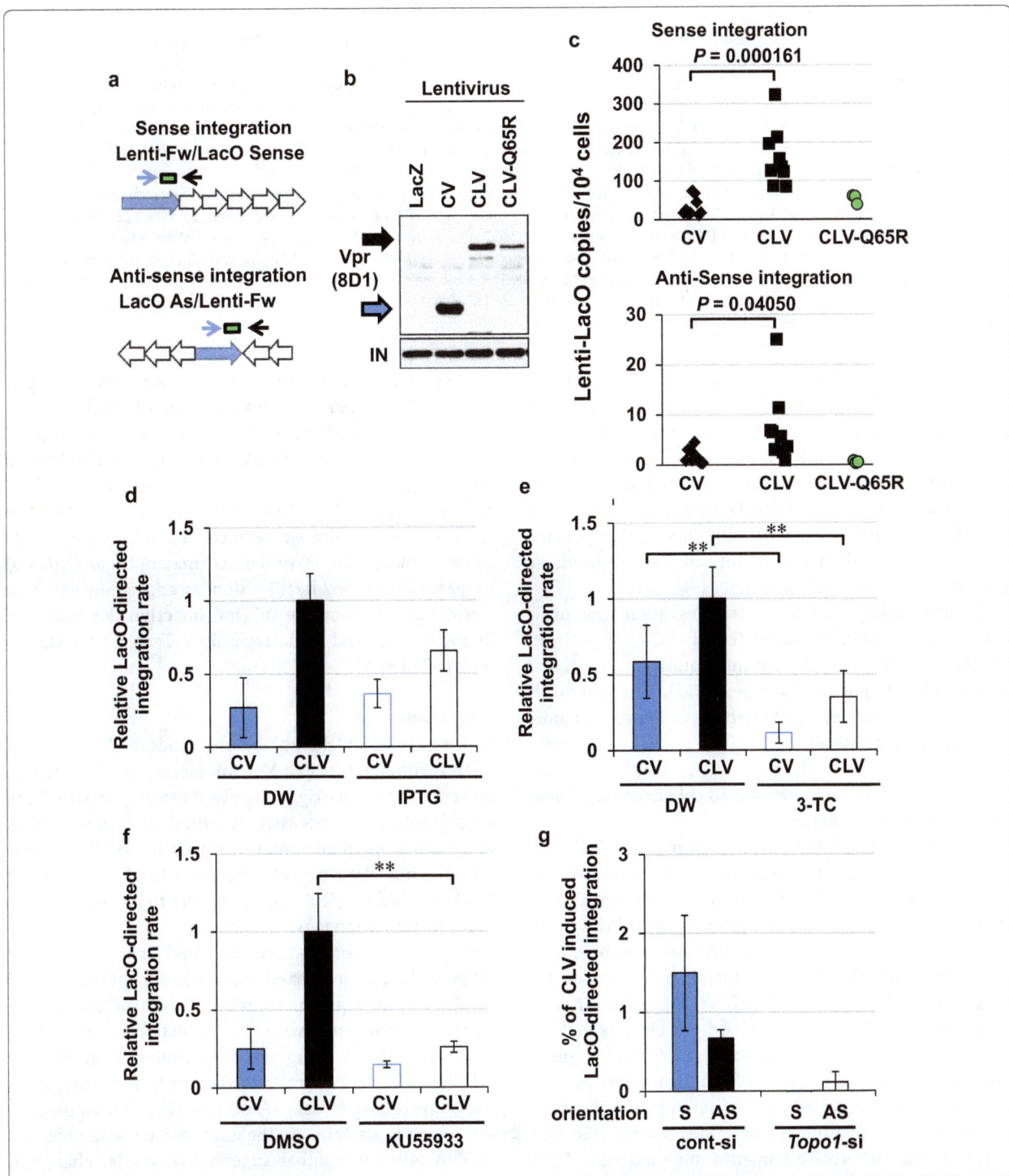

virus was infected, the frequency of proviral DNA integration into the LacO repeats significantly increased without marked effects on the overall viral infectivity (Fig. 7c and Additional file 12: Figure S11). In striking contrast, the infection of CLV-Q65R virus, a lentivirus with Cherry-LacR fused to Vpr mutant of Q65R, did not induce the LacO-directed integration, indicating that Vpr-induced ubiquitination and DSB is required for these integrations (Fig. 7b, c). The frequency of Vpr-induced LacO-directed integration was reduced by isopropyl β-D-1-thiogalactopyranoside (IPTG), which blocks LacO/LacR binding (Fig. 7d), as well as

(See figure on previous page.)

Fig. 7 Proviral DNA integration in Vpr-accumulated sites. **a** Schematic of LacO-directed integration of proviral DNA. The qPCR analysis of the copy number of LacO-integrated proviral DNA was performed using PCR primers targeting the 3′-LTR (blue arrow) and LacO repeat (red arrow). The green box indicates the position of the TaqMan probe for the 3′-LTR (nucleotide sequence is shown in Additional file 20: Table S3). **b** Production of lentiviral particles with CV, CLV, and CLV-Q65R. Integrase (IN) was detected as an internal control. *LacZ*-coding lentivirus (LacZ) was included as a negative control. **c** Site-specific integration of proviral DNA. CV, CLV, and CLV-Q65R incorporated lentivirus was infected into U2OS/2-6-3 cells and subjected to qPCR analysis (Fig. 7a) at 2dpi (n = 9, 9, 3 for CV, CLV, and CLV-Q65R, respectively). Similar infectivity of each virus was confirmed by colony-formation assay (Additional file 12; Figure S11). **d** Effects of LacO/LacR inhibition on site-specific integration of proviral DNA. Cells were pretreated with IPTG (15 mM, 1 h) prior to the lentivirus infection. Error bars indicate ± SEM. Data were obtained from more than three independent experiments. **e** A reverse transcriptase inhibitor blocked the infection. Cells were pretreated with 3-TC (50 μM, 1 h) prior to lentivirus infection. **P < 0.05. **f** Site-specific integration of proviral DNA depended on ATM activity. ATM inhibitor, KU55933 (10 μM) was added to culture medium 1 h before infection. **g** Topo1 is important for site-specific integration of proviral DNA. A U2OS/2-6-3 subclone transduced with pCAL-loxP-CLV (263/loxP-CLV) was infected with Cre- or LacZ-expressing adenovirus for 2 days under down-regulation of *Topo1*. The cells were then infected with NL4-3/D64A/R− virus and subjected to qPCR analysis at 2dpi. The overall integration rate was quantitated by *Alu-gag* two-step nested qPCR (Additional file 11: Figure S10) to estimate the percentage of LacO-directed integration. *S* sense integration, *AS* anti-sense integration

by the reverse-transcriptase inhibitor 2′,3′-dideoxy-3′-thiacytidine (3-TC) (Fig. 7e). In addition, these site-directed integrations were abrogated by the treatment with an ATM inhibitor (KU55933) (Fig. 7f), which is consistent with the results of a previous work showing that ATM activity is required for DSB-directed integration [8]. Moreover, RNAi experiment indicated that proviral DNA is integrated in the vicinity of Vpr-accumulated sites in a Topo1-dependent manner (Fig. 7g).

We also explored the lentiviral integration sites using linear amplification mediated (LAM)-PCR for estimating the frequency of selective integration into the LacO repeats (Additional file 13: Figure S12). Two out of 96 analysed samples (2%) contained LacO-dependent integrations in the genome.

Topo1 requirement for Vpr-mediated enhancement of viral infection in non-dividing cells

Lastly, we examined the role of Vpr-induced DSB and Topo1 in the viral infection of resting macrophages. First, we prepared Vpr-proficient (R+) and deficient (R−) viruses, infected them into MonoMac-6 (MM-6) cells and applied the cells to neutral comet assay. In this experiment, we used IN-D64A mutant virus to exclude the effects of IN-dependent DSB [47, 48]. MM-6 is a monocyte leukaemia-derived macrophage-like cell line that can differentiate into resting macrophages following phorbol 12-myristate 13-acetate (PMA) treatment. A neutral comet assay revealed that infection of the R+ virus provoked DSBs in differentiated MM-6 cells (Fig. 8a). Furthermore, RNAi experiments revealed that DSB induction by the R+ virus was Topo1-dependent (Fig. 8b and Additional file 4: Table S1 for knockdown efficiency). Moreover, the addition of rVpr in the culture medium of MM-6 cells also induced DSBs that depended on *Topo1*, *DDB1* and *SLX4* (Fig. 8c). Notably, down-regulation of *Topo1* significantly suppressed the viral infectivity of the R+ virus, although the originally low infectivity of R− was unaffected (Fig. 8d, R+, P < 0.0001; R−, P = 0.78

and Additional file 14: Figure S13 for other sets of Topo1 siRNA). Vpr-dependent upregulation of viral infectivity was confirmed using luciferase assay (Additional file 15: Figure S14a) and EGFP expression (Additional file 15: Figure S14b). Similarly, down-regulation of *DDB1* and *SLX4* also led to decrease in the viral infectivity of the R+ virus. Finally, we performed similar experiments using primary monocyte-derived macrophages (MDMs) prepared from two healthy donors and confirmed that Vpr-dependent increase in viral infection depended on Topo1 (Fig. 8e and Additional file 4: Table S1 for knockdown efficiency).

Discussion

Studies aimed at elucidating the mode of Vpr-induced DDR identified multiple Vpr-interacting cellular factors; however, the initial triggering event remains elusive. Here we presented evidence that structural alteration of DNA is the most upstream event of Vpr-induced DDR. Interestingly, our data suggest that structural alteration of DNA also induce DSB and contribute to HIV-1 infection in resting macrophages.

First, AFM observations revealed that supercoiled DNA shifted to a relaxed form when rVpr was added to DNA in an aqueous solution. This structural alteration was confirmed with the detection of negatively supercoiled DNA using the supercoiling assay with *E. coli* Topo1. Previous reports demonstrating that negative supercoiling of dsDNA occurs when RNA polymerase unwinds dsDNA or the nucleosome assembles on dsDNA [49, 50] together suggest that similar change in the topological configuration of dsDNA was induced by Vpr. This idea was also supported by Vpr-dependent loading of the ssDNA-binding proteins onto dsDNA.

Vpr-induced structural alteration of DNA was also observed in vivo in an experimental series using the LacO/LacR system in U2OS/2-6-3 cells. When a chimeric fusion protein of Vpr and LacR accumulated on the LacO region, we observed the formation of activated

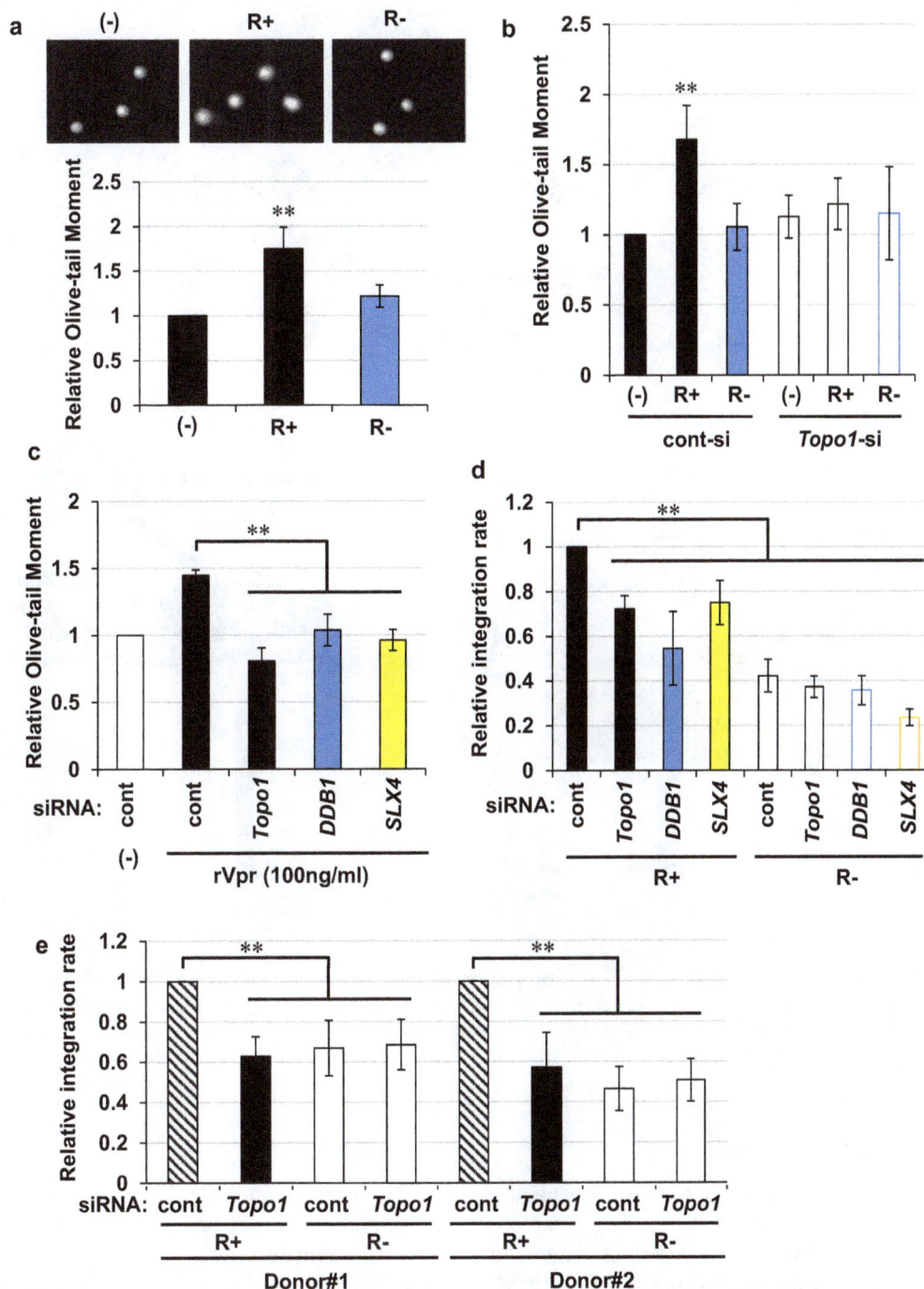

Fig. 8 Vpr-induced DSB stimulates viral infection in resting macrophages. **a** Vpr induced DSBs in resting macrophages. Differentiated MM-6 cells were infected with NL4-3/D64A virus for 1 day, and then subjected to neutral comet assay. Representative images of each comet are shown (upper panel). The relative Olive-tail moment was evaluated (lower panel). Error bars indicate ± SEM calculated based on data obtained from more than three independent experiments. Data from non-infected cells (−), Vpr-proficient virus (R+), and Vpr-deficient virus (R−) are shown. **P < 0.05. **b** Involvement of Topo1 in Vpr-induced DSB. Neutral comet assay was performed as in **a** after 3 days of Topo1 targeting siRNA transfection. **c** DSB induced by rVpr was blocked by down-regulation of Topo1. Three days after transfection of indicated siRNA, cells were treated with rVpr (100 ng/ml, 16 h). **d** Integration of proviral DNA was blocked by down-regulation of Topo1. MM-6 cells were infected with Vpr-proficient (R+) or deficient (R−) NL4-3 virus after transfection with siRNA, and the integration rate was quantitated by Alu-gag two-step nested qPCR at 2dpi; relative integration rates are shown. **e** Vpr-dependent increase of viral infectivity required Topo1 in MDMs. MDMs from two healthy donors were infected with Vpr-proficient (R+) or deficient (R−) NL4-3 virus 2 days after transfection with Topo1 targeting siRNA, and the integration rates were quantitated as in **d** at 2dpi

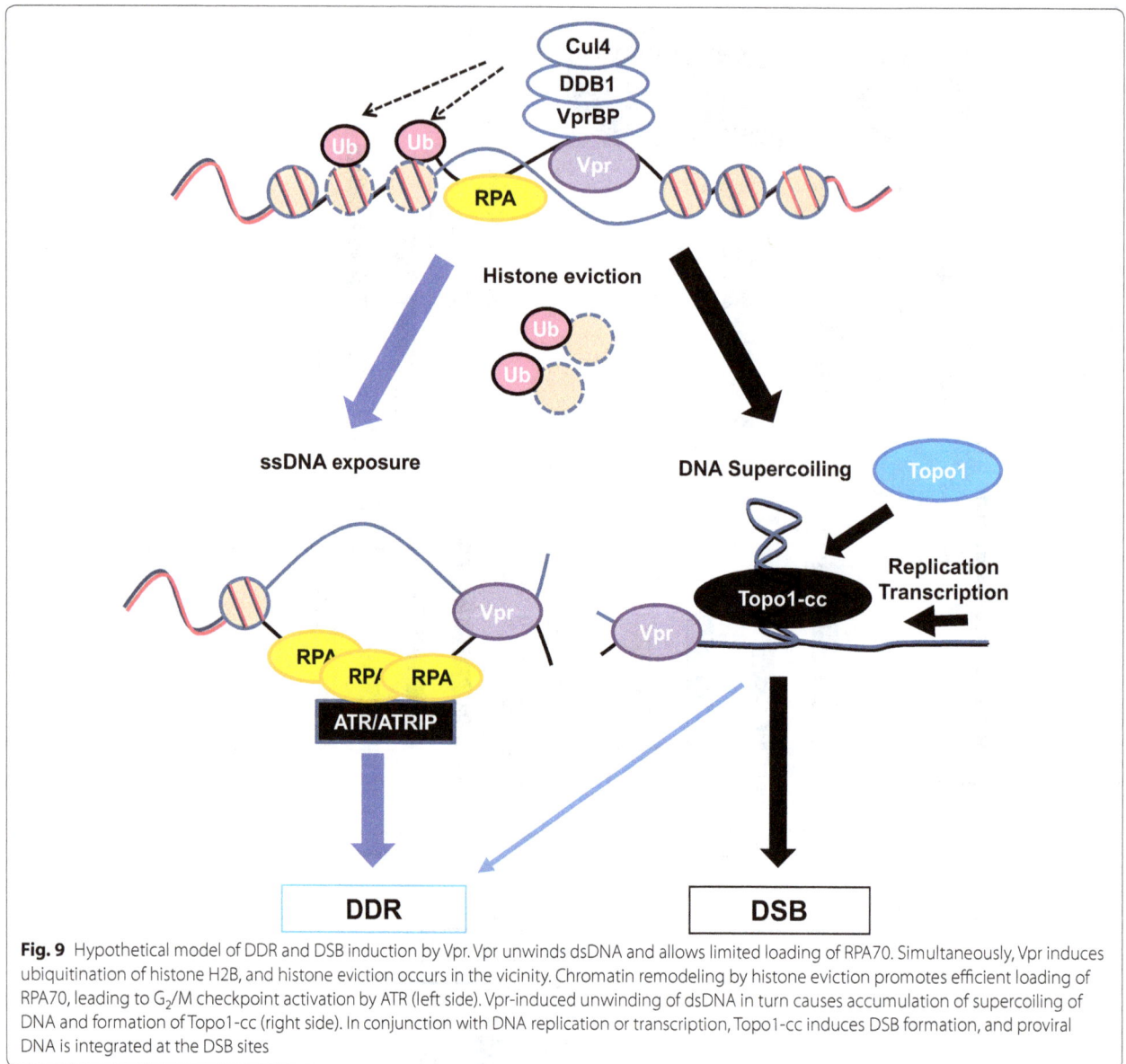

Fig. 9 Hypothetical model of DDR and DSB induction by Vpr. Vpr unwinds dsDNA and allows limited loading of RPA70. Simultaneously, Vpr induces ubiquitination of histone H2B, and histone eviction occurs in the vicinity. Chromatin remodeling by histone eviction promotes efficient loading of RPA70, leading to G_2/M checkpoint activation by ATR (left side). Vpr-induced unwinding of dsDNA in turn causes accumulation of supercoiling of DNA and formation of Topo1-cc (right side). In conjunction with DNA replication or transcription, Topo1-cc induces DSB formation, and proviral DNA is integrated at the DSB sites

forms of multiple DDR-related molecules, chromatin loading of RPA70, accumulation of negative supercoiling, generation of Topo1-cc and DSBs in the same region foci (Fig. 5 and Additional file 6: Figure S5). RPA70 loading onto chromatin by Vpr-induced unwinding of dsDNA effectively explains the mechanism of Vpr-induced DDR.

Notably, our data suggested that Vpr-induced RPA70 loading was modulated at least two steps (Fig. 9). In the first step, the DNA-binding activity of Vpr changes the superhelicity of the DNA and partially unwinds dsDNA. This function was demonstrated using in vitro experiments (Fig. 1c, d), which also revealed the importance of the positively charged amino acids in the C-terminal

stretch. In the second step, Vpr-mediated ubiquitination is required for chromatin remodelling, which enables the recruitment of cellular factors, including RPA70, to chromatin. This step was demonstrated via experiments using well-characterised Q65R mutant, which is defective in the ubiquitination process [21, 22]. Intriguingly, when the Q65R mutant was forced to accumulate on the LacO repeats, it could not stimulate RPA70 loading (Fig. 5d), although the RPA70 loading defect of the Q65R mutant was complemented by TSA (Figs. 5e, 6e). To elucidate this phenomenon, we investigated whether Vpr modulated chromatin remodelling and induced ubiquitination of histone H2B [51, 52]. Interestingly, the FRAP assay revealed that the recovery of H2B after photo-bleaching was more rapid in cells expressing Vpr-Wt than in those expressing the Q65R mutant. Similarly, a non-ubiquitinated H2B mutant exhibited reduced mobility in the Vpr-expressing cells. Moreover, the ubiquitination of H2B was promoted by Vpr-Wt, but not by the Q65R mutant. Considering that Cul4 regulates H2B ubiquitination for facilitating the DDR [53] and that the Q65R mutant is ubiquitination-defective due to its inability to bind DDB1/VprBP [21, 22], it is plausible that H2B is a target of Vpr-mediated ubiquitination, which is critical for Vpr-induced RPA70 loading. In addition to histone H2B, the association of Vpr with several chromatin modification factors, including p300, SNF2 h, NuRD and HDAC1 [38, 54–56], may also contribute to the efficient reorganization of chromatin. Our data suggested that the concerted actions of structural alteration of DNA and chromatin remodelling are required for efficient RPA70 loading by Vpr.

Notably, we found that Vpr-induced structural alteration of DNA could induce both DDR activation and DSB formation. In the latter process, Topo1 played a key role in creating DNA breaks (Figs. 4f, 8b, c; Additional file 8: Figure S7d), albeit its subtle contribution to Vpr-induced DDR activation (Fig. 4d). We also detected Vpr-induced DSB in resting macrophages in a Topo1-dependent manner (Fig. 8b, c), which suggested that Topo1-cc-mediated DSB could also arise in non-proliferating cells through interference with transcription [28]. Here, although we focussed on Topo1, we could not exclude the possibility of involvement of the other DNA structure modification factors such as Topo2, structure-specific nucleases including SLX4-Mus81/Eme1, and nucleotide excision repair (NER) factors in the processing of Vpr-induced aberrant DNA structures. Consistent with this possibility, we observed that the down-regulation of SLX4 or XPG (a nuclease acting in NER) by siRNA suppressed Vpr-induced DSB (Fig. 4f and Additional file 16: Figure S15c, d). In addition, these factors also function in Topo1-mediated DSB induction. SLX4 causes DSBs through Topo1-bound DNA strand incision during the replication process [57, 58] and XPG induces DSBs through the processing of R-loops (DNA/RNA hybrids), which are formed when Topo1 inhibition blocks the transcription [59, 60]. In resting macrophages, it is plausible that R-loop formation is a major trigger event of Vpr-induced DSBs. Consistently, we observed an increase in R-loops at the Vpr-accumulated region (Additional file 17: Figure S16) and a decrease in Vpr-induced γH2AX-positive cells by the over-expression of RNaseH1, an RNase that degrades R-loops (Additional file 5: Figure S4).

We confirmed the requirement of SLX4 for Vpr-induced DDR, which was in concordance with the report of Laguette et al. [14], but in contrast with another study that reported SLX4 to be dispensable [61]. These discrepant observations are attributable to the different levels of residual activity of SLX4 under down-regulation by siRNA and gene disruption. In addition, differentially reorganised DNA repair pathway in SLX4 deficient cells leads to different cellular responses to Vpr.

Several lines of evidence indicate that DSBs increase the efficiency of HIV-1 infection, especially in resting cells [8, 18, 62, 63]. The finding that Vpr-induced DSBs are important for viral infection in resting macrophages effectively explains the previous observations that Vpr is required for the infection of resting cells [5–8]. Furthermore, the observation that DSB sites are directly targeted by proviral DNA integration supports the relevance of Vpr-induced DSB in viral infection [8].

The mechanism by which Vpr induces structural alteration of DNA remains unclear. In this study, we analysed DNA supercoiling using recombinant Vpr and Vpr-derived peptides, which suggested the necessity of C-terminal stretch of Vpr for DNA unwinding. Notably, we also detected that a higher concentration of Vpr-derived peptides (0.15–1.5 Vpr-peptides/bp) resulted in strongly underwound DNA (Additional file 18: Figure S17) in the DNA supercoiling assay. In a previous electron microscopic study, higher concentrations of Vpr (at least 4.5 Vpr-peptides/bp) induced the aggregation of DNA [26]. Because plectonemic or toroidal DNA structures are the compacted forms of negatively supercoiled DNA, it is possible that our current findings reflect the same phenomena as that reported in a previous study [26]. Siddiqui et al. [64] reported that Vpr-induced DDR required helical domain II (37–50 aa), but not the C-terminal region. These contradictory observations in the function of the C-terminal region of Vpr could be derived from the methods adopted for evaluating the Vpr-induced DNA damages. Siddiqui et al. [64] assessed the chromosomal abnormalities as Vpr-induced DNA damages, whereas we measured DSB itself by neutral comet assay and LM-PCR (Figs. 4f, 5f).

HIV treatment with cART can effectively suppress viral replication. However, complete eradication of HIV has not been successfully achieved, largely due to long-lived reservoir cells [1]. Recent observations indicate that viral sanctuary sites are distributed in various organs, including in the gut-associated lymphoid tissue and the central nervous system, in which persistent infections are observed [2, 3]. Vpr has reportedly been detected in the cerebrospinal fluid of HIV-positive patients [65, 66]. Notably, Topo1-mediated DNA damage is responsible for several neurodegenerative disorders [67], suggesting that Vpr may be involved in the development of HIV associated neurocognitive disorder

[68] by exacerbating Topo1 insults. Our results provide a rationale for developing anti-Vpr compounds, which can significantly contribute to the improvement of the therapeutic regimen for HIV-positive patients under the current cART.

Conclusions

We discovered that Vpr induces DNA structural alteration as an initial trigger of DDR and DSB. Notably, Vpr modulates chromatin remodelling by ubiquitinating histone H2B, and it facilitates RPA70 loading on unwound supercoiled DNA. We believe that our findings provide an answer to the long-standing question on how Vpr facilitates the infection of HIV-1 into macrophages.

Methods

Key resources (cell lines, chemicals, reagents, antibodies, recombinant DNA)

List of resources is included in Additional file 19: Table S2.

Cell lines and cell culture

Cell lines used were MonoMac-6 (MM-6) (DSMZ), HEK293T (RIKEN Cell Bank), HT1080 (the Healthy Science Research Resources Bank), ΔVpr, Mit-23 (derived from HT1080) [38], U2OS/2-6-3 (provided by Dr. David Spector, Cold Spring Harbor Laboratory, Cold Spring Harbor) [40], U2OS/2-6-3+pCAL-loxP-CLV (263/loxP-CLV), HT1080vRxt (retroviral RetroX-tet-ONE)-Luc or -Vpr, Mit-23+H2B-GFP and HT1080vRxt-Vpr+H2B-GFP. We confirmed no contamination of mycoplasma by periodically checking with Hoechst-33258 (Sigma-Aldrich) staining. MM-6 cells were cultured in RPMI 1640 with 10% fetal bovine serum (FBS) (Gibco) supplemented with 1% NEAA (Gibco) and 1% OPI media (Sigma). For differentiating into macrophage-like state, MM-6 cells were treated for 3 days with 50 nM of PMA. HEK293T and HT1080 cells were cultured in DMEM with 10% FBS, and ΔVpr and Mit-23 cells were cultured in DMEM with 10% tetracycline free FBS (Hyclone) supplemented with HygromycinB (12.5 µg/ml) and G418 (100 µg/ml). U2OS/2-6-3 cells were cultured in DMEM with 10% FBS supplemented with HygromycinB (12.5 µg/ml). 263/loxP-CLV cells, U2OS/2-6-3 derived newly established cell line stably transduced with pCAL-loxP-CLV, were cultured in DMEM with 10% FBS supplemented with HygromycinB (12.5 µg/ml) and G418 (100 µg/ml). HT1080vRxt-Luc or -Vpr cells, HT1080 derived newly established cell lines stably transduced with retroviral RetroX-tet-ONE-Luc or -Vpr, were cultured in DMEM with 10% tetracycline free FBS supplemented with puromycin (1 µg/ml). All cell lines stably transduced with pEF-Bos-H2B-GFP (+H2B-GFP) were maintained in BlasticidineS (2 µg/ml) containing

medium. All cells were grown at 37 °C in humidified atmosphere containing 5% CO_2.

Preparation of monocyte derived macrophages (MDMs)

Experimental procedures were approved by the internal review board. Peripheral blood mononuclear cells (PBMCs) of healthy volunteers who gave informed consent were isolated by Ficoll density gradient separation using Lymphoprep (Axis-Shield). Monocytes were isolated using monocyte isolation kit II (Miltenyi) by depletion of non-monocytes. For preparation of MDMs, isolated monocytes were cultured for 7 days in RPMI1640 supplemented with 10% FBS in the presence of 25–50 ng/ml of recombinant human macrophage-colony stimulating factor (rhM-CSF) (R&D).

Bacterial strains

DH5α chemical competent *E. coli* (TOYOBO) was used for standard transformation. For the transformation of retrovirus, lentivirus, and HIV-1 vector DNA, Stbl3 chemically competent *E. coli* (Life Technologies) was used. In the case of protein expression, BL21DE3 (Stratagene) was used for transformation.

rVpr purification from Wheat germ extract

By Wheat germ extract (WGE) cell free transcription/translation system (CellFree Sciences), FLAG-Strep-tag2 (F/S) fused to the N-terminus of Vpr (pNL4-3, GenBank: AF324493.2) was expressed by pEU-F/S-Vpr as template. After the protein synthesis, WGE was diluted in 3× volume of StA binding Buffer (50 mM Tris–Cl [pH 8.0], 500 mM NaCl, 1 mM EDTA, 1% NP40, 0.5% Brij-35) supplemented with RNaseA (100 µg/ml). After the incubation with Strep-Tactin agarose beads overnight at 4 °C on rotating platform, beads were washed with StA binding buffer, and eluted by 1×SA elution buffer (Calbiochem) supplemented with 1% NP40. The eluate was incubated with FLAG-M2 agarose beads overnight at 4 °C on rotating platform. The beads were extensively washed with phosphate buffer saline (PBS) (−), and eluted by 0.1 M HEPES [pH 2.5] and immediately neutralized by 1 M HEPES [pH 8.0], and adjusted to 50 mM of NaCl. The concentration of Vpr in the eluted fraction was determined by α-Vpr ELISA (MBL) [13] or Coomassie Brilliant Blue (CBB) gel staining compared to known amounts of Bovine serum albumin (BSA). The rVpr produced by WGE was used in experiments except Figs. 1c, 2c. Comparable activity of F/S-Vpr with rVpr from *E. coli* was confirmed by neutral comet assay.

Purification of rVpr from *E. coli*

rVpr was purified as previously reported [13] with some modification. Briefly, BL21DE3 codon plus was transformed with pGEX-Vpr, in which Vpr was fused to C-terminus of GST followed by PreScission protease cleavage site, and cultured in 2×YTG supplemented with 100 µg/ml Ampicillin (2×YTG-Amp) over night at 30 °C. On the next day, the culture was inoculated to 1:50 ratio into fresh 2×YTG-Amp, and incubated at 37 °C until OD600 reached to 0.8. And then, 1 mM of IPTG was added to the bacterial culture medium, and further incubated for 3 h at 25 °C. Collected pellet from 500 ml culture was suspended in 20 ml of Binding buffer (20 mM sodium-phosphate buffer [pH 7.6], 150 mM NaCl, 0.5% TritonX-100, 10% glycerol) supplemented with 1 mM PMSF. After sonication and centrifugation, lysate was filtered through 5 µm filter and incubated with 500 µl of glutathione Sepharose (GSH) beads overnight at 4 °C on rotating platform. On the next day, beads were sequentially washed with Binding buffer supplemented with 500 mM NaCl or 1% TritonX-100, and Cleavage buffer (50 mM Tris–HCl [pH 7.0], 150 mM NaCl, 1 mM EDTA, 10% glycerol) twice, and then suspended in Cleavage buffer supplemented with 1 mM dithiothreitol (DTT) and 20 µl of PreScission protease. After overnight incubation on rotating platform at 4 °C, GSH beads were collected (Vpr remains bound to GSH beads), and washed with Binding buffer. Then, Vpr protein was eluted with Binding buffer supplemented with 0.1% TritonX-100. The eluate was incubated with new GSH beads to remove the un-cleaved GST-Vpr and PreScission protease for 1 h, and then supernatant was incubated with α-Vpr-antibody (8D1) conjugated CNBr-agarose beads overnight at 4 °C on rotating platform. The beads were extensively washed with PBS (−), and Vpr was eluted by 0.1 M HEPES [pH 2.5] and immediately neutralized by 1 M HEPES [pH 8.0]. The concentration of Vpr in eluted fraction was determined by α-Vpr ELISA [13]. The rVpr expressed in bacteria was used in experiments for Figs. 1c and 2c.

rRPA70 purification

BL21DE3 was transformed with pET15-6×His-RPA70 (in which hRPA70 was tagged with hexa-histidine followed by PreScission protease cleavage site on N-terminus) and cultured in 2×YTG-Amp overnight at 30 °C. On the next day, the culture was inoculated to 1:50 ratio into fresh 2×YTG-Amp, and incubated at 37 °C until OD600 reached to 0.8. And then, 1 mM of IPTG was added to bacterial culture medium, further incubated overnight at 16 °C. Collected pellet from 500 ml culture was suspended in 20 ml of Buffer-A (50 mM Tris–HCl [pH 7.5], 500 mM NaCl, 0.5% TritonX-100, 10 mM mercaptoethanol, 10% glycerol) supplemented with 1 mM PMSF. After sonication and centrifugation, lysate was filtered through 5 µm filter and incubated with 10 ml of Affi-gel Blue resin (BioRad) overnight at 4 °C on rotating platform. Beads

were washed with 20 ml of Buffer-A twice, and eluted with 10 ml of lysis buffer supplemented with 2.5 M NaCl. Eluate was diluted by 4-fold volume of Buffer-B (50 mM Tris–HCl [pH 8.0], 0.5% TritonX-100, 0.625% Empigen, 10% glycerol, 10 mM mercaptoethanol, 12.5 mM imidazole), followed by overnight incubation with Ni–NTA beads (Invitrogen). Beads were washed with Buffer-C (50 mM Tris–HCl [pH 8.0], 1 M NaCl, 0.5% Empigen, 0.5% TritonX-100, 10 mM mercaptoethanol, 10% glycerol, 10 mM imidazol) and Buffer-D (50 mM Tris–HCl [pH 8.0], 150 mM NaCl, 1% TritonX-100, 0.5% Empigen, 10% glycerol). Subsequently, beads were further washed with Buffer-E (50 mM Tris–HCl [pH 7.0], 150 mM NaCl, 0.1% Empigen, 10% glycerol) twice, and suspend in Buffer-E supplemented with 1 mM DTT, 1 mM EDTA, and 20 µl of PreScission protease. After overnight incubation on rotating platform at 4 °C, GSH beads were added to the eluate to remove the PreScission protease, and mixed for 1 h, and then supernatant was used as purified rRPA70 fraction. The concentration of RPA70 was estimated on CBB gel staining compared to known amounts of BSA.

Sample preparation for AFM analysis

Fifty ng of pUC18 was incubated with 5 mM of Chlq or 0.5 µM of rVpr (1000-fold excess amount of Vpr to pUC18; 0.37 Vpr molecule/bp) in 50 µl of AFM reaction buffer (10 mM Tris–HCl [pH 8.0], 50 mM NaCl, 1 mM MgCl$_2$) for 30 min at 37 °C. Prior to the binding of DNA, freshly cleaved mica were treated with AFM binding buffer (AFM reaction buffer supplemented with 5 mM NiCl$_2$) for at least 10 min, and quickly blew out by N$_2$ gas just before sample loading. And then, appropriate amounts of DNA sample (typically 10 µl) was dropped on the Ni^{2+}-treated mica surface and placed for 10 min. Following quick washes of mica surface with AFM binding buffer twice, 100 µl of AFM binding buffer was loaded on mica for in liquid AFM observation.

AFM measurement in aqueous solution

All measurements were carried out with a JPK NanoWizard ULTRA Speed AFM (JPK Instruments) on inverted microscope (IX71, Olympus) equipped with acoustic hood and active vibration isolation (Micro40, Accurion). Ultrashort cantilever (USC-F0.3-k0.3, NanoWorld) was used with 110–120 kHz drive frequency for high-speed, high-resolution imaging in liquid environment. The images were scanned in an intermittent contact mode (AC mode) for 2.0 µm × 2.0 µm area (512 × 512 pixels) at scan rate of 2.0 Hz, Z-range of 1.3 µm. Data processing was performed by JPK SPM Data Processing software (JPK Instruments). For processing images, the same parameters were used for all samples analysed in the same day. To obtain a root mean square of roughness (Rq) value, DNA molecule was manually surrounded by the minimal rectangle. For each treatment, at least 30 randomly selected DNA molecules were subjected to Rq value measurements, and independent experiments were performed more than three times.

RPA70 Pull down assay by DNA-bound beads

At first, 10 pmol of biotinylated 80-mer ss/dsDNA was incubated with 10 μl of Dynabeads M280 Streptavidine (SA-beads) in SA binding buffer (10 mM Tris–HCl [pH 8.0], 1 M NaCl, 1 mM EDTA) at room temperature on rotating platform. After 15 min, beads were washed with SA binding buffer three times, and kept in IP buffer (50 mM Tris–HCl [pH 8.0], 150 mM NaCl, 1 mM EDTA, 1% NP40). Subsequently, 10 pmol of rRPA70 and rVpr was added to suspension of DNA-bound beads, and incubated for 1 h at 4 °C on the rotating platform. Beads were washed with IP buffer three times, and proteins recovered by pull-down procedures (pulled-down proteins) were analysed by WB.

T4gp32 Pull down assay by DNA-bound beads

The beads bound with ss/dsDNA was prepared as above, and beads were suspended in 1×CutSmart buffer (NEB) supplemented with 1% NP40. Subsequently, 50 pmol of T4gp32 (NEB) and 100 pmol of C45 or C45D18 peptide was added to suspension of DNA-bound beads, and incubated for 1 h at room temperature on rotating platform. Beads were washed by 1×CutSmart buffer supplemented with 1% NP40 three times. Pulled-down proteins were separated on SDS-PAGE, followed by staining with Oriole fluorescent gel staining (BioRad), and visualized by LAS400 with UV transilluminator.

Supercoiling assay

Supercoiled plasmid DNA, pBluescriptII (500 ng, Fig. 2b) or pUC18 (100 ng, Fig. 2c), was incubated in 20 μl of 1×CutSmart buffer with 0.025 U of E. coli Topoisomerase1 (NEB) and increasing amounts of rVpr (0.71, 2.36, 7.1 pmol and 0.63, 2, 6.32 pmol for Fig. 2b, c, respectively) for 30 min at 37 °C. After that, samples were heat-inactivated for 20 min at 80 °C, and incubated for 20 min at 55 °C with 0.5% SDS and Proteinase K (1 mg/ml) for deproteinisation. Following phenol–chloroform extraction, purified DNA was separated on 0.8% agarose gel, and stained with ethidium bromide or 1×SyBr Gold (Life technologies) (Fig. 2b, c, respectively). Images were captured by GelDoc Ez (BioRad), and the intensity of each topoisomers was analysed by Image Lab software (BioRad).

Immunohistochemistry (IHC)

Immunohistochemistry was performed as a standard protocol. Briefly, cells were fixed with 4%

paraformaldehyde, and permeabilized with 0.5% TritonX-100. For the staining of Topo1, we performed pre-extraction with following buffer (20 mM HEPES [pH 7.5], 50 mM NaCl, 300 mM sucrose, 0.1% TritonX-100, 3 mM $MgCl_2$) before fixing. After blocking with 5% skim milk/TBS with 0.1% Tween20, indicated antibodies were used. After that, optimal α-IgG antibody conjugated with Alexa fluorescent dye was used as a secondary antibody. Nuclei were stained by 1 μM of Hoechst-33258 and observed with fluorescent microscope (BX51, Olympus; BZ-X710, Keyence).

DNA–protein covalent complex recovery (RADAR)

DNA–protein covalent complex was recovered according to a protocol previously reported [40]. Briefly, Mit-23 cells were treated with Dox (3 μg/ml) for 1 day or CPT (20 μM) for 1 h. In the case of MG-132 treatment, MG-132 (50 μM) was added to the culture medium 2 h prior to recovery. After treatment, cells were directly lysed in Buffer-M (6 M guanidine thiocyanate, 10 mM Tris–HCl [pH 6.5], 20 mM EDTA, 4% TritonX-100, 1% N-lauroylsarcosine, 1% DTT), and ethanol precipitation was performed by addition of half volume of 99% ethanol and centrifugation. Following washing with 70% ethanol twice, pellets were dissolved and sonicated in 8 mM NaOH solution. Amounts of DNA were quantitated by Picogreen (Invitrogen) with InfiniteM1000 PRO plate reader. For slot-blotting, equal amounts of DNA were absorbed to nitrocellulose membrane (BioRad) by BioDot-SF microfiltration apparatus (BioRad) with TBS buffer (10 mM Tris [pH 7.5], 150 mM NaCl). Topo1-cc or dsDNA were detected by respective antibodies.

Immunoprecipitation (IP)

Immunoprecipitation for detecting post-translational modifications of Topo1, Mit-23 cells were transfected with 3×FLAG/6×His-tagged ubiquitin or SUMO-1 expression vector. On the next day, cells were suspended in medium with or without of Dox (3 μg/ml) and incubated for 1 day. Then, MG-132 (50 μM) was added to all samples for 2 h. For CPT-treatment, cells were treated for 1 h before recovery. For detecting the ubiquitination, cells were lysed in 0.5×RIPA buffer (50 mM Tris–HCl [pH 8.0], 150 mM NaCl, 1 mM EDTA, 1% NP40, 0.25% sodium deoxychorate (DOC), 0.05% SDS) supplemented with 1× protease inhibitor cocktail (Roche) and 10 mM N-ethylmaleimide (NEM), and subjected to sonication. After that, samples were incubated with 50 U of Benzonase and 2.5 mM $MgCl_2$ for 1 h at 16 °C. Following centrifugation, equal amounts of supernatant were incubated for 16 h with α-Topo1 polyclonal antibody or Rabbit-IgG at 4 °C. Immunocomplex was recovered by Dyna-Beads ProteinA and washed with 0.5×RIPA buffer, and subjected to WB analysis. For detecting SUMO-1 modification, cells were boiled in Hot-Lysis buffer (10 mM Tris–HCl [pH 8.0], 150 mM NaCl, 2% SDS) supplemented with 1× protease inhibitor cocktail and 10 mM NEM for 10 min, and diluted in 2-fold volume of Hot-Lysis Dilution buffer (10 mM Tris–HCl [pH 8.0], 150 mM NaCl, 1 mM EDTA, 1% TrironX-100) supplemented with 10 mM NEM. After the sonication, samples were incubated for 1 h with 50 U of Benzonase and 2.5 mM MgCl$_2$ at 16 °C. Following centrifugation, samples were further diluted in 19-fold volume of Hot-Lysis Dilution buffer (at this time concentration of SDS was 0.05%), and equal amounts of supernatant were incubated for 16 h with α-Topo1 monoclonal antibody or Mouse-IgM at 4 °C. Immunocomplex was recovered by ProteinL magnetic beads (Thermo Scientific) and washed with Hot Lysis Wash buffer (10 mM Tris–HCl [pH 8.0], 250 mM NaCl, 1 mM EDTA, 1% NP40), and subjected to WB analysis.

Flow cytometry (FCM) analysis

Two days before Dox treatment, Mit-23 cells were transfected with indicated siRNA (50 nM) or plasmid DNA by Lipofectamine RNAiMax or Lipofectamine 2000 transfection reagent, respectively. After culturing cells in the presence of Dox (3 µg/ml) for 1 day, we harvested cells and suspended in freshly prepared 70% ethanol. Recovered cells were kept for 2 h at −20 °C. After that, cells were suspended in FCM buffer [PBS (+) supplemented with 4% FBS and 0.1% TritonX-100] and left at 4 °C for 30 min. For γH2AX-staining, cells were incubated with 100 µl of FCM buffer supplemented with 0.5 µg of α-γH2AX-antibody FITC conjugated (Millipore). After incubation for 2 h at 4 °C, samples were washed three time with FCM buffer, and then nuclear staining was achieved by propidium iodide (1 µg/ml)/PBS (−) supplemented with RNaseA (200 µg/ml). After treatment for 1 h at room temperature in the dark place, FCM analysis was performed by FACSCalibur on at least 10,000 cells.

Neutral comet assay

Neutral comet assay was performed following the manufacturer's instruction (Trevigen) with some modification. Briefly, Mit-23 cells were harvested by 2 mM EDTA/PBS (−). Differentiated MM-6 cells were detached by Accutase (Innovative Cell Technologies) and collected. After resuspension in PBS (−), cells were embedded in Low-Melting Agarose (Trevigen), spread and solidified over the Comet Slides (Trevigen) on ice. The slides were immersed in Lysis Buffer (Trevigen) for at least 1 h, and then incubated in neutral electrophoresis buffer (0.1 M Tris-Ac [pH 9.0], 0.3 M NaOAc·3H$_2$O) for 30 min at 4 °C. After electrophoresis for 1 h at 0.75 V/cm at 4 °C, samples were fixed in precipitation buffer (1 M NH$_4$Ac, 85%

ethanol) and 70% ethanol. After staining nuclei by SyBr gold, images were captured by (BZ-X710, Keyence) with 20× objectives utilizing function of Z-stacks and image stitching for obtaining with high resolution image of large field. Integrated images were analysed by Comet Assay IV software (Perceptive Instruments) using "Olive-tail moment" as a parameter of extent of DSB. Olive-tail moment generally indicate the extent of DNA damages, which calculated by product of the tail length and the fraction of total DNA in the tail. In Comet Assay IV software (Perceptive Instruments), "Olive-tail moment" is defined as: the product of the proportion of tail intensity and the displacement of tail center of mass relative to the center of the head. In all experiments, at least 80 nuclei were subjected to analysis.

Pull-down assay of negative supercoiled DNA

U2OS/2-6-3 cells were transfected with indicated plasmid DNA by Viafect transfection reagent (Promega). After 2 days of transfection, 5 × 10^6 cells were suspended in 250 µl of RSB (10 mM Tris [pH 7.5], 10 mM NaCl, 3 mM MgCl$_2$) and combined with 3.5 ml of RSB with 0.1% NP40. After gentle mixing, cells were centrifuged at 500×g for 10 min at 4 °C. Nuclear pellet was suspended in PBS (−) supplemented with 5 µM of Ez-Link Psoralen-PEG$_3$-Biotin (bPso) (Thermo scientific) for 30 min at 4 °C. After centrifugation at 500×g at 4 °C for 10 min, pellet was suspended in 100 µl of PBS (−) and removed to 96-well plate. For cross-linking the bPso to DNA, 365 nm wavelength of UV (UVL-21, UVP) was irradiated for 30 min on ice, and then collected nuclei were lysed in sonication buffer (50 mM Tris [pH 7.5], 140 mM NaCl, 1 mM EDTA, 1 mM EGTA, 1% TritonX-100, 0.1% DOC, 0.1% SDS) supplemented with 1× protease inhibitor cocktail. To obtain the DNA fragment with average size of 250 bp, sonication was carried out following conditions: 20 cycles of 30 s-ON/30 s-OFF, using Bioruptor UCD-250 (Cosmo Bio). After that, samples were centrifuged at 16,000×g for 30 min at 4 °C, and obtained supernatants was gently mixed with SA-beads blocked with 0.5% BSA and 100 µg/ml salmon sperm DNA at least 12 h. SA-beads were sequentially washed with RIPA buffer (50 mM Tris–HCl [pH 8.0], 150 mM NaCl, 1 mM EDTA, 1% NP40, 0.5% DOC, 0.1% SDS) for 10 min, High salt wash buffer (50 mM Tris–HCl [pH 8.0], 500 mM NaCl, 1 mM EDTA, 1% NP40, 0.5% DOC, 0.1% SDS) for 15 min, LiCl wash buffer (50 mM Tris–HCl [pH 8.0], 250 mM LiCl, 1 mM EDTA, 1% NP40, 0.5% DOC) for 15 min, and 1×TE buffer (10 mM Tris–HCl [pH 8.0], 1 mM EDTA) for 10 min twice. All processes were performed at 4 °C on rotating platform. After washing, SA-beads was treated with RNaseA (1 mg/ml) in 1×TE buffer for 30 min at 37 °C, and ProteinaseK (100 µg/ml) with 0.5% SDS for 1 h at 55 °C.

And then supernatant was purified by phenol–chloroform extraction (fraction-1). Furthermore, residual DNA on SA-beads was further extracted by 95% formamide with 10 mM EDTA for 10 min at 90 °C (fraction-2). Combined fractions were purified by ethanol precipitation, and purified DNA was dissolved in 1×TE buffer and subjected to qPCR analysis with SyBr Premix ExTaq Tli RNaseH plus (TaKaRa) by StepOne Real-time PCR system. Oligonucleotides used in this procedure are listed in (Additional file 20: Table S3).

Chromatin immunoprecipitation (ChIP)

U2OS/2-6-3 cells were transfected with indicated plasmid DNA by Viafect transfection reagent. After the 2 days of transfection, cells were cross-linked with 1% paraformaldehyde for 10 min, followed by quenching with 0.125 M glycine for 5 min at room temperature. After washing with PBS (−) twice, cells were suspended in Buffer-1 (10 mM HEPES [pH 7.5], 10 mM EDTA, 0.5 mM EGTA, 0.75% TritonX-100) supplemented with 1×protease inhibitor cocktail and incubated for 10 min on ice. After the centrifugation at 1700×g for 10 min at 4 °C, collected cells were resuspended in Buffer-2 (10 mM HEPES [pH 7.5], 200 mM NaCl, 1 mM EDTA, 0.5 mM EGTA) supplemented with 1× protease inhibitor cocktail and incubated for 5 min on ice. Subsequently, cells were recovered by centrifugation (1700×g for 10 min at 4 °C), and lysed in SDS lysis buffer (50 mM Tris–HCl [pH 8.0], 10 mM EDTA, 1% SDS) supplemented with 1× protease inhibitor cocktail. After fragmentation to average length of 250 bp, samples were centrifuged at 16,000×g for 30 min at 4 °C, and obtained supernatants were diluted in 9-fold volume of ChIP Dilution buffer (50 mM Tris–HCl [pH 8.0], 167 mM NaCl, 1.1% TritonX-100, 0.11% DOC). After pre-clearing with ProteinG Sepharose beads and IgG Sepharose beads, 2 µg of α-RPA70 monoclonal-antibody or mouse-IgG were added to each aliquot of chromatin lysate, and incubated on rotating platform for over 12 h at 4 °C. Immunocomplex was recovered by Dynabeads ProteinG blocked with 0.5% BSA and 100 µg/ml salmon sperm DNA. After 1 h incubation, beads were extensively washed as described in "Pull-down assay of negative supercoiled DNA", and incubated for 6 h at 65 °C in 1×TE buffer supplemented with 250 mM NaCl and 0.5% SDS, and treated with RNaseA (1 mg/ml) for 30 min at 37 °C, and ProteinaseK (100 µg/ml) for 1 h at 55 °C. At this time, input DNA was treated as same way. For eluting DNA, beads were incubated with 0.1 M NaHCO₃ and 1% SDS for 30 min at 65 °C, and recovered DNA was purified by phenol–chloroform extraction and ethanol precipitation. Purified DNA was dissolved in 1×TE

buffer and subjected to qPCR analysis. Oligonucleotides used in this procedure are listed in (Additional file 20: Table S3).

Native-ChIP

For detecting Topo1-cc (covalent complex of Topo1 and DNA), ChIP assay without cross-linking was performed. U2OS/2-6-3 cells were transfected with indicated plasmid DNA by Viafect transfection reagent. After 2 days of transfection, cells were treated with MG-132 (50 µM) for 2 h, and directly lysed in Buffer-M. DNA–protein covalent complex was recovered by ethanol precipitation as described. Pellets were dissolved in SDS lysis buffer supplemented with 1× protease inhibitor cocktail and sonicated. Following dilution, immunoprecipitation was performed with α-Topo1 polyclonal-antibody or Rabbit IgG. Immunocomplex was recovered by DynaBeads ProteinA blocked with 0.5% BSA and 100 µg/ml salmon sperm DNA, and washed as with the ChIP protocol. Collected beads were incubated in 1×TE with RNaseA (1 mg/ml) for 30 min at 37 °C, ProteinaseK (100 µg/ml) with 0.5% SDS for 1 h at 55 °C, and 0.1 M NaHCO₃ with 1% SDS for 30 min at 65 °C. Eluted DNA was purified, and analysed by qPCR as in standard ChIP assay. Oligonucleotides used in this procedure are listed in (Additional file 20: Table S3).

DNA/RNA hybrids immunoprecipitation (DRIP)

Genomic DNA was purified by DNeasy Blood & Tissue Kit (Qiagen) or Buffer-M according to RADAR protocol [39]. Following sonication, samples were treated with or without of RNaseH (20 U, NEB) in 1×RNaseH Reaction buffer overnight at 37 °C. After purification, DNA pellets were dissolved in DRIP buffer (50 mM Tris–HCl [pH 8.0], 150 mM NaCl, 1 mM EDTA, 0.05% TritonX-100), and incubated with S9.6 antibody (KeraFast) or mouse IgG for 12 h at 4 °C on rotating platform. Following processes were performed as with Native-ChIP, and analysed by qPCR as in standard ChIP assay. The promotor and terminator regions of *Actin* gene were analysed by the qPCR analysis, as negative and positive control of DRIP assay, respectively [69]. Oligonucleotides used in this procedure are listed in (Additional file 20: Table S3).

Ligation-mediated (LM)-PCR

LM-PCR experiments were performed according to a protocol previously reported [41] with some modifications. In brief, after 2 days of transfection, cells were directly lysed in HMW buffer (10 mM Tris–HCl [pH 7.5], 100 mM NaCl, 1 mM EDTA, 0.5% SDS) supplemented with ProteinaseK (200 µg/ml), and incubated overnight at 55 °C without agitation. After phenol–chloroform extraction, same volume of isopropanol was added to sample, and DNA was gently picked up and rinsed with 70% ethanol. Recovered DNA was suspended in $1 \times$ TE supplemented with RNaseA (100 µg/ml). Equal amounts of DNA was treated with Quick-Blunting Kit (NEB) and ligated with blunt-end linkers (JW-Linker: annealed JW102 with JW103). Following purification, equal amounts of DNA were subjected to qPCR analysis with LacO-Rev and JW102 primers using SyBr Premix ExTaq Tli RNaseH plus. For estimating the amounts of LacO/JW-linker junction, corresponding DNA fragment was cloned into pMD20, and used as standard sample. The qPCR against to *β-globin* was carried out in parallel to normalize the amounts of input DNA. Oligonucleotides used in this procedure are listed in (Additional file 20: Table S3).

Fluorescence recovery after photobleaching (FRAP) assay

For FRAP assay, newly established cell lines: Mit-23 with H2B(Wt)-GFP or H2B(K120R)-GFP, HT1080vRxt-Vpr-Wt or -Q65R with H2B(Wt)-GFP, in which pEF-Bos-H2B-GFP was stably transduced to Mit-23 or HT1080vRxt-Vpr, were treated with Dox (3 µg/ml) for 1.5 days. Images were obtained by a Leica TCS SP5 confocal microscope with a Leica HCX APO $100 \times /1.40$–0.60 oil immersion lens, and obtained data were analysed by Leica LAS AF Lite software (Leica). For GFP excitation, we used the 488 nm line of an Argon laser and fluorescence emission was collected between 500 and 530 nm. All experiments were done on warmed stage at 37 °C. In experiments, pre-bleach image was acquired by three consecutive images. Then a single square on the nucleus was bleached with five times of laser pulses of 1.318 s at 100% power. Images were then collected at 10 s intervals for 180 s. For calculating the rate of FRAP, the background signals (ROI^B) were subtracted from the region of interest for bleached area (ROI^+) and un-bleached area (ROI^-). The corrected signal of ROI^+ was normalized by ROI^- at each time point, and relative signal intensity compared to pre-bleaching (ROI^0) was used to evaluate the change of GFP intensity, according to the equation;

$$\text{Relative signal intensity}$$
$$= \{(ROI^+ - ROI^B) \div (ROI^- - ROI^B)\}$$
$$\div (ROI^0 - ROI^B)$$

The recovery of GFP signal intensity was expressed by subtracting the relative signal intensity of immediately after bleaching from that of each time point. In all experiments, at least 10 cells were subjected to analysis.

Production of pseudotyped HIV-1

For production of Vesicular Stomatitis Virus Glycoprotein (VSV-G) pseudotyped HIV-1, HEK293T cells were co-transfected with pNL4-3/E- and pHIT-VSV-G using FuGENE6 transfection reagent (Promega). On the next day, culture medium was changed to DMEM supplemented with 0.1% FBS. On the day 2 after transfection, culture supernatant containing the virus were recovered and filtered through a 0.45 µm-filter, and viral titer was determined by p24 ELISA kit (Zeptometrics). NL4-3-Luc/E- and NL4-3-EGFP/E-, which contains *Luciferase* and *EGFP* in-frame of *Nef*, were prepared as same manner. Viral samples were treated with DNase I (Takara) before infection.

Lentivirus production

Lentivirus was produced using Virapower Lentiviral packaging mix (Invitrogen) according to a manufacturer's instruction with some modification. Briefly, HEK293T cells were co-transfected with pLenti6, pLP1-D64A, pLP2, and pLP-VSV-G using Lipofectamine 2000 transfection reagent. Culture medium was replaced to fresh medium at 16 h after transfection. On the day 2 after transfection, culture supernatant containing the virus was filtered through a 0.45 µm-filter and ultra-centrifuged at 40,000 rpm for 1 h at 4 °C (Optima TLX ultracentrifuge, Beckman Coulter). After removing supernatant, viral pellet was dissolved in Opti-MEM (Life technologies), and viral titer was determined by p24 ELISA kit. Viral samples were treated with DNase I before infection.

HIV-1 infection to MM-6 cells

For pseudotyped HIV-1 infection, 2.5×10^5 MM-6 cells were differentiated by 50 nM of PMA for 3 days in 12-well plate. In RNAi experiments, cells were transfected with 300 nM of indicated siRNA by Nucleofector Kit-V and suspended in PMA containing medium. After 3 days, NL4-3 viral solution (p24, 50 ng) was added, and incubated for 2 h. Following washing twice with prewarmed medium, cells were cultured in PMA containing medium for additional 1 or 2 days, for neutral comet assay or *Alu-gag* two-step nested qPCR analysis, respectively. For luciferase assay, cell cultures (50,000 cells/well, in 96well plate) at 3 days post-infection (dpi) were directly lysed in equal volume of One-Glo Luciferase assay system (Promega) solution, and relative light units (RLU) were measured by microplate luminometer (Veritas). For FCM analysis of EGFP, cells were fixed with 1% paraformaldehyde at least 30 min at room temperature at 3dpi, and analysed by FACSCalibur on at least 10,000 cells.

HIV-1 infection to MDMs

For pseudotyped HIV-1 infection, 2.5×10^5 MDMs were differentiated by 25–50 ng/ml of rhM-CSF for 5 days in 12-well plate. In RNAi experiments, cells were transfected with 50 nM of indicated siRNA by Lipo-fectamine RNAiMax transfection reagent for 4 h and replaced to rhM-CSF containing medium. After 2 days of transfection, NL4-3 viral solution (p24, 12.5 ng) was added, and incubated for 2 h. Following washing twice with pre-warmed medium, cells were cultured in rhM-CSF containing medium. *Alu-gag* two-step nested qPCR analysis was performed at 2dpi.

HIV-1 infection to U2OS/2-6-3 cells and analysis of LacO-directed integration

U2OS/2-6-3 cells of 5×10^5 were transfected with indi-cated plasmid DNA by Viafect transfection reagent. After 2 days of transfection, cells were incubated with NL4-3 viral solution (p24, 100 ng) for 2 days, and subjected to qPCR analysis. Genomic DNA was extracted using Quickgene Nucleic acid isolation system (KURABO). The qPCR was done with LacO-(sense or antisense), Lenti-5237F, and TaqMan probe (pLenti6-LTR probe) using SsoAdvance universal probe Supermix by StepOne Real-time system. To measure copy numbers of inte-grated viral DNA that possessed the LacO/proviral DNA junction, corresponding DNA fragment was cloned into pMD20 and used as standard samples. In parallel, qPCR for *β-globin* was performed for normalization of input DNA. At this time, *Alu-gag* two-step nested qPCR was performed and measuring the overall infectivity. Oligo-nucleotides used in this procedure are listed in (Addi-tional file 20: Table S3).

Alu-gag two-step nested qPCR
Genomic DNA was extracted using Quickgene Nucleic acid isolation system, and 100 ng of DNA was subjected to 12 cycles of *Alu-gag* 1st PCR using AmpliTaq gold 360 with Alu-F/R and 1st-gag-R. And then, qPCR was per-formed with 2-LTR-S and 2nd tag-R, and TaqMan probe (Probe-2). For determining the frequency of the integra-tion, gDNA containing 0.485 copies of HIV integration/cell [8] was subjected to amplification at the same time. The qPCR against to *β-globin* was carried out in paral-lel to normalizing the amounts of input DNA. Oligonu-cleotides used in this procedure are listed in (Additional file 20: Table S3).

Lentivirus infection to U2OS/2-6-3 cells and analysis of LacO-directed integration
Lentiviral solution (p24, 100 ng) was infected to 2.5×10^5 U2OS/2-6-3 cells for 2 days. To quantitate the LacO-directed integration, gDNA was subjected to qPCR analysis with LacO-(sense or antisense)/Lenti-5237F, and TaqMan probe (pLenti6-LTR probe). For measuring the overall infectivity, cells were cultured in the presence of BlasticidineS (10 µg/ml) for 2 weeks. For normalizing

the plating efficiency, colonies were formed in normal culture medium. Colonies were fixed with 70% ethanol and stained with Giemsa's staining solution, and enumer-ated. Oligonucleotides used in this procedure are listed in (Additional file 20: Table S3).

Cre mediated expression of Cherry-LacR-Vpr
U2OS/2-6-3+pCAL-loxP-CLV (263/loxP-CLV), in which expression of LacR-fused Vpr was switched on when Cre-recombinase was expressed, were first established by G418 selection. Then, cells were infected with adeno-virus for LacZ (control) or Cre (inducing CLV expres-sion) expression at multiplicity of infection (MOI) of 100 for 2 days, and subjected to live cell imaging and ChIP assay for Vpr (Additional file 8: Figure S7a, b). For siRNA experiments, 2.5×10^5 cells were transfected with control or *Topo1* siRNA (50 nM) by Lipofectamine RNAiMax transfection reagent. After 1.5 days of siRNA transfection, adenovirus was infected for 2 days, and cells were subjected to following analysis; LacO-directed inte-gration, native-ChIP assay for Topo1-cc and LM-PCR (Fig. 7g and Additional file 8: Figure S7c, d, respectively). Oligonucleotides used in this procedure are listed in (Additional file 20: Table S3).

Linear amplification mediated-PCR
LAM-PCR was performed, as previously described [8] with some modification. Briefly, 1st liner PCR was per-formed using biotinylated-Lenti-5203F primer by two round of amplification with 50 cycles using Taq poly-merase (Qiagen). After purification by SA-beads, dsDNA was synthesized with Klenow fragment (NEB) with ran-dom hexamer. Following extensive washes, dsDNA on SA-beads were digested with *Msp*I or *Nla*III, and ligated with corresponding dsDNA linker cassettes (LC). After that, 1st PCR was performed with biotinylated-M667/LC1, followed by SA-beads purification. And then, 2nd exponential PCR was performed with EV984/LC2. Size selection of amplified DNA was performed on agarose gel, and cloned into pGEM-T Easy vector. Sequenc-ing was carried out by ABI3130x (Applied Biosystems), and integration sites were determined. Oligonucleotides used in this procedure are listed in (Additional file 20: Table S3).

Quantitative reverse-transcription-PCR (qRT-PCR)
Total RNA was purified by RNeasy kit (Qiagen), and cDNA was generated by HighCapacity cDNA reverse transcription kit (Invitrogen). Quantitative-PCR was per-formed using SyBr premix ExTaq Tli RNaseH plus. The expression levels of each gene were normalized by the relative amounts of *β-Actin*. The primers used for qRT-PCR are listed in (Additional file 21: Table S4).

Additional files

Additional file 1: Figure S1. Vpr induces structural alteration of DNA. **a** Representative AFM images of dsDNA in 1.0 μm × 1.0 μm field. **b** Representative raw data of Rq values of dsDNA. The Rq values of each dsDNA are shown as a plot, and the medians are indicated by red bars. **c** Relative Rq values of Vpr mutants. C-terminal mutants of Vpr were defective in DNA structural alteration. Data were obtained from more than three independent experiments. Error bar indicates ± SEM. In Fig. 1b, data of Buffer, Chlq, Wt, ΔC12 and Ct4RA are depicted.

Additional file 2: Figure S2. The interaction between Vpr and RPA70 (a) or T4gp32 (b) was not detected. **a** FLAG-Strep-Vpr (0.1, 0.317. 1.0 pmol) was incubated with rRPA70 (1.0 pmol), and pulled-down with Streptavidine M280 beads. Proteins were analysed by WB with indicated antibodies. **b** FLAG-Strep-Vpr (1, 3.17, 10 pmol) was incubated with T4gp32 (100 pmol), and pulled-down with Streptavidine M280 beads. Proteins were visualized by Oriole fluorescent gel staining.

Additional file 3: Figure S3. Vpr provokes Topo1 stress. **a** RADAR analysis detecting covalently bound DNA and Topo1. HEK293T cells were transfected with indicated Topo1-HA construct. Y723F is a catalytically inactive mutant of Topo1. A covalent complex of Topo1 and DNA was formed in the cells that were first transduced with Topo1-Wt, and then treated with CPT (20 μM, 1 h) or paraformaldehyde (PFA; 1 mM, 2 h), whereas the complex was only detected in cells with Topo1-Y723F when treated with PFA, but not with CPT. The same membrane was reprobed with α-dsDNA antibody after stripping. **b** Different amounts of DNA were blotted in the RADAR analysis.

Additional file 4: Table S1. Knockdown efficiency of siRNA target genes. Relative expression levels compared to cont-si (100%: shaded) are shown. Data were obtained from at least three independent experiments.

Additional file 5: Figure S4. Vpr-induced DNA damages are suppressed by TDP1 or RNaseH1 expression. **a** Exogenous expression of RNaseH1 (RNH1) and TDP1. Mit-23 cells were transfected with indicated vector (pFLAG-CMV2 based vector), and whole cell extracts were subjected to WB analysis. Arrowhead (black), TDP1; arrow, RNaseH1; arrowhead (red), Vpr; asterisk, non-specific bands. **b** RNH1 and TDP1 suppresses Vpr induced DDR. Mit-23 cells transfected with RNH1 or TDP1 showed reduced level of Vpr-induced phosphorylation of H2AX. A representative result out of two independent experiments is depicted.

Additional file 6: Figure S5. Forced accumulation of Vpr induced DDR in the vicinity of chromatin. **a–e** Forced accumulation of Vpr induces phosphorylation of H2AX at Ser139 (a), ATM at Ser1981 (b), RPA32 at Ser33 (c), Rad17 at Ser645 (d), and accumulation of mono- and poly-ubiquitin conjugates (e), on surrounding region.

Additional file 7: Figure S6. LM-PCR for detecting DSB-ends in the LacO repeats. **a**. Schematic of LM-PCR. Genomic DNA samples prepared from cells, which were transduced with LacR-construct were treated with T4 polymerase and T4 PNK for blunting the DSB ends, and ligated with blunt-end JW-linkers. LacO/JW-linker junctions were amplified by specific primers, shown in (b). **b**. Diagram of LacO/JW-linker amplification product. Arrows above the box indicate the PCR primers for JW-linker and LacO. **c** Sequencing chromatogram of LacO/JW-linker junction. Black arrow and red arrow indicate JW-linker and LacO repeats, respectively. **d** Representative amplification plot of LacO/JW-qPCR. Cherry-LacR fused-OVA, Black; -Fok1, blue; -Vpr, red curve. Gray curve show the standard samples with indicated copy numbers.

Additional file 8: Figure S7. Topo1 is involved in Vpr-induced DDR and DSB. **a** Live cell imaging of CLV inducible cell line. To confirm effect of Vpr on Topo1-cc formation, we transfected pCAL-loxP-CLV to U2OS/2-6-3 cells, and obtained a cell line (263/loxP-CLV), in which expression of a Cherry-LacR fused Vpr (CLV) can be switched on after Cre expression. In the experiment, 263/loxP-CLV cells were infected with adenoviruses expressing LacZ (Ad-LacZ) or Cre (Ad-Cre) for 2 days at MOI of 100. Single focus of mCherry was distinctly observed in Ad-Cre infected cells (lower panel), suggesting that CLV was expressed in Cre-dependent manner. Scale bar indicates 20 μm. **b** Specific accumulation of CLV on the LacO repeats.

ChIP assay with α-Vpr antibody (8D1) was performed in 263/loxP-CLV cells infected with Ad-LacZ or -Cre at 2dpi. **c** Down regulation of *Topo1* reduces Vpr induced Topo1-cc on the LacO repeats. After downregulation of *Topo1*, 263/loxP-CLV cells, which were infected with Ad-Cre, was subjected to native-ChIP assay with α-Topo1 antibody. A representative result out of two independent experiments is depicted. **d** Topo1 is required for Vpr-induced DSB on the LacO repeats. After downregulation of *Topo1*, 263/loxP-CLV cells were infected with Ad-LacZ or -Cre, and subjected to LM-PCR analysis to measure the extent of DSB on the LacO repeats. Vpr-induced DSB was calculated by subtracting the amounts of DSB observed in Ad-LacZ infected cells from those observed in Ad-Cre infected cells. Data were obtained from three independent experiments.

Additional file 9: Figure S8. Representative data of Lenti-LacO qPCR for detecting the LacO-directed integration. **a, b** Amplification plots of sense integration (a) and anti-sense integration (b), respectively. Blue (light blue ~ dark blue) and red (pink ~ red) curves show CV- and CLV-virus infected samples with different MOIs shown by amounts of p24, respectively. Gray curves indicate standard samples with indicated copy numbers. **c, d** Sequencing chromatograms of sense (c) and anti-sense (d) integration product. Blue arrows and red arrows indicate 3'-LTR and LacO repeats, respectively.

Additional file 10: Figure S9. Proviral integration in the vicinity of Vpr-induced DSB sites. Targeting of HIV-1 proviral DNA to CLV-induced DSB sites. U2OS/2-6-3 cells were first transfected with indicated construct, and then infected with NL-4-3/D64A/R− virus. The percentages of LacO directed integration per overall integration (*Alu-gag* two-step qPCR) are shown. Data were obtained from three independent experiments. Error bar indicates ± SEM. In Cherry-Vpr, Cherry-LacR-Vpr, and Fok1-Cherry-LacR, the *P*-value was 0.37, 0.051, and 0.015 for sense integration, respectively. The *P*-value for antisense-integration was 0.44, 0.001, and 5.21×10^{-5}, respectively.

Additional file 11: Figure S10. Schematic of *Alu-gag* two-step nested qPCR. First PCR to amplify *Alu*-proviral DNA junction was performed using PCR primers targeting the *Alu* (black arrow) and *gag* (pink arrows). Red wavy line fused to *gag*-primer indicates the tag-sequence for 2nd qPCR primer binding. In second qPCR, viral DNA fragments were amplified by LTR primer (blue arrow) and tag-primer (red arrow). The green box indicates the position of the TaqMan probe for *gag*.

Additional file 12: Figure S11. Incorporation of Cherry-LacR-Vpr does not affect overall viral infectivity. U2OS/2-6-3 cells infected with indicated lentivirus, which had Blasticidine-resistance gene, were subjected to Blasticidine (Bsd) selection. The infected cells obtain Bsd resistance by the successful lentiviral integration. Data were obtained from three independent experiments. Error bar indicates ± SEM.

Additional file 13: Figure S12. A representative sequencing chromatogram of the LacO/proviral DNA junction, obtained by the LAM-PCR. Blue arrows and red arrows indicate 3'-LTR and LacO repeats, respectively.

Additional file 14: Figure S13. Topo1 is required for Vpr-dependent upregulation of viral infection. **a** MM-6 cells were infected with Vpr proficient (R+) or deficient (R−) NL4-3 viruses under down-regulation of *Topo1* by three species of siRNAs. The integration rate was quantitated by *Alu-gag* two-step nested qPCR at 2dpi; relative integration rates are shown. Data were obtained from more than three independent experiments. Error bar indicates ± SEM. **P < 0.05 **b** Knockdown efficiency of each siRNA. Relative levels of *Topo1* expression are shown. Topo1 siRNA#3 was used in other experiments.

Additional file 15: Figure S14. Vpr upregulates viral infection in differentiated MM-6 cells. **a** MM-6 cells were infected with Vpr proficient (R+) or deficient (R−) NL4-3-Luc/E- viruses. Luciferase assay was performed at 3dpi. Data were obtained from more than three independent experiments. Error bar indicates ± SEM. **b** MM-6 cells were infected with Vpr proficient (R+) or deficient (R−) NL4-3-EGFP/E- viruses. Percentage of EGFP positive cells was determined by FCM at 3dpi. Representative FCM data are shown in bottom panels. Green colored plots were gated as EGFP positive cells.

Additional file 16: Figure S15. XPG is required for Vpr-induced DDR and DSB. **a, b** Effects of downregulation of XPG on Vpr-induced DDR. The expression of *XPG* in Mit-23 cells was first downregulated by siRNA, and then Vpr expression was initiated on day 2 after introduction of *XPG* targeting siRNA. On day 1 after Vpr expression was started, phosphorylation of H2AX (a) and G$_2$/M checkpoint activation (b) was analysed by flow cytometry. Downregulation of *XPG* significantly reduced Vpr-induced phosphorylation of H2AX ($P = 4.4 \times 10^{-5}$), and the G$_2$/M arrest ($P = 0.025$). Data were obtained from three independent experiments. Error bar indicates ± SEM. **c** XPG is required for Vpr-induced DSBs. Neutral comet assay was performed using Mit-23 cell, the *XPG* expression of which was down-regulated. Data were obtained from three independent experiments. Error bar indicates ± SEM. $P = 0.037$. **d** XPG is required for rVpr-induced DSB in resting macrophages. Differentiated MM-6 cells were treated with 100 ng/ml of rVpr under the down-regulation of *XPG*, and subjected to neutral comet assay. Data were obtained from three independent experiments. Error bar indicates ± SEM. $P = 0.001$. **e** XPG is required for Vpr-induced upregulation of viral infection in resting macrophages. Differentiated MM-6 cells were infected with Vpr proficient (R+) or deficient (R−) NL4-3 viruses after transfection of siRNA, and the integration rate was quantitated by *Alu-gag* two-step nested qPCR; relative integration rates are shown. A representative result out of two independent experiments is depicted.

Additional file 17: Figure S16. Forced accumulation of Vpr increases formation of R-loops. **a** U2OS/2-6-3 cells were transfected with indicated LacR fused constructs. Two days after transfection, DNA samples were prepared and subjected to DRIP assay. DRIP assay was done with α-DNA/RNA hybrids antibody (S9.6). RNaseH treatments were performed to confirm the specificity of DRIP assay. Analysis of promotor (green column) and terminator (yellow column) regions of *Actin* gene were included in the qPCR analysis, as negative and positive control of DRIP assay, respectively. A representative result out of two independent experiments is depicted. **b** 263/loxP-CLV cells were infected with Ad-LacZ or -Cre. DNA samples were prepared and subjected to DRIP assay at 2dpi. Data were obtained from more than three independent experiments. Error bar indicates ± SEM.

Additional file 18: Figure S17. C-terminus of Vpr is required for topoisomer induction activity. DNA supercoiling assay was performed with increasing amounts of peptides (1, 10, 100 pmol; 0.015, 0.15, 1.5 Vpr molecules/bp). In the presence of C45, faster migrating topoisomers appeared.

Additional file 19: Table S2. List of resources used in this study.

Additional file 20: Table S3. List of oligonucleotides used in this study.

Additional file 21: Table S4. List of primers for qRT-PCR.

Abbreviations
AFM: atomic force microscopy; ATR: ataxia-telangiectasia and Rad3-related; cART: combined antiretroviral therapy; ChIP: chromatin immunoprecipitation; CPT: camptothecin; DDR: DNA damage response; DSB: DNA double-strand break; FRAP: fluorescence recovery after photo-bleaching; HIV-1: human immunodeficiency virus-1; LM-PCR: ligation-mediated (LM)-PCR; MDMs: monocyte derived macrophages; MOI: multiplicity of infection; RADAR: rapid approach to DNA adducts recovery; RPA70: replication protein A 70-kDa subunit; SSB: DNA single-strand break; Topo1: topoisomerase 1; Topo1-cc: Topo1-covalent complex; Vpr: viral protein R.

Authors' contributions
KI conducted all experiments, and JK performed FRAP analysis. KI and YI designed the experiments and wrote the paper. All authors read and approved the final manuscript.

Author details
[1] Department of Intractable Diseases, National Center for Global Health and Medicine, 1-21-1 Toyama, Shinjuku-ku, Tokyo 162-8655, Japan. [2] Department of Genome Repair Dynamics, Radiation Biology Center, Kyoto University, Yoshidakonoe-cho, Sakyo-ku, Kyoto 606-8501, Japan.

Acknowledgements
We thank Dr. Mari Shimura for Mit-23 cells, Dr. David Spector for U2OS/2-6-3 cells, Dr. Evi Soutoglou for the Cherry-LacR construct, and Dr. Kenzo Tokunaga for the pNL4-3 vector. FRAP and AFM analyses were supported by the Radiation Biology Center Cooperative Research Program (Kyoto University), and One-stop Sharing Facility Center for Future Drug Discovery (The University of Tokyo), respectively.

Competing interests
The authors declare that they have no competing interests.

Funding
This work was supported in part by JSPS KAKENHI Grant Number JP26860313, Grant for National Center for Global Health and Medicine (21A-129), Grant-in-Aid for Research on HIV/AIDS Project from the Ministry of Health, Labor and Welfare of Japan, and the National Center for Global Health and Medicine (25A-108).

References
1. Trono D, Van Lint C, Rouzioux C, Verdin E, Barré-Sinoussi F, Chun TW, et al. HIV persistence and the prospect of long-term drug-free remissions for HIV-infected individuals. Science. 2010;329:174–80.
2. Iglesias-Ussel MD, Romerio F. HIV reservoirs: the new frontier. AIDS Rev. 2011;13:13–29.
3. Abbas W, Tariq M, Iqbal M, Kumar A, Herbein G. Eradication of HIV-1 from the macrophage reservoir: an uncertain goal? Viruses. 2015;7:1578–98.
4. Cohen EA, Dehni G, Sodroski JG, Haseltine WA. Human immunodeficiency virus vpr product is a virion-associated regulatory protein. J Virol. 1990;64:3097–9.
5. Balliet JW, Kolson DL, Eiger G, Kim FM, McGann KA, Srinivasan A, et al. Distinct effects in primary macrophages and lymphocytes of the human immunodeficiency virus type 1 accessory genes vpr, vpu, and nef: mutational analysis of a primary HIV-1 isolate. Virology. 1994;200:623–31.
6. Connor RI, Chen BK, Choe S, Landau NR. Vpr is required for efficient replication of human immunodeficiency virus type-1 in mononuclear phagocytes. Virology. 1995;206:935–44.
7. Eckstein DA, Sherman MP, Penn ML, Chin PS, De Noronha CM, Greene WC, et al. HIV-1 Vpr enhances viral burden by facilitating infection of tissue macrophages but not nondividing CD4+ T cells. J Exp Med. 2001;194:1407–19.
8. Koyama T, Sun B, Tokunaga K, Tatsumi M, Ishizaka Y. DNA damage enhances integration of HIV-1 into macrophages by overcoming integrase inhibition. Retrovirology. 2013;10:21.
9. Guenzel CA, Hérate C, Benichou S. HIV-1 Vpr-a still "enigmatic multitasker". Front Microbiol. 2014;5:127.
10. Roshal M, Kim B, Zhu Y, Nghiem P, Planelles V. Activation of the ATR-mediated DNA damage response by the HIV-1 viral protein R. J Biol Chem. 2003;278:25879–86.
11. Zimmerman ES, Chen J, Andersen JL, Ardon O, Dehart JL, Blackett J, et al. Human immunodeficiency virus type 1 Vpr-mediated G2 arrest requires Rad17 and Hus1 and induces nuclear BRCA1 and gamma-H2AX focus formation. Mol Cell Biol. 2004;24:9286–94.
12. Lai M, Zimmerman ES, Planelles V, Chen J. Activation of the ATR pathway by human immunodeficiency virus type 1 Vpr involves its direct binding to chromatin in vivo. J Virol. 2005;79:15443–551.
13. Nakai-Murakami C, Shimura M, Kinomoto M, Takizawa Y, Tokunaga K, Taguchi T, et al. HIV-1 Vpr induces ATM-dependent cellular signal with enhanced homologous recombination. Oncogene. 2007;26:477–86.
14. Laguette N, Brégnard C, Hue P, Basbous J, Yatim A, Larroque M, et al. Premature activation of the SLX4 complex by Vpr promotes G2/M arrest and escape from innate immune sensing. Cell. 2014;156:134–45.

15. Morellet N, Bouaziz S, Petitjean P, Roques BP. NMR structure of the HIV-1 regulatory protein VPR. J Mol Biol. 2003;327:215–27.

16. Tachiwana H, Shimura M, Nakai-Murakami C, Tokunaga K, Takizawa Y, Sata T, et al. HIV-1 Vpr induces DNA double-strand breaks. Cancer Res. 2006;66:627–31.

17. Shimura M, Tanaka Y, Nakamura S, Minemoto Y, Yamashita K, Hatake K, et al. Micronuclei formation and aneuploidy induced by Vpr, an accessory gene of human immunodeficiency virus type 1. FASEB J. 1999;6:621–37.

18. Groschel B, Bushman F. Cell cycle arrest in G2/M promotes early steps of infection by human immunodeficiency virus. J Virol. 2005;79:5695–704.

19. Zimmerman ES, Sherman MP, Blackett JL, Neidleman JA, Kreis C, Mundt P, et al. Human immunodeficiency virus type 1 Vpr induces DNA replication stress in vitro and in vivo. J Virol. 2006;80:10407–18.

20. Zou L, Elledge SJ. Sensing DNA damage through ATRIP recognition of RPA-ssDNA complexes. Science. 2003;300:1542–8.

21. DeHart JL, Zimmerman ES, Ardon O, Monteiro-Filho CM, Argañaraz ER, Planelles V. HIV-1 Vpr activates the G2 checkpoint through manipulation of the ubiquitin proteasome system. Virol J. 2007;4:57.

22. Belzile JP, Duisit G, Rougeau N, Mercier J, Finzi A, Cohen EA. HIV-1 Vpr-mediated G2 arrest involves the DDB1-CUL4AVPRBP E3 ubiquitin ligase. PLoS Pathog. 2007;3:e85.

23. Belzile JP, Richard J, Rougeau N, Xiao Y, Cohen EA. HIV-1 Vpr induces the K48-linked polyubiquitination and proteasomal degradation of target cellular proteins to activate ATR and promote G2 arrest. J Virol. 2010;84:3320–30.

24. Tan L, Ehrlich E, Yu XF. DDB1 and Cul4A are required for human immuno-deficiency virus type 1 Vpr-induced G2 arrest. J Virol. 2007;81:10822–30.

25. Kichler A, Pages JC, Leborgne C, Druillennec S, Lenoir C, Coulaud D, et al. Efficient DNA transfection mediated by the C-terminal domain of human immunodeficiency virus type 1 viral protein R. J Virol. 2000;74:5424–31.

26. Lyonnais S, Gorelick RJ, Heniche-Boukhalfa F, Bouaziz S, Parissi V, Mouscadet JF, et al. A protein ballet around the viral genome orches-trated by HIV-1 reverse transcriptase leads to an architectural switch: from nucleocapsid-condensed RNA to Vpr-bridged DNA. Virus Res. 2013;171:287–303.

27. Pommier Y, Sun Y, Huang SN, Nitiss JL. Roles of eukaryotic topoisomerases in transcription, replication and genomic stability. Nat Rev Mol Cell Biol. 2016;17:703–21.

28. Sordet O, Redon CE, Guirouilh-Barbat J, Smith S, Solier S, Douarre C, et al. Ataxia telangiectasia mutated activation by transcription- and topoisomerase I-induced DNA double-strand breaks. EMBO Rep. 2009;10:887–93.

29. Eldin P, Chazal N, Fenard D, Bernard E, Guichou JF, Briant L. Vpr expression abolishes the capacity of HIV-1 infected cells to repair uracilated DNA. Nucleic Acids Res. 2014;42:1698–710.

30. Lahouassa H, Blondot ML, Chauveau L, Chougui G, Morel M, Leduc M, et al. HIV-1 Vpr degrades the HLTF DNA translocase in T cells and mac-rophages. Proc Natl Acad Sci USA. 2016;113:5311–6.

31. Murphy PJ, Shannon M, Goertz J. Visualization of recombinant DNA and protein complexes using atomic force microscopy. J Vis Exp. 2011;53:3061.

32. Mizoguchi I, Ooe Y, Hoshino S, Shimura M, Kasahara T, Kano S, et al. Improved gene expression in resting macrophages using an oligopep-tide derived from Vpr of human immunodeficiency virus type-1. Biochem Biophys Res Commun. 2005;338:1499–506.

33. Shamoo Y, Friedman AM, Parsons MR, Konigsberg WH, Steitz TA. Crystal structure of a replication fork single-stranded DNA binding protein (T4 gp32) complexed to DNA. Nature. 1995;376:362–6.

34. Jose D, Weitzel SE, Baase WA, von Hippel PH. Mapping the interactions of the single-stranded DNA binding protein of bacteriophage T4 (gp32) with DNA lattices at single nucleotide resolution: gp32 monomer bind-ing. Nucleic Acids Res. 2015;43:9276–90.

35. Nitiss JL, Soans E, Rogojina A, Seth A, Mishina M. Topoisomerase assays. Curr Protoc Pharmacol. 2012;3:3.3.1–3.27.

36. Desai SD, Zhang H, Rodriguez-Bauman A, Yang JM, Wu X, Gounder MK, et al. Transcription-dependent degradation of topoisomerase I-DNA covalent complexes. Mol Cell Biol. 2003;23:2341–50.

37. Steinacher R, Osman F, Lorenz A, Bryer C, Whitby MC. Slx8 removes Pli1-dependent protein-SUMO conjugates including SUMOylated topoi-somerase I to promote genome stability. PLoS ONE. 2013;8:e71960.

38. Shimura M, Toyoda Y, Iijima K, Kinomoto M, Tokunaga K, Yoda K, et al. Epi-genetic displacement of HP1 from heterochromatin by HIV-1 Vpr causes premature sister chromatid separation. J Cell Biol. 2011;194:721–35.

39. Kiianitsa K, Maizels N. A rapid and sensitive assay for DNA-protein cova-lent complexes in living cells. Nucleic Acids Res. 2013;41:e104.

40. Janicki SM, Tsukamoto T, Salghetti SE, Tansey WP, Sachidanandam R, Prasanth KV, et al. From silencing to gene expression: real-time analysis in single cells. Cell. 2004;116:683–98.

41. Soutoglou E, Dorn JF, Sengupta K, Jasin M, Nussenzweig A, Ried T, Danuser G, Misteli T. Positional stability of single double-strand breaks in mammalian cells. Nat Cell Biol. 2007;9:675–82.

42. Soutoglou E, Misteli T. Activation of the cellular DNA damage response in the absence of DNA lesions. Science. 2008;320:1507–10.

43. Naughton C, Avlonitis N, Corless S, Prendergast JG, Mati IK, Eijk PP, et al. Transcription forms and remodels supercoiling domains unfolding large-scale chromatin structures. Nat Struct Mol Biol. 2013;20:387–95.

44. Anders L, Guenther MG, Qi J, Fan ZP, Marineau JJ, Rahl PB, et al. Genome-wide localization of small molecules. Nat Biotechnol. 2014;32:92–6.

45. Kimura H, Cook PR. Kinetics of core histones in living human cells: little exchange of H3 and H4 and some rapid exchange of H2B. J Cell Biol. 2001;153:1341–53.

46. Tóth KF, Knoch TA, Wachsmuth M, Frank-Stöhr M, Stöhr M, Bacher CP, et al. Trichostatin A-induced histone acetylation causes decondensation of interphase chromatin. J Cell Sci. 2004;117:4277–87.

47. Daniel R, Ramcharan J, Rogakou E, Taganov KD, Greger JG, Bonner W, et al. Histone H2AX is phosphorylated at sites of retroviral DNA integration but is dispensable for postintegration repair. J Biol Chem. 2004;279:45810–4.

48. Cooper A, García M, Petrovas C, Yamamoto T, Koup RA, Nabel GJ. HIV-1 causes CD4 cell death through DNA-dependent protein kinase during viral integration. Nature. 2013;498:376–9.

49. Beard P, Hughes M, Nyfeler K, Hoey M. Unwinding of the DNA helix in simian virus 40 chromosome templates by RNA polymerase. Eur J Bio-chem. 1984;143:39–45.

50. Sekulic N, Bassett EA, Rogers DJ, Black BE. The structure of (CENP-A-H4)₂ reveals physical features that mark centromeres. Nature. 2010;467:347–51.

51. Pavri R, Zhu B, Li G, Trojer P, Mandal S, Shilatifard A, et al. Histone H2B monoubiquitination functions cooperatively with FACT to regulate elongation by RNA polymerase II. Cell. 2006;125:703–17.

52. Nakamura K, Kato A, Kobayashi J, Yanagihara H, Sakamoto S, Oliveira DV, et al. Regulation of homologous recombination by RNF20-dependent H2B ubiquitination. Mol Cell. 2011;41:515–28.

53. Zeng M, Ren L, Mizuno K, Nestoras K, Wang H, Tang Z, et al. CRL4(Wdr70) regulates H2B monoubiquitination and facilitates Exo1-dependent resec-tion. Nat Commun. 2016;7:11364.

54. Taneichi D, Iijima K, Doi A, Koyama T, Minemoto Y, Tokunaga K, et al. Iden-tification of SNF2 h, a chromatin-remodeling factor, as a novel binding protein of Vpr of human immunodeficiency virus type 1. J Neuroimmune Pharmacol. 2011;6:177–87.

55. Maudet C, Sourisce A, Dragin L, Lahouassa H, Rain JC, Bouaziz S, et al. HIV-1 Vpr induces the degradation of ZIP and sZIP, adaptors of the NuRD chromatin remodeling complex, by hijacking DCAF1/VprBP. PLoS ONE. 2013;8:e77320.

56. Romani B, Baygloo NS, Hamidi-Fard M, Aghasadeghi MR, Allahbakhshi E. HIV-1 Vpr protein induces proteasomal degradation of chromatin-associated class I HDACs to overcome latent infection of macrophages. J Biol Chem. 2016;291:2696–711.

57. Deng C, Brown JA, You D, Brown JM. Multiple endonucleases function to repair covalent topoisomerase I complexes in Saccharomyces cerevisiae. Genetics. 2005;170:591–600.

58. Kim Y, Spitz GS, Veturi U, Lach FP, Auerbach AD, Smogorzewska A. Regula-tion of multiple DNA repair pathways by the Fanconi anemia protein SLX4. Blood. 2013;121:54–63.

59. Sollier J, Stork CT, García-Rubio ML, Paulsen RD, Aguilera A, Cimprich KA. Transcription-coupled nucleotide excision repair factors promote R-loop-induced genome instability. Mol Cell. 2014;56:777–85.

60. Sollier J, Cimprich KA. Breaking bad: R-loops and genome integrity. Trends Cell Biol. 2015;25:514–22.

61. Fregoso OI, Emerman M. Activation of the DNA damage response is a conserved function of HIV-1 and HIV-2 Vpr that is independent of SLX4 recruitment. MBio. 2016;7:e01433-16.

62. Smith JA, Daniel R. Up-regulation of HIV-1 transduction in nondividing cells by double-strand DNA break-inducing agents. Biotechnol Lett. 2011;33:243–52.
63. Ebina H, Kanemura Y, Suzuki Y, Urata K, Misawa N, Koyanagi Y. Integrase-independent HIV-1 infection is augmented under conditions of DNA damage and produces a viral reservoir. Virology. 2012;427:44–50.
64. Siddiqui K, Del Valle L, Morellet N, Cui J, Ghafouri M, Mukerjee R, et al. Molecular mimicry in inducing DNA damage between HIV-1 Vpr and the anticancer agent, cisplatin. Oncogene. 2008;27:32–43.
65. Levy DN, Refaeli Y, MacGregor RR, Weiner DB. Serum Vpr regulates productive infection and latency of human immunodeficiency virus type 1. Proc Natl Acad Sci USA. 1994;91:10873–7.
66. Power C, Hui E, Vivithanaporn P, Acharjee S, Polyak M. Delineating HIV-associated neurocognitive disorders using transgenic models: the neuropathogenic actions of Vpr. J Neuroimmune Pharmacol. 2012;7:319–31.
67. Katyal S, Lee Y, Nitiss KC, Downing SM, Li Y, Shimada M, et al. Aberrant topoisomerase-1 DNA lesions are pathogenic in neurodegenerative genome instability syndromes. Nat Neurosci. 2014;17:813–21.
68. Saylor D, Dickens AM, Sacktor N, Haughey N, Slusher B, Pletnikov M, et al. HIV-associated neurocognitive disorder—pathogenesis and prospects for treatment. Nat Rev Neurol. 2016;12:234–48.
69. Skourti-Stathaki K, Kamieniarz-Gdula K, Proudfoot NJ. R-loops induce repressive chromatin marks over mammalian gene terminators. Nature. 2014;516:436–9.

7

Super-resolution fluorescence microscopy studies of human immunodeficiency virus

Jakub Chojnacki[1][*] (ID) and Christian Eggeling[1,2,3] (ID)

Abstract

Super-resolution fluorescence microscopy combines the ability to observe biological processes beyond the diffraction limit of conventional light microscopy with all advantages of the fluorescence readout such as labelling specificity and non-invasive live-cell imaging. Due to their subdiffraction size (< 200 nm) viruses are ideal candidates for super-resolution microscopy studies, and Human Immunodeficiency Virus type 1 (HIV-1) is to date the most studied virus by this technique. This review outlines principles of different super-resolution techniques as well as their advantages and disadvantages for virological studies, especially in the context of live-cell imaging applications. We highlight the findings of super-resolution based HIV-1 studies performed so far, their contributions to the understanding of HIV-1 replication cycle and how the current advances in super-resolution microscopy may open new avenues for future virology research.

Keywords: Human immunodeficiency virus, HIV-1, Super-resolution microscopy, Nanoscopy, Fluorescence

Background

The direct observation studies of biological systems via fluorescence microscopy (FM) is an invaluable tool of scientific discovery thanks to its ability for dynamic analysis of multiple specifically labelled molecules of interest. In the field of virology, fluorescence microscopy has enabled researchers to track the virus particle movements through the cells and probe for the co-localisation with cellular components greatly contributing to our understating of the virus replication cycles. However due to the fundamental physical barrier associated with the diffraction limit of visible light the resolution of conventional fluorescence microscope is theoretically limited to ~ 200 nm in the focal plane (xy) and ~ 600 nm along the optical axis (z) [1] and in fact it is often even lower in non-ideal conditions of actual experiments [2]. Hence the analysis of objects smaller than this limit by conventional FM cannot yield any information about their details. Since viruses are mostly smaller than 200 nm, this makes the studies of virus architecture and the distribution

and dynamics of molecules within the individual sites of virus-cell interactions impossible using this method. Therefore for many decades visualisation of subviral details was performed solely via electron microscopy (EM) based methods which became a de facto gold standard for virus imaging. EM and in particular the advanced implementation of EM such as cryo electron tomography (cryo-ET) has yielded invaluable insights into the minute details of virus structures. These are discussed in the accompanying review by Mak and de Marco [3]. However, as is the case with all scientific tools, EM studies carry specific drawbacks. In particular, EM approaches require laborious preparation of biological samples (fixation or freezing) thus making it unsuitable for study of dynamic processes during virus-cell interactions.

This technological impasse for virology studies has changed dramatically with the development of super-resolution fluorescence microscopy (SRFM) or nanoscopy techniques that work around the diffraction limit of light to improve the resolution (for in-depth reviews please refer to [4–6]). While these techniques can now routinely offer a spatial resolution of 10–100 nm the field is constantly evolving with most recent advances indicating that a resolution of down to 1 nm is now achievable [7]. These capabilities represent a powerful approach that

*Correspondence: jakub.chojnacki@rdm.ox.ac.uk
[1] MRC Human Immunology Unit, Weatherall Institute of Molecular Medicine, University of Oxford, Oxford OX3 9DS, UK
Full list of author information is available at the end of the article

combines increased resolution that can resolve virus sub-structures with all advantages of FM. These include labelling specificity, non-invasive live-cell imaging and higher throughput making SRFM an ideal tool for in-depth studies of subviral architecture and virus-cell interactions.

SRFM studies have provided a number of ground breaking insights into retroviral replication cycle. However, to date these studies have almost exclusively focussed on Human Immunodeficiency Virus Type 1 (HIV-1) (Fig. 1). This is due the fact that over 30 years of intense research into this important human pathogen has already provided a detailed understanding of virus replication cycle. This, in turn, provided guidance and well characterised reagents towards the design of SRFM studies aiming to fill the gaps in the knowledge of HIV-1 biology. In this review we outline the principles of SRFM techniques, and guide the reader through their advantages and disadvantages for virological studies especially in the context of the live cell imaging. Finally, we highlight the findings of SRFM-based HIV-1 studies performed to date, how they have contributed to our understanding of HIV-1 replication cycle and spread and discuss possible future directions in this field.

SFRM techniques in virus research

Multiple SRFM approaches have evolved over the years that offer improved spatial resolution over conventional wide-field or laser scanning confocal microscopes (Fig. 2). Approaches such as structured illumination (SIM) [8], image scanning [9], multifocal structured illumination [10], Airyscan [11], or re-scan [12] microscopy achieve a 1.5–2-fold improvement in resolution (down to 100–150 nm). While these approaches offer distinct advantages such as their straightforward applicability to conventionally prepared samples their modest resolution increase has prevented their widespread use in the virus research, where studied virus structures are even smaller. Instead, to date, most of HIV-1 SRFM studies have utilised techniques such as Stimulated Emission Depletion (STED) microscopy [13] or Photo-Activation Localization Microscopy [(f)PALM] [14, 15] and (direct) Stochastic Optical Reconstruction Microscopy [(d)STORM] [16, 17], that offer spatial resolution below 100 nm and thus enable for the analysis of the details of virus architecture as well as interactions between viruses and cell components during virus replication and spread. In the next sections we will introduce the reader into the principles and some technical details of these SRFM approaches, highlighting their advantages as well as disadvantages.

SIM and related techniques

As highlighted, SIM and related techniques such as image scanning, multifocal structured illumination,

Airyscan, or re-scan microscopy achieve a 1.5–2-fold improvement in spatial resolution compared to conventional optical microscopes (down to 100–150 nm). These approaches usually make use of optical properties of the microscope (such as heterogeneity or patterns in the detected signal) in conjunction with distinct image analyses. For example, SIM takes advantage of Moiré pattern effect (Fig. 2c) to reveal sub-diffraction sized information about the sample structures. This is achieved by illuminating a wide field of the sample with a high frequency striped pattern (Fig. 2c—"Excitation"). This light pattern creates the Moiré pattern interference with structures in the sample (Fig. 2c—"Read-out"). A series of camera images (typically more than 9) is obtained by scanning and rotating the illumination pattern. These raw images, in conjunction with distinct image analysis, are then used to reconstruct the final image containing high-resolution information (Fig. 2c—"Processing" and "Final Image") [8]. The spatio-temporal resolution, ease-of-use, versatility, and reliability (specifically with respect to possible artefacts from the required image analysis) of this approach have been further increased by operating it with Total Internal Reflection Fluorescence illumination (TIRF), which reduces the excitation in axial z-direction to ~ 100 nm above the sample coverslip surface [18]. Other improvements include the use of different illumination patterns such as multiple spots instead of stripes [10], adapting principles principles of SIM to confocal setups (Airyscan or re-scan microscopy) [11, 12] or by introducing control measures on the final reconstructed image [19]. Despite their still limited spatial resolution, these approaches are very versatile, offering 3D and live-cell imaging capability that works well with conventional microscopy fluorophores and FPs. Thus they are ideally suited for studies that would benefit even from a modest resolution increase. Unfortunately (as previously indicated), this only modest resolution increase has prevented the widespread use of these approaches in areas such as virus research, which usually require sub-100 nm resolution.

Sub-100 nm resolution SRFM approaches

Sub-100 nm resolution SRFM approaches achieve sub-diffraction scales by switching the fluorescent labels between bright and dark states with only a small subset of all fluorophores being allowed to fluoresce and thus be individually distinguished at any given moment. Combined with the knowledge of the precise position of these fluorescing molecules, this allows for the generation of an image that is no longer restricted by the light diffraction limit [20]. The main difference between switching-based SRFM techniques relates to how the knowledge of the fluorophore position is generated and they can be put

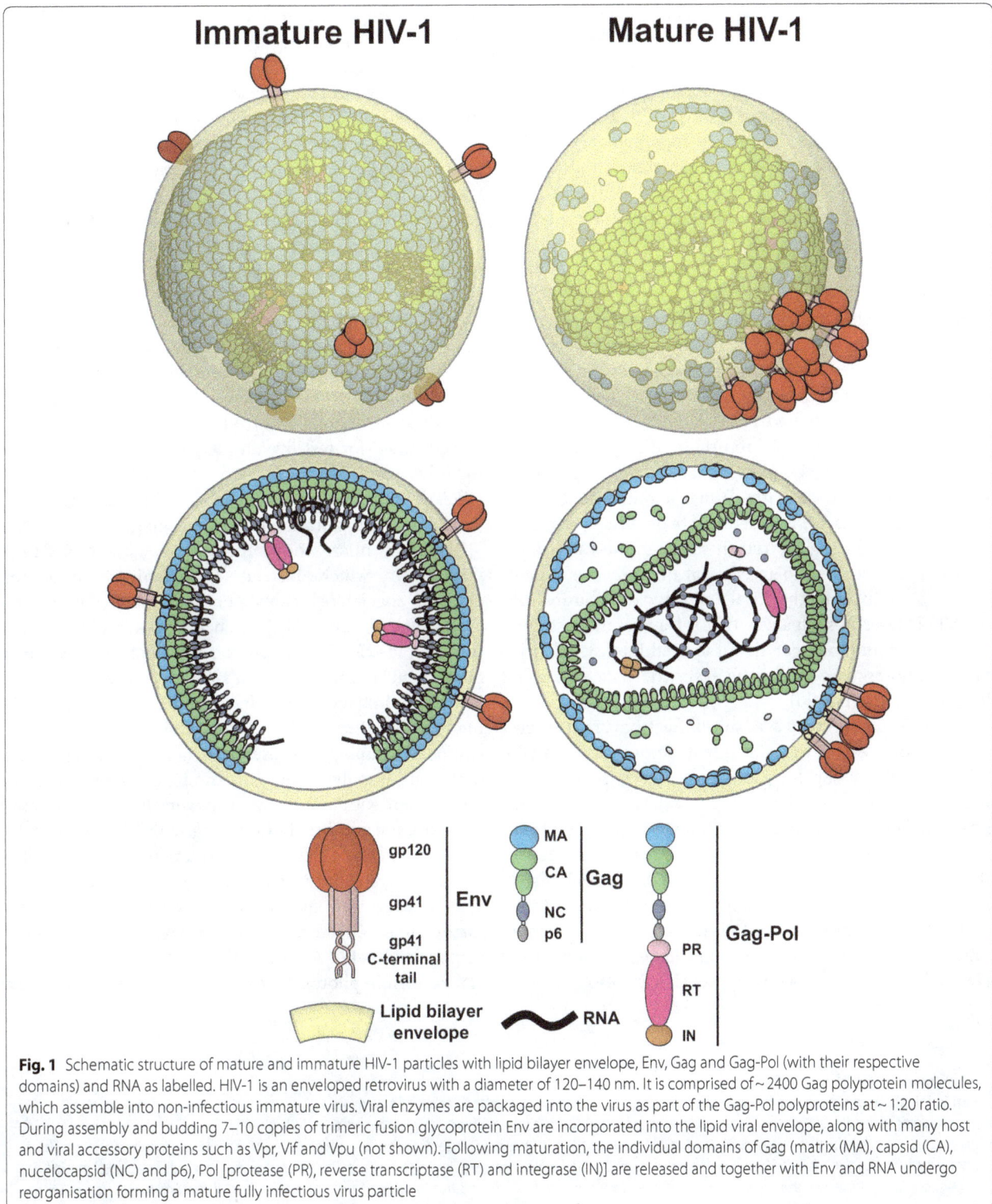

Fig. 1 Schematic structure of mature and immature HIV-1 particles with lipid bilayer envelope, Env, Gag and Gag-Pol (with their respective domains) and RNA as labelled. HIV-1 is an enveloped retrovirus with a diameter of 120–140 nm. It is comprised of ~ 2400 Gag polyprotein molecules, which assemble into non-infectious immature virus. Viral enzymes are packaged into the virus as part of the Gag-Pol polyproteins at ~ 1:20 ratio. During assembly and budding 7–10 copies of trimeric fusion glycoprotein Env are incorporated into the lipid viral envelope, along with many host and viral accessory proteins such as Vpr, Vif and Vpu (not shown). Following maturation, the individual domains of Gag (matrix (MA), capsid (CA), nucelocapsid (NC) and p6), Pol [protease (PR), reverse transcriptase (RT) and integrase (IN)] are released and together with Env and RNA undergo reorganisation forming a mature fully infectious virus particle

into two groups: 1. Targeted shift of excited fluorophore into the dark state at the fringes of a precisely positioned fluorescence excitation spot. This strategy is employed by STED microscopy [13], as well as the related Reversible Saturable Optical (Fluorescence) Transition (RESOLFT) microscopy [21, 22] variant. 2. Stochastic switching of fluorescing molecules in the entire field of view followed by their precise localisation. Techniques based on this approach [here collectively called Single Molecule Switching Microscopy (SMSM)] include (f)PALM [14, 15] and (d)STORM [16, 17], as well as variants thereof such as Ground State Depletion microscopy followed by Individual Molecule return (GSDIM) [23], Point Accumulation for Imaging in Nanoscale Topography (PAINT) [24], or Super-resolution Optical Fluctuation Imaging (SOFI) [25]. The following sections introduce the principles behind these techniques and highlight their advantages as well as disadvantages.

STED microscopy

STED SRFM relies on driving excited fluorophores (i.e. in their fluorescent bright state) back into their dark ground state via a non-destructive process employing stimulated emission using additional laser light. Specifically, laser excitation puts fluorophores into their excited state from where they spontaneously return to the ground state emitting a fluorescence photon that can be registered by the microscope detector. When a red-shifted laser (so-called STED laser) is added it acts on already excited fluorophore inducing the return to the ground non-fluorescent state leading to an efficient fluorescence depletion. By modulating the focal intensity distribution of the STED laser in such a way that it features at least one intensity minimum (e.g. a donut-shaped intensity distribution) fluorescence is depleted everywhere except at the local minimum (Fig. 2d).

This effectively creates a sub-diffraction sized excitation spot, which when scanned across the sample (Fig. 2d—"Excitation") creates an image with sub-diffraction spatial resolution [13, 26, 27] (Fig. 2d—"Final image"). Since the efficiency of fluorescence depletion scales with the intensity of the STED laser, the size of the effective scanning spot and thus the spatial resolution can be tuned accordingly from diffraction limited (i.e. ~200 nm with STED laser off) to in principle unlimited scale (usually <50–60 nm in cellular imaging) [28, 29]. STED microscopy approach can also provide

resolution improvement both in lateral and axial directions with <100 nm axial resolution demonstrated in biological samples [29–32]. Here, a unique property of STED microscopy is the flexibility in designing an experiment by straightforwardly tuning the spatial resolution along all spatial directions. Another advantage of STED microscopy lies in the ability to create a direct image without the need of post processing thus simplifying the acquisition process and avoiding potential post-processing induced image artefacts. While the requirement for high STED laser intensities (GW cm^{-2}) raises concerns over increased photobleaching and phototoxicity, this drawback has been efficiently mitigated through improved sample preparation and image acquisition protocols thus making STED microscopy suitable for live-cell observations [33–38]. Overall, due to its ability to directly acquire super-resolved images STED microscopy is well suited for fast live and fixed imaging studies. On the other hand, due to the high laser powers required for efficient fluorophore depletion this technique may not be suitable for long duration live cell imaging.

RESOLFT microscopy represents a variant of STED microscopy which instead of organic fluorophores employs special reversibly photoswitchable fluorescent labels such as reversibly switchable fluorescent proteins (rsFPs) [20–22]. These labels are switched between a fluorescent/bright and a dark state by light induced conformational changes [39]. In a similar fashion to STED microscopy, RESOLFT is also usually employed on a confocal scanning microscope, where switching to the dark state is only induced at the focal periphery using a laser spot with a local intensity zero (such as a donut-shaped intensity distribution) (Fig. 2d). Because switching between the different conformational states requires low laser intensities (~1 kW cm^{-2}), RESOLFT has been shown to be well suited for live-cell imaging [21, 40], further improved through optimized image acquisition protocols [41–43]. Although the requirement to use special reversible photoswitchable labels can be considered

(See figure on next page.)
Fig. 2 Principles of different super-resolution fluorescence microscopy methods and a comparison of their resolution capabilities. "Excitation" and "Read-out" panels refer to the fluorophore excitation and signal acquisition at a single point in time as the final image is built either by laser scanning (indicated by the arrows) or wide-field illumination of the imaged field of view. Some microscopy techniques require additional post-processing of the acquired "Read-out" snapshots to build the final image, as indicated by the "Processing" panels. For a detailed explanation of each technique please see the corresponding sections. **a** A hypothetical ground truth image of 140 nm mature and immature virus particles with fluorescently tagged Env molecules. Image depth (z) has been ignored for the sake of clarity. **b** A standard confocal microscopy delivering a blurred diffraction-limited resolution image. **c** Structured Illumination Microscopy (SIM) ("SIM and related techniques" section). **d** Stimulated Emission Depletion (STED) and Reversible Saturable Optical Fluorescence Transitions (RESOLFT) microscopy ("STED microscopy" section). **e** Single Molecule Switching Microscopy (SMSM) ("Single molecule switching microscopy (SMSM)" section). **f** Light-sheet microscopy. Please note that this technique by itself does not provide much improvement in the spatial resolution, but it is often combined with other super-resolution microscopy techniques due to the general improvements it brings to the imaging of cellular structures ("Light-sheet microscopy" section). **g** Scanning Stimulated Emission Depletion Fluorescence Correlation Spectroscopy (sSTED-FCS) ("Imaging speed" section)

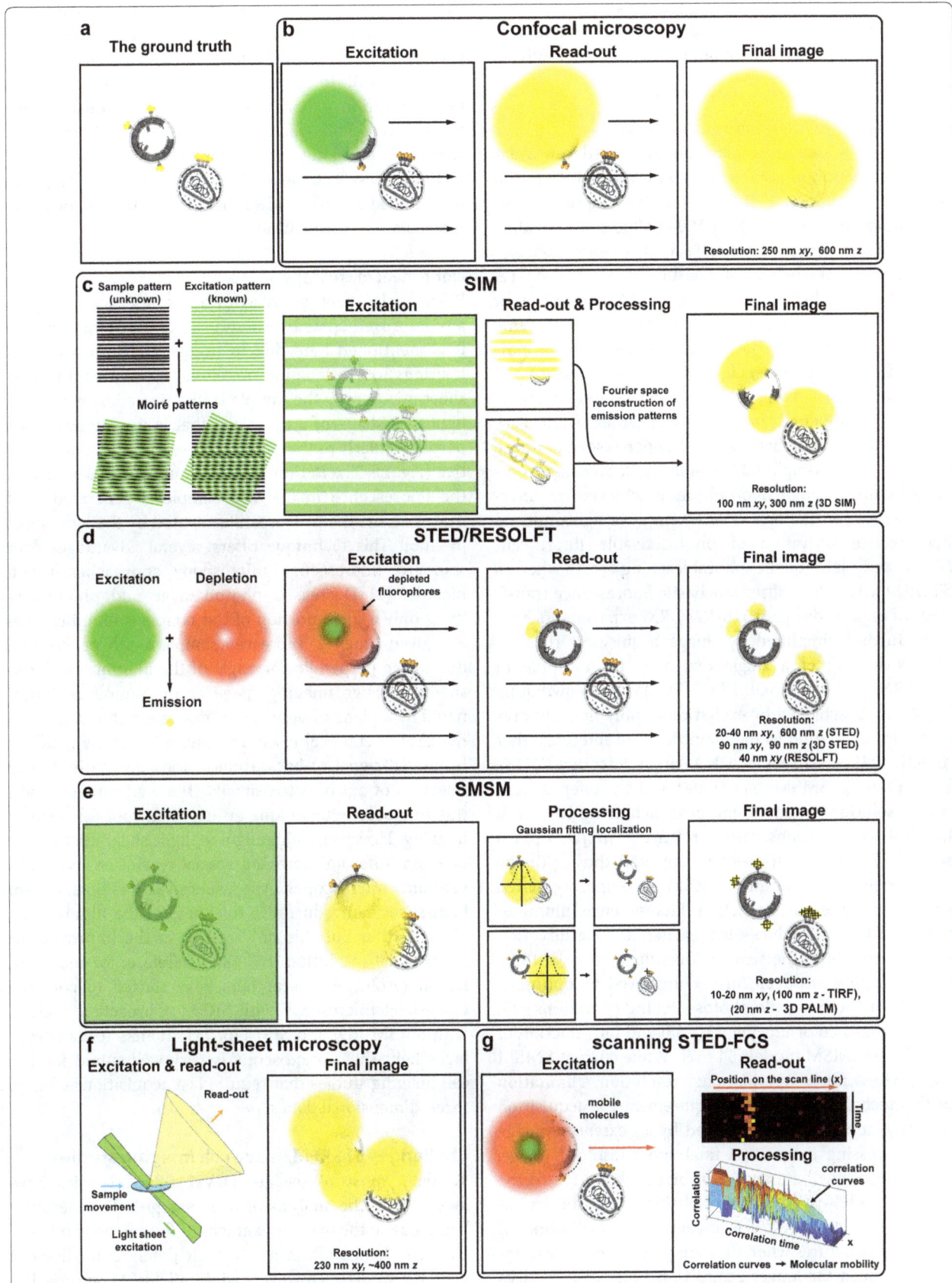

a The ground truth

b Confocal microscopy
Excitation — Read-out — Final image
Resolution: 250 nm xy, 600 nm z

c SIM
Sample pattern (unknown) + Excitation pattern (known)
Moiré patterns
Excitation — Read-out & Processing — Fourier space reconstruction of emission patterns — Final image
Resolution: 100 nm xy, 300 nm z (3D SIM)

d STED/RESOLFT
Excitation Depletion + Emission
Excitation — depleted fluorophores — Read-out — Final image
Resolution: 20-40 nm xy, 600 nm z (STED); 90 nm xy, 90 nm z (3D STED); 40 nm xy (RESOLFT)

e SMSM
Excitation — Read-out — Processing — Gaussian fitting localization — Final image
Resolution: 10-20 nm xy, (100 nm z - TIRF), (20 nm z - 3D PALM)

f Light-sheet microscopy
Excitation & read-out — Read-out — Sample movement — Light sheet excitation — Final image
Resolution: 230 nm xy, ~400 nm z

g scanning STED-FCS
Excitation — mobile molecules — Read-out — Position on the scan line (x) — Time — Processing — correlation curves — Correlation — Correlation time — x
Correlation curves → Molecular mobility

a drawback for this technique, there are already multiple label variants available in several colours [21, 41, 42] and suitable photoswitchable organic dyes are currently in development [44–46].

Single molecule switching microscopy (SMSM)

SMSM-based approaches are usually based on wide-field illumination in combination with camera detection (Fig. 2e—"Excitation"). They rely on building a sub-diffraction image from a cycle of 100–10,000 s of individual camera frames where only small subsets of individual isolated fluorescent labels are stochastically switched-on, i.e. allowed in their bright on-state, and a different subset of individual labels is on for each subsequent camera frame (Fig. 2e—"Read-out"). The spatial positions of the individual fluorescing molecules are precisely determined from their recorded blurred fluorescence spots, and positions of all individual labels across all camera frames are then used to construct the final super-resolved image (Fig. 2e—"Processing" and "Final image"). Stochastic on–off switching of single fluorophores is achieved via different means. For example, PALM employs light-induced fluorescence activation of photoactivable fluorescent labels and subsequent photobleaching [15] whereas STORM originally utilised stochastic fluorescence transitions of organic dye pairs [16]. STORM experiments have been further simplified by image acquisition through photoswitching of a single dye only, for example in dSTORM [17] and GSDIM [23]. Finally, photoswitching in PAINT is achieved by excitation of only fluorophores that transiently bind to the membranes of interest either directly [24] or via specific DNA-target detection (DNA-PAINT) [47]. SMSM techniques usually offer a very high resolution enhancement, often achieving 10-20 nm localisation precisions, using relatively simple optical setups. To reduce out-of-focus light and thus optimize single-molecule localisation SMSM is commonly paired with Total Internal Reflection Fluorescence illumination (TIRF) that reduces the excitation in z-direction to ~ 100 nm above the sample coverslip surface. SMSM-based imaging has been further improved by optimisations in single-molecule photoswitching conditions [17, 48–50], multi-color imaging [51–53] and introduction of various 3D SMSM modes [54–57]. While current SMSM approaches offer a superior image resolution, a limitation of this technique lies in the requirement for acquisition of many camera frames followed by an extensive image post-processing to create a final super-resolved image. These steps may be a source of bias such as due to the imperfect photoswitching or labelling (see for example [58]) which may cause incomplete visualisation of observed structures when they are present in a low number. The need for longer acquisition times also reduces

the time resolution and thus applicability to resolve live-cell dynamics. However, this issue is mitigated by the use of optimised image acquisition and processing protocols [59–63]. In summary, SMSM currently offers the best resolution enhancement out of all popular super-resolution techniques. However, this comes at the cost of several second-long acquisition times thus making this technique less suitable for live cell imaging but very useful for fixed sample studies that require highest possible, molecular level resolution.

Light-sheet microscopy

While light-sheet microscopy does not per-se supply any improved spatial resolution (Fig. 2f—"Final image") it is mentioned here due to the general improvements it brings to the imaging of cellular structures. In light-sheet microscopy the sample is illuminated by a beam of light in a shape of a flat plane that is usually generated perpendicularly to the optical axis of the detection objective (Fig. 2f—"Excitation and read-out"). In this approach the fluorescence image of a sample is generated as it moves across the thin area illuminated by the light-sheet [64–66]. This technique offers several advantages over standard fluorescence microscopy approaches which include: (1) Decreased photodamage and phototoxicity as only a small portion of the sample is illuminated at any given time; (2) Increased sample depth penetration due to the perpendicular angle of the illuminating light-sheet; (3) High imaging speed as the sample is illuminated by a plane of light rather than a point source (as is the case in confocal laser scanning microscopy); and (4) Improved signal-to-background ratios due to improved rejection of out-of-focus signals. These advantages make this microscopy technique an excellent tool for live-cell imaging. However, as highlighted, light-sheet microscopy does not offer an increased spatial resolution over conventional microscopes. Approaches such as Bessel beam light-sheet can reduce the thickness of the illumination plane further but this only results in the improvement to the axial resolution [67, 68]. Therefore, for increased lateral resolution, researchers have started to combine light-sheet microscopy with SRFM approaches, such as with SMSM [69] and SIM [70, 71]. Thanks to its advantages light-sheet microscopy is very well suited for live cell imaging studies that require fast acquisitions of large three-dimensional data sets.

Challenges of SRFM in live cell imaging studies

To date, most of to-date HIV-1 SRFM studies have focussed on the analysis of fixed samples. On the other hand, one of the main advantages of fluorescence microscopy and hence SRFM lies in their potential for live-cell imaging studies. However, while all SRFM approaches can be used to observe live fluorescently labelled samples, the choice of the most suitable technique for virology studies in live conditions must consider not only their resolution capabilities but also imaging speed, sample depth penetration, photobleaching and phototoxicity, as well as accurate labelling.

Imaging speed

Imaging speed is critical for acquisition of dynamic events in cells and viruses. While SMSM techniques offer a very high spatial resolution this comes at a cost of imaging speed as thousands of photoswitching cycles are required to build up the final image. Although with improvements in hardware and localisation algorithms [59–63] the time resolution has been improved to 0.5–2 s (albeit at the cost of reduced spatial resolution) it might still not be optimal for the live imaging of molecular details of virus-cell interactions. This is because processes such as molecular diffusion and clustering dynamics typically occur within milliseconds at the nanometre scales. Similarly, to SMSM techniques, SIM imaging speed is limited by the time required to acquire fluorescent signal from multiple illumination pattern configurations. While a single-color 2D image of a cell can be acquired at 0.1–1 s resolution [72] this may still be non-ideal for live-cell imaging of fast dynamic processes.

Imaging speeds are faster in STED microscopy. As a laser scanning technique its imaging speed chiefly depends on the imaged field of view i.e. the smaller image, the faster the acquisition. STED-microscopy based studies of HIV-1 uptake into HeLa cells have demonstrated a maximum temporal resolution of 5–10 ms, when employing ultrafast beam-scanners on small regions of interest [73]. On the other hand, parallelized scanning approaches have also been developed to increase imaging speed in large fields of view [74–76].

The temporal resolution can be further increased by combing SRFM with single-molecule-based spectroscopic tools such as single-particle tracking (SPT) or fluorescence correlation spectroscopy (FCS). For example, combining SPT with the principle of photoswitching [77] such as in spt-PALM enabled the single-molecule based monitoring of molecular diffusion patterns of HIV-1 Gag and tsO45 proteins from vesicular stomatitis virus G (VSVG) [78]. On the other hand, FCS measurements enable for the determination of not only molecular mobility but also anomalies in diffusion [79, 80]. This is achieved by recording of the fluorescence signal over time as tagged molecules diffuse in and out of the observation spot. The correlation of these fluctuations is then used to determine the molecular transit times of molecules through the observation area and allows calculation of a value of the diffusion coefficient (Fig. 2g—"Processing").

When combined with STED microscope, (STED–)FCS enables for the determination of molecular diffusion modes of individual molecules with high spatial and temporal resolution [81]. In combination with fast line-scanning, STED-FCS [or scanning STED-FCS (sSTED-FCS)] allows for the observation of multiple positions at once (Fig. 2g—"Excitation and read-out") and has been applied to study molecular trapping sites at 80-nm spatial resolution in the plasma membrane of living cells [82, 83]. sSTED-FCS has recently been utilised to determine the molecular mobility of proteins on the surface of individual HIV-1 particles [84] as well as molecular dynamics in the interior of the live HeLa and CHO cells [85]. In summary, this technique has high potential for studies of molecular interaction dynamics at cell surfaces such as at virus assembly and fusion sites.

Sample depth penetration

Sample depth penetration in fluorescence microscopy imaging is generally limited by light scattering and optical aberrations due to refractive index mismatches. This leads to deterioration of image resolution and contrast as well as reduction of signal-to-noise levels, especially in SFRM [86, 87]. Such deteriorating effects can, for example, be addressed through 2-photon-based excitation to reduce scattering [88–90] or the use of microscope objective lenses with a better matching of the sample's refractive index (such as a glycerol-immersion objective) [86]. Ultimately, this issue is solved by the use of adaptive optics to reduce bias from optical aberrations [91], which has already been shown to significantly improve image quality and resolution in STED microscopy [87].

Photobleaching and phototoxicity

Laser light exposure, especially at high laser intensities, may lead to the generation of reactive species (such as radicals or singlet oxygen) that cause photobleaching and phototoxicity in living systems resulting in cell death. Consequently, these deteriorating effects have to be considered in any (especially live) fluorescence imaging experiments, thus also in SFRM: (1) SIM: Photobleaching and phototoxicity becomes an issue through the requirement of recording multiple raw images for one final image. This limitation is mitigated by optimization of the optical path and illumination scheme, enabling live-cell recordings even in 3D (for a review see [92]) (2) SMSM: Despite the use of low illumination intensities (kW cm^{-2}), the UV laser irradiation often required for photoswitching is a cause of pronounced phototoxicity. This can be minimized through far-red illumination schemes (>640 nm) or minimization of activation light through the application of distinct labels and buffers (for an overview see [93]). (3) STED/RESOLFT microscopy:

STED microscopy typically utilises high-intensity (GW cm^{-2}) laser light that may lead to phototoxic effects. On the other hand, optimized sample preparation protocols, fast beam-scanning and the adaptation of the wavelength of the STED-laser have proven STED microscopy as viable tool for live-cell investigations, even when employing fluorescent proteins [33, 34]. Moreover, the aforementioned tunability of the STED microscope enables weighing spatial resolution against high laser intensity (for a review see [4]). RESOLFT microscopy uses much lower laser intensities than STED microscopy, but photobleaching or phototoxicity may still be a problem due to the usually employed near-UV laser light and imperfect photoswitching efficiency of fluorescent labels [94]. Nevertheless, live-cell RESOLFT microscopy has successfully been performed using fast, repetitive, parallelized and/or optimized image acquisition schemes [40, 43].

Labelling

In general with all SRFM approaches greater care has to be taken with respect to labelling and sample preparations as well as data acquisition and analysis approaches, since the increased resolution of SFRM also enhances sensitivity to artefacts such as background staining or stressed cells. While certain imperfections might be forgiven in conventional microscopy, they are usually not in SRFM [4]. Furthermore, a great care has to be taken when using larger fluorescent tags such as antibodies (as employed in immunolabelling), since spatial resolutions of < 20–30 nm are achieved in some SRFM experiments. Consequently, the size of the tags start to bias the image and thus the determination of the spatial position and organization of the tagged molecules. This caveat makes the use of smaller tags such as nanobodies or click chemistry necessary in SRFM studies (for an overview see [5]).

Live-cell SRFM studies of HIV-1 face further unique issues associated with labelling of virus components with technique compatible fluorophores while maintaining a minimal effect on virus morphology and functions. Although convenient, fluorescence tagging via antibodies or nanobodies has only a limited usability in live-cell imaging since it restricts studies to virus or cell external surfaces only. However, effective strategies based on fluorescence proteins have already been developed for HIV-1 studies via conventional microscopy [95–97] and these can be adopted for live-cell SRFM. Organic-dye compatible HIV-1 tagging strategies via non-fluorescent tags such as tetracysteine (TC) tag [98], SNAP-tag [99], CLIP-tag [100] or artificial amino acids and click chemistry [101] can also offer a viable strategies for conducting live-cell SRFM studies of virus replication cycle. For an in-depth review of HIV-1 fluorescent labelling strategies please refer to the work by Sakin et al. [102].

SFRM studies of HIV-1

While SRFM technologies outlined above undergo constant development their application has already provided many novel insights into the previously unexplored details of HIV-1 replication cycle (Fig. 3). The following sections outline how these studies have contributed to the knowledge of HIV-1 replication taking the assembly of a new virus particle as a starting point.

Assembly

HIV-1 assembles initially as immature particles on the plasma membrane of the infected cells [103]. This process is driven by the virus structural polyprotein Gag as it binds to the inner leaflet of the plasma membrane via matrix (MA) domain and forms hexameric protein shell bound by intermolecular interactions of capsid (CA) domain. Gag is also responsible for the recruitment of other virus and host cell components to the budding site. These include genomic RNA, Gag-Pol polyprotein which also encodes viral enzymes, fusion glycoprotein Env, Viral protein R (Vpr) as well as components of endosomal sorting complex required for transport (ESCRT) machinery [104], which are needed for HIV-1 release. Virus assembly has been very extensively studied via a variety of methods including electron microscopy (EM) and conventional fluorescence microscopy [103]. Well characterised nature of Gag mediated HIV-1 assembly made it a good candidate for a proof-of-concept study of PALM conducted by Betzig and co-workers. This and subsequent SRFM studies [14, 78, 99, 105–109] revealed an existence of 100–200 nm Gag clusters on the surface of COS-7, 293T, HeLa and A3.01 cells. Moreover, a quantitative PALM study has shown that tagged Gag protein clusters are indistinguishable from the mixed clusters of tagged and unmodified Gag suggesting that they represent a true virus assembly sites in the context of Gag transfected COS-7 cells [110]. Finally, 15 nm resolution obtained in a dSTORM study allowed for a visualisation of a ring-like Gag distribution representing a 2D projection of a semi-spherical structure of the HIV-1 Gag shell in A3.01 T cell line (Fig. 3a) [105]. A similar Gag distribution has also been obtained in SRFM imaging of immature virus particle (see "Maturation" section).

In addition to just confirming Gag assembly models derived from previous EM-based studies, SRFM experiments also described novel aspects of Gag assembly inaccessible to conventional light microscopy or EM. Specifically, a spt-PALM live-cell study tracked individual Gag molecules on the plasma membrane of COS-7 cells and demonstrated an existence of two distinct Gag populations; a larger immobile pool of Gag clusters representing virus assembly sites and a more mobile population of individual Gag molecules [78]. Two Gag populations forming either large (at the virus assembly site) or small clusters were also observed in A3.01 cells by a study utilising dSTORM [105]. Finally, the analysis of Gag clusters by quantitative PALM demonstrated that small (< 100 Gag molecules) clusters comprise ~ 40% of all detected Gag clusters suggesting that transition from small-sized clusters to a growing assembly site may represent a rate-limiting step for HIV-1 particle formation in Gag-transfected COS-7 cells [107].

Multi-colour SRFM provides a possibility to study spatial and temporal relationships between virus and cell proteins recruited to the individual virus assembly sites. One of the targets of interest is the fusion glycoprotein Env. Env traffics to the plasma membrane separately from Gag and becomes incorporated into assembled virus via interactions of MA domain of Gag and the cytoplasmic tail of Env (EnvCT) [111]. However, the exact mechanism of incorporation into the virus particle remains unknown. SRFM imaging using (d)STORM in fixed samples has determined Env distribution in the proximity of Gag assembly sites. It demonstrated the existence of large Env clusters at Gag assembly sites in HeLa cells transfected with replication incompetent pCHIV construct that expresses all HIV-1 proteins except Nef (Fig. 3b) [109]. Interestingly, the majority of Env molecules did not colocalize with the assembly site itself but rather was observed in its immediate vicinity. These findings are consistent with

7–10 Env molecules observed via EM and SRFM in budded HIV-1 particles [112, 113]. Furthermore they suggest that, rather than by random incorporation, Env is recruited to the virus budding site via mechanisms that may involve factors other than direct Gag-Env interactions to exclude most of Env from the nascent virus particle [109]. Dynamics of Env incorporation have been studied by Fluorescence Recovery After Photobleaching (FRAP) indicating that Env molecules are immobile in the areas corresponding to Gag structures [114]. Here, SRFM approaches will also be beneficial for, for example, studying the dynamics of Env or Gag at individual (sub-diffraction sized) virus assembly sites. For example, sSTED-FCS was recently used to study diffusion properties of Env on individual virus particles and in the plasma membrane of Env-transfected HeLa cells [84].

Another so far unexplored aspect of virus assembly is the behaviour of lipids at the individual virus assembly sites. Lipidome studies of virus particles revealed a modified lipid content compared to the host-cell membrane, especially an enrichment in saturated lipids, sphingolipids and cholesterol [115–117], indicating sorting of lipids and proteins at the virus assembly site, i.e. viruses potentially arise from so-called "lipid rafts" [118]. However, the exact lipid distribution and their dynamics as Gag assembles on the plasma membrane remain unclear. Experiments with cholera toxin capped GM1 via dSTORM have shown that GM1 does not colocalize with Gag assembly

(See figure on next page.)

Fig. 3 Super-resolution fluorescence microscopy studies and their contribution to the understanding of HIV-1 replication cycle (illustrated in the lower panel). Virus Assembly: **a** dSTORM imaging of cell surface Gag distribution (green) showing representative virus-sized clusters (upper panel) and their fluorescence intensity line profiles (lower panel). Scale bar: 200 nm [105]. The density distributions of Gag protein localizations was found to be similar to the ring-like arrangement of Gag found in immature virus (see panel **f**). **b** dSTORM imaging of Env distribution (red) around cell surface Gag clusters (green). Env molecules (right panels—dots) appear to be largely excluded from the sites of Gag assembly (right panels—circle). Scale bar: 100 nm [109]. Release: **c.** Distribution of Gag (green) and ESCRT protein Tsg101 (red) within budding viruses imaged by dSTORM. Protein localization densities indicate the accumulation of ESCRT proteins at the neck of the virus buds [122]. **d** Distribution of Gag (red) and ESCRT protein Tsg101 (green) within a budding virus imaged by 3D PALM. In this study protein localization densities indicate the existence of ESCRT components within the virus particle. Scale bar: 50 nm [104]. **e** Tetherin clusters (red) at Gag assembly sites (green) imaged by dSTORM Scale bar: 200 nm [108]. Virus architecture and maturation: **f** STED imaging of Gag distribution (red) in immature and mature virus particles showing a 2D projection of ring-like Gag lattice in immature and a central condensed accumulation in mature virus particles (left panels). HIV-1 maturation kinetics was estimated by time-lapse imaging of Gag structures and quantifying the percentage of HIV-1 particles with ring-like distributions over time (right panel). Scale bar: 100 nm [100]. **g** STED imaging of Env distribution (red) on individual eGFP.Vpr tagged virus particles (green) with multi-clustered Env distribution in immature non-infectious particles (PR-) coalescing into a single cluster in mature fully infectious virus (wt) (right panel). Scale bar: 100 nm [112]. **h** sSTED-FCS measurements of Env mobility on individual mature and immature virus particles by fast line-scanning (red line) over individual eGFP.Vpr tagged virus particles (green) and determination of diffusion characteristics at each line pixel using FCS. Representative FCS correlation curve data for Env in mature (red), immature (blue) and fixed (purple) viruses with faster decay indicating increased mobility (right panel). Env was found to undergo maturation-induced increase in mobility indicating its diffusion as one of the causes for Env clustering. Scale bar: 200 nm [84]. Cell-to-cell transfer: **i** Visualising individual virus positions (red/yellow, identified by Gag) by STED microscopy at the contact sites between the infected macrophages (blue cell border in inset) and astrocytes (labelled via glial fibrillary acidic protein (GFAP), green) Scale bar: 500 nm. Inset scale bar: 3 μm [133]. Entry and post-entry: **j.** STED imaging of Env (red) and CD4 (blue) distributions in cell-attached eGFP.Vpr labelled HIV-1 (green) showing a single contact point between Env and CD4. Scale bar: 100 nm [112]. **k** dSTORM image of MA clusters (red) and eGFP.Vpr labelled viruses (green) after their attachment to cells. MA cluster sizes were found to be larger than those in cell-free virus particles. Scale bar: 2 μm [136]. **l** PALM/dSTORM image of RTC/PIC [viral DNA (red), CA (blue) and IN (green)] in the cytoplasm of infected macrophage. Scale bar: 100 nm [138]. Images were modified from indicated references with permission

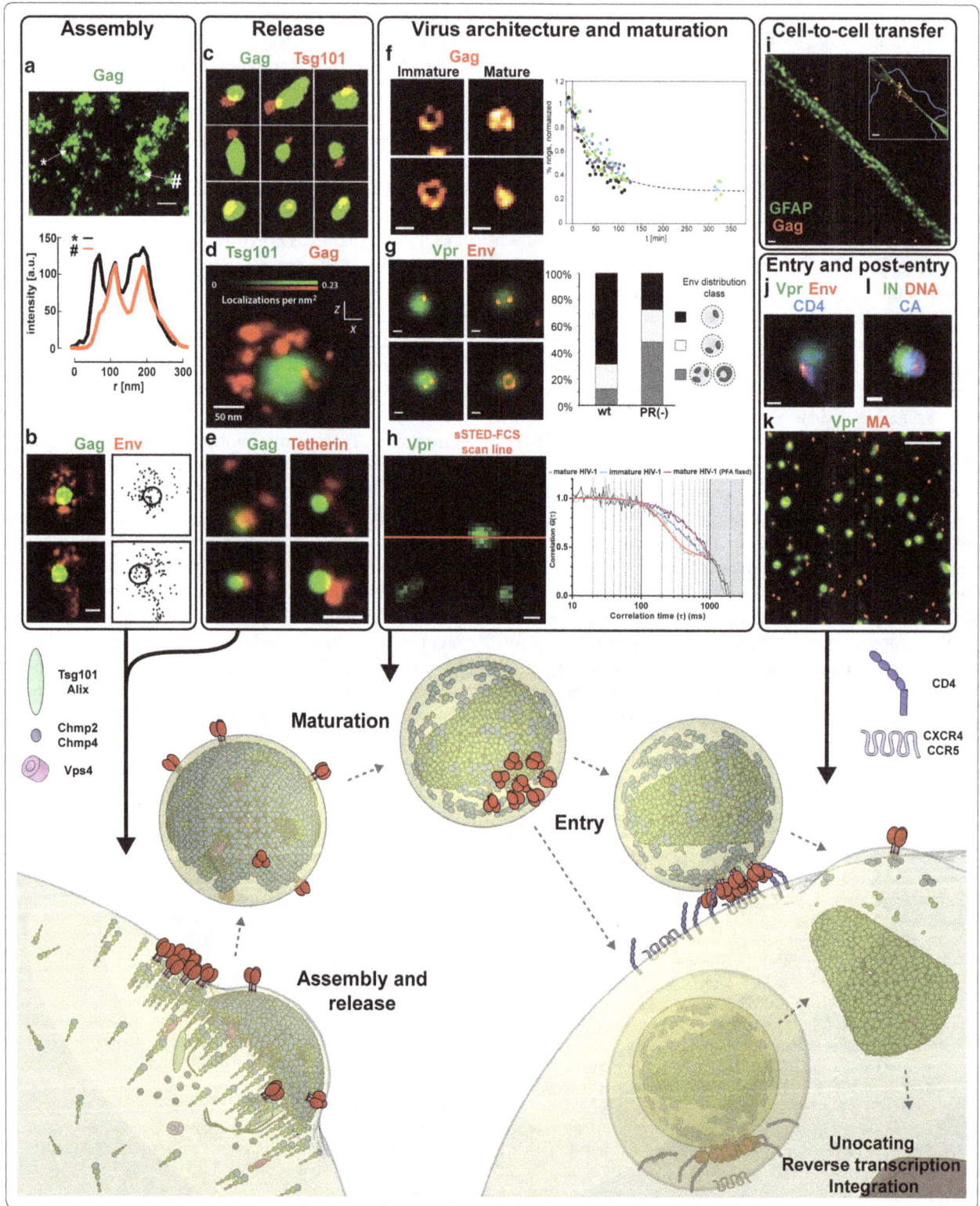

Assembly

a Gag

b Gag Env

Release

c Gag Tsg101

d Tsg101 Gag

Localizations per nm²

50 nm

e Gag Tetherin

Virus architecture and maturation

f Gag
Immature Mature

g Vpr Env

Env distribution class

wt PR(-)

h Vpr sSTED-FCS scan line

mature HIV-1 — immature HIV-1 — mature HIV-1 (PFA fixed)

Cell-to-cell transfer

i

GFAP Gag

Entry and post-entry

j Vpr Env CD4

l IN DNA CA

k Vpr MA

Tsg101 Alix

Chmp2 Chmp4

Vps4

CD4

CXCR4 CCR5

Maturation

Entry

Assembly and release

Uncoating
Reverse transcription
Integration

sites in fixed HeLa cells [108], and details of lipid dynamics at individual HIV-1 assembly sites are currently under investigation via (s)STED-FCS.

Release

The ESCRT machinery is responsible for mediating intracellular fission events such as cytokinesis and the formation of multi-vesicular bodies. HIV-1 hijacks elements of this machinery in order to separate (or bud off) from the plasma membrane of the infected cell [103, 104]. This is achieved by recruiting ESCRT proteins Tsg101 and Alix via p6 domain of Gag which, in turn, recruit further proteins such as Chmp2, Chmp4 and Vps4. While the conventional microscopy studies have provided invaluable insights into the kinetics of the recruitment of ESCRT proteins [119, 120], SRFM has enabled for a closer look at the distribution of ESCRT components within the individual virus budding site. A SMSM-based analysis of ESCRT proteins at the plasma membrane of Gag producing HeLa cells revealed an accumulation of ESCRT proteins in areas of 45–60 nm in diameter at the neck of the budding virus (Fig. 3c). This observation supports a model in which ESCRT proteins accumulate at the plasma membrane below the neck to mediate the scission of the budding virus [121, 122]. However, these observations are inconsistent with the results of a 3D-PALM study in COS-7 cells which indicated that the ESCRT protein machinery accumulated at the head of the budding virus. This study supports a different model where ESCRT filaments grow away from the viral head towards the plasma membrane to mediate scission (Fig. 3d) [123].

SRFM-based experiments have also provided new details of the tetherin (CD317)-mediated restriction of HIV-1 release restriction. Tetherin prevents HIV-1 release from the cell surface by forming a physical link between the budded virus and the plasma membrane [124, 125]. This tetherin-mediated restriction pathway is counteracted by the viral protein U (Vpu), which removes tetherin from the plasma membrane. Quantitative dSTORM analysis of tetherin at Vpu-negative virus assembly sites in HeLa cells highlighted that each site contained 4-7 theterin dimers (Fig. 3e) [108].

Maturation

Concurrently with virus budding, the viral protease (PR) cleaves the Gag protein lattice inside the virus in a series of tightly regulated steps to release individual proteins, namely MA (matrix), CA (capsid), NC (nucleocapsid) and p6. This PR activity reorganises the virus architecture from an immature and non-infectious into a mature and fully infectious form, characterised by a conical capsid (Fig. 1). This process is termed maturation and it is a critical step in HIV-1 replication cycle as it primes newly produced virus particles for infection of other cells. The architecture of both mature and immature virus particles has been extensively studied by EM based approaches [103]. However, with the ability for the determination of the relative distribution of fluorescently tagged viral proteins and studying

dynamic properties of maturation, SRFM-based studies have contributed with essential novel insights into this stage of virus replication.

SRFM has been used to study the distribution and dynamics of virus internal structures during maturation. A PALM study introduced an approach for discriminating between VSV-G pseudotyped mature and immature HIV-1 particles. It relies on the statistical analysis of the signal intensity distributions detected from labelled integrase enzyme domain (IN) of Gag-Pol polyprotein [126]. Immature viruses displayed compact clusters, while mature viruses were characterized by more elongated spots, which were interpreted as conical viral capsids. However, dynamic analysis of virus maturation was infeasible in this study due to the insufficient temporal resolution of the PALM experiments. This limitation was addressed in a STED microscopy study of virus maturation, where the semi-spherical Gag lattice of the immature replication incompetent pCHIV virus particle was visualized and accurately distinguished from the condensed protein distribution found in fully mature virus. The use of a photodestructible viral protease inhibitor enabled for the synchronisation of the virus maturation process, allowing for time-resolved observations of the disassembly of Gag lattice (Fig. 3f) [100]. A detailed analysis of the data revealed a maturation kinetics half-time of ~ 30 min and demonstrated that proteolysis directly induces morphological conversion without further delay, thus making it a rate-limiting step in HIV-1 maturation. This study represented the first time-lapse visualisation of maturation induced reorganisations within individual HIV-1 particles.

Previous EM-based study has suggested an irregular Env distribution on virus surface [113]. Thanks to higher throughput and specific labelling, STED microscopy based experiments allowed for imaging of Env distribution on a large number of individual virus particles generated from 293T cells transfected with replication incompetent pCHIV construct [112]. Env distribution analysis revealed that the surface of immature HIV-1 particles is characterized by multiple separated Env molecules while that of mature particles by only a single Env cluster (Fig. 3g) [112]. This study thus demonstrated the existence of a novel "inside-out" mechanism where PR-induced disassembly of the Gag lattice inside the virus and allows for multi-clustered Env to coalesce into a single cluster in fully infectious mature particles. As multiple Env trimers are required for virus fusion [127, 128] this mechanism ensures that immature virus particles with a broad distribution of single Env molecules are unable to fuse with the target cell membrane until the virus reaches morphological maturity with multiple Env molecules gathered into a single cluster.

The above study has suggested that Gag lattice disassembly mediated clustering of Env molecules may result from an increase in Env mobility upon maturation. Measurements of Env molecular mobility on the surface of individual virus particles via sSTED-FCS have confirmed that Env mobility is dependent on the virus maturation status in pCHIV particles (Fig. 3h) [84]. This study has also demonstrated that the virus surface is generally a very low-mobility environment, where protein mobility is two orders of magnitude slower than on the plasma member of the cell. This is thought to be mainly due to the highly packed lipid environment stemming from the large portion of saturated lipids in the viral membrane [84, 115, 116]. These sSTED-FCS measurements provided, for the first time, information on the dynamic properties of molecules within subdiffraction sized highly curved virus envelopes.

Spread and persistence

HIV-1 has evolved many mechanisms to facilitate efficient spread and persistence in the infected hosts. These mechanisms include direct cell-to-cell transfer via virological synapses [129], establishment of virus reservoirs [130], and the modulation of the infected cell via HIV accessory proteins [131]. However, to date, only few SRFM studies have targeted these aspects of HIV-1 infection. For example, SRFM was used to track the position of HIV-1 accessory protein Nef in transfected HeLa cells. Nef promotes HIV-1 immune evasion by downregulating immune signalling molecules such as MHC-I in infected cells. Here, SRFM was used for high precision localisation of Nef/MHC-I complexes in individual early and late endosome vesicles as well as in the Trans-Golgi network [132]. A recent STED microscopy study also tracked the trapping and sequestration of fully infectious macrophage produced virus particles inside astrocytes (Fig. 3i) [133]. Astrocytes are one of the HIV-1 reservoirs in the brain but it is currently unclear whether these cells support virus replication or only act as passive HIV-1 reservoirs. The multicolour STED analysis of individual HIV-1 particles sequestered inside astrocytes highlighted that they do not fuse with the astrocytes plasma membrane and therefore do not infect them [133]. Rather, astrocytes act only as a passive reservoir of HIV-1 particles. While challenging, SRFM studies of cell-to-cell transmission and virus reservoirs have the potential to provide novel details on the distribution and dynamics of the molecules involved thus contributing to the analysis of HIV-1 replication and spread.

Virus entry

HIV-1 entry into the target cell is mediated by binding of Env to cell surface or endocytosed CD4 receptors and CXCR4/CCR5 chemokine co-receptors. Attachment of individual pCHIV particles to cluster of CD4 receptors has been observed via STED microscopy in SupT1R5 cells [112]. Images have shown single clusters of Env oriented towards CD4 clusters on the cell surface indicating direct interactions between Env and CD4 clusters (Fig. 3j). This study has also demonstrated that the cell contact can induce reclustering of mobile Env molecules on the virus surface, presumably through progressive capture of individual Env trimers by virus facing CD4 molecules. These findings are in agreement with cryo-ET studies that proposed the existence of an "entry claw" structure that connects viruses and cell membranes [134]. In another application of SRFM to HIV-1 entry studies, 3D STORM imaging was used for high resolution visualisation of the exposure of neutralizing and non-neutralizing epitopes on single HIV-1$_{JRFL}$ pseudoviruses bound to TZM-bl CD4 T cells [135].

SRFM has also been used to study possible rearrangements of virus internal proteins during attachment and entry. A dSTORM study has visualised the distribution of MA and CA proteins in unbound and cell-attached fully infectious virus particles, highlighting an increase in cluster sizes of MA and CA in virus particles after cellular internalization, suggesting that virus internal structures undergo rearrangments during the entry (Fig. 3k) [136]. A subsequent study using a combination of EM and SRFM imaging indicated that the reported increase in size of mature HIV-1 particles is solely triggered by CD4-Env attachment and therefore it is independent of virus fusion [137]. The observed virus expansion may thus be a manifestation of a novel mechanism that primes HIV-1 for fusion. However, it is currently unclear what virus-intrinsic mechanism may be responsible for the remodelling of the virus envelope membrane, which would be required for such an event.

Post-entry events

Following entry of the HIV-1 capsid into the cell cytoplasm, the virus genomic RNA is transcribed into double stranded DNA by reverse transcriptase (RT) and integrated into the cellular genome by the viral integrase (IN). The so called reverse transcription complex (RTC) and pre-integration complex (PIC), which are comprised of viral genome and proteins, facilitate reverse transcription, trafficking and nuclear import. Despite the fact that the subdiffraction size and transient occurrence of these complexes makes an analysis of their structural details and dynamics well suited for SRFM studies, these post-entry events are still the least understood phase of the virus replication cycle. Nevertheless, PALM was already used to compare the architecture of fluorescent IN labelled structures in VSV-G pseudotyped cell free virions and post entry HIV-1 subviral complexes [126]. Analysis of the spatial distribution of labelled IN revealed that structures resembling IN complex are mainly present in the cell cytoplasm with only smaller IN structures detected in the cell nucleus. This study has also reported the presence of CA molecules in these cytoplasmic complexes. This result is consistent with findings of another dSTORM/PALM study that visualised fully infectious HIV-1-derived proteins in dsDNA containing post entry RTC/PIC complexes (Fig. 3l). Here, CA was also found in cytoplasmic RTC/PICs and in nuclear PICs, but only in primary human macrophages and not in HeLa cells [138]. The presence of CA was also detected in nuclear PICs of CHO cells imaged by SIM [139]. These findings suggest that there are host cell dependent differences in the degree of capsid disassembly as HIV-1 post-entry complexes travel towards the nucleus.

Conclusions

Since their introduction, SRFM methods have now reached a high state of maturity, and with the increasing availability of commercial turn-key systems they have the potential to become a standard approach for bioimaging. However, it is clear that there is no one-fits-all approach, and as highlighted each technique comes with a unique set of advantages and disadvantages. On top of that SRFM technology is continuously evolving, with the refinement of existing techniques and combinatorial approaches allowing to mitigate disadvantages of each technique.

Virus research with its clear reason to look beyond the diffraction barrier took an early advantage of this field, and SRFM studies have already provided many novel insights into the understating of the HIV-1 replication cycle. Yet, arguably these are still early days of SRFM imaging with many more aspects of HIV-1 that still await investigation. Moreover, to date most of SRFM HIV-1 studies have been performed in the context of fixed viruses and in vitro cell cultures. On the other hand, SRFM approaches are particularly suitable to study the dynamic behaviour of individual subviral structures and their interactions with cell components in the context of live cells or tissues, and it is in this area where they hold the most potential for future improvements in the understanding of virus replication cycle.

Abbreviations

FM: Fluorescence microscopy; EM: Electron microscopy; cryo-ET: cryo electron tomography; SRFM: Super-resolution fluorescence microscopy; HIV-1: Human immunodeficiency virus type 1; SIM: Structured illumination microscopy; STED: Stimulated emission depletion microscopy; RESOLFT: Reversible saturable optical fluorescence transition microscopy; SMSM: Single molecule switching microscopy; PALM: Photo-activation localization microscopy; (d)STORM: (direct) Stochastic optical reconstruction microscopy; GSDIM: Ground state depletion microscopy followed by individual molecule return; PAINT: Point accumulation for imaging in nanoscale topography; MINFLUX: Minimal emission fluxes microscopy; TIRF: Total internal reflection fluorescence; SPT: Single particle tracking; FCS: Fluorescence Correlation spectroscopy; sSTED-FCS: Scanning stimulated emission depletion fluorescence correlation spectroscopy; MA: Matrix; CA: Capsid; NC: Nucelocapsid; PR: Protease; RT: Reverse transcriptase; IN: Integrase; ESCRT: Endosomal sorting complex required for transport; FRAP: Fluorescence recovery after photobleaching; GFAP: Glial fibrillary acidic protein.

Authors' contributions
JC and CE wrote the manuscript. JC prepared the figures. Both authors read and approved the final manuscript.

Author details
[1] MRC Human Immunology Unit, Weatherall Institute of Molecular Medicine, University of Oxford, Oxford OX3 9DS, UK. [2] Institute of Applied Optics, Friedrich-Schiller-University Jena, Max-Wien Platz 4, 07743 Jena, Germany. [3] Leibniz Institute of Photonic Technology e.V., Albert-Einstein-Straße 9, 07745 Jena, Germany.

Acknowledgements
We would like to thank Sergi Padilla-Parra for helpful suggestions and critical review of our manuscript.

Competing interests
The authors declare no competing financial interests.

Funding
J.C. and C.E. are supported by the MRC (grant number MC_UU_12010/unit programs G0902418 and MC_UU_12025), MRC/BBSRC/EPSRC (grant MR/K01577X/1), Wellcome Trust [Grant 104924/14/Z/14 and Strategic Award 091911 (Micron)], Deutsche Forschungsgemeinschaft (Research unit 1905 "Structure and function of the peroxisomal translocon"), and Oxford internal funds (EPA Cephalosporin Fund and John Fell Fund).

References
1. Abbe E. Beiträge zur Theorie des Mikroskops und der mikroskopischen Wahrnehmung. Arch Für Mikrosk Anat. 1873;9:413–68.
2. Nieuwenhuizen RPJ, Lidke KA, Bates M, Puig DL, Grünwald D, Stallinga S, et al. Measuring image resolution in optical nanoscopy. Nat Methods. 2013;10:557–62.
3. Mak J, de Marco A. Recent advances in retroviruses via cryo-electron microscopy. Retrovirology. 2018;15(1):23.
4. Eggeling C, Willig KI, Sahl SJ, Hell SW. Lens-based fluorescence nanoscopy. Q Rev Biophys. 2015;48:178–243.
5. Hell SW, Sahl SJ, Bates M, Zhuang X, Heintzmann R, Booth MJ, et al. The 2015 super-resolution microscopy roadmap. J Phys Appl Phys. 2015;48:443001.
6. Sahl SJ, Hell SW, Jakobs S. Fluorescence nanoscopy in cell biology. Nat Rev Mol Cell Biol. 2017;18:685–701.

7. Balzarotti F, Eilers Y, Gwosch KC, Gynnå AH, Westphal V, Stefani FD, et al. Nanometer resolution imaging and tracking of fluorescent molecules with minimal photon fluxes. Science. 2017;355:606–12.

8. Gustafsson MG. Surpassing the lateral resolution limit by a factor of two using structured illumination microscopy. J Microsc. 2000;198:82–7.

9. Müller CB, Enderlein J. Image scanning microscopy. Phys Rev Lett. 2010;104:198101.

10. York AG, Parekh SH, Nogare DD, Fischer RS, Temprine K, Mione M, et al. Resolution doubling in live, multicellular organisms via multifocal structured illumination microscopy. Nat Methods. 2012;9:749–54.

11. Korobchevskaya K, Lagerholm B, Colin-York H, Fritzsche M. Exploring the potential of airyscan microscopy for live cell imaging. Photonics. 2017;4:41.

12. De Luca GMR, Breedijk RMP, Brandt RAJ, Zeelenberg CHC, de Jong BE, Timmermans W, et al. Re-scan confocal microscopy: scanning twice for better resolution. Biomed Opt Express. 2013;4:2644.

13. Hell SW, Wichmann J. Breaking the diffraction resolution limit by stimulated emission: stimulated-emission-depletion fluorescence microscopy. Opt Lett. 1994;19:780–2.

14. Betzig E, Patterson GH, Sougrat R, Lindwasser OW, Olenych S, Bonifacino JS, et al. Imaging intracellular fluorescent proteins at nanometer resolution. Science. 2006;313:1642–5.

15. Hess ST, Girirajan TPK, Mason MD. Ultra-high resolution imaging by fluorescence photoactivation localization microscopy. Biophys J. 2006;91:4258–72.

16. Rust MJ, Bates M, Zhuang X. Sub-diffraction-limit imaging by stochastic optical reconstruction microscopy (STORM). Nat Methods. 2006;3:793–6.

17. Heilemann M, van de Linde S, Schüttpelz M, Kasper R, Seefeldt B, Mukherjee A, et al. Subdiffraction-resolution fluorescence imaging with conventional fluorescent probes. Angew Chem Int Ed. 2008;47:6172–6.

18. Li D, Shao L, Chen B-C, Zhang X, Zhang M, Moses B, et al. Extended-resolution structured illumination imaging of endocytic and cytoskeletal dynamics. Science. 2015;349:aab3500.

19. Ball G, Demmerle J, Kaufmann R, Davis I, Dobbie IM, Schermelleh L. SIM-check: a toolbox for successful super-resolution structured illumination microscopy. Sci Rep. 2015;5:15915.

20. Hell SW, Jakobs S, Kastrup L. Imaging and writing at the nanoscale with focused visible light through saturable optical transitions. Appl Phys Mater Sci Process. 2003;77:859–60.

21. Grotjohann T, Testa I, Leutenegger M, Bock H, Urban NT, Lavoie-Cardinal F, et al. Diffraction-unlimited all-optical imaging and writing with a photochromic GFP. Nature. 2011;478:204–8.

22. Hofmann M, Eggeling C, Jakobs S, Hell SW. Breaking the diffraction barrier in fluorescence microscopy at low light intensities by using reversibly photoswitchable proteins. Proc Natl Acad Sci. 2005;102:17565–9.

23. Fölling J, Bossi M, Bock H, Medda R, Wurm CA, Hein B, et al. Fluorescence nanoscopy by ground-state depletion and single-molecule return. Nat Methods. 2008;5:943–5.

24. Sharonov A, Hochstrasser RM. Wide-field subdiffraction imaging by accumulated binding of diffusing probes. Proc Natl Acad Sci. 2006;103:18911–6.

25. Dertinger T, Colyer R, Iyer G, Weiss S, Enderlein J. Fast, background-free, 3D super-resolution optical fluctuation imaging (SOFI). Proc Natl Acad Sci. 2009;106:22287–92.

26. Klar TA, Jakobs S, Dyba M, Egner A, Hell SW. Fluorescence microscopy with diffraction resolution barrier broken by stimulated emission. Proc Natl Acad Sci USA. 2000;97:8206–10.

27. Klar TA, Engel E, Hell SW. Breaking Abbe's diffraction resolution limit in fluorescence microscopy with stimulated emission depletion beams of various shapes. Phys Rev E. 2001;64:066613.

28. Westphal V, Hell SW. nanoscale resolution in the focal plane of an optical microscope. Phys Rev Lett. 2005;94:143903.

29. Harke B, Keller J, Ullal CK, Westphal V, Schönle A, Hell SW. Resolution scaling in STED microscopy. Opt Express. 2008;16:4154.

30. Osseforth C, Moffitt JR, Schermelleh L, Michaelis J. Simultaneous dual-color 3D STED microscopy. Opt Express. 2014;22:7028.

31. Schmidt R, Wurm CA, Jakobs S, Engelhardt J, Egner A, Hell SW. Spherical nanosized focal spot unravels the interior of cells. Nat Methods. 2008;5:539–44.

32. Hell SW, Schmidt R, Egner A. Diffraction-unlimited three-dimensional optical nanoscopy with opposing lenses. Nat Photonics. 2009;3:381–7.

33. Bottanelli F, Kromann EB, Allgeyer ES, Erdmann RS, Wood Baguley S, Sirinakis G, et al. Two-colour live-cell nanoscale imaging of intracellular targets. Nat Commun. 2016;7:10778.

34. Nagerl UV, Willig KI, Hein B, Hell SW, Bonhoeffer T. Live-cell imaging of dendritic spines by STED microscopy. Proc Natl Acad Sci. 2008;105:18982–7.

35. Westphal V, Rizzoli SO, Lauterbach MA, Kamin D, Jahn R, Hell SW. Video-rate far-field optical nanoscopy dissects synaptic vesicle movement. Science. 2008;320:246–9.

36. Vicidomini G, Moneron G, Han KY, Westphal V, Ta H, Reuss M, et al. Sharper low-power STED nanoscopy by time gating. Nat Methods. 2011;8:571–3.

37. Staudt T, Engler A, Rittweger E, Harke B, Engelhardt J, Hell SW. Far-field optical nanoscopy with reduced number of state transition cycles. Opt Express. 2011;19:5644.

38. Heine J, Reuss M, Harke B, D'Este E, Sahl SJ, Hell SW. Adaptive-illumination STED nanoscopy. Proc Natl Acad Sci. 2017;114:9797–802.

39. Andresen M, Wahl MC, Stiel AC, Grater F, Schafer LV, Trowitzsch S, et al. Structure and mechanism of the reversible photoswitch of a fluorescent protein. Proc Natl Acad Sci. 2005;102:13070–4.

40. Testa I, Urban NT, Jakobs S, Eggeling C, Willig KI, Hell SW. Nanoscopy of living brain slices with low light levels. Neuron. 2012;75:992–1000.

41. Lavoie-Cardinal F, Jensen NA, Westphal V, Stiel AC, Chmyrov A, Bierwagen J, et al. Two-color RESOLFT nanoscopy with green and red fluorescent photochromic proteins. ChemPhysChem. 2014;15:655–63.

42. Tiwari DK, Arai Y, Yamanaka M, Matsuda T, Agetsuma M, Nakano M, et al. A fast- and positively photoswitchable fluorescent protein for ultralow-laser-power RESOLFT nanoscopy. Nat Methods. 2015;12:515–8.

43. Masullo L, Boden A, Pennacchietti F, Coceano G, Ratz M, Testa I. Enhanced photon collection enables four dimensional fluorescence nanoscopy of living systems. 2018; Available from http://biorxiv.org/lookup/doi/10.1101/248880.

44. Kwon J, Hwang J, Park J, Han GR, Han KY, Kim SK. RESOLFT nanoscopy with photoswitchable organic fluorophores. Sci Rep. 2016;5:17804.

45. Roubinet B, Bossi ML, Alt P, Leutenegger M, Shojaei H, Schnorrenberg S, et al. Carboxylated photoswitchable diarylethenes for biolabeling and super-resolution RESOLFT microscopy. Angew Chem Int Ed. 2016;55:15429–33.

46. Xiong Y, Vargas Jentzsch A, Osterrieth JWM, Sezgin E, Sazanovich IV, Reglinski K, et al. Spironaphthoxazine switchable dyes for biological imaging. Chem Sci. 2018;9:3029–40.

47. Jungmann R, Avendaño MS, Woehrstein JB, Dai M, Shih WM, Yin P. Multiplexed 3D cellular super-resolution imaging with DNA-PAINT and Exchange-PAINT. Nat Methods. 2014;11:313–8.

48. Vogelsang J, Cordes T, Forthmann C, Steinhauer C, Tinnefeld P. Controlling the fluorescence of ordinary oxazine dyes for single-molecule switching and superresolution microscopy. Proc Natl Acad Sci. 2009;106:8107–12.

49. Dempsey GT, Vaughan JC, Chen KH, Bates M, Zhuang X. Evaluation of fluorophores for optimal performance in localization-based super-resolution imaging. Nat Methods. 2011;8:1027–36.

50. van de Linde S, Endesfelder U, Mukherjee A, Schüttpelz M, Wiebusch G, Wolter S, et al. Multicolor photoswitching microscopy for subdiffraction-resolution fluorescence imaging. Photochem Photobiol Sci. 2009;8:465.

51. Shroff H, Galbraith CG, Galbraith JA, White H, Gillette J, Olenych S, et al. Dual-color superresolution imaging of genetically expressed probes within individual adhesion complexes. Proc Natl Acad Sci. 2007;104:20308–13.

52. Bock H, Geisler C, Wurm CA, von Middendorff C, Jakobs S, Schönle A, et al. Two-color far-field fluorescence nanoscopy based on photoswitchable emitters. Appl Phys B. 2007;88:161–5.

53. Bates M, Huang B, Dempsey GT, Zhuang X. Multicolor super-resolution imaging with photo-switchable fluorescent probes. Science. 2007;317:1749–53.

54. Huang B, Wang W, Bates M, Zhuang X. Three-dimensional super-resolution imaging by stochastic optical reconstruction microscopy. Science. 2008;319:810–3.

55. Juette MF, Gould TJ, Lessard MD, Mlodzianoski MJ, Nagpure BS, Bennett BT, et al. Three-dimensional sub–100 nm resolution fluorescence microscopy of thick samples. Nat Methods. 2008;5:527–9.

56. Shtengel G, Galbraith JA, Galbraith CG, Lippincott-Schwartz J, Gillette JM, Manley S, et al. Interferometric fluorescent super-resolution microscopy resolves 3D cellular ultrastructure. Proc Natl Acad Sci. 2009;106:3125–30.

57. Pavani SRP, Thompson MA, Biteen JS, Lord SJ, Liu N, Twieg RJ, et al. Three-dimensional, single-molecule fluorescence imaging beyond the diffraction limit by using a double-helix point spread function. Proc Natl Acad Sci. 2009;106:2995–9.

58. Durisic N, Laparra-Cuervo L, Sandoval-Álvarez Á, Borbely JS, Lakadamyali M. Single-molecule evaluation of fluorescent protein photoactivation efficiency using an in vivo nanotemplate. Nat Methods. 2014;11:156–62.

59. Jones SA, Shim S-H, He J, Zhuang X. Fast, three-dimensional super-resolution imaging of live cells. Nat Methods. 2011;8:499–505.

60. Huang F, Hartwich TMP, Rivera-Molina FE, Lin Y, Duim WC, Long JJ, et al. Video-rate nanoscopy using sCMOS camera–specific single-molecule localization algorithms. Nat Methods. 2013;10:653–8.

61. Min J, Vonesch C, Kirshner H, Carlini L, Olivier N, Holden S, et al. FALCON: fast and unbiased reconstruction of high-density super-resolution microscopy data. Sci Rep. 2015;4:4577.

62. Cox S, Rosten E, Monypenny J, Jovanovic-Talisman T, Burnette DT, Lippincott-Schwartz J, et al. Bayesian localization microscopy reveals nanoscale podosome dynamics. Nat Methods. 2012;9:195–200.

63. Gustafsson N, Culley S, Ashdown G, Owen DM, Pereira PM, Henriques R. Fast live-cell conventional fluorophore nanoscopy with ImageJ through super-resolution radial fluctuations. Nat Commun. 2016;7:12471.

64. Power RM, Huisken J. A guide to light-sheet fluorescence microscopy for multiscale imaging. Nat Methods. 2017;14:360–73.

65. Voie AH, Burns DH, Spelman FA. Orthogonal-plane fluorescence optical sectioning: three-dimensional imaging of macroscopic biological specimens. J Microsc. 1993;170:229–36.

66. Huisken J. Optical sectioning deep inside live embryos by selective plane illumination microscopy. Science. 2004;305:1007–9.

67. Chen B-C, Legant WR, Wang K, Shao L, Milkie DE, Davidson MW, et al. Lattice light-sheet microscopy: Imaging molecules to embryos at high spatiotemporal resolution. Science. 2014;346:1257998.

68. Planchon TA, Gao L, Milkie DE, Davidson MW, Galbraith JA, Galbraith CG, et al. Rapid three-dimensional isotropic imaging of living cells using Bessel beam plane illumination. Nat Methods. 2011;8:417–23.

69. Cella Zanacchi F, Lavagnino Z, Perrone Donnorso M, Del Bue A, Furia L, Faretta M, et al. Live-cell 3D super-resolution imaging in thick biological samples. Nat Methods. 2011;8:1047–9.

70. Gao L, Shao L, Higgins CD, Poulton JS, Peifer M, Davidson MW, et al. Noninvasive imaging beyond the diffraction limit of 3D dynamics in thickly fluorescent specimens. Cell. 2012;151:1370–85.

71. Chang B-J, Perez Meza VD, Stelzer EHK. csiLSFM combines light-sheet fluorescence microscopy and coherent structured illumination for a lateral resolution below 100 nm. Proc Natl Acad Sci. 2017;114:4869–74.

72. Kner P, Chhun BB, Griffis ER, Winoto L, Gustafsson MGL. Super-resolution video microscopy of live cells by structured illumination. Nat Methods. 2009;6:339–42.

73. Schneider J, Zahn J, Maglione M, Sigrist SJ, Marquard J, Chojnacki J, et al. Ultrafast, temporally stochastic STED nanoscopy of millisecond dynamics. Nat Methods. 2015;12:827–30.

74. Schwentker MA, Bock H, Hofmann M, Jakobs S, Bewersdorf J, Eggeling C, et al. Wide-field subdiffraction RESOLFT microscopy using fluorescent protein photoswitching. Microsc Res Tech. 2007;70:269–80.

75. Chmyrov A, Keller J, Grotjohann T, Ratz M, d'Este E, Jakobs S, et al. Nanoscopy with more than 100,000 "doughnuts". Nat Methods. 2013;10:737–40.

76. Yang B, Przybilla F, Mestre M, Trebbia J-B, Lounis B. Large parallelization of STED nanoscopy using optical lattices. Opt Express. 2014;22:5581.

77. Eggeling C, Hilbert M, Bock H, Ringemann C, Hofmann M, Stiel AC, et al. Reversible photoswitching enables single-molecule fluorescence fluctuation spectroscopy at high molecular concentration. Microsc Res Tech. 2007;70:1003–9.

78. Manley S, Gillette JM, Patterson GH, Shroff H, Hess HF, Betzig E, et al. High-density mapping of single-molecule trajectories with photoactivated localization microscopy. Nat Methods. 2008;5:155–7.

79. Magde D, Elson E, Webb WW. Thermodynamic fluctuations in a reacting system—measurement by fluorescence correlation spectroscopy. Phys Rev Lett. 1972;29:705–8.

80. Schwille P, Korlach J, Webb WW. Fluorescence correlation spectroscopy with single-molecule sensitivity on cell and model membranes. Cytometry. 1999;36:176–82.

81. Eggeling C, Ringemann C, Medda R, Schwarzmann G, Sandhoff K, Polyakova S, et al. Direct observation of the nanoscale dynamics of membrane lipids in a living cell. Nature. 2009;457:1159–62.

82. Honigmann A, Mueller V, Ta H, Schoenle A, Sezgin E, Hell SW, et al. Scanning STED-FCS reveals spatiotemporal heterogeneity of lipid interaction in the plasma membrane of living cells. Nat Commun. 2014;5:5412.

83. Benda A, Ma Y, Gaus K. Self-calibrated line-scan STED-FCS to quantify lipid dynamics in model and cell membranes. Biophys J. 2015;108:596–609.

84. Chojnacki J, Waithe D, Carravilla P, Huarte N, Galiani S, Enderlein J, et al. Envelope glycoprotein mobility on HIV-1 particles depends on the virus maturation state. Nat Commun. 2017;8:545.

85. Lanzanò L, Scipioni L, Di Bona M, Bianchini P, Bizzarri R, Cardarelli F, et al. Measurement of nanoscale three-dimensional diffusion in the interior of living cells by STED-FCS. Nat Commun. 2017;8:65.

86. Urban NT, Willig KI, Hell SW, Nägerl UV. STED nanoscopy of actin dynamics in synapses deep inside living brain slices. Biophys J. 2011;101:1277–84.

87. Gould TJ, Burke D, Bewersdorf J, Booth MJ. Adaptive optics enables 3D STED microscopy in aberrating specimens. Opt Express. 2012;20:20998.

88. Takasaki KT, Ding JB, Sabatini BL. Live-cell superresolution imaging by pulsed STED two-photon excitation microscopy. Biophys J. 2013;104:770–7.

89. Moneron G, Hell SW. Two-photon excitation STED microscopy. Opt Express. 2009;17:14567.

90. Fölling J, Belov V, Riedel D, Schönle A, Egner A, Eggeling C, et al. fluorescence nanoscopy with optical sectioning by two-photon induced molecular switching using continuous-wave lasers. ChemPhysChem. 2008;9:321–6.

91. Booth MJ. Adaptive optical microscopy: the ongoing quest for a perfect image. Light Sci Appl. 2014;3:e165.

92. Heintzmann R, Huser T. Super-resolution structured illumination microscopy. Chem Rev. 2017;117:13890–908.

93. Wäldchen S, Lehmann J, Klein T, van de Linde S, Sauer M. Light-induced cell damage in live-cell super-resolution microscopy. Sci Rep. 2015;5:15348.

94. Xiong Y, Rivera-Fuentes P, Sezgin E, Vargas Jentzsch A, Eggeling C, Anderson HL. Photoswitchable spiropyran dyads for biological imaging. Org Lett. 2016;18:3666–9.

95. Hubner W, McNerney GP, Chen P, Dale BM, Gordon RE, Chuang FYS, et al. Quantitative 3D video microscopy of HIV transfer across T cell virological synapses. Science. 2009;323:1743–7.

96. Ivanchenko S, Godinez WJ, Lampe M, Kräusslich H-G, Eils R, Rohr K, et al. Dynamics of HIV-1 assembly and release. Mothes W, editor. PLoS Pathog. 2009;5:e1000652.

97. Nakane S, Iwamoto A, Matsuda Z. The V4 and V5 variable loops of HIV-1 envelope glycoprotein are tolerant to insertion of green fluorescent protein and are useful targets for labeling. J Biol Chem. 2015;290:15279–91.

98. Pereira CF, Ellenberg PC, Jones KL, Fernandez TL, Smyth RP, Hawkes DJ, et al. Labeling of multiple HIV-1 proteins with the biarsenical-tetracysteine system. Aiyar A, editor. PLoS ONE. 2011;6:e17016.

99. Eckhardt M, Anders M, Muranyi W, Heilemann M, Krijnse-Locker J, Müller B. A SNAP-tagged derivative of HIV-1—a versatile tool to study virus-cell interactions. Ambrose Z, editor. PLoS ONE. 2011;6:e22007.

100. Hanne J, Göttfert F, Schimer J, Anders-Össwein M, Konvalinka J, Engelhardt J, et al. Stimulated emission depletion nanoscopy reveals time-course of human immunodeficiency virus proteolytic maturation. ACS Nano. 2016;10:8215–22.

101. Sakin V, Hanne J, Dunder J, Anders-Össwein M, Laketa V, Nikić I, et al. A versatile tool for live-cell imaging and super-resolution nanoscopy

studies of HIV-1 env distribution and mobility. Cell Chem Biol. 2017;24(635–645):e5.

102. Sakin V, Paci G, Lemke EA, Müller B. Labeling of virus components for advanced, quantitative imaging analyses. FEBS Lett. 2016;590:1896–914.

103. Freed EO. HIV-1 assembly, release and maturation. Nat Rev Microbiol. 2015;13:484–96.

104. Lippincott-Schwartz J, Freed EO, van Engelenburg SB. A consensus view of ESCRT-mediated human immunodeficiency virus Type 1 abscission. Annu Rev Virol. 2017;4:309–25.

105. Malkusch S, Muranyi W, Müller B, Kräusslich H-G, Heilemann M. Single-molecule coordinate-based analysis of the morphology of HIV-1 assembly sites with near-molecular spatial resolution. Histochem Cell Biol. 2013;139:173–9.

106. Helma J, Schmidthals K, Lux V, Nüske S, Scholz AM, Kräusslich H-G, et al. Direct and dynamic detection of HIV-1 in living cells. Marcello A, editor. PLoS ONE. 2012;7:e50026.

107. Gunzenhäuser J, Olivier N, Pengo T, Manley S. Quantitative super-resolution imaging reveals protein stoichiometry and nanoscale morphology of assembling HIV-gag virions. Nano Lett. 2012;12:4705–10.

108. Lehmann M, Rocha S, Mangeat B, Blanchet F, Uji-i H, Hofkens J, et al. Quantitative multicolor super-resolution microscopy reveals tetherin HIV-1 interaction. Kräusslich H-G, editor. PLoS Pathog. 2011;7:e1002456.

109. Muranyi W, Malkusch S, Müller B, Heilemann M, Kräusslich H-G. Super-resolution microscopy reveals specific recruitment of HIV-1 envelope proteins to viral assembly sites dependent on the envelope C-terminal tail. Trkola A, editor. PLoS Pathog. 2013;9:e1003198.

110. Gunzenhäuser J, Wyss R, Manley S. A quantitative approach to evaluate the impact of fluorescent labeling on membrane-bound HIV-gag assembly by titration of unlabeled proteins. Saad J, editor. PLoS ONE. 2014;9:e115095.

111. Tedbury PR, Freed EO. The role of matrix in HIV-1 envelope glycoprotein incorporation. Trends Microbiol. 2014;22:372–8.

112. Chojnacki J, Staudt T, Glass B, Bingen P, Engelhardt J, Anders M, et al. Maturation-dependent HIV-1 surface protein redistribution revealed by fluorescence nanoscopy. Science. 2012;338:524–8.

113. Zhu P, Chertova E, Bess J, Lifson JD, Arthur LO, Liu J, et al. Electron tomography analysis of envelope glycoprotein trimers on HIV and simian immunodeficiency virus virions. Proc Natl Acad Sci. 2003;100:15812–7.

114. Roy NH, Chan J, Lambele M, Thali M. Clustering and mobility of HIV-1 env at viral assembly sites predict its propensity to induce cell-cell fusion. J Virol. 2013;87:7516–25.

115. Brugger B, Glass B, Haberkant P, Leibrecht I, Wieland FT, Kräusslich H-G. The HIV lipidome: a raft with an unusual composition. Proc Natl Acad Sci. 2006;103:2641–6.

116. Lorizate M, Sachsenheimer T, Glass B, Habermann A, Gerl MJ, Kräusslich H-G, et al. Comparative lipidomics analysis of HIV-1 particles and their producer cell membrane in different cell lines: Lipidomics of HIV-1 particles and producer plasma membranes. Cell Microbiol. 2013;15:292–304.

117. Chan R, Uchil PD, Jin J, Shui G, Ott DE, Mothes W, et al. Retroviruses human immunodeficiency virus and murine leukemia virus are enriched in phosphoinositides. J Virol. 2008;82:11228–38.

118. Sezgin E, Levental I, Mayor S, Eggeling C. The mystery of membrane organization: composition, regulation and roles of lipid rafts. Nat Rev Mol Cell Biol. 2017;18:361–74.

119. Jouvenet N, Zhadina M, Bieniasz PD, Simon SM. Dynamics of ESCRT protein recruitment during retroviral assembly. Nat Cell Biol. 2011;13:394–401.

120. Baumgärtel V, Ivanchenko S, Dupont A, Sergeev M, Wiseman PW, Kräusslich H-G, et al. Live-cell visualization of dynamics of HIV budding site interactions with an ESCRT component. Nat Cell Biol. 2011;13:469–74.

121. Prescher J, Baumgärtel V, Ivanchenko S, Torrano AA, Bräuchle C, Müller B, et al. Super-resolution imaging of ESCRT-proteins at HIV-1 assembly sites. Aiken C, editor. PLoS Pathog. 2015;11:e1004677.

122. Bleck M, Itano MS, Johnson DS, Thomas VK, North AJ, Bieniasz PD, et al. Temporal and spatial organization of ESCRT protein recruitment during HIV-1 budding. Proc Natl Acad Sci. 2014;111:12211–6.

123. Van Engelenburg SB, Shtengel G, Sengupta P, Waki K, Jarnik M, Ablan SD, et al. Distribution of ESCRT machinery at HIV assembly sites reveals virus scaffolding of ESCRT subunits. Science. 2014;343:653–6.

124. Neil SJD, Zang T, Bieniasz PD. Tetherin inhibits retrovirus release and is antagonized by HIV-1 Vpu. Nature. 2008;451:425–30.

125. Van Damme N, Goff D, Katsura C, Jorgenson RL, Mitchell R, Johnson MC, et al. The interferon-induced protein BST-2 restricts HIV-1 release and is downregulated from the cell surface by the viral vpu protein. Cell Host Microbe. 2008;3:245–52.

126. Lelek M, Di Nunzio F, Henriques R, Charneau P, Arhel N, Zimmer C. Superresolution imaging of HIV in infected cells with FlAsH-PALM. Proc Natl Acad Sci. 2012;109:8564–9.

127. Brandenberg OF, Magnus C, Rusert P, Regoes RR, Trkola A. Different infectivity of HIV-1 strains is linked to number of envelope trimers required for entry. Emerman M, editor. PLoS Pathog. 2015;11:e1004595.

128. Brandenberg OF, Magnus C, Regoes RR, Trkola A. The HIV-1 entry process: a stoichiometric view. Trends Microbiol. 2015;23:763–74.

129. Sattentau QJ. Cell-to-cell spread of retroviruses. Viruses. 2010;2:1306–21.

130. Battistini A, Sgarbanti M. HIV-1 latency: an update of molecular mechanisms and therapeutic strategies. Viruses. 2014;6:1715–58.

131. Malim MH, Emerman M. HIV-1 accessory proteins—ensuring viral survival in a hostile environment. Cell Host Microbe. 2008;3:388–98.

132. Dirk BS, Pawlak EN, Johnson AL, Van Nynatten LR, Jacob RA, Heit B, et al. HIV-1 Nef sequesters MHC-I intracellularly by targeting early stages of endocytosis and recycling. Sci Rep. 2016;6:37021.

133. Russell RA, Chojnacki J, Jones DM, Johnson E, Do T, Eggeling C, et al. Astrocytes resist HIV-1 fusion but engulf infected macrophage material. Cell Rep. 2017;18:1473–83.

134. Sougrat R, Bartesaghi A, Lifson JD, Bennett AE, Bess JW, Zabransky DJ, et al. Electron tomography of the contact between T cells and SIV/HIV-1: implications for viral entry. PLoS Pathog. 2007;3:e63.

135. Mengistu M, Ray K, Lewis GK, DeVico AL. Antigenic properties of the human immunodeficiency virus envelope glycoprotein Gp120 on virions bound to target cells. Aiken C, editor. PLoS Pathog. 2015;11:e1004772.

136. Pereira CF, Rossy J, Owen DM, Mak J, Gaus K. HIV taken by STORM: super-resolution fluorescence microscopy of a viral infection. Virol J. 2012;9:84.

137. Pham S, Tabarin T, Garvey M, Pade C, Rossy J, Monaghan P, et al. Cryo-electron microscopy and single molecule fluorescent microscopy detect CD4 receptor induced HIV size expansion prior to cell entry. Virology. 2015;486:121–33.

138. Peng K, Muranyi W, Glass B, Laketa V, Yant SR, Tsai L, et al. Quantitative microscopy of functional HIV post-entry complexes reveals association of replication with the viral capsid. eLife. 2014;3:e04114.

139. Hulme AE, Kelley Z, Foley D, Hope TJ. Complementary assays reveal a low level of CA associated with viral complexes in the nuclei of HIV-1-infected cells. Ross SR, editor. J Virol. 2015;89:5350–61.

8

Reconstruction of a replication-competent ancestral murine endogenous retrovirus-L

Daniel Blanco-Melo[1,3] ⓘ, Robert J. Gifford[2] and Paul D. Bieniasz[1]* ⓘ

Abstract

Background: About 10% of the mouse genome is composed of endogenous retroviruses (ERVs) that represent a molecular fossil record of past retroviral infections. One such retrovirus, murine ERV-L (MuERV-L) is an *env*-deficient ERV that has undergone episodic proliferation, with the most recent amplification occurring ~2 million years ago. MuERV-L related sequences have been co-opted by mice for antiretroviral defense, and possibly as promoters for some genes that regulate totipotency in early mouse embryos. However, MuERV-L sequences present in modern mouse genomes have not been observed to replicate.

Results: Here, we describe the reconstruction of an ancestral MuERV-L (ancML) sequence through paleovirological analyses of MuERV-L elements in the modern mouse genome. The resulting MuERV-L (ancML) sequence was synthesized and a reporter gene embedded. The reconstructed MuERV-L (ancML) could replicate in a manner that is dependent on reverse transcription and generated de novo integrants. Notably, MuERV-L (ancML) exhibited a narrow host range. Interferon-α could reduce MuERV-L (ancML) replication, suggesting the existence of interferon-inducible genes that could inhibit MuERV-L replication. While mouse APOBEC3 was able to restrict the replication of MuERV-L (ancML), inspection of endogenous MuERV-L sequences suggested that the impact of APOBEC3 mediated hypermutation on MuERV-L has been minimal.

Conclusion: The reconstruction of an ancestral MuERV-L sequence highlights the potential for the retroviral fossil record to illuminate ancient events and enable studies of the impact of retroviral elements on animal evolution.

Background

Uniquely among animal viruses, retroviruses integrate into the genome of the host cell as an obligate step in their replication cycle. Because the target cells of some retroviruses can include cells of the germ line, proviruses can occasionally become vertically inherited [1]. A subset of these inherited proviruses can become fixed in the population through genetic drift, or sometimes by providing an evolutionary advantage to the host. Inherited proviruses are termed endogenous retroviruses (ERVs) and are present in all animal species that have been examined, accounting for approximately 8 and 10% of the

human and mouse genomes, respectively [2]. In nearly every case, however, fixed proviruses have inactivating mutations that prevent their further spread.

The vast array of ERVs represent an extensive viral fossil record that provides an opportunity to study the biology of ancient or extinct retroviruses, and the effects that these viruses have had on the evolution of their hosts [3]. Previously, we and others have reconstructed a full-length infectious human ERV (HERV-K) [4, 5], functional capsid proteins of endogenous chimpanzee gammaretroviruses (CERV 1 and 2) [6, 7], and lentiviruses, PSIV and RELIK [8], as well as functional envelope proteins from CERV2 and HERV-T [9, 10]. These reconstruction experiments have enabled the identification of ancient virus receptors [9, 10] and demonstrated the ancient origin of cyclophilin A-lentiviral capsid interactions [8].

*Correspondence: pbieniasz@rockefeller.edu
[1] Laboratory of Retrovirology and Howard Hughes Medical Institute, The Rockefeller University, New York, NY, USA
Full list of author information is available at the end of the article

Additionally, these studies have shown that the replication of HERV-K, CERV1 and CERV2 was affected by the APOBEC3 cytidine deaminases [5, 6, 11]. Overall these "paleovirological" studies have provided previously inaccessible insights into the co-evolution of viruses and hosts.

Murine ERV-L (MuERV-L) is an abundant mouse ERV that is transcriptionally active at an early (2-cell) stage of the mouse embryo [12–15]. Previous analyses have established that MuERV-L underwent two amplification bursts, one after the divergence of the *Mus* and *Rattus* genera around ~10 million years ago (MYA), and a more recent and prolific burst about 2 MYA, which is distinguished by the presence of a 33nt in-frame deletion in the 5' half of the *gag* ORF (Fig. 1a) [16]. These amplifications led to the deposition of thousands of MuERV-L derived sequences in the mouse genome. Moreover, MuERV-L belongs to a larger family of ERV-L elements that have been active throughout the evolution of mammals [17–19]. In contrast to their human counterparts, many MuERV-L elements have complete coding potential, encoding open reading frames (ORFs) for *gag* and *pol* (Fig. 1a) [20]. However, like other ERV-L elements, MuERV-L is characterized by the complete absence of an *env* gene that, coupled with its highly restricted early transcription profile, suggests an entirely intracellular retrotransposon-like replication cycle [21]. Indeed, MuERV-L transcripts are able to give rise to intracellular viral-like particles that accumulate in the endoplasmic reticulum [13] but are not thought to be replication competent.

MuERV-L related or derived sequences appear to have been co-opted for two distinct biological activities in the mouse. The antiretroviral restriction factor Fv1, which inhibits infection by MuLV and certain other retroviruses is derived from MuERV-L-like Gag sequences and appeared in the mouse genome at least 5 MYA [22–24]. Additionally, recent studies have suggested that the propensity of MuERV-L to be transcriptionally active only at the two-cell stage of mouse embryogenesis may have led to the co-option of its long terminal repeats (LTRs), as promoters of genes involved in the zygotic genome activation [14, 15]. Transcriptional activity of MuERV-L LTRs in two-cell mouse embryos may drive the expression of hundreds of genes that contribute to the totipotency of the blastomeres, but also results in the expression of MuERV-L Gag–Pol polyprotein and the formation of intracellular viral-like particles [13–15]. As development progresses, MuERV-L LTRs appear to be silenced [14, 25, 26]. The expression of MuERV-L at the two-cell stage does not induce an increase in their copy numbers, suggesting that the expressed proviruses do not have the potential to re-integrate into the genome [25].

In fact, no extant copy of MuERV-L has been demonstrated to be capable of completing a replication cycle. Therefore, we set out to derive a replication-competent MuERV-L, based on the premise that an ancestral reconstruction would deliver a sequence that most closely resembles that of a functional ancestor. Herein, we describe the analysis of MuERV-L elements in the mouse genome, a successful reconstruction of a ~2MY old replication-competent ancestral sequence and an analysis of its replication and its interaction with the components of the host intrinsic/innate immune systems.

Methods

Bioinformatic analyses and ancestral reconstruction

Screening for MuERV-L elements was performed using amino acid and nucleotide sequences from the MuERV-L reference sequence (MuERV-L[ref], GenBank: Y12713) [20] as probes for tBLASTn (*gag* and *pol*) and BLASTn (LTR) [27] searches of two mouse genome assemblies: Mm_Celera (NCBI: GCF_000002165.2) [28] and GRCm38/mm10 (UCSC: mm10) [29]. To avoid the identification of sequences from related but distinct retroviruses, BLAST hits with an e-value $\leq$ 1e−10 were used as probes for a second round of BLASTx or BLASTn searches against a previously constructed database of endogenous and exogenous class III retroviral sequences. Results from these BLAST searches were imported into a relational database to facilitate the management of the screening process and analysis of hits. Reciprocal hits to MuERV-L[ref] were first ordered by chromosome and orientation and then adjacent or overlapping hits were assembled into proviral loci by comparison with the MuERV-L[ref] sequence, allowing for insertions no longer than 10,000 nucleotides. The resulting MuERV-L loci were annotated as genomic features of GRCm38 (downloaded from Ensembl [30] using BioMart) by comparison of their chromosome location using in-house Perl scripts.

Dates of integration for MuERV-L elements were estimated by determining the divergence (K) to a consensus sequence (for solo LTRs) or between paired LTRs (for provirus-containing loci) using PAUP* [31], divided by 2× the mouse neutral substitution rate (r) of 4.5×10^{-9} substitutions per site per year [29] (K/2r) [32, 33]. The mean sequence identity between the consensus LTR sequence and each of the solo LTRs was 95.43%, with very few outliers (1.5% of solo LTRs showed less than 80% identity), suggesting that the consensus sequence is adequate to perform these estimations. Nevertheless, the estimated ages derived using this method represent approximations to the integration dates and should be treated as such.

Statistical analyses of the positions of MuERV-L elements relative to mouse genomic features were

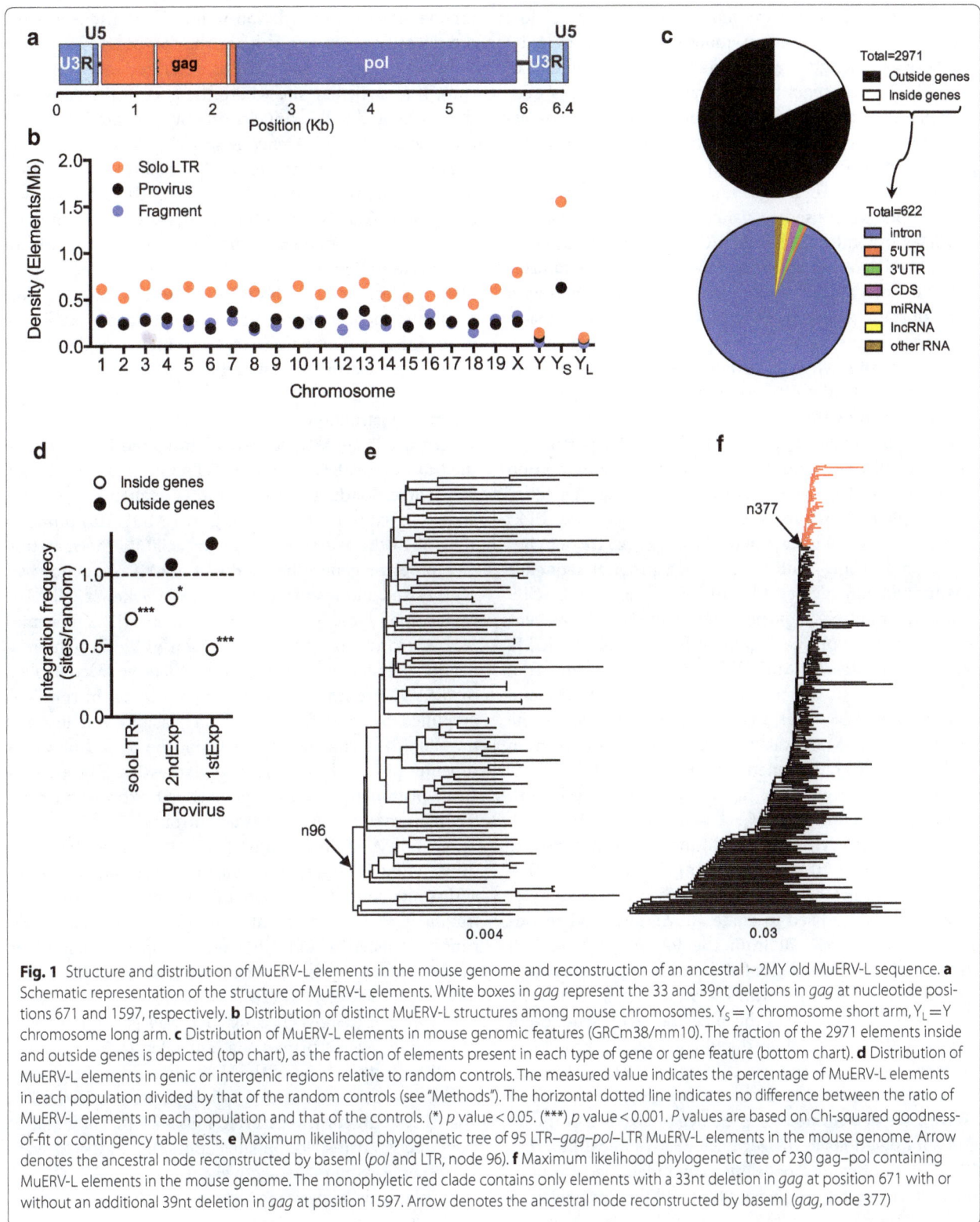

Fig. 1 Structure and distribution of MuERV-L elements in the mouse genome and reconstruction of an ancestral ~ 2MY old MuERV-L sequence. **a** Schematic representation of the structure of MuERV-L elements. White boxes in *gag* represent the 33 and 39nt deletions in *gag* at nucleotide positions 671 and 1597, respectively. **b** Distribution of distinct MuERV-L structures among mouse chromosomes. Y_S = Y chromosome short arm, Y_L = Y chromosome long arm. **c** Distribution of MuERV-L elements in mouse genomic features (GRCm38/mm10). The fraction of the 2971 elements inside and outside genes is depicted (top chart), as the fraction of elements present in each type of gene or gene feature (bottom chart). **d** Distribution of MuERV-L elements in genic or intergenic regions relative to random controls. The measured value indicates the percentage of MuERV-L elements in each population divided by that of the random controls (see "Methods"). The horizontal dotted line indicates no difference between the ratio of MuERV-L elements in each population and that of the controls. (*) *p* value < 0.05. (***) *p* value < 0.001. *P* values are based on Chi-squared goodness-of-fit or contingency table tests. **e** Maximum likelihood phylogenetic tree of 95 LTR–*gag*–*pol*–LTR MuERV-L elements in the mouse genome. Arrow denotes the ancestral node reconstructed by baseml (*pol* and LTR, node 96). **f** Maximum likelihood phylogenetic tree of 230 gag–pol containing MuERV-L elements in the mouse genome. The monophyletic red clade contains only elements with a 33nt deletion in *gag* at position 671 with or without an additional 39nt deletion in *gag* at position 1597. Arrow denotes the ancestral node reconstructed by baseml (*gag*, node 377)

performed using the Pearson's Chi-squared test for count data (chisq.test) implemented in R. As controls, two sets of random coordinates in the mouse genome were computationally generated using in-house Perl scripts and the runif function implemented in R. For solo LTR comparisons, 10,000 random mouse sequences of 500 nucleotides in length were generated. For proviral loci comparisons, 5000 random mouse sequences of 6500 nucleotides in length were generated. The coordinates of both MuERV-L integrations and random sequences were then mapped to the GRCm38 genome assembly to determine overlapping genomic features (intergenic regions, genes, common repeats and others) using in-house Perl scripts. For ancML integration comparisons, in-house Perl scripts were used to generate controls, consisting of 1000 randomly selected EcoRV-containing fragments (of 1000 nucleotides in length) from the Chinese hamster genome. Each ancML integration site was matched with three of these genomic sequences such that control sites were equidistant from an EcoRV site as was each ancML integration site, as described in [34]. These sites were then mapped to the Chinese hamster genome (criGri1) [35] to determine the overlapping genomic features.

Ancestral reconstruction of MuERV-L was performed using two distinct sequence sets. For the reconstruction of the ancestral *pol* gene and the LTRs, we used a set of 95 complete proviral sequences (LTR–*gag*–*pol*–LTR) identified by default-parameter based BLASTn searches of GRCm38 using MuERV-L^{ref}. Each proviral sequence was individually aligned to MuERV-L^{ref} using MUSCLE [36] and a multiple sequence alignment (MSA) was generated using the profile alignment function of MUSCLE. Insertions relative to MuERV-L^{ref} were eliminated from the MSA, except a 6nt insertion at position 298 and 6249 in both LTRs that was shared between 25% of the sequences. The MSA was used to construct a maximum likelihood (ML) phylogenetic tree using raxML [37] with the following parameters: rapid bootstrap analysis with 1000 replicates under GTRCAT followed by a ML search under GTRGAMMA to evaluate the final tree topology (-m GTRCAT -# 1000 -x 13 -k -f a). Thereafter, the tree was midpoint rooted. The MSA together with the phylogenetic tree were used to guide an ML ancestral reconstruction using baseml from the PAML package [38] (model: REV, initial values of alpha and kappa were calculated on the MSA by jmodeltest [39], branch lengths were used as initial values). For the ancestral reconstruction of the *gag* ORF we first aligned and constructed a phylogenetic tree using 230 *gag*–*pol* containing sequences (identified by our screening of the mouse genome described above). We determined the presence or absence of the 33 and 39nt deletions in the *gag* ORF relative to MuERV-L^{ref} (that does not show any deletion) and identified a monophyletic clade of 40 sequences that had the 33nt deletion in *gag* (irrespective of the status of the 39nt deletion). Thereafter, reconstruction of the ancestral *gag* sequence corresponding to the internal node for this monophyletic clade was performed as described above. A correction for the effect of methylation-induced mutations at CpG dinucleotides was applied on both strands of all three sequences (*gag*, *pol* and LTR) as described in [8]. Specifically, if a particular site where the ancestral reconstruction estimated a TG dinucleotide but at least 10% of the sequences in the MSA encoded a CG at that position, the TG state was considered to be the result of methylation-induced mutation and the sequence at this position was assigned as CG. The resulting sequences were combined to produce the sequence from which ancML was derived.

Hypermutation analysis and statistics were performed using Hypermut 2.0 [40] on the set of 230 *gag*–*pol* containing sequences used to reconstruct an ancestral *gag*, using either default parameters or with exclusion of sites with a 5′ C next to the mutated G.

Plasmid construction

To construct ancML, sequences from the U3 region of the MuERV-L 5′LTR 5′ to the TATA box were substituted with corresponding CMV promoter sequences. We also added an extra 12nt containing two MluI sites immediately 3′ to the *pol* stop codon to facilitate the insertion of a reporter gene. The modified ancML sequence was synthesized and inserted into pUC57 (Genewiz, NJ). The replication dependent LINE-1 element (L1.3 plasmid) [41] was kindly provided by Dr. John V. Moran. The replication dependent *neo* cassette (a *neo* gene controlled by a SV40 promoter and interrupted by an intron) was amplified by PCR from the L1.3 plasmid and inserted into ancML using the MluI sites at the 3′ end of *pol*. A separate pCR3.1 based plasmid, expressing GFP (from a CMV promoter) and a *neo* gene (NEO, expressed from a SV40 promoter) was used as a control.

The ancML-RTmut construct was created by using overlapping PCR and primers that annealed to the RT active site with four nucleotide mismatches, the PCR fragment was inserted into ancML using unique surrounding BstZ17I and NheI restriction sites contained in the outmost primers, generating an ancML with a mutated RT active site (YIDD to AIAA).

The ancMLΔGAAGT construct was generated using PCR and a reverse primer that annealed to the 5′ end of the PBS and the 3′ end of the U5 region of the 5′LTR, and lacked the intervening 5nt linker sequence (GAAGT). The PCR fragment was inserted into ancML using unique AgeI and KpnI restriction sites contained in the forward and reverse primers, respectively.

A plasmid expressing mouse APOBEC3 (mA3, C57BL/6J strain) was kindly provided by Rachel Liberatore (unpublished). A C-termini HA-tagged version of mA3 was produced by PCR using primers containing two HA tags and a 15nt linker sequence, following previously published functional human HA-tagged APOBEC3 proteins [42, 43]. This construct was introduced into the retroviral expression plasmid LBCX using unique SfiI sites. A retroviral vector (LBCX) expressing Fv1^{bbn} was kindly provided by Dr. Theodora Hatziioannou [44].

Cell culture

Cell lines (except CHO-K1 and pgsA cells) were maintained in Dulbecco's Modified Eagle Medium (DMEM), Eagle's Minimum Essential Medium (EMEM) or Roswell Park Memorial Institute medium (RPMI) supplemented with 10% FBS and gentamycin (2 µg/ml, Gibco) according to ATCC instructions. CHO-K1 and pgsA cells were maintained in Ham's F-12 media supplemented with 10% FBS, 1 mM of L-glutamine and 2 µg/ml of gentamycin. All cells were incubated at 37 °C, except DF-1 cells that were incubated at 39 °C.

Generation of CHO cell lines expressing murine APOBEC3

293T cells were transfected (using polyethylenimine) with plasmids expressing MuLV gag–pol, and VSV-G, along with an LBCX based retroviral vector expressing HA-tagged mA3 or Fv1^{bbn}. Viral stocks were harvested and filtered (0.22 µm) 2 days after transfection, and were used to transduce CHO-K1 cells (seeded in 24 well plates). Transduced cells were expanded in 10 cm dishes with media supplemented with 5 µg/ml of blasticidin (Thermo Fisher Scientific Inc.). Single cell clones expressing mA3 were isolated by seeding blasticidin resistant cells at 0.5 cells per well in a 96 well plate. Three distinct single clones that expressed mA3 in 100% of the cells (tested by immunofluorescence) were used in ancML replication assays.

Immunofluorescence assay

Individual clones of CHO cells expressing murine APOBEC3 were fixed with 4% paraformaldehyde (PFA) for 30 min followed by treatment with 10 mM glycine (diluted in PBS) for another 30 min. Cells were permeabilized with a buffer containing 0.1% of Triton X-100 and 5% goat serum (diluted in PBS) for 15 min. Cells were then washed 2 times with PBS before being treated with mouse monoclonal anti-HA antibody (Covance) diluted in a buffer containing 0.1% Tween-20 and 5% goat serum (diluted in PBS) for 2 h at room temperature. Cells were washed three times with PBS before being treated with goat anti-mouse secondary antibody (Alexa Fluor 488 dye, ThermoFisher) diluted in a buffer containing 0.1% Tween-20 and 5% goat serum (diluted in PBS) for 1 h at room temperature. Cells were washed three more times with PBS and fluorescent microscopy images were analyzed using the EVOS FL Cell Imaging System.

MuLV infection assay

293T cells were transfected (using polyethylenimine) with plasmids expressing N-tropic or B-tropic MuLV gag–pol, and VSV-G, along with a CNCG based retroviral vector expressing GFP [45]. Viral stocks were harvested 2 days after transfection, filtered (0.22 µm) and were used to infect control or Fv1^{bbn}-expressing CHO cells. Two days post infection the percentage of GFP positive population was quantified using the Guava EasyCyte flow cytometer (Millipore).

MuERV-L(ancML) replication assays

The cell lines listed in Table 2 were seeded in 12 well plates 1 day before being transfected with 700 ng of plasmids containing L1.3, ancML or a plasmid expressing *gfp* and a *neo* gene, using 4 µl of Lipofectamine 2000 (Thermo Fisher Scientific Inc.) according to manufacturer instructions. Two days after transfection, cells were plated in 6-well plates with G418 selection media (containing concentrations of G418 that were previously calibrated for each cell type). Ten days later, surviving cells were fixed with 4% PFA and colonies were stained using 0.3% crystal violet in 20% ethanol for counting.

Subsequently, the ancML replication assays were routinely done using CHO-K1 cells as follows. CHO-K1 cells were seeded at 3×10^5 cells per well in a 12 well plate. One day later the cells were transfected with 1 µg of plasmid DNA, using 3 µl of Transit-CHO supplemented with 0.5 µl of CHO-mojo reagent (Mirus) diluted in Opti-MEM (Gibco). One day later, the cells were expanded on a 10 cm dish with media supplemented with or without AZT (obtained through the NIH AIDS Reagent Program, Division of AIDS, NIAID, NIH) or mouse IFNα (Pestka Biomedical Laboratories, Inc.). Two days later, cells were plated in a 15 cm dish or three 96 well plates (for analysis of single cell clones) with media supplemented with 1 µg/ml of G418. For controls, 1/1000 of the cells transfected with the NEO plasmid were plated in the 15 cm dish with selection media. Cells in 15 cm dishes were cultured under selection for 10 days before treatment with 4% PFA and colonies were stained with 0.3% crystal violet in 20% ethanol for counting. Single colonies in 96 well plates were monitored and expanded until reaching confluence in a 10 cm dish. Genomic DNA (gDNA) was extracted from 5×10^6 cells using QIAmp DNA mini kit (QIAGEN) for analysis of ancML integration (see below).

To determine the fate of the intron interrupting the *neo* gene during ancML replication, gDNA extracted from CHO pools of cells transfected with a plasmid expressing ancML, ancMLΔGAAGT or an empty vector, was used as template for PCR analysis. Forward and reverse primers were design to anneal to the extreme 5′ and 3′ ends of the *neo* gene. For all PCRs performed in this study we used Phusion High-Fidelity DNA Polymerase (Thermo Fisher Scientific Inc.).

Integration site analyses

Sites of ancML integration were determined using a universal Genome Walker kit (Clontech). Briefly, gDNA was extracted from expanded single cell clones of CHO cells following transfection with a plasmid containing ancML and selected in G418. The gDNA was digested with EcoRV (New England Biolabs) and ligated to adaptors. Nested PCRs were performed using forward primers that were designed to anneal to the R region of the 3′LTR and the reverse primers to the adaptor sequence, thereby amplifying 3′ flanking sequences. Bands from second round PCR reactions were gel purified and inserted into pCR-Blunt II-TOPO using the Zero Blunt TOPO PCR cloning Kit (Life technologies) for sequencing. To amplify and sequence the 5′ flanking site we use reverse primers specific to the 5′ LTR and designed forward primers that would specifically anneal to the predicted integration site, based on the previously sequenced 3′ flanking sequence. The resulting CHO gDNA sequences were mapped to the CHO genome (criGri1) using BLAT [46] searches on the UCSC genome browser [47]. To account for biases due to location and density of EcoRV restriction sites, we compared the distribution of the 26 ancML integration sites to matched random controls consisting of three random genomic locations that were at the same distance from an EcoRV site as the site found in the flanking CHO DNA sequence for each MuERV-L integration site [34] (see above).

Results

Bioinformatic screens for MuERV-L elements in the mouse genome

To construct a replication-competent MuERV-L sequence we first catalogued the diversity of MuERV-L related sequences in the mouse genome. Currently, there are two available complete mouse genome assemblies: the Mouse Genome Reference Consortium build 38 (GRCm38 also known as mm10) corresponding to the C57BL/6J strain [29], and the whole genome shotgun (WGS) assembly (Celera) that corresponds to a mixture of 5 strains (129X1/SvJ, 129S1/SvImJ, DBA/2J, A/J and C57BL/6J) [28]. We mined both genome assemblies using BLASTn and tBLASTn [27] searches with separate *gag*,

pol and LTR probes from a MuERV-L reference sequence (GenBank: Y12713) [20]. The resulting hits were defragmented by merging contiguous hits that mapped to the same locus, representing individual elements.

Overall, we found nearly 3000 MuERV-L elements in the mouse genome that had three major types of structures (Table 1, Fig. 1b, Additional file 1: Table S1). One type comprised complete or near complete proviruses, consisting of an internal *gag–pol* region flanked by two LTRs. The frequency with which this structure occurred was highly discrepant in the two genome assemblies, with 220 proviruses being present in the Celera assembly and 719 in GRCm38 (Table 1). It is unclear whether this discrepancy is due to the different mouse strains or the assembly methods used in each genome project. A second type of MuERV-L elements were solo LTRs that typically arise from recombination between the LTRs flanking a provirus, resulting in the complete excision of the internal sequence. This type of element represents the single most abundant ERV type in animal genomes and accounts for >50% of the MuERV-L elements in the mouse genome (Table 1). The third type of MuERV-L structures, representing ~25% of all elements, were composed of internal sequences with or without a single associated LTR (Table 1).

Because the GRCm38 assembly was better supported by external and internal annotations we utilized this data source to analyze the distribution of MuERV-L elements in the genome (Fig. 1b–d). MuERV-L elements were roughly evenly distributed across mouse chromosomes (Fig. 1b), with the exception of the Y chromosome in which MuERV-L was underrepresented. Indeed, there were only a few elements in the Y chromosome. This finding was surprising, given that other ERVs, (e.g. HERV-K) are enriched in the human Y chromosome [48]. However, in contrast to human Y chromosome, the long arm of the mouse Y chromosome is a highly dynamic gene rich region that has frequently expanded and undergone rearrangement over the past ~3 MY [49]. The distribution of MuERV-L elements in this mouse chromosome shows a clear discrepancy between the short and long arms (Fig. 1b). This finding is likely explained by the low recombination rate of the short arm of the mouse Y chromosome, resulting in an enrichment of mobile DNA elements, while recent gene amplification and

Table 1 MuERV-L sequences identified in mouse genome assemblies

Assembly	Strain	References	Total	soloLTR	Provirus	Fragments
GRCm38	C57BL/6J	[29]	2971	1588	719	664
Mm_Celera	Mixture	[28]	2768	1775	220	773

rearrangement events in the long arm may have inhibited the fixation of MuERV-L elements.

The majority (79%) of MuERV-L elements were found in intergenic regions (Fig. 1c). About ~ 19.5% of elements were found inside introns (Fig. 1c), of which the majority (65%) were found in antisense orientation relative to of the corresponding gene, as previously documented for Intracisternal A particles (IAPs) [50]. The remaining elements (1.5%) were found primarily in non-coding RNA genes and untranslated exons (UTRs, Fig. 1c). Only 10 LTRs were found overlapping coding exons. This distribution differs significantly compared to randomized controls ($p < 0.001$). This enrichment of elements outside genes was also apparent if analysis was confined to solo LTRs (p value < 0.001, Fig. 1d) or if proviruses from the 2MYA or 10MYA expansions were analyzed separately (p values < 0.05, Fig. 1d). Overall, these observations are consistent with an expected selective pressure against retention of MuERV-L elements in genes, which was less evident for younger loci (2nd expansion, Fig. 1d). Interestingly, 10.13% of proviruses implicated in the 10MYA expansion have lost a recognizable ORF (either *gag* or *pol*), in contrast to integrations implicated in the 2MYA expansion where only 5.02% have lost an ORF, consistent with the notion that a modest selection to purge MuERV-L sequences is ongoing.

Reconstruction of an ancestral MuERV-L

To reconstruct the ancestral MuERV-L LTRs and the *pol* ORF, we selected 95 complete (LTR–*gag*–*pol*–LTR) proviruses that were most closely related to a reference MuERV-L sequence (defined by BLAST searches), as this sequence has retained coding potential for both ORFs, has almost identical LTRs, and contained recognizable functional motifs [20]. These sequences were used to guide a maximum likelihood (ML) reconstruction of the root node (*pol* n96) and a pair of identical LTRs (Fig. 1e).

For reconstruction of the Gag gene we took a slightly different approach. As the 2nd expansion was the most prolific and we expected that younger integrations would be less divergent from a functional ancestor than older integrations, we selected *gag* sequences that were specific to the most recent expansion (based on the presence of the 33nt in-frame deletion in *gag*). After aligning 230 *gag*–*pol* containing loci that were present in both Celera and GRCm38 assemblies to the reference sequence (that does not exhibit the deletion), we identified a monophyletic clade of 40 elements that all contained a 33nt in-frame deletion in the 5′ half of their *gag* ORFs (Fig. 1f). The *gag* sequences in this clade were selected to guide a ML reconstruction of this internal node (*gag* n377). Thereafter, the combined ancestral LTR, *gag* and *pol* ancestral sequences were corrected for probable errors

derived from deamination of methylated CpG dinucleotides to create a ~ 2 MY ancestral MuERV-L sequence (ancML, Fig. 2 and Additional file 2) (see "Methods").

ancML is replication-competent and its replication is dependent on a functional reverse transcriptase

To assess the potential replication competence of the reconstructed ancestral MuERV-L sequence, we inserted the full-length ancML sequence into a plasmid vector, replacing the U3 region of the 5′ LTR by a CMV promoter to overcome the highly restricted promoter activity of the MuERV-L LTR (Fig. 3a). This design allows for the loss of the CMV promoter sequence after transcription, reverse transcription and integration, resulting in two identical flanking LTRs. A replication-dependent reporter gene, consisting of a *neo* gene controlled by a separate SV40 promoter and interrupted by an intron, was inserted between *pol* and the 3′ LTR (Fig. 3a). While the SV40p-*neo* cassette is in reverse orientation relative to ancML transcription, the splice donor and acceptor sites of the intron are in the same orientation as the ancML transcription. Thus, only if ancML undergoes splicing, reverse transcription and integration in the host cell genome the intron is removed and a functional Neo (G418 resistance) protein is expressed. This approach has been used previously to monitor the intracellular replication of retrotransposons [51].

We determined whether transfection of a plasmid harboring ancML could produce G418 resistant colonies in cultured cell lines. For this purpose we tested a set of 13 cell lines: 6 of primate origin, 5 from rodents, 1 from a carnivore and 1 from an avian species (Table 2). Despite efficient transfection in the majority of the cells tested, and the abundant formation of G418-resistant colonies using a control plasmid, the ancML expression plasmid was able to generate G418 resistant colonies only in Chinese hamster ovary K1 (CHO) cells, CHO-derived pgsA cells, and (to a greatly reduced extent) in Vero cells (Table 2 and Fig. 3b). Surprisingly, a control plasmid expressing a LINE1 element containing the same replication dependent *neo* resistant gene (L1.3 plasmid) [41] failed to produce G418 resistant colonies in 4 of the cells tested, including Vero (Table 2). Conversely, all the cell lines tested generated G418 resistant colonies when transfected with a control plasmid expressing an intact *neo* gene.

To determine whether the ancML-associated G418 resistant colonies had arisen as a result of ancML replication, we mutated the predicted ancML reverse transcriptase (RT) active site from YIDD to AIAA (Fig. 2). This mutation completely abolished the production of G148 resistant colonies following ancML transfection (Fig. 3c). Additionally, we found that the formation

```
1     TGTAGTGGCTATTCCTGGTTGTCAACTTGACAATATTTGGAATGAACTACAATCCGGAATTGGAAGGCTCACCAGTGACCCTTATCTGGAGGCTTGGAGATCCTTATCTGGATCTTGGTATGGAGATCT
130   TGAGCCATAGTGGCTATGGATTCCAGAAGATTGAATCTCCGAGTTTAAGGAACACACCTTTAATCTGGGCTACGCCTTTCATCTGGGATTAAAGGTGTGGTGGAACACACCTTTAATCTGGGCTACACC
259   TTCTGCTGGAGACAATATAAGGACATTGGAAGAAGGGAGTCTAGCTCTAGCTCTTGCTCTTGCTCCTTCGCCTGCTTGCTGCGTGAGACTGAGTAACTGCTAGATCCTTGGACTTCCATTCACAGCTGC
388   GACTGAACAATTGTTGGGAATTGGGCTGCCGACTGTAAGTCATCAATAAATTCCTTTACTATCTAGAGACTATCCATAAGTTCTGTGACTCTAGAGAACCCTGACTAATACAGAAGTTGGTACCAGGAG
517   TGGTTCTAGAGTAACAGAAGTACAAGGATGAATCTTTTAAAATTCTGGAATTGGCTTGTTGATCCACCAGCACTTTCAACTATTGAAACCTCTCCAGATTCTCTCCCTCCTGGGAGCTCAGAGAATTTT
1                                      M  N  L  L  K  F  W  N  W  L  V  D  P  P  A  L  S  T  I  E  T  S  P  D  S  L  P  P  G  S  S  E  N  F
646   GAAGACCCATGGTTGAAACTATATTCCGAACTTAAAGAAGCTAATGCCCTTGATTTTCTTAATGAATTAGGTGATTCAGTGCACAAAGCTTTCTACAAGATGGGGAAAAAATCGAAAAATGATTTTACT
35     E  D  P  W  L  K  L  Y  S  E  L  K  E  A  N  A  L  D  F  L  N  E  L  G  D  S  V  H  K  A  F  Y  K  M  G  K  K  S  K  N  D  F  T
775   GGCTGGCTGCTCTTAGTATCTGTGGAAAAAATGATGAATGAAAGGAAGGAGTTGTGTGATAAAATCGAAAGGCTCCAGACACAAGTAAACGATCTAAAAGTTGCTAAGTGTGTCCTTGAGGAGAATCTT
78     G  W  L  L  L  V  S  V  E  K  M  M  N  E  R  K  E  L  C  D  K  I  E  R  L  Q  T  Q  V  N  D  L  K  V  A  K  C  V  L  E  E  N  L
904   CTCTCTTGTAGCAATAGAGCTCAAGTTGCAGAAAATCAAACAGAAACTCTCATTGTAAGGTTGGCTGAACTACAGCGAAAATTCAAGTCTCAGCCTCAGAGTGTGTCGACAGTTAAAGTAAGGGCTCTA
121    L  S  C  S  N  R  A  Q  V  A  E  N  Q  T  E  T  L  I  V  R  L  A  E  L  Q  R  K  F  K  S  Q  P  Q  S  V  S  T  V  K  V  R  A  L
1033  ATTGGCAAAGAATGGGATCCTACAACATGGGACGGGGATGTGTGGGAAGACCATGTTGAAGCTGAGAATTTTGAATCCTCAGATTCTCAAGGGTTTGCCCCACCTGAGGAAGTAGTACCCTCAGCCCCA
164    I  G  K  E  W  D  P  T  T  W  D  G  D  V  W  E  D  H  V  E  A  E  N  F  E  S  S  D  S  Q  G  F  A  P  P  E  E  V  V  P  S  A  P
1162  CCTCTTGAAATAATGCCTTCCCCACATGAGGAAATTAATTTTGCAGAGTCTGCTCACGGCCCACCAATAGTTTCTTCTAGACCTGTAACCAGACTCAAAGCAAAACAGGCTCCTAGAGGGGAGGTAGAA
207    P  L  E  I  M  P  S  P  H  E  E  I  N  F  A  E  S  A  H  G  P  P  I  V  S  S  R  P  V  T  R  L  K  A  K  Q  A  P  R  G  E  V  E
1291  AGTGTAGTCCATGAGGAAATTCGCTACACTACTAAGGAGCTTAATGAGTTTGCTAATTCATTCAAGCAGAAACCTGGTGAATATGTGTGGGAATGGATTTTAAGGGTGTGGGATAAGGGTGGAAGGAAC
250    S  V  V  H  E  E  I  R  Y  T  T  K  E  L  N  E  F  A  N  S  F  K  Q  K  P  G  E  Y  V  W  E  W  I  L  R  V  W  D  K  G  G  R  N
1420  ATAAAACTAGAGCAGGCTGAGTTTATTGACATGGGTCCTCTGAGTAGAGATTCTAGGTTTAATACGGAAGCTCGCATAGTTAAAAAAGGTGTCAAAAGTTTGTTTGAATGGTTGGCTGAGGTGTTTATC
293    I  K  L  E  Q  A  E  F  I  D  M  G  P  L  S  R  D  S  R  F  N  T  E  A  R  I  V  K  K  G  V  K  S  L  F  E  W  L  A  E  V  F  I
1549  AAAAGATGGCCTACTGGAAATGACTTGGAGATGCCTGATATTCCGTGGCTTAGTGTTGATGAAGGGATTTTAAGACTTAGGGAAATTGCAATGCTAGAGTGGATATATTGTGTAAAGCATAATTGTCCA
336    K  R  W  P  T  G  N  D  L  E  M  P  D  I  P  W  L  S  V  D  E  G  I  L  R  L  R  E  I  A  M  L  E  W  I  Y  C  V  K  H  N  C  P
1678  CAATGGGAAGGTCCAGAAGATATGCCTTTCACCAGCTCTATAAGACGCAAATTGGTGAGAGGGGCACCAGCACATTTGAAGGGTTTTGTTCTTTCCCTTTTCCTTGTGCCAGATCTTAGCATTGGAGAT
379    Q  W  E  G  P  E  D  M  P  F  T  S  S  I  R  R  K  L  V  R  G  A  P  A  H  L  K  G  F  V  L  S  L  F  L  V  P  D  L  S  I  G  D
1807  GCTTCTGCTCAATTAGATGAATTAAATTCACTGGGTTTAGTTGGATTCCGAGGTAACAAGGGCCAGGTGGCAGCATTGAATCGCCCGAGACAAGGTGATTCTAGTTATTATAATGGACAGCGTAGACAA
422    A  S  A  Q  L  D  E  L  N  S  L  G  L  V  G  F  R  G  N  K  G  Q  V  A  A  L  N  R  P  R  Q  G  D  S  S  Y  Y  N  G  Q  R  R  Q
1936  AAGAATGTTTATAATAACATACCCAGTAATGGTCAGCACAGGAGAGGTGAAATTTATAATGGCATGACTCGGTTGGACCTTTGGTACTGGCTAACCAATCATGGTGTTTCCAGGAATGAAATACATAGG
465    K  N  V  Y  N  N  I  P  S  N  G  Q  H  R  R  G  E  I  Y  N  G  M  T  R  L  D  L  W  Y  W  L  T  N  H  G  V  S  R  N  E  I  H  R
2065  AAGCCTACTGCATATTTGTTTGATCTGTATAAGCAGAAAAATTCTCAAACAAATGAAAGAAAGGCTACATTAGATCGTGGTAAACAGACAAATGAAAGAAAGGCTACATTAGATCGTGGTAAACAGCAA
508    K  P  T  A  Y  L  F  D  L  Y  K  Q  K  N  S  Q  T  N  E  R  K  A  T  L  D  R  G  K  Q  T  N  E  R  K  A  T  L  D  R  G  K  Q  Q
2194  TCTCGGCCAGTGAATCAATTTCCAGACTTGAGACAGTTTGCAGATCCAGAACCCCTTGAATGAAGGGGTGGCCAGGTTCCGCTGAGGAAGGATCTTGATAAGACACTCAAAGGTTTTGCTGTTACCCTT
551    S  R  P  V  N  Q  F  P  D  L  R  Q  F  A  D  P  E  P  L  E  *  R  G  G  Q  V  P  L  R  K  D  L  D  K  T  L  K  G  F  A  V  T  L
2323  TCTCCAGTTCTTCCCCAGAGGGACCTACGGCCTTTTACAAGGGTAACTGTACACTGGGGAAAAGGAAATAATCAGACTTTTCGGGGTCTGCTGGATACTGGTTCTGAGTTGACACTGATCCCAGGGGAT
594    S  P  V  L  P  Q  R  D  L  R  P  F  T  R  V  T  V  H  W  G  K  G  N  N  Q  T  F  R  G  L  L  D  T  G  S  E  L  T  L  I  P  G  D
2452  CCCAAGAAACATTGTGGCCCTCCAGTTAAAGTAGGGGCTTATGGAGGGCAGGTGATTAATGGAGTTTTGACTGATGTCCGACTCACAGTAGGTCCAGTAGGTCCCCGGACACATCCTGTGGTGATTTCC
637    P  K  K  H  C  G  P  P  V  K  V  G  A  Y  G  G  Q  V  I  N  G  V  L  T  D  V  R  L  T  V  G  P  V  G  P  R  T  H  P  V  V  I  S
2581  CCAGTTCCAGAATGTATAATTGGGATAGATATACTCAGAAATTGGCAGAATTCTCATATTGGTTCCCTGAACTGTAGAGTGAGGGCTATTATGGTTGGAAAGGCCAAATGGAAGCCTTTAGAGTTGCCT
680    P  V  P  E  C  I  I  G  I  D  I  L  R  N  W  Q  N  S  H  I  G  S  L  N  C  R  V  R  A  I  M  V  G  K  A  K  W  K  P  L  E  L  P
2710  CTGCCAAAGAAAATAGTGAATCAAAAACAGTATCGTATTCCTGGAGGAATTGCAGAAATTACTGCCACTATCAAGGACTTGAAAGATGCAGGGGTGGTGGTTCCCACCACATCTCCGTTTAACTCTCCT
723    L  P  K  K  I  V  N  Q  K  Q  Y  R  I  P  G  G  I  A  E  I  T  A  T  I  K  D  L  K  D  A  G  V  V  V  P  T  T  S  P  F  N  S  P
2839  ATCTGGCCAGTGCAGAAAACAGATGGATCATGGAGAATGACAGTTGATTATCGAAAACTAAATCAGGTAGTAACTCCAATTGCAGCTGCTGTACCAGATGTAGTTTCGTTACTTGAGCAAATTAACACA
766    I  W  P  V  Q  K  T  D  G  S  W  R  M  T  V  D  Y  R  K  L  N  Q  V  V  T  P  I  A  A  A  V  P  D  V  V  S  L  L  E  Q  I  N  T
2968  TCTCCTGGCACCTGGTATGCGGCTATTGATCTGGCAAATGCCTTCTTCTCAGTACCTGTCCATAAGGACCACCAGAAGCAATTTGCTTTCAGTTGGCAAGGCCAACAGTATACCTTCACAGTTTTGCCT
809    S  P  G  T  W  Y  A  A  I  D  L  A  N  A  F  F  S  V  P  V  H  K  D  H  Q  K  Q  F  A  F  S  W  Q  G  Q  Q  Y  T  F  T  V  L  P
3097  CAAGGATATATTAACTCTCCTGCCCTGTGTCATAATTTAGTTAGAAGGGATCTTGATCGTTTGGATCTTCCACAAAATATCACATTGGTGCACTATATTGATGACATTATGCTGATTGGACCAAGTGAG
852    Q  G  Y  I  N  S  P  A  L  C  H  N  L  V  R  R  D  L  D  R  L  D  L  P  Q  N  I  T  L  V  H  Y  I  D  D  I  M  L  I  G  P  S  E
3226  CAGGAAGTAGCAACCACTTTGGACTCATTGGTAACACATATGCGTATCAGAGGATGGGAAATAAATCCAACCAAAATTCAAGGACCATCTACCTCAGTGAAATTCTTAGGAGTCCAGTGGTGTGGGGCA
895    Q  E  V  A  T  T  L  D  S  L  V  T  H  M  R  I  R  G  W  E  I  N  P  T  K  I  Q  G  P  S  T  S  V  K  F  L  G  V  Q  W  C  G  A
3355  TGCAGAGATATTCCTTCTAAGGTGAAAGATAAGTTATTGCACCTGGCCCCTCCTACAACCAAGAAAGAAGCACAACGTTTAGTGGGTCTATTTGGATTCTGGAGACAACACATCCCTCACTTGGGTGTG
938    C  R  D  I  P  S  K  V  K  D  K  L  L  H  L  A  P  P  T  T  K  K  E  A  Q  R  L  V  G  L  F  G  F  W  R  Q  H  I  P  H  L  G  V
3484  TTACTTAGGCCTATTTACCAAGTGACTCGGAAAGCTGCTAGCTTTGTGTGGGGCCTGGAACAGGAGAAGGCCCTTCAACAGGTCCAGGCTGCTGTGCAGGCTGCTCTACCACTTGGACCATATGACCCA
981    L  L  R  P  I  Y  Q  V  T  R  K  A  A  S  F  V  W  G  L  E  Q  E  K  A  L  Q  Q  V  Q  A  A  V  Q  A  A  L  P  L  G  P  Y  D  P
3613  GCAGACCCGATGGTACTTGAGGTGTCTGTGGCTGATAGAGATGCTGTTTGGAGCCTCTGGCAGGCCCCTGTAGGTGAATCACAGAAAAGACCTTTGGGATTTTGGAGCAAAGCTCTACCATCATCTGCA
1024   A  D  P  M  V  L  E  V  S  V  A  D  R  D  A  V  W  S  L  W  Q  A  P  V  G  E  S  Q  K  R  P  L  G  F  W  S  K  A  L  P  S  S  A
3742  GACAACTATTCTCCCTTTGAAAAACAGCTCTTGGCCTGCTATTGGGCCTTAGTGGAAACTGAACGTTTGACAATAGGACACCAAGTTACTATGCGACCTGAACTACCCATCATGAGCTGGGTACTATCA
1067   D  N  Y  S  P  F  E  K  Q  L  L  A  C  Y  W  A  L  V  E  T  E  R  L  T  I  G  H  Q  V  T  M  R  P  E  L  P  I  M  S  W  V  L  S
3871  GACCCTGCAAGTCATAAAGTGGGACGCGCACAGCAGCAGTCTATTATCAAATGGAAGTGGTATATACGTGATCGGGCCAGAGCAGGTCCTGAAGGCACAAGCAAGTTACATGAAGAAGTTGCTCAAATG
1110   D  P  A  S  H  K  V  G  R  A  Q  Q  Q  S  I  I  K  W  K  W  Y  I  R  D  R  A  R  A  G  P  E  G  T  S  K  L  H  E  E  V  A  Q  M
4000  CCTATGGTTTCTACTCCTGTTACAATGCCATCTGCTGCCAAGCATGCGCCTATAGCCTCATGGGGTGTTCCCTATGATCAACTGACCGAAGAGGAGAAGACTAGAGCCTGGTTTACTGATGGCTCTGCA
1153   P  M  V  S  T  P  V  T  M  P  S  A  A  K  H  A  P  I  A  S  W  G  V  P  Y  D  Q  L  T  E  E  E  K  T  R  A  W  F  T  D  G  S  A
4129  CGTTATGCAGGCACCACCCAGAAGTGGACAGCTGCAGCATTACAACCCCTTTCTGGGACAACCTTGAAAGACACAGGTGAAGGGAAATCTTCACAGTGGGCAGAACTTCGGGCAGTACACATGGTATTA
1196   R  Y  A  G  T  T  Q  K  W  T  A  A  A  L  Q  P  L  S  G  T  T  L  K  D  T  G  E  G  K  S  S  Q  W  A  E  L  R  A  V  H  M  V  L
4258  CAGTTTGTTTGCAAGAAGAAATGGCCAGATGTACGATTATTCACTGACTCATGGGCTGTAGCCAATGGATTGGCTGGATGGTCAGGGACTTGGAAAGATCACAATTGGAAAATTGGTGAGAAAGACATC
1239   Q  F  V  C  K  K  K  W  P  D  V  R  L  F  T  D  S  W  A  V  A  N  G  L  A  G  W  S  G  T  W  K  D  H  N  W  K  I  G  E  K  D  I
4387  TGGGGAAGAAGTATGTGGATAGATCTCTCCAAATGGGCAAAGGATGTGAAGATATTTGTGTCCCATGTAAATGCTCACCAAAAGGTGACTTCAGCCGAGGAGGAGTTCAATAATCAAGTGGATAAGATG
1282   W  G  R  S  M  W  I  D  L  S  K  W  A  K  D  V  K  I  F  V  S  H  V  N  A  H  Q  K  V  T  S  A  E  E  E  F  N  N  Q  V  D  K  M
4516  ACCCGTTCTGTGGACAGTCAGCCTCTCTCCCCAGCCATCCCTGTCATTGCTCAATGGGCACATGAACAAAGTGGCCATGGTGGTCGAGATGGAGGTTATGCTTGGGCTCAGCAACACGGGCTTCCACTC
1325   T  R  S  V  D  S  Q  P  L  S  P  A  I  P  V  I  A  Q  W  A  H  E  Q  S  G  H  G  G  R  D  G  G  Y  A  W  A  Q  Q  H  G  L  P  L
4645  ACCAAGGCTGACCTGGCTACAGCTGCTGCTGATTGCCAGATCTGCCAACAGCAGAAACCAACACTGAGCCCCAGATATGGCACCATTCCTCGAGGTGACCAGCCAGCAACCTGGTGGCAGGTTGACTAC
1368   T  K  A  D  L  A  T  A  A  A  D  C  Q  I  C  Q  Q  Q  K  P  T  L  S  P  R  Y  G  T  I  P  R  G  D  Q  P  A  T  W  W  Q  V  D  Y
4774  ATTGGACCACTTCCTTCGTGGAAAGGACAGCGTTTTGTTCTTACTGGAGTAGATACTTATTCTGGTTATGGATTTGCCTTTCCTGCACGTAATGCCTCTGCTAAAACCACCATTCACGGACTGACAGAA
1411   I  G  P  L  P  S  W  K  G  Q  R  F  V  L  T  G  V  D  T  Y  S  G  Y  G  F  A  F  P  A  R  N  A  S  A  K  T  T  I  H  G  L  T  E
4903  TGCCTTATCTATCGTCATGGTATTCCACACAGTATTGCTTCTGACCAAGGAACTCATTTCACAGCCAGAGAAGTACGACAGTGGGCCCACGATCATGGAATTCACTGGTCTTACCACATTCCCCATCAT
1454   C  L  I  Y  R  H  G  I  P  H  S  I  A  S  D  Q  G  T  H  F  T  A  R  E  V  R  Q  W  A  H  D  H  G  I  H  W  S  Y  H  I  P  H  H
5032  CCTGAAGCAGCTGGTCTGATAGAAAGATGGAATGGCCTTTTGAAGACGCAGTTACAGCGCCAATTAGGTGGTAACAGCTTGGAAGGCTGGGGCAGAGTTCTTCAGAAGGCAGTATATGCTTTGAATCAG
1497   P  E  A  A  G  L  I  E  R  W  N  G  L  L  K  T  Q  L  Q  R  Q  L  G  G  N  S  L  E  G  W  G  R  V  L  Q  K  A  V  Y  A  L  N  Q
5161  CGCTCGATATATGGTACAGTTTCACCCATAGCCAGGATTCATGGGTCCAGGAATCAAGGGGTGGAAAACGGAATAGTTCCACTTACTATCACTCCTAGTGACCCTCTAGGAAAATTTTTGCTTCCTGTC
1540   R  S  I  Y  G  T  V  S  P  I  A  R  I  H  G  S  R  N  Q  G  V  E  N  G  I  V  P  L  T  I  T  P  S  D  P  L  G  K  F  L  L  P  V
5290  CCCATAACTCTAGGTTCTGCTGGCCTAGAAGTTTTGGCTCCAGAGAGGGGAGTGCTCCTACCAGGAGCTACAACAAACATTCCATTGAACTGGAAGCTCAGACTTCCCCCTGGTCATTTTGGGCTTCTA
1583   P  I  T  L  G  S  A  G  L  E  V  L  A  P  E  R  G  V  L  L  P  G  A  T  T  N  I  P  L  N  W  K  L  R  L  P  P  G  H  F  G  L  L
5419  ATGCCCTTAAACCAACAGGCTAAAAAAGGAATAACAGTGTTAGGAGGGGTGATAGATCCAGATTACCATGGGGAAATTGGATTACCTCTTCACAATGGTGGTAAGCAAGATTATGTCTGGAGTGTAGGA
1626   M  P  L  N  Q  Q  A  K  K  G  I  T  V  L  G  G  V  I  D  P  D  Y  H  G  E  I  G  L  P  L  H  N  G  G  K  Q  D  Y  V  W  S  V  G
5548  GATCCCTTAGGGCGTCTCTTAGTACTACCATGTCCTGTGATTAAAGTCAATGGGAAACTACAACAGCCTAATCCAAGCAGGATGACAAAGGACGCAGACCCATCAGGAATGAAGGTATGGGTCAATCCT
1669   D  P  L  G  R  L  L  V  L  P  C  P  V  I  K  V  N  G  K  L  Q  Q  P  N  P  S  R  M  T  K  D  A  D  P  S  G  M  K  V  W  V  N  P
5677  CCAGGAAAAGAGCCAAGACCTGCTGAGGTGCTGGCTGAAGGTGAAGGAAATACAGAATGGGTAGTAGAGGAAGGTAGTTATAAATACCAATTAAGGCCACGTAACCAGTTGCAGAAACGAGGATTATAA
1712   P  G  K  E  P  R  P  A  E  V  L  A  E  G  E  G  N  T  E  W  V  V  E  E  G  S  Y  K  Y  Q  L  R  P  R  N  Q  L  Q  K  R  G  L  *
5806  AGTAATATGAATGCCCCATTGTAAATTTACAAATGCGTTTGCGATTGTACGAGGGATAGTTATATCATGTTAGGCGTATTTACAACCTTGTTATTGTTTCATGTGAACATGAGATATTATTTGTGTCAA
5935  GTTGACAAGGGGTGGATTGTAGTGGCTATTCCTGGTTGTCAACTTGACAATATTTGGAATGAACTACAATCCGGAATTGGAAGGCTCACCAGTGACCCTTATCTGGAGGCTTGGAGATCCTTATCTGGA
6064  TCTTGGTATGGAGATCTTGAGCCATAGTGGCTATGGATTCCAGAAGATTGAATCTCCGAGTTTAAGGAACACACCTTTAATCTGGGCTACGCCTTTCATCTGGGATTAAAGGTGTGGTGGAACACACCT
6193  TTAATCTGGGCTACACCTTCTGCTGGAGACAATATAAGGACATTGGAAGAAGGGAGTCTAGCTCTAGCTCTTGCTCTTGCTCCTTCGCCTGCTTGCTGCGTGAGACTGAGTAACTGCTAGATCCTTGGA
6322  CTTCCATTCACAGCTGCGACTGAACAATTGTTGGGAATTGGGCTGCCGACTGTAAGTCATCAATAAATTCCTTTACTATCTAGAGACTATCCATAAGTTCTGTGACTCTAGAGAACCCTGACTAATACA
```

(See figure on previous page.)

Fig. 2 Nucleotide sequence and translation products of a reconstructed ancestral MuERV-L. LTR sequences are shown in bold italics. Nucleotide and protein sequence of *gag* and *pol* are indicated in red and blue, respectively (amino acid single letter code, (*) represents stop codons). The 33nt deletion in gag is shown with a magenta triangle. The position of the 39nt that are deleted in some MuERV-Ls is highlighted in magenta. The RT active site is highlighted in yellow. The PBS is indicated in violet, the polypurine tract in red, the TATA box in green and the polyadenylation site in bright blue

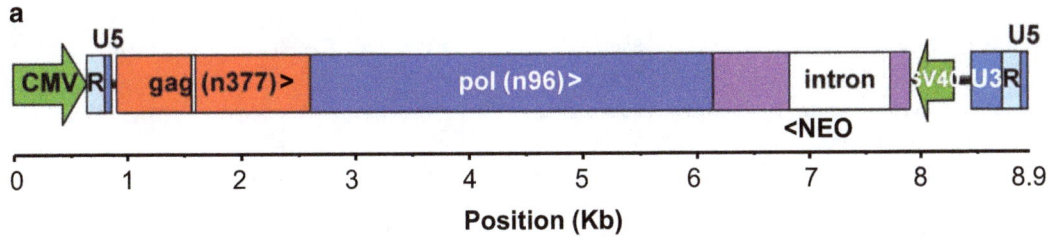

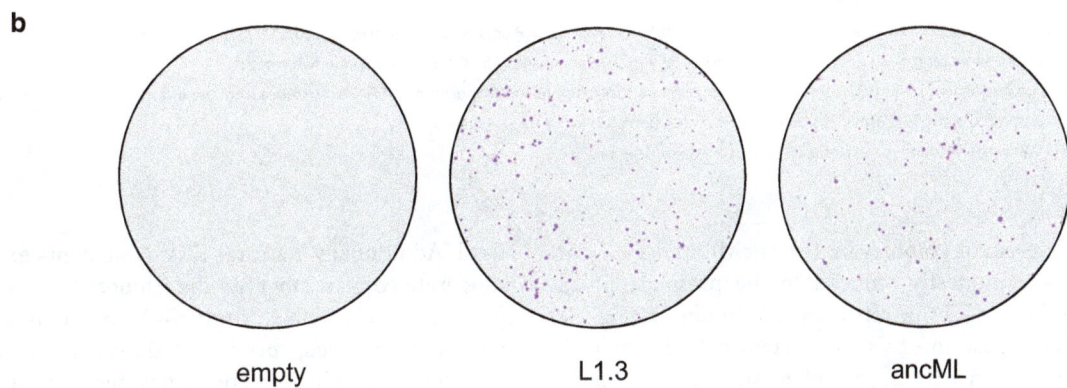

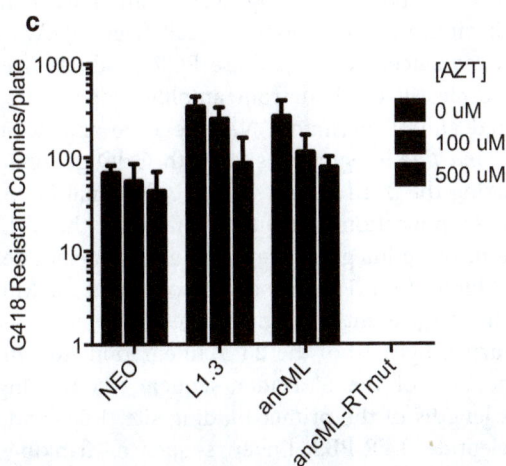

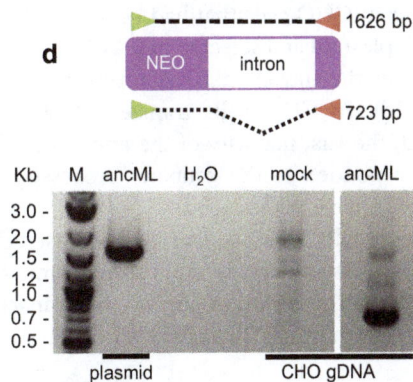

Fig. 3 Reverse transcription-dependent ancML replication. **a** Organization of the ancML construct. Green arrows indicate promoter sequences. NEO: *neo* gene in reverse orientation relative to ancML transcription. Chevrons indicate the orientation for each ORF (>: forward, <: reverse). A white box indicates a 33nt deletion in *gag* at position 671. **b** G418 resistant colonies on 15 cm cell culture plates derived from CHO cells transfected with plasmids expressing ancML, L1.3 or an empty vector. **c** Quantification of G418 resistant CHO cell colonies following transfection and treatment in the presence or absence AZT. CHO cells were transfected with plasmids expressing a *neo* gene (NEO), L1.3, ancML or an ancML construct with inactivating mutations in the RT active site (ancML-RTmut). AZT treatment was applied for 2 days before G418 selection. Data are mean ± SD from 3 independent experiments. **d** PCR amplification of the *neo* gene in genomic DNA (gDNA) extracted from CHO cells following transfection with a plasmid expressing ancML or an empty vector. A scheme of the PCR amplification strategy is shown on top. The use of template DNA from plasmid or from CHO gDNA as well as a water control is indicated. M: molecular weight ladder

Table 2 Cell lines tested for replication of ancML

Cell Line	Organism	Lineage	GFP[#]	NEO[a]	L1.3[b]	ancML[c]
DF-1	*Gallus gallus*	Aves	***	+++	++	−
CRFK	*Felis catus*	Carnivora	**	+++	+	−
CV-1	*Cercopithecus aethiops*	Primates	*	++	+	−
Vero	*Cercopithecus aethiops*	Primates	***	+++	−	+
HT1080	*Homo sapiens*	Primates	**	++	+	−
HOS	*Homo sapiens*	Primates	*	++	−	−
Huh7.5	*Homo sapiens*	Primates	*	++	−	−
HeLa	*Homo sapiens*	Primates	***	+++	++	−
pgsA745	*Cricetulus griseus*	Rodentia	**	++	+	++
CHO-K1	*Cricetulus griseus*	Rodentia	**	++	+	++
MusDunni	*Mus dunni*	Rodentia	***	+++	+	−
SC-1	*Mus musculus*	Rodentia	**	++	−	−
NIH3T3	*Mus musculus*	Rodentia	**	++	++	−

All cell lines were transfected using lipofectamine 2000

[#] A plasmid expressing GFP was utilized as a transfection control. Percentage of GFP positive cells: (−) 0%, (*) < 10%, (**) 10–50%, (***) > 50%

[a] A pCR3.1 plasmid expressing a *neo* gene from a SV40 promoter was used as a control for G418 resistant colony formation

[b] The replication dependent LINE1 (L1.3) plasmid [41] was used as a control for retrotransposition and G418 resistance from the interrupted NEO reporter cassette

[c] ancML correspond to a pUC57 plasmid containing the cassette depicted in Fig. 3a

Number of G418 resistant colonies: (−) None, (+) ≤ 10, (++) > 10, (+++) > 50

of G418 resistant colonies by the ancML and L1.3 constructs was modestly reduced in the presence of azidothymidine (AZT), a retroviral RT inhibitor (Fig. 3c), while the formation of G418 resistant colonies by CHO cells transfected with a control plasmid expressing the *neo* gene was nearly unaffected. We isolated genomic DNA (gDNA) from CHO cells that had been transfected with the ancML plasmid and selected in G418, and determined the fate of the intron in DNA forms of ancML by PCR (Fig. 3d). In CHO cells transfected with the ancML plasmid, the vast majority of the amplified DNA sequences corresponded to the properly processed *neo* gene, with the intron excised (Fig. 3d).

Overall, these results indicate that the reconstructed ancestral MuERV-L sequence is replication competent and able to undergo transcription and reverse transcription upon transfection into CHO cells.

Analysis of ancML integration in CHO cells

We next determined whether ancML underwent bona fide integration into CHO cell DNA. For this purpose we used an adapter ligation-PCR technique (Genome Walker kit, Clontech) to amplify integration sites using primers specific to the MuERV-L LTR and an adaptor sequence. The risk of amplifying CHO genomic DNA from hamster ERV-L LTR sequences was minimal as these LTR sequences are quite divergent from those of ancML (only 55.8% of sequence identity) with indels and substitutions in the annealing sites for the primer sets

used. Additionally, hamster ERV-L elements exist only in moderate copy numbers in the Chinese hamster genome [52]. Therefore, DNA from G418-resistant single cell clones of CHO cells, previously transfected with ancML, was digested with restriction enzymes, ligated to linkers and subjected to nested PCR reactions. This procedure revealed bands of varying sizes, sometimes consistent with multiple integrations per cell (Fig. 4a). We cloned and sequenced some of these PCR products. Although some clearly resulted from amplification of the transfected ancML plasmid DNA, we were able to identify 26 *bona-fide* integration sites with CHO genomic DNA flanking the 3′ LTR (Fig. 4b and Additional file 3: Table S2). Amplification of sequences flanking the 5′ LTR for one of these integrants revealed a five-nucleotide target site duplication (Fig. 4b), as was observed for MuERV-L sequences present in the mouse genome.

Surprisingly, 10 of the 26 3′ integration sites included a portion of the 5′ leader sequence containing various lengths of the primer-binding site (PBS) and a five-nucleotide LTR-PBS linker sequence, flanking CHO DNA (Fig. 4b). This separation of LTR and PBS is uncommon in exogenous retroviruses and has only previously been observed in another ERV, HERV-E [53]. Elimination of these five nucleotides in the ancML sequence resulted in a ~4 fold reduction in the number of G418 resistant colonies, suggesting an enhancing, but nonessential role for the five nucleotide linker in MuERV-L replication (Fig. 4c). Intriguingly, ~6.5% of the complete

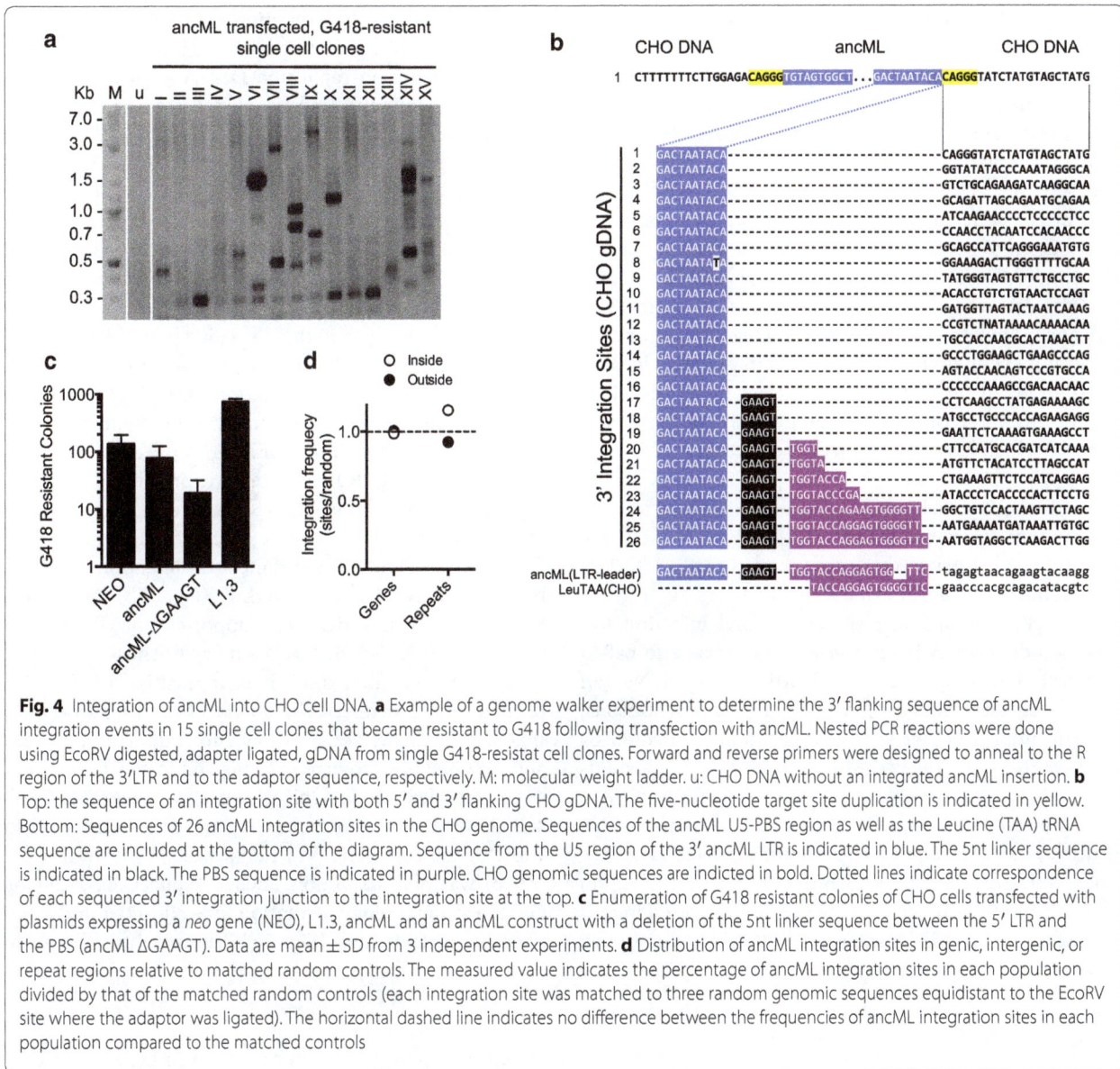

Fig. 4 Integration of ancML into CHO cell DNA. **a** Example of a genome walker experiment to determine the 3′ flanking sequence of ancML integration events in 15 single cell clones that became resistant to G418 following transfection with ancML. Nested PCR reactions were done using EcoRV digested, adapter ligated, gDNA from single G418-resistat cell clones. Forward and reverse primers were designed to anneal to the R region of the 3′LTR and to the adaptor sequence, respectively. M: molecular weight ladder. u: CHO DNA without an integrated ancML insertion. **b** Top: the sequence of an integration site with both 5′ and 3′ flanking CHO gDNA. The five-nucleotide target site duplication is indicated in yellow. Bottom: Sequences of 26 ancML integration sites in the CHO genome. Sequences of the ancML U5-PBS region as well as the Leucine (TAA) tRNA sequence are included at the bottom of the diagram. Sequence from the U5 region of the 3′ ancML LTR is indicated in blue. The 5nt linker sequence is indicated in black. The PBS sequence is indicated in purple. CHO genomic sequences are indicted in bold. Dotted lines indicate correspondence of each sequenced 3′ integration junction to the integration site at the top. **c** Enumeration of G418 resistant colonies of CHO cells transfected with plasmids expressing a *neo* gene (NEO), L1.3, ancML and an ancML construct with a deletion of the 5nt linker sequence between the 5′ LTR and the PBS (ancML ΔGAAGT). Data are mean ± SD from 3 independent experiments. **d** Distribution of ancML integration sites in genic, intergenic, or repeat regions relative to matched random controls. The measured value indicates the percentage of ancML integration sites in each population divided by that of the matched random controls (each integration site was matched to three random genomic sequences equidistant to the EcoRV site where the adaptor was ligated). The horizontal dashed line indicates no difference between the frequencies of ancML integration sites in each population compared to the matched controls

(LTR–*gag*–*pol*–LTR) proviruses in the mouse genome also contain similar sequences (5-nt linker/PBS) at the end of the 3′ LTR, thus showing that this phenomenon also occurred during ancient MuERV-L replication events (Additional file 1: Table S1). During reverse transcription, after the synthesis of the plus-strand strong-stop DNA (+sssDNA), RNase H should remove the primer tRNA, thereby exposing sequences on the +sss-DNA that are complementary to the minus strand PBS which will guide the second strand transfer [54, 55]. Inefficient removal of the tRNA primer might result in the synthesis of +sssDNA that includes additional sequences 3′ to the PBS. Such a scenario might explain the unusual

integration site structure that we observed for some MuERV-L and ancML insertions (Fig. 4b).

We mapped the position of the 26 ancML integration sites to the Chinese hamster genome using the UCSC genome browser (Fig. 4d) [35, 47]. The Chinese hamster genome (CriGri_1.0) is currently assembled to the scaffold level and has been annotated by distinct de novo, expression-based and homology gene prediction systems [35]. The majority of the ancML integration sites (19/26 sites) corresponded to intergenic regions, 5/26 sites corresponded to introns and one corresponded to exon 3 of *Znf462*. The single remaining site could not be classified as intergenic or in genes because it mapped to multiple scaffolds. Of the 26 integration sites, 10 were in elements corresponding to SINE (4), LINE (4) and ERV-L (2) elements. This distribution of ancML integration sites, i.e. within genes versus intergenic regions, as well as within versus outside repetitive sequences, did not differ significantly from matched randomized controls (p value $= 0.97$ and 0.56 respectively) (Fig. 4d). Although the distribution of the sequenced ancML integration sites and the distribution of MuERV-L elements in the mouse genome appeared different (Figs. 1d and 4b), our ancML integration site dataset was too small to establish statistical significance. Nonetheless, our results suggest that ancML integration sites are random (or close to random) in their distribution in CHO DNA, in contrast to the distribution of MuERV-L proviruses that are found in the mouse genome which have been subject to selection.

ancML is sensitive to innate host antiviral defenses
In response to exogenous microbial threats, hosts have evolved sets of genes that sense, and directly interfere with replication of pathogens. One class of such genes which are expressed in response to viral infection following induction by interferons (IFNs), cause a so-called antiviral state [56]. It is not known whether IFNs can inhibit the intracellular replication of retrotransposons. To determine whether ancML replication is affected by type-I IFNs, we transfected CHO cells with plasmids expressing ancML, L1.3 or a *neo* gene and cultured them with media containing varying amounts of murine IFNα (mIFNα) for 2 days prior to selection in G418 (Fig. 5a). The replication of L1.3 was reduced by ~4 fold upon mIFN-α treatment, and there was a larger, dose dependent effect on ancML, reaching a ~20-fold reduction in

G418 resistant colony formation with 50U/ml of mIFNα (Fig. 5a). Notably, generation of G418-resistant colonies by transfected, non-replicated DNA was not affected by mIFNα. Previous studies have observed that mouse IFNα can stimulate an antiviral state in CHO cells [57–60] and promote the induction of hamster ISGs [61]. Thus, these experiments suggest that IFNα is able to inhibit one or more steps in MuERV-L replication. Interestingly pluripotent stem cells have been shown to express a subset of ISGs [62], and suppression of ERV replication may be one impetus for the acquisition of this property.

We also tested whether specific candidate innate immune effectors could inhibit ancML replication. We first tested if the murine restriction factor Fv1 (thought to have been co-opted from a MuERV-L-like element) could have had an impact on MuERV-L replication. For this we constructed CHO cells stably expressing a chimeric form of Fv1 that shows an expanded resistance to different MuLVs (Fv1bbn) [63]. As expected, Fv1bbn-expressing CHO cells exhibited resistance to infection by both N-tropic and B-tropic MuLV (Fig. 5b). However, Fv1bbn-expressing CHO cells supported ancML, or L1.3 replication (Fig. 5c), at levels similar to those of control cells, indicating that ancML is insensitive to this Fv1 protein. We also tested the ability of mouse APOBEC3, that has been previously shown to inhibit endogenous and exogenous retroviruses (reviewed in [64]), to inhibit ancML replication. For this purpose, we generated CHO cell clones that stably expressing the mouse *Apobec3* in 100% of the cells (Fig. 5d). Remarkably, mouse *Apobec3* (mA3) was able to inhibit ancML replication, reducing G418 resistant colony formation by ~30-fold, but did not affect L1.3 replication (Fig. 5e). The inability of mA3 to

(See figure on next page.)

Fig. 5 MuERV-L(ancML) replication can be inhibited by innate immune effectors. **a** Enumeration of G418 resistant colonies generated in the presence of increasing amounts of mouse IFNα. CHO cells were transfected with plasmids expressing a *neo* gene (NEO), L1.3, or ancML and cultured with increasing amounts of mouse IFNα for 2 days before G418 selection. Data are mean ± SD from 3 independent experiments. **b** Infectivity of MuLV on CHO cells expressing Fv1bbn. Percentage of MuLV infected (GFP positive) cells in CHO cells stably expressing Fv1bbn (red) or an empty vector (black). Circles and triangles indicate infection by N-tropic or B-tropic MuLV, respectively. **c** Enumeration of G418 resistant colonies of CHO cells expressing Fv1bbn or an empty vector were transfected with plasmids expressing a *neo* gene (NEO), L1.3, or ancML. Data are mean ± SD from 2 independent experiments. **d** Representative images of Immunofluorescence assays on CHO cells stably expressing an HA-tagged version of mouse APOBEC3 or an empty vector. CHO cells were fixed with 4% PFA and stained with anti-HA antibodies. **e** Enumeration of G418 resistant colonies of CHO cells expressing mouse APOBEC3. Three clones of CHO cells expressing HA-tagged mA3 or an empty vector were transfected with plasmids expressing a *neo* gene (NEO), L1.3, or ancML. Data are mean ± SD from 3 experiments with independent single cell clones. **f** and **g** Analysis of MuERV-L elements using Hypermut 2.0. Ratio of G to A mutations at preferred mA3 editing sites (RD 3′ to a G) (Y-axis) plotted against ratio of G to A mutations at disfavored mA3 editing sites (YN|RC 3′ to a G) (control ratio, X-axis). No 5′ context was imposed (**f**), or sites with a 5′ C to the mutated G were excluded (**g**). 230 gag–pol containing MuERV-L elements in the mouse genome were compared to their consensus sequence. Data points in red and orange indicate MuERV-L sequences that were statistically significantly enriched in putative mA3 induced mutations (p value < 0.05). Data points in orange represent MuERV-L elements that are statistically significantly enriched mA3-induced mutations in both analyses (p value < 0.01). **h** Profile of G to A transitions in two putatively mA3-edited MuERV-L proviral sequences compared to a consensus sequence. The profile of the reference MuERV-L sequence is shown for comparison (MLref, non significantly mA3 edited). Lines in red and cyan represent putative mA3-derived G to A transitions, not accounting for the +2 position (dinucleotide changes from GG to AG and GA to AA respectively), whereas lines in green and magenta represent non mA3-derived G to A transitions (GC to AC and GT to AT respectively). Lines in yellow indicate gaps compared to the consensus sequence

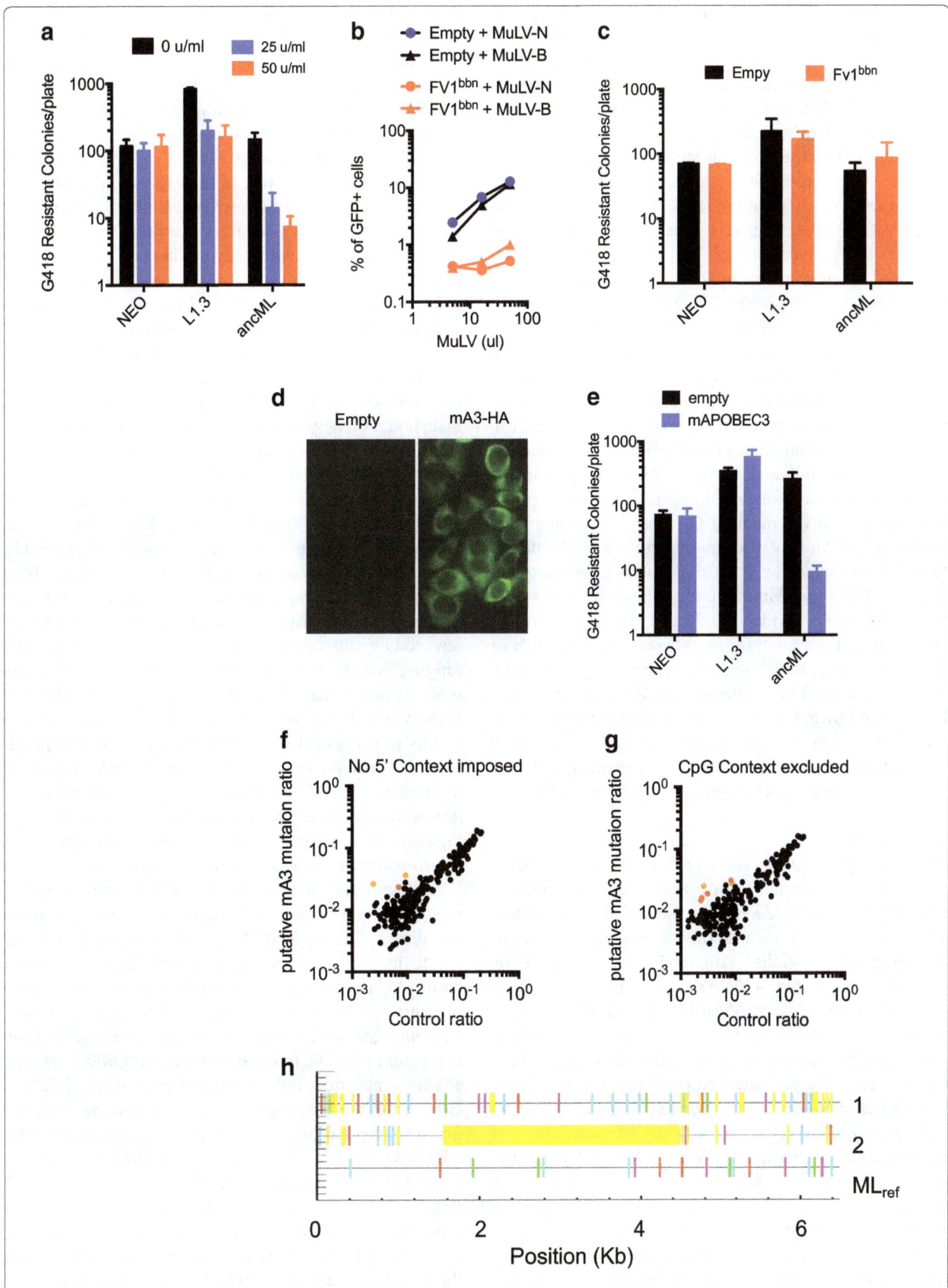

restrict human L1.3 retrotransposition has been previously documented [65], while some human APOBEC3 proteins inhibit L1.3 retrotransposition [42, 66, 67], suggesting that species-dependent differences exist in the ability of APOBEC3 proteins to inhibit the replication of endogenous retroelements.

Because mA3 clearly inhibited ancML replication, and therefore might have affected MuERV-L sequence or replication in vivo, we inspected the 230 gag–pol containing MuERV-L elements that were used to derive ancML *gag* (Fig. 1f) using Hypermut 2.0 [40] (Fig. 5f–h). For each MuERV-L element we compared the number of G to A transitions in mA3-preferred motifs (5′ G(A|G)(A|G|T) 3′) with those in control sites (5′ G(C|T)N 3′ or 5′ G(A|G) C 3′) relative to a consensus sequence (Additional file 4: Table S3). Only three MuERV-L elements showed significant ($p < 0.05$) evidence of mA3 dependent hypermutation when no 5′ context was enforced (Fig. 5f). Because spontaneous deamination of methylated CpG dinucleotides can also produce G to A transitions, we performed the same analysis after excluding sites containing a C nucleotide 5′ to the mutated G. When these sites were excluded, 10 MuERV-L elements showed a significant ($p < 0.05$) evidence for mA3 dependent hypermutation (Fig. 5g). Only two MuERV-L elements exhibited statistically significant evidence of mA3 dependent hypermutation in both analyses (p value < 0.01), and both of these elements carried a relatively low mutational burden (Fig. 5f–h). Thus, although ancML replication can be inhibited by mA3, analysis of MuERV-L proviruses in the mouse genome suggests that MuERV-L either rarely encountered mA3, or is inhibited in a manner that prevents the deposition of hypermutated proviruses.

Discussion

Here, we report the successful reconstruction of a ~ 2MY old replication competent ancestral MuERV-L sequence, through the analysis of a recently expanded subset of fossilized MuERV-L elements in the mouse genome. According to previous studies [16], and corroborated here, MuERV-L originated ~ 10 MYA, after the *Rattus–Mus* split and underwent a prolific expansion ~ 2 MYA. In fact, almost 65% of solo LTRs and MuERV-L proviruses identified herein have an estimated integration date of < 3 MYA. Furthermore, the estimated dates of solo LTRs follow a bimodal distribution (a major one centered ~ 3MYA and the other ~ 8MYA) consistent with the estimated times of both expansions (Additional file 1: Table S1). A combination of homology searches and defragmentation methods provided the material for the estimation of the sequence of the ~ 2MY old replication-competent ancestor.

Other highly abundant *env*-defective ERVs typically appear to be derived from closely related elements that possess an *env* gene. While other closely related elements do possess an *env* gene, there are no documented ERV-L elements that encode an *env*. It is likely, therefore, that an ancestral ERV-L element lacked an *env* gene. Thus, the bulk of MuERV-L replication likely occurred through entirely intracellular retrotransposon-like mechanisms [21]. Moreover, the bulk of MuERV-L replication likely occurred in early embryos, as the expression of MuERV-L elements appears to be restricted to the 2-cell embryo, although It is unknown whether this property is confined to the subset of elements that proliferated ~ 2MYA. It is possible that the early embryonic environment is also necessary in some other way for MuERV-L replication given its apparently restricted tropism in cell lines. In particular, it is intriguing that (and as yet unexplained why) MuERV-L only replicated with reasonable efficiency in Chinese hamster ovary cells, even when provided with a promoter that should drive its expression in nearly any cell type.

MuERV-L belongs to an ancient mammalian ERV family (which originated > 100 MYA [18]) that is distantly related to spumaviruses. Therefore, modern functional viral sequences are therefore not useful for attempts to increase the replicative efficiency of ancML. Remarkably, there is a high number of MuERV-L proviruses that have retained their coding potential, and share a high degree of sequence similarity to the functional ancML (with only few coding differences and overall nucleotide identity ranging from 96.16 to 99.31%). However, currently there is no evidence that the ongoing expression of MuERV-L elements at the two-cell stage of the mouse embryo results in successful re-integration, although it is possible that MuERV-L replication and reintegration occurs in modern mouse embryos at some very low rate. Nevertheless, examination of recent *bona fide* integrations might highlight important residues that might be altered to improve ancML replication and/or integration.

We found that mouse IFNα was able to inhibit ancML replication, suggesting that interferon stimulated genes can directly inhibit MuERV-L replication, possibly leading to its recent extinction as a replication competent entity. Alternatively, early embryos may express antiviral proteins that inhibit re-integration of modern MuERV-L elements that would otherwise be intrinsically replication competent [62]. We found that mouse APOBEC3 inhibits ancML replication, but mutational profiles of MuERV-L elements in the mouse genome provide minimal evidence for mA3-dependent hypermutation as a mechanism for inhibition in vivo. During mouse development, mA3 is expressed at the two-cell stage, increasing at the four-cell stage to become one of the top 30% most highly expressed genes [68]. Thus, it is at least possible that mA3 may have acted on replicating MuERV-L elements, perhaps in part through deaminase-independent mechanisms [69].

Despite the apparently random integration pattern of ancML, the analysis of fixed MuERV-L elements showed that there has been a selective pressure to eliminate MuERV-L integrations from genes. Conversely, MuERV-L related sequences (Fv1) have clearly been positively selected to provide defense against retroviral infection [22–24] and recent studies have suggested that regulatory elements of MuERV-L LTRs may have been co-opted to regulate the expression of numerous genes during embryogenesis [14, 15]. While Fv1 arose at least ~5–7 MYA, it is unclear whether the potential exaptation of MuERV-L regulatory sequences occurred during the 10MYA expansion or the more recent ~2 MYA expansion. Nonetheless, there appears to be both a benefit (co-option for antiviral defense and regulation of embryogenesis) and cost (disruption of gene function) associated with the presence of MuERV-L elements in the mouse genome.

MuERV-L appears to be the only member of the ERV-L family that seems to have been reactivated in recent evolutionary times. It is particularly intriguing that the recent expansion is characterized by an in-frame deletion in *gag*, as it could be this deletion the responsible for releasing some MuERV-L elements from the deleterious effects of a hypothetical inhibitory factor ~2MYA. Recent studies have shown the fundamental role that some endogenous retroviral sequences may play in mammalian development and protection from exogenous retroviral infection [15, 23, 24, 70–73]. Indeed one report has suggested that knockdown of MuERV-L transcripts impacts embryonic development [74]. Nevertheless, it remains to be determined whether the current presence of MuERV-L transcripts, proteins and virus-like particles at the two-cell stage of the mouse embryo might be beneficial or deleterious to the mouse.

Conclusions

The reconstruction of an ancestral MuERV-L sequence highlights the potential for the retroviral fossil record to illuminate ancient events and represents a unique opportunity to study ERV-L biology and reactivation, the role of MuERV-L in mouse development and potentially uncover new roles for ERVs in mammalian biology.

Additional files

Additional file 1: Table S1. MuERV-L loci identified in mouse genome assemblies.

Additional file 2. ancML sequence in FASTA format.

Additional file 3: Table S2. ancML integration sites cloned from CHO gDNA.

Additional file 4: Table S3. Analysis for hypermutation in MuERV-L elements in the mouse genome.

Authors' contributions
DBM performed all the experimental work and analysis. RG supervised the computational work and PDB supervised the experimental work. All authors wrote, read and approved the final manuscript.

Author details
[1] Laboratory of Retrovirology and Howard Hughes Medical Institute, The Rockefeller University, New York, NY, USA. [2] MRC-University of Glasgow Centre for Virus Research, Glasgow, UK. [3] Present Address: Department of Microbiology, Icahn School of Medicine at Mount Sinai, New York, NY, USA.

Acknowledgements
We thank Dr. John V. Moran for kindly sharing the L1.3 plasmid (JM101), Theodora Hatziioannou for the plasmid expressing Fv1[bbn], and Rachel Liberatore for the plasmid expressing mouse APOBEC3. We also thank all the members of the Bieniasz lab for their help and suggestions on the project.

Competing interests
The authors declare that they have no competing interests.

Funding
This work was supported by a grant from the National Institute of Allergy and Infectious diseases (R3764003 to PDB) and a grant from the UK Medical Research Council (MC_UU_12014/10 to RJG).

References
1. Weiss RA. The discovery of endogenous retroviruses. Retrovirology. 2006;3:67.
2. Lander ES, Linton LM, Birren B, Nusbaum C, Zody MC, Baldwin J, Devon K, Dewar K, Doyle M, FitzHugh W, et al. Initial sequencing and analysis of the human genome. Nature. 2001;409(6822):860–921.
3. Emerman M, Malik HS. Paleovirology—modern consequences of ancient viruses. PLoS Biol. 2010;8(2):e1000301.
4. Dewannieux M, Harper F, Richaud A, Letzelter C, Ribet D, Pierron G, Heidmann T. Identification of an infectious progenitor for the multiple-copy HERV-K human endogenous retroelements. Genome Res. 2006;16(12):1548–56.
5. Lee YN, Bieniasz PD. Reconstitution of an infectious human endogenous retrovirus. PLoS Pathog. 2007;3(1):e10.
6. Perez-Caballero D, Soll SJ, Bieniasz PD. Evidence for restriction of ancient primate gammaretroviruses by APOBEC3 but not TRIM5alpha proteins. PLoS Pathog. 2008;4(10):e1000181.
7. Kaiser SM, Malik HS, Emerman M. Restriction of an extinct retrovirus by the human TRIM5alpha antiviral protein. Science. 2007;316(5832):1756–8.
8. Goldstone DC, Yap MW, Robertson LE, Haire LF, Taylor WR, Katzourakis A, Stoye JP, Taylor IA. Structural and functional analysis of prehistoric lentiviruses uncovers an ancient molecular interface. Cell Host Microbe. 2010;8(3):248–59.
9. Soll SJ, Neil SJ, Bieniasz PD. Identification of a receptor for an extinct virus. Proc Natl Acad Sci USA. 2010;107(45):19496–501.
10. Blanco-Melo D, Gifford RJ, Bieniasz PD. Co-option of an endogenous retrovirus envelope for host defense in hominid ancestors. Elife. 2017;6:e22519.
11. Lee YN, Malim MH, Bieniasz PD. Hypermutation of an ancient human retrovirus by APOBEC3G. J Virol. 2008;82(17):8762–70.
12. Kigami D, Minami N, Takayama H, Imai H. MuERV-L is one of the earliest transcribed genes in mouse one-cell embryos. Biol Reprod. 2003;68(2):651–4.
13. Ribet D, Louvet-Vallee S, Harper F, de Parseval N, Dewannieux M, Heidmann O, Pierron G, Maro B, Heidmann T. Murine endogenous retrovirus MuERV-L is the progenitor of the "orphan" epsilon viruslike particles of the early mouse embryo. J Virol. 2008;82(3):1622–5.
14. Macfarlan TS, Gifford WD, Agarwal S, Driscoll S, Lettieri K, Wang J, Andrews SE, Franco L, Rosenfeld MG, Ren B, et al. Endogenous retroviruses and neighboring genes are coordinately repressed by LSD1/KDM1A. Genes Dev. 2011;25(6):594–607.

15. Macfarlan TS, Gifford WD, Driscoll S, Lettieri K, Rowe HM, Bonanomi D, Firth A, Singer O, Trono D, Pfaff SL. Embryonic stem cell potency fluctuates with endogenous retrovirus activity. Nature. 2012;487(7405):57–63.

16. Costas J. Molecular characterization of the recent intragenomic spread of the murine endogenous retrovirus MuERV-L. J Mol Evol. 2003;56(2):181–6.

17. Benit L, Lallemand JB, Casella JF, Philippe H, Heidmann T. ERV-L elements: a family of endogenous retrovirus-like elements active throughout the evolution of mammals. J Virol. 1999;73(4):3301–8.

18. Lee A, Nolan A, Watson J, Tristem M. Identification of an ancient endogenous retrovirus, predating the divergence of the placental mammals. Philos Trans R Soc Lond B Biol Sci. 2013;368(1626):20120503.

19. Cordonnier A, Casella JF, Heidmann T. Isolation of novel human endogenous retrovirus-like elements with foamy virus-related pol sequence. J Virol. 1995;69(9):5890–7.

20. Benit L, De Parseval N, Casella JF, Callebaut I, Cordonnier A, Heidmann T. Cloning of a new murine endogenous retrovirus, MuERV-L, with strong similarity to the human HERV-L element and with a gag coding sequence closely related to the Fv1 restriction gene. J Virol. 1997;71(7):5652–7.

21. Magiorkinis G, Gifford RJ, Katzourakis A, De Ranter J, Belshaw R. Env-less endogenous retroviruses are genomic superspreaders. Proc Natl Acad Sci USA. 2012;109(19):7385–90.

22. Best S, Le Tissier P, Towers G, Stoye JP. Positional cloning of the mouse retrovirus restriction gene Fv1. Nature. 1996;382(6594):826–9.

23. Yan Y, Buckler-White A, Wollenberg K, Kozak CA. Origin, antiviral function and evidence for positive selection of the gammaretrovirus restriction gene Fv1 in the genus Mus. Proc Natl Acad Sci USA. 2009;106(9):3259–63.

24. Yap MW, Colbeck E, Ellis SA, Stoye JP. Evolution of the retroviral restriction gene Fv1: inhibition of non-MLV retroviruses. PLoS Pathog. 2014;10(3):e1003968.

25. Guallar D, Perez-Palacios R, Climent M, Martinez-Abadia I, Larraga A, Fernandez-Juan M, Vallejo C, Muniesa P, Schoorlemmer J. Expression of endogenous retroviruses is negatively regulated by the pluripotency marker Rex1/Zfp42. Nucleic Acids Res. 2012;40(18):8993–9007.

26. Rowe HM, Trono D. Dynamic control of endogenous retroviruses during development. Virology. 2011;411(2):273–87.

27. Camacho C, Coulouris G, Avagyan V, Ma N, Papadopoulos J, Bealer K, Madden TL. BLAST+: architecture and applications. BMC Bioinformatics. 2009;10:421.

28. Mural RJ, Adams MD, Myers EW, Smith HO, Miklos GL, Wides R, Halpern A, Li PW, Sutton GG, Nadeau J, et al. A comparison of whole-genome shotgun-derived mouse chromosome 16 and the human genome. Science. 2002;296(5573):1661–71.

29. Mouse Genome Sequencing Consortium, Waterston RH, Lindblad-Toh K, Birney E, Rogers J, Abril JF, Agarwal P, Agarwala R, Ainscough R, Alexandersson M, et al. Initial sequencing and comparative analysis of the mouse genome. Nature. 2002;420(6915):520–62.

30. Hubbard T, Barker D, Birney E, Cameron G, Chen Y, Clark L, Cox T, Cuff J, Curwen V, Down T, et al. The Ensembl genome database project. Nucleic Acids Res. 2002;30(1):38–41.

31. Swofford DL. PAUP*. Phylogenetic analysis using parsimony (*and other methods). Version 4. Sunderland: Sinauer Associates; 2002.

32. Lebedev YB, Belonovitch OS, Zybrova NV, Khil PP, Kurdyukov SG, Vinogradova TV, Hunsmann G, Sverdlov ED. Differences in HERV-K LTR insertions in orthologous loci of humans and great apes. Gene. 2000;247(1–2):265–77.

33. Subramanian RP, Wildschutte JH, Russo C, Coffin JM. Identification, characterization, and comparative genomic distribution of the HERV-K (HML-2) group of human endogenous retroviruses. Retrovirology. 2011;8:90.

34. Marshall HM, Ronen K, Berry C, Llano M, Sutherland H, Saenz D, Bickmore W, Poeschla E, Bushman FD. Role of PSIP1/LEDGF/p75 in lentiviral infectivity and integration targeting. PLoS ONE. 2007;2(12):e1340.

35. Xu X, Nagarajan H, Lewis NE, Pan S, Cai Z, Liu X, Chen W, Xie M, Wang W, Hammond S, et al. The genomic sequence of the Chinese hamster ovary (CHO)-K1 cell line. Nat Biotechnol. 2011;29(8):735–41.

36. Edgar RC. MUSCLE: multiple sequence alignment with high accuracy and high throughput. Nucleic Acids Res. 2004;32(5):1792–7.

37. Stamatakis A. RAxML version 8: a tool for phylogenetic analysis and post-analysis of large phylogenies. Bioinformatics. 2014;30(9):1312–3.

38. Yang Z. PAML: a program package for phylogenetic analysis by maximum likelihood. Comput Appl Biosci. 1997;13(5):555–6.

39. Darriba D, Taboada GL, Doallo R, Posada D. jModelTest 2: more models, new heuristics and parallel computing. Nat Methods. 2012;9(8):772.

40. Rose PP, Korber BT. Detecting hypermutations in viral sequences with an emphasis on G → A hypermutation. Bioinformatics. 2000;16(4):400–1.

41. Moran JV, DeBerardinis RJ, Kazazian HH Jr. Exon shuffling by L1 retrotransposition. Science. 1999;283(5407):1530–4.

42. Kinomoto M, Kanno T, Shimura M, Ishizaka Y, Kojima A, Kurata T, Sata T, Tokunaga K. All APOBEC3 family proteins differentially inhibit LINE-1 retrotransposition. Nucleic Acids Res. 2007;35(9):2955–64.

43. Mariani R, Chen D, Schrofelbauer B, Navarro F, Konig R, Bollman B, Munk C, Nymark-McMahon H, Landau NR. Species-specific exclusion of APOBEC3G from HIV-1 virions by Vif. Cell. 2003;114(1):21–31.

44. Hatziioannou T, Cowan S, Bieniasz PD. Capsid-dependent and -independent postentry restriction of primate lentivirus tropism in rodent cells. J Virol. 2004;78(2):1006–11.

45. Soneoka Y, Cannon PM, Ramsdale EE, Griffiths JC, Romano G, Kingsman SM, Kingsman AJ. A transient three-plasmid expression system for the production of high titer retroviral vectors. Nucleic Acids Res. 1995;23(4):628–33.

46. Kent WJ. BLAT—the BLAST-like alignment tool. Genome Res. 2002;12(4):656–64.

47. Kent WJ, Sugnet CW, Furey TS, Roskin KM, Pringle TH, Zahler AM, Haussler D. The human genome browser at UCSC. Genome Res. 2002;12(6):996–1006.

48. Brady T, Lee YN, Ronen K, Malani N, Berry CC, Bieniasz PD, Bushman FD. Integration target site selection by a resurrected human endogenous retrovirus. Genes Dev. 2009;23(5):633–42.

49. Soh YQ, Alfoldi J, Pyntikova T, Brown LG, Graves T, Minx PJ, Fulton RS, Kremitzki C, Koutseva N, Mueller JL, et al. Sequencing the mouse Y chromosome reveals convergent gene acquisition and amplification on both sex chromosomes. Cell. 2014;159(4):800–13.

50. Qin C, Wang Z, Shang J, Bekkari K, Liu R, Pacchione S, McNulty KA, Ng A, Barnum JE, Storer RD. Intracisternal A particle genes: distribution in the mouse genome, active subtypes, and potential roles as species-specific mediators of susceptibility to cancer. Mol Carcinog. 2010;49(1):54–67.

51. Moran JV, Holmes SE, Naas TP, DeBerardinis RJ, Boeke JD, Kazazian HH Jr. High frequency retrotransposition in cultured mammalian cells. Cell. 1996;87(5):917–27.

52. Lewis NE, Liu X, Li Y, Nagarajan H, Yerganian G, O'Brien E, Bordbar A, Roth AM, Rosenbloom J, Bian C, et al. Genomic landscapes of Chinese hamster ovary cell lines as revealed by the Cricetulus griseus draft genome. Nat Biotechnol. 2013;31(8):759–65.

53. Repaske R, Steele PE, O'Neill RR, Rabson AB, Martin MA. Nucleotide sequence of a full-length human endogenous retroviral segment. J Virol. 1985;54(3):764–72.

54. Coffin JM, Hughes SH, Varmus H. Retroviruses. Plainview, NY: Cold Spring Harbor Laboratory Press; 1997.

55. Champoux JJ, Schultz SJ. Ribonuclease H: properties, substrate specificity and roles in retroviral reverse transcription. FEBS J. 2009;276(6):1506–16.

56. Schoggins JW, Wilson SJ, Panis M, Murphy MY, Jones CT, Bieniasz P, Rice CM. A diverse range of gene products are effectors of the type I interferon antiviral response. Nature. 2011;472(7344):481–5.

57. Zwarthoff EC, Bosveld IJ, Vonk WP, Trapman J. Constitutive expression of a murine interferon alpha gene in hamster cells and characterization of its protein product. J Gen Virol. 1985;66(Pt 4):685–91.

58. Van Heuvel M, Bosveld IJ, Mooren AA, Trapman J, Zwarthoff EC. Properties of natural and hybrid murine alpha interferons. J Gen Virol. 1986;67(Pt 10):2215–22.

59. Trapman J, van Heuvel M, de Jonge P, Bosveld IJ, Klaassen P, Zwarthoff EC. Structure-function analysis of mouse interferon alpha species: MuIFN-alpha 10, a subspecies with low antiviral activity. J Gen Virol. 1988;69(Pt 1):67–75.

60. Van Heuvel M, Bosveld IJ, Klaassen P, Zwarthoff EC, Trapman J. Structure-function analysis of murine interferon-alpha: antiviral properties of novel hybrid interferons. J Interferon Res. 1988;8(1):5–14.

61. van Heuvel M, Govaert-Siemerink M, Bosveld IJ, Zwarthoff EC, Trapman J. Interferon-alpha-(IFN) producing CHO cell lines are resistant to the antiproliferative activity of IFN: a correlation with gene expression. J Cell Biochem. 1988;38(4):269–78.

62. Wu X, Dao Thi VL, Huang Y, Billerbeck E, Saha D, Hoffmann HH, Wang Y, Silva LAV, Sarbanes S, Sun T, et al. Intrinsic immunity shapes viral resistance of stem cells. Cell. 2018;172(3):423–38.

63. Bock M, Bishop KN, Towers G, Stoye JP. Use of a transient assay for studying the genetic determinants of Fv1 restriction. J Virol. 2000;74(16):7422–30.

64. Rehwinkel J. Mouse knockout models for HIV-1 restriction factors. Cell Mol Life Sci. 2014;71(19):3749–66.

65. Lovsin N, Peterlin BM. APOBEC3 proteins inhibit LINE-1 retrotransposition in the absence of ORF1p binding. Ann N Y Acad Sci. 2009;1178:268–75.

66. Muckenfuss H, Hamdorf M, Held U, Perkovic M, Lower J, Cichutek K, Flory E, Schumann GG, Munk C. APOBEC3 proteins inhibit human LINE-1 retrotransposition. J Biol Chem. 2006;281(31):22161–72.

67. Stenglein MD, Harris RS. APOBEC3B and APOBEC3F inhibit L1 retrotransposition by a DNA deamination-independent mechanism. J Biol Chem. 2006;281(25):16837–41.

68. Xie D, Chen CC, Ptaszek LM, Xiao S, Cao X, Fang F, Ng HH, Lewin HA, Cowan C, Zhong S. Rewirable gene regulatory networks in the preimplantation embryonic development of three mammalian species. Genome Res. 2010;20(6):804–15.

69. MacMillan AL, Kohli RM, Ross SR. APOBEC3 inhibition of mouse mammary tumor virus infection: the role of cytidine deamination versus inhibition of reverse transcription. J Virol. 2013;87(9):4808–17.

70. Lavialle C, Cornelis G, Dupressoir A, Esnault C, Heidmann O, Vernochet C, Heidmann T. Paleovirology of 'syncytins', retroviral env genes exapted for a role in placentation. Philos Trans R Soc Lond B Biol Sci. 2013;368(1626):20120507.

71. Wang J, Xie G, Singh M, Ghanbarian AT, Rasko T, Szvetnik A, Cai H, Besser D, Prigione A, Fuchs NV, et al. Primate-specific endogenous retrovirus-driven transcription defines naive-like stem cells. Nature. 2014;516(7531):405–9.

72. Lu X, Sachs F, Ramsay L, Jacques PE, Goke J, Bourque G, Ng HH. The retrovirus HERVH is a long noncoding RNA required for human embryonic stem cell identity. Nat Struct Mol Biol. 2014;21(4):423–5.

73. Armezzani A, Varela M, Spencer TE, Palmarini M, Arnaud F. "Menage a trois": the evolutionary interplay between JSRV, enJSRVs and domestic sheep. Viruses. 2014;6(12):4926–45.

74. Huang Y, Kim JK, Do DV, Lee C, Penfold CA, Zylicz JJ, Marioni JC, Hackett JA, Surani MA. Stella modulates transcriptional and endogenous retrovirus programs during maternal-to-zygotic transition. Elife. 2017;6:e22345.

9

HIV-1 cell-to-cell transmission and broadly neutralizing antibodies

Jérémy Dufloo[1,2], Timothée Bruel[1,2,3] and Olivier Schwartz[1,2,3]*

Abstract

HIV-1 spreads through contacts between infected and target cells. Polarized viral budding at the contact site forms the virological synapse. Additional cellular processes, such as nanotubes, filopodia, virus accumulation in endocytic or phagocytic compartments promote efficient viral propagation. Cell-to-cell transmission allows immune evasion and likely contributes to HIV-1 spread in vivo. Anti-HIV-1 broadly neutralizing antibodies (bNAbs) defeat the majority of circulating viral strains by binding to the viral envelope glycoprotein (Env). Several bNAbs have entered clinical evaluation during the last years. It is thus important to understand their mechanism of action and to determine how they interact with infected cells. In experimental models, HIV-1 cell-to-cell transmission is sensitive to neutralization, but the effect of antibodies is often less marked than during cell-free infection. This may be due to differences in the conformation or accessibility of Env at the surface of virions and cells. In this review, we summarize the current knowledge on HIV-1 cell-to-cell transmission and discuss the role of bNAbs during this process.

Keywords: HIV-1, bNAbs, Cell-to-cell transmission, Neutralization

Background

Human Immunodeficiency Virus (HIV-1) is the etiological agent of AIDS [1]. Identification of molecular mechanisms governing the replication of HIV-1 allowed the design of potent antiretroviral treatment (ART). Combined ART restored the life expectancy of patients, transforming a fatal infection into a manageable chronic disease. However, limited access to therapy in many regions of the world and the existence of a viral reservoir insensitive to treatment urge the need for novel antiviral strategies.

HIV-1 infects cells by multiple mechanisms, either as cell-free or cell-associated particles [2, 3]. HIV-1 infection is more efficient when the virus is transmitted through direct cell contacts. HIV-1 follows different routes of cell-to-cell transmission [4]. One main mechanism involves a structure called the Virological Synapse (VS). It allows the polarized delivery of newly formed viral particles [5, 6]. Its organization requires both

cellular and viral proteins. The virus also hijacks other cellular pathways to spread, such as nanotubes, filopodia, phagocytic or endocytic compartments.

As part of the immune response, infected individuals rapidly develop anti-HIV-1 antibodies, as soon as one week following initial viral exposure [7]. These early-produced antibodies do not neutralize the virus [7]. The first neutralizing antibodies are detected two to three months later [8]. These antibodies are inefficient against heterologous viral strains and are rapidly escaped by mutation of the autologous virus [9, 10]. Some patients called elite neutralizers develop antibodies with broad neutralization potency [11]. Deconvolution of their polyclonal response enabled the identification of several monoclonal bNAbs (reviewed in [12]). Potent bNAbs present peculiar molecular features, such as intensive hypermutation and often long CDRH3 regions (reviewed in [13]). bNAbs target conserved regions on the viral Env spike, called sites of vulnerability [13]. These include the CD4 binding site (CD4bs), the N-glycans of V1/V2 and V3 loops, the gp41 membrane proximal external region (MPER), and the gp120/gp41 interface, which comprises a recently described epitope composed of the fusion peptide at the N-terminus of gp41 and the N88 glycan on gp120

*Correspondence: schwartz@pasteur.fr
[1] Virus and Immunity Unit, Department of Virology, Institut Pasteur, Paris, France
Full list of author information is available at the end of the article

[14–16]. bNAbs are often screened and selected with assays that use cell-free virus. The capacity of bNAbs to suppress cell-to-cell transmission has been thus often under-evaluated. In vitro, bNAbs neutralize cell-free infection by many viral strains and trigger Fc-mediated effector mechanisms, including antibody-dependent cellular cytotoxicity (ADCC) [17]. In animal models, bNAbs display both prophylactic [18] and therapeutic efficacy (reviewed in [19]). They clear HIV-infected cells and modulate host immune responses [20, 21]. These findings suggest that bNAbs could target the latent HIV reservoir and contribute to long-term remission of HIV-1 infection in humans.

Phase 1 studies of bNAbs targeting the CD4bs (3BNC117 and VRC01) and the V3 loop (10-1074) demonstrated their safety and efficacy (reviewed in [22]). Infusion of single bNAbs induced a transient decline in viremia of approximately 1.5 $\log_{10}$ copies/ml, followed by selection of escape variants [23–25]. Of note, the half-life of 10-1074 (24 days) was higher than that of 3BNC117 and VRC01 (around 15 days). In ART-treated patients pre-screened for their susceptibility to 3BNC117, infusion of this antibody delayed viral rebound after ART cessation by an average of 8 weeks [26]. Moreover, 3BNC117 potentiated subsequent anti-HIV-1 host antibody responses, demonstrating an immunomodulatory potential that is not fully understood [27]. Thus, understanding the molecular and cellular bases of bNAbs antiviral activity is critical to optimize their in vivo efficacy.

In this review, we first summarize the current knowledge on HIV cell-to-cell transmission. We discuss the mechanisms that may account for the differences observed in neutralization of cell-free and cell-associated HIV-1. We then detail how bNAbs bound at the cell surface neutralize viral propagation but also destroy infected cells by ADCC and other mechanisms.

HIV-1 cell-to-cell transmission

The virological synapse between infected an uninfected T cells

Early studies reported secretion of HIV-1 particles and relocalization of adhesion molecules at the contact zone between infected and uninfected T cells [28–30]. The precise mechanisms of viral cell-to-cell transmission were initially described with another retrovirus, Human T cell Leukemia Virus type 1 (HTLV-I) [31]. Upon cell–cell contacts, HTLV-I Env, Gag and the viral genome accumulate at cell–cell junctions, allowing polarized budding of viral particles and their transfer to the target cells in a confined area. Igakura and colleagues named this structure the "virological synapse" (VS) due to its similarities with the immunological synapse that forms between T lymphocytes and Dendritic Cells (DCs) during antigen

presentation [32]. The VS was then observed during HIV-1 spread in T cells [5]. The HIV-1 VS displayed similar features: recruitment of Env and Gag at the interface on the producer cell side and of the cytoskeleton on the target side [5] (Fig. 1a). An infected cell can generate more than one VS, allowing simultaneous transfer of HIV-1 to multiple targets [33].

HIV-1 drives the organization of the VS. The VS is initiated by interactions between Env on the donor and CD4 on the target cell [5]. Env-mediated fusion seems to be regulated at the VS to decrease or slow down the formation of syncytia. The interaction between the Env cytoplasmic domain and the underlying immature Gag (p55) lattice reduces Env fusogenicity [34]. Fusion is also impaired by cellular proteins, such as tetraspanins or ezrin that accumulate at the VS [35, 36]. Co-receptor (CCR5 or CXCR4) engagement is not necessary for VS formation and transfer of virions [37]. However, co-receptors are required for subsequent productive infection [38].

After initial CD4/Env interactions, cellular adhesion molecules such as LFA-1, ICAM-1 and ICAM-3 are recruited to stabilize the VS [33, 39]. These adhesins are not mandatory, as blocking ICAM-1/3 and LFA-1 by antibodies does not inhibit the creation of cell conjugates and viral transfer [40]. Whether the recruitment of adhesion molecules to the VS is involved in its stabilization or has other functions is not fully understood. The cytoskeleton plays a predominant role during HIV-1 cell-to-cell transmission. The formation of the VS depends on actin and tubulin [5, 41, 42], and is associated with a relocalization of the MTOC towards the site of cell–cell contact, which contributes to the trafficking of viral and cellular proteins to the VS [31, 43, 44]. However, viral transfer can occur simultaneously to multiple targets, even if the MTOC is localized towards a single recipient cell [43]. Lipid rafts also promote Gag and Env clustering at the synapse [45].

Various viral and cellular proteins modulate positively or negatively HIV-1 cell-to-cell transfer. The viral protein Nef promotes the accumulation of Gag below the cellular membrane, increasing the transfer of mature HIV-1 virions and productive infection of target cells [46]. BST2/Tetherin, an interferon-induced gene that restricts HIV-1, accumulates with Gag and actin at the VS in infected donor cells and limits viral cell-to-cell spread [47, 48]. However, the inhibitory effect of tetherin is debated [49]. IFITM3, another interferon-stimulated gene with antiviral activities, also impairs cell-to-cell transfer of HIV-1 when expressed on either donor and target cells [50] and may act by infiltrating budding viral particles [50, 51].

Following VS formation, depending on the cell types used, newly produced viral particles can either fuse directly at the target cell plasma membrane [5] or be

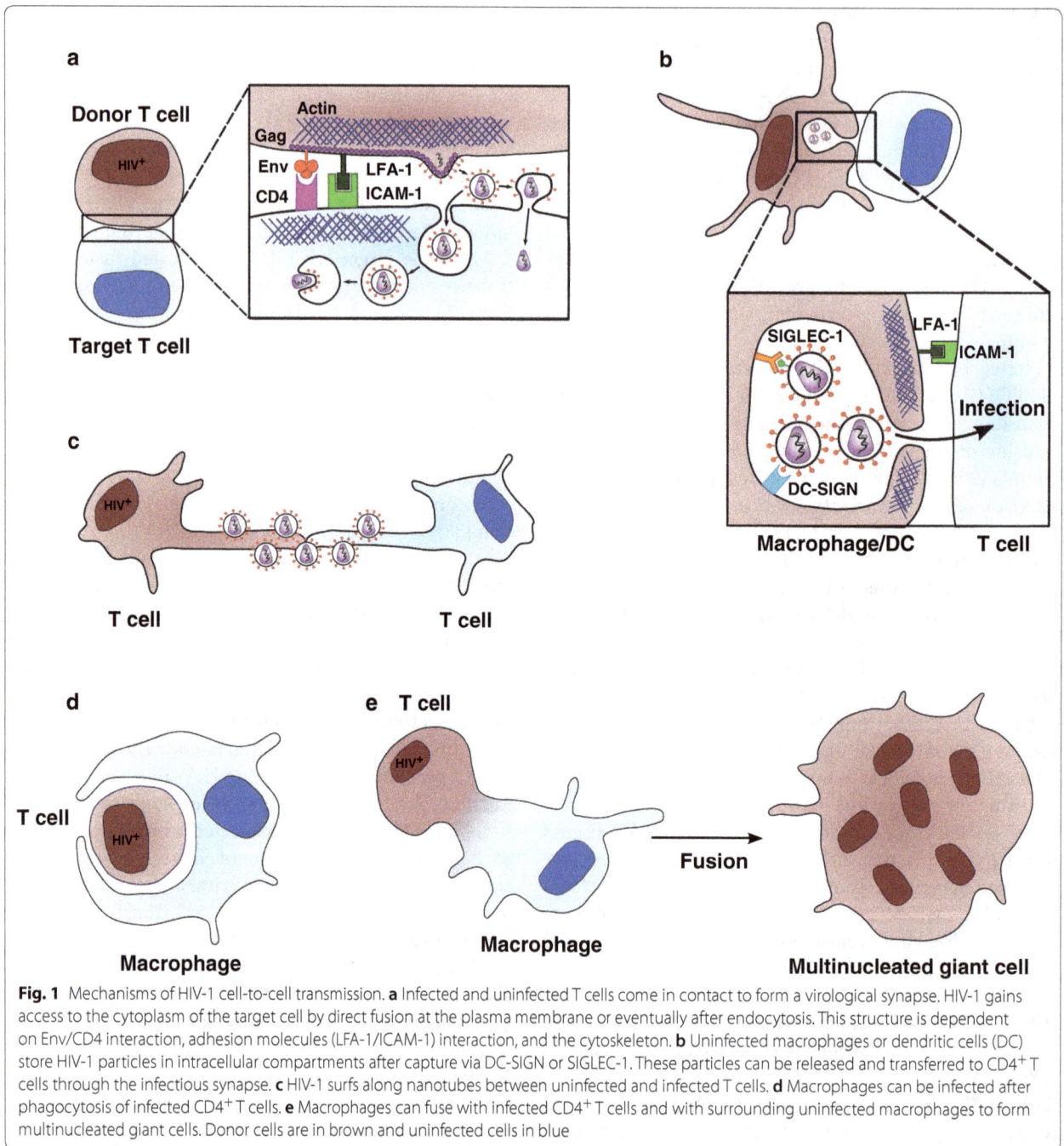

Fig. 1 Mechanisms of HIV-1 cell-to-cell transmission. **a** Infected and uninfected T cells come in contact to form a virological synapse. HIV-1 gains access to the cytoplasm of the target cell by direct fusion at the plasma membrane or eventually after endocytosis. This structure is dependent on Env/CD4 interaction, adhesion molecules (LFA-1/ICAM-1) interaction, and the cytoskeleton. **b** Uninfected macrophages or dendritic cells (DC) store HIV-1 particles in intracellular compartments after capture via DC-SIGN or SIGLEC-1. These particles can be released and transferred to CD4+ T cells through the infectious synapse. **c** HIV-1 surfs along nanotubes between uninfected and infected T cells. **d** Macrophages can be infected after phagocytosis of infected CD4+ T cells. **e** Macrophages can fuse with infected CD4+ T cells and with surrounding uninfected macrophages to form multinucleated giant cells. Donor cells are in brown and uninfected cells in blue

endocytosed by the acceptor T cell in a clathrin- and dynamin-dependent manner [38, 52, 53] (Fig. 1a). It has been proposed that HIV-1 viral particles transferred through the VS may undergo maturation after endocytosis [54]. However, this route of entry has not been observed during cell-free infection [55]. Whatever the entry route, polarized HIV-1 budding leads to a massive release of viral particles into the cytoplasm of the target cell. This high multiplicity of infection (MOI) leads to a

two to three log increase in the efficiency of transmission for cell-associated HIV-1 compared to cell-free virus [37, 56, 57]. It also enhances the number of integrated proviruses [58, 59], and accelerates viral gene expression and spread [60].

VS formation has been observed in vivo by intravital imaging of mice infected with the Friend murine leukemia virus [61]. This study confirmed the role of Env for VS formation and the polarization of Gag at the sites of cell–cell contact in vivo. HIV-1 spread has also been studied in humanized mouse models. HIV-1-infected T cells migrate to lymph nodes, where they bind to target cells, transfer the virus, and also form syncytia [62, 63]. Tomographic analyses identified HIV-1 budding at sites of close cell–cell contact through LFA-1- and ICAM-1-positive structures [64]. Furthermore, the observation of Env-dependent stable contacts between infected and uninfected CD4$^+$ T cells, co-transmission of multiple viral genotypes, and foci of viral replication suggests that cell-to-cell transmission occurs in lymphoid organs of humanized mice [65].

Thus, T cell-to-T cell transmission of HIV-1 is highly efficient in vitro and likely contributes to viral dissemination in vivo.

The infectious synapse between DCs/macrophages and T cells

DCs and macrophages transmit HIV-1 to T cells through different routes, namely *cis*- and *trans*-infections. During *cis*-infection, DCs and macrophages are productively infected and transmit HIV-1 to CD4$^+$ T cells through a VS-like structure [66–68]. However, DCs are relatively resistant to productive infection [69]. They express SAMHD1, which inhibits reverse transcription [70–72] and regulates immune sensing and host responses [73–75]. These cells express low levels of HIV-1 receptor and co-receptors [76, 77]. Macrophages can be productively infected by HIV-1, which buds and accumulates into intracellular tetraspanin-rich compartments termed Virus Containing Compartments (VCCs) [78–80]. VCCs are connected to the cell membrane and release virus to neighboring cells [80].

DCs or macrophages that have captured viral particles but are not productively infected also transmit HIV-1 to CD4$^+$ T cells [81]. This *trans*-infection mechanism is thought to play a role in vivo (reviewed in [82]). DCs and macrophages may capture HIV-1 in a CD4-independent manner. Different cellular proteins bind HIV-1 particles. Env interacts with the C-type lectin DC-SIGN prior to internalization into VCCs [83–86]. In mature DCs, Siglec-1 capture virions in an Env-independent manner by binding to gangliosides present on the viral membrane, also leading to internalization into VCCs [87–90]. After capture, HIV-1 is transferred to T cells through a structure reminiscent of the VS: the Infectious Synapse (IS) [91] (Fig. 1b). In contrast to the VS, CD4 and Env are dispensable for the formation of the IS, but are necessary for viral fusion and productive infection of T cells [92]. IS formation and subsequent viral transfer require the cortical actin cytoskeleton, which is stabilized by tetraspanin-7 and dynamin-2 in DCs [93]. Interactions between LFA-1 and ICAM-1, and between MHC and TCR

modulate DC-to-T cell *trans*-infection [91]. Exosomes released by DCs may also facilitate viral transfer [94]. Recent multidimensional techniques have revealed that the myeloid compartment is more complex than initially thought and comprises at least four monocyte and six DC subsets, including novel pre-DC and plasmacytoid DC (pDC) populations [95, 96]. It will be of interest to determine the sensitivity to HIV-1 infection and the ability to transfer the virus across the spectrum of DC subsets [97].

Other modes of cell-to-cell transmission of HIV-1

Various additional modes of cell-associated HIV-1 transfer have been reported. HIV-1 can use close-ended membrane protrusions called tunneling nanotubes (TNTs) that form between infected and uninfected T cells to spread in a receptor-dependent manner [98] (Fig. 1c). A similar usage of TNTs was observed in macrophages and it has been proposed that Nef induces these TNTs [99, 100]. HIV-1 is contained within endosomes during TNT-mediated transfer in macrophages [101, 102]. Actin-rich membrane protrusions called filopodia are also induced in DCs after interaction between HIV-1 and DC-SIGN, in a Cdc42- [103] and Diaph2-dependent manner [93, 104], facilitating HIV-1 transfer to CD4$^+$ T cells.

Macrophages also engulf living or dying HIV-1-infected T cells allowing their productive infection [105] (Fig. 1d). The impact of the most potent bNAbs on this mode of transmission has not been assessed yet. A two-step process for transfer of HIV-1 from infected CD4$^+$ T cells to macrophages has been described [106]. First, CD4$^+$ T cells establish a contact with macrophages and fuse. This macrophage-T cell hybrid will then fuse with surrounding uninfected macrophages, spreading the infection via multinucleated giant cells (Fig. 1e). CD4$^+$ T cells can also form a VS-like structure with epithelial cells from the genital mucosa, which leads to transcytosis of HIV-1 through the epithelium and subsequent infection of stromal macrophages [107, 108].

Overall, HIV-1 hijacks various pathways to spread across cells that contact each other. This likely contributes to inter- and intra-individual viral propagation. Thus, efficacious antiviral agents must block both cell-free and cell-to-cell infection.

bNAbs and cell-to-cell transmission of HIV-1
Inhibition of HIV-1 transmission through the virological synapse

Before the discovery of bNAbs, several studies investigated the capacity of antibodies to block HIV-1 cell-to-cell transmission. Some sera from infected patients lost their neutralizing activity when the source of HIV-1 was cell-associated [57, 109, 110]. The ability of patients' sera

(See figure on next page.)
Fig. 2 Neutralization potency of bNAbs against cell-free and cell-to-cell transmission of various viral strains. Cell-free (**a**) and cell-to-cell (**b**) neutralization IC50s of different bNAbs against several viral strains were compiled from the indicated studies (Malbec et al. [116]; Reh et al. [117], Gombos et al. [118], and Li et al. [119]). IC50s are color-coded with a heat map ranging from 0 (green) to 15 µg/ml and more (red). *x* not effective, no IC50 could be determined; *ND* not done; *Lab-a* lab-adapted

to maintain activity against cell-associated HIV-1 was patient-dependent and correlated with the neutralization breadth [111]. First generation neutralizing monoclonal antibodies, such as the anti-MPER 2F5 and 4E10, the anti-V3 antibody 257-D, and the anti-CD4bs b12 were also tested in cell–cell assays, but results were conflicting, and no clear pattern could be determined [112–114].

The development of second generation bNAbs allowed a more comprehensive examination of the role of antibodies during T cell-to-T cell transfer of HIV-1 (Fig. 2). The epitope targeted may influence the efficacy of a given antibody [115]. It has been shown that some CD4bs-directed antibodies were less potent neutralizers during cell-to-cell transmission than during cell-free transfer, with IC50s that were 10 times higher in intercellular systems [115]. Our laboratory tested the ability of 15 bNAbs targeting different Env epitopes to inhibit cell-to-cell transmission of both lab-adapted and Transmitted/Founder (T/F) HIV-1 strains [116]. We confirmed the relative neutralization resistance of cell-associated HIV-1. However, we identified bNAbs that were potent neutralizers of cell-associated virus in primary CD4$^+$ T cells and pDCs. The most active bNAbs were targeting the CD4bs (NIH45-46 and 3BNC60) or the glycan/V3 loop (10-1074 and PGT121). They significantly decreased the formation of clusters and syncytia between uninfected and infected T cells, and the transfer of viral material through the VS. The efficacy of bNAbs against cell-associated HIV-1 was also dependent on the viral strain studied, indicating that the antibody breadth may be different against virions and infected cells. Another study analyzed the activity of 16 bNAbs during cell-free and cell-to-cell transmission of 11 viral strains [117]. Again, the neutralizing activity of bNAbs was generally decreased in cell-to-cell assays. Some bNAbs maintained a high level of inhibition against various viral strains, but no single bNAb was potent for all strains tested [117]. Combinating bNAbs may overcome this problem. For instance, a combination of PG9 and VRC01 demonstrated improved ability to neutralize cell-associated HIV-1 compared to individual antibodies [118]. Recently, a study focused on the maximum neutralization capacity of bNAbs during cell-to-cell transmission rather than on the IC50 [119]. During cell-to-cell transmission of two T/F strains, most of the tested bNAbs failed to reach 100% of neutralization, even at high concentrations. This phenomenon was not

observed with two lab-adapted strains. This residual replication may allow the virus to keep spreading and may lead to the apparition of escape mutations. Whether the ability of primary HIV-1 isolates to spread by cell-to-cell transmission differs from lab-adapted strains, and how this may impair neutralization efficacy of bNAbs are still unresolved questions.

Antibodies interfere with HIV-1 cell-to-cell transmission through different mechanisms. For instance, b12 (a first generation anti-CD4bs antibody) inhibits the formation of the VS while 2F5 or 4E10 (anti-MPER) rather act later, by inhibiting viral fusion [114, 120]. Other bNAbs targeting the gp120, such as NIH45-46, 3BNC60, VRC01, 10-1074, or PGT121 also inhibit the formation of conjugates between infected and target CD4$^+$ T cells [116]. Antibody efficacy varies depending on their time of addition in the co-culture [120]. For instance, b12 impairs VS formation, but does not disrupt an existing one [120]. Therefore, depending on the epitopes, bNAbs may either impair formation of cell conjugates and VS, transfer of viral material to target cells, or fusion.

Inhibition of HIV-1 transfer from DCs and macrophages
HIV-1 transiting through a macrophage/T cell VS is inhibited by anti-gp120 bNAbs, but less sensitive to some anti-gp41 antibodies [68]. Early studies showed that neutralizing antibodies 2F5, 2G12 and b12 inhibited HIV-1 transfer from infected DCs to T cells without impairing the formation of the IS [121, 122]. The role of bNAbs on *trans*-infection is debated. 2F5-, 4E10- and 2G12-opsonized HIV-1 particles are captured more efficiently by DCs in a DC-SIGN-dependent manner, probably because DC-SIGN also binds IgG [123]. The particles recover their infectivity after internalization, probably due to antigen–antibody dissociation, leading to enhanced *trans*-infection. However, some bNAbs were also shown to inhibit infection or *trans*-infection from monocyte-derived or plasmacytoid dendritic cells to CD4$^+$ T cells and vice versa [116, 124, 125]. In another study, gp120-targeting antibodies (b12, VRC01, PG16 and 2G12) had a higher IC50 against DC-associated virus, whereas anti-MPER 4E10 and 2F5 maintained their potency during DC-to-T cell transmission [126].

Therefore, some bNAbs inhibit *trans*-infection and transmission from DCs or macrophages to lymphocytes. Discrepancies have been reported for the same

a Cell-free

Malbec et al (2013)

	Lab-adapted		Primary	
	NL4.3	NLAD8	WITO	SUMA
VRC01	0,2	0,3	ND	ND
NIH45-46	0,06	0,2	ND	ND
3BNC60	0,05	0,1	ND	ND
10-1074	x	0,1	ND	ND
PGT121	x	0,1	ND	ND
PG16	0,7	0,05	ND	ND
8ANC195	4	5,7	ND	ND
3BC176	0,7	>15	ND	ND
4E10	4,3	>15	ND	ND
10E8	0,1	1,1	ND	ND

Li et al (2017)

	Lab-adapted	Primary		
	NL4.3	JR-FL	RHPA	QH0692
VRC01	0,17	0,04	1,3	0,28
HJ16	0,02	x	0,004	0,56
2G12	0,1	0,3	x	2,24
PGT126	x	0,1	0,013	0,003
10-1074	x	0,01	0,021	0,02
PGT121	x	0,04	0,013	0,058
PG9	0,36	x	5,1	x
35O22	0,01	0,002	x	0,002
4E10	0,3	1	1,3	0,1
2F5	0,06	0,03	0,13	0,008

Gombos et al (2015)

	Lab-a	Primary		
	BAL	WITO	CH040	CH077
VRC01	0,055	0,13	0,49	0,27
CH101	x	0,13	x	0,33
PGT126	0,072	2,03	x	0,005
PG9	x	0,005	x	0,003
4E10	3,06	2,69	x	3,36
10E8	1,62	0,77	1,86	0,82

Reh et al (2015)

	Subtype A				Subtype B					Subtype C		
	Primary		Lab-adapted		Primary							
	BG505	BG505 N332	JR-FL	JR-CSF	SF162	DH123	PVO.4	REJO	THRO	ZM53	ZM109	ZM214
b12	x	x	0,007	0,009	0,008	0,035	x	4,484	0,041	x	x	0,017
VRC01	0,135	0,050	0,017	0,188	0,318	0,193	0,357	0,046	1,533	1,600	0,168	0,171
NIH45-46	0,014	0,003	0,007	0,033	0,026	0,060	x	0,003	0,259	x	x	0,040
PGV04	0,023	0,036	0,039	0,056	0,024	0,049	0,211	0,025	x	0,841	0,023	0,344
3BNC117	0,010	0,012	0,002	0,013	0,015	0,041	0,028	0,011	0,226	0,133	0,102	0,071
PGT121	0,257	0,006	0,049	0,044	0,002	0,003	0,161	33,10	x	0,005	x	0,368
PGT125	0,008	0,002	0,017	0,003	0,001	0,009	0,020	x	x	x	x	x
PGT128	1,928	0,002	0,164	0,019	0,026	0,184	0,047	x	x	x	x	x
PGT135	x	x	x	0,042	0,016	x	x	x	x	x	x	x
PGT145	0,034	0,004	x	0,001	x	0,006	0,167	0,000	0,007	1,832	0,104	x
PG9	0,045	0,016	x	0,007	x	0,181	x	0,015	x	0,092	0,437	x
PG16	0,021	0,007	x	0,000	x	2,128	x	0,105	5,065	0,010		x
2G12	x	0,467	0,411	0,889	0,436	x	0,880	x	x	x	x	x
2F5	0,310	0,015	0,103	0,040	0,228	1,239	x	0,034	10,77	x	x	x
10E8	0,035	0,014	0,020	0,016	0,017	0,073	0,308	0,010	0,019	0,343	0,035	0,093
4E10	0,215	0,125	0,444	0,651	1,872	1,405	x	0,201	0,090	2,687	0,145	x

b Cell-to-cell

Malbec et al (2013)

	Lab-adapted		Primary	
	NL4.3	NLAD8	WITO	SUMA
VRC01	7,2	12,1	14,3	x
NIH45-46	1,2	2,5	3,1	13,9
3BNC60	0,9	2,3	3,4	3,3
10-1074	x	1,6	1,8	1,9
PGT121	x	1,3	ND	ND
PG16	>15	0,5	0,05	0,3
8ANC195	x	x	x	3,7
3BC176	x	x	x	x
4E10	x	>15	ND	ND
10E8	6,7	>15	9,4	>15

Li et al (2017)

	Lab-adapted	Primary		
	NL4.3	JR-FL	RHPA	QH0692
VRC01	2,1	0,5	4,6	12,60
HJ16	0,9	x	0,17	34,80
2G12	3,6	0,7	x	83,00
PGT126	x	0,07	>25	0,30
10-1074	x	0,09	>25	0,14
PGT121	x	0,03	0,16	0,10
PG9	2,5	x	>50	x
35O22	0,07	1	x	6,90
4E10	5,9	9,2	146	7,40
2F5	4,5	1,4	9,5	2,80

Gombos et al (2015)

	Lab-a	Primary		
	BAL	WITO	CH040	CH077
VRC01	0,22	1,3	3,19	2,23
CH101	x	1,09	x	1,88
PGT126	0,18	3,16	x	1,34
PG9	x	0,071	x	0,35
4E10	3,1	3,74	x	0,62
10E8	1,23	1,67	0,82	2,29

Reh et al (2015)

	Subtype A				Subtype B					Subtype C		
	Primary		Lab-adapted		Primary							
	BG505	BG505 N332	JR-FL	JR-CSF	SF162	DH123	PVO.4	REJO	THRO	ZM53	ZM109	ZM214
b12	x	x	0,44	5,06	>1	>1	x	370,5	82,88	x	x	>30
VRC01	2,52	1,08	0,80	4,26	6,08	7,77	9,87	2,13	>100	31,28	2,66	>40
NIH45-46	0,63	0,38	0,25	0,57	0,70	0,88	x	0,10	29,91	x	x	3,34
PGV04	0,17	0,15	0,90	0,59	0,78	0,70	2,33	0,53	x	11,32	0,30	>10
3BNC117	0,45	0,28	0,08	0,36	0,84	1,06	0,94	0,40	53,37	3,60	0,67	>5
PGT121	1,73	0,28	1,09	0,96	0,20	0,08	2,91	45,86	x	0,11	x	>10
PGT125	0,19	0,11	0,34	0,08	0,13	0,32	0,42	x	x	x	x	x
PGT128	2,80	0,07	2,64	0,44	0,58	2,32	1,07	x	x	x	x	x
PGT135	x	x	x	0,44	0,31	x	x	x	x	x	x	x
PGT145	0,09	0,04	x	0,02	x	0,17	3,26	0,04	0,14	0,15	0,26	x
PG9	0,98	0,35	x	0,10	x	1,64	x	0,81	x	1,06	7,04	x
PG16	0,20	0,15	x	0,02	x	0,56	x	6,27	2,80	0,11	x	x
2G12	x	0,36	1,83	1,84	8,61	x	6,31	x	x	x	x	x
2F5	1,51	0,51	1,62	0,63	3,33	12,20	x	1,12	>100	x	x	x
10E8	0,34	0,29	0,24	0,41	0,46	2,18	2,89	0,20	0,57	0,23	0,34	0,82
4E10	5,81	2,61	8,46	2,99	16,62	62,63	x	2,67	8,97	2,39	6,38	x

0 µg/ml   >15 µg/ml

antibodies in different studies. These discrepant results likely depend on the DC subtype used, which may express different levels of molecules such as DC-SIGN, Siglec-1, or Env, at the surface or within intracellular compartments.

Potential explanations for the increased resistance of cell-associated HIV-1 to neutralization by bNAbs

Different non-mutually exclusive mechanisms may account for the increased resistance of cell-to-cell HIV-1 transmission to bNAbs. They include steric hindrance at the VS, the MOI associated to this mode of viral propagation, the accessibility and conformation of Env at the cell surface, and the stability of Env-Ab complexes at the cell surface.

Steric hindrance at the VS and in other cellular compartments

The VS involves a physical proximity of the membranes of donor and target T cells and may imply a low accessibility of bNAbs to the VS (Fig. 3a). However, some bNAbs like b12, NIH45-46 or 3BNC60 successfully accumulate at the VS between T cells [116, 120]. It will be of interest to determine whether access to the VS correlates with the inhibitory activity of each antibody. It is also possible that some antibodies bind to Env outside of the synapse, and will then be transported to the VS as a complex with their antigens. The virus may also be endocytosed after transmission through the VS [54], limiting the time frame of access of bNAbs. A llama antibody termed J3 is a potent neutralizer of cell-to-cell HIV-1 transmission [127]. The small size of the llama VHH compared to the human Fc may enable a better access to the VS. However, recombinant J3 with a human Fc display the same potency of neutralization against HIV-1 cell-to-cell transmission [127]. Thus, the size of the antibody does not seem to be a limiting factor in that case. The situation may be different in DCs or macrophages. A full-size 10E8 was less potent in these cells but 10E8 Fab, smaller in size, had more comparable neutralization IC50s during cell-free and cell-associated transmission [68]. This is consistent with the observation that bNAbs do not easily access virus contained within VCCs in macrophages [128]. This is also the case in DCs, where HIV-1 virions present in VCCs are protected from recognition by bNAbs, even if these compartments are connected to the extracellular milieu [89].

Thus, steric hindrance may impact neutralization of cell–cell transmission by some bNAbs and depends on the cell type and the antibody used. The most potent antibodies gain access to the VS and impair its function.

Cell-to-cell HIV-1 transmission is associated with higher MOIs

The VS leads to an elevated concentration of viral particles in the synaptic cleft, which most likely increases the MOI during cell-to-cell transmission [37, 56–60] (Fig. 3b). Increased amounts of virus would then require more antibody, thus increasing IC50s. However, with some antibodies, differences in IC50s are still observed when cell-free and cell-associated viral inputs are normalized [126]. With the most potent bNAbs, such as 10-1074 and 3BNC117, the IC50s remain low in coculture systems [116, 117, 119]. Thus, differences between cell-to-cell and cell-free modes of transmission are not only a matter of quantity of transferred virus.

Composition of cell-free particles and virions produced at the VS

Cell-free neutralization assays mostly use virus produced by transfection of 293T cells. Cell-to-cell assays generally rely on CD4 T cell lines or primary cells as the source of virus. Some HIV-1 strains are more susceptible to bNAbs when produced in 293T compared to primary cells [129]. This might be due to the content of cellular molecules in viral particles, as HIV-1 incorporates host membrane when budding. Thus, comparison between cell-free and cell-associated neutralization may be biased by the cell types in which the virus was produced. In addition, the composition of viral particles may vary at the VS (Fig. 3c). For example, HIV-1 virions can incorporate ICAM-1 that will increase infectivity, especially if the target cell expresses LFA-1 [130, 131]. ICAM-1-bearing virions are more resistant to neutralization by HIV-1-infected patients' sera or neutralizing anti-gp120 antibodies [132]. Given that adhesion molecules accumulate at the VS, they could be more incorporated in viral particles budding at this site. The lipid component of VS-budding virions may be also different, since synapses are known to be enriched in rafts, and this may also impact sensitivity to neutralizing antibodies. Even though technically challenging, a characterization of the cellular composition of virions produced at the VS will give insights into the mechanisms underlying the resistance of cell-to-cell transmission to some bNAbs.

Conformation and amount of Env at the cell surface and at the VS

The conformation and oligomerization states of Env are probably more heterogeneous at the plasma membrane than at the surface of virions, that contain a very limited number of Env trimers [133]. At the plasma membrane, a high amount of Env monomers and trimers, at different stages of maturation and glycosylation, are present.

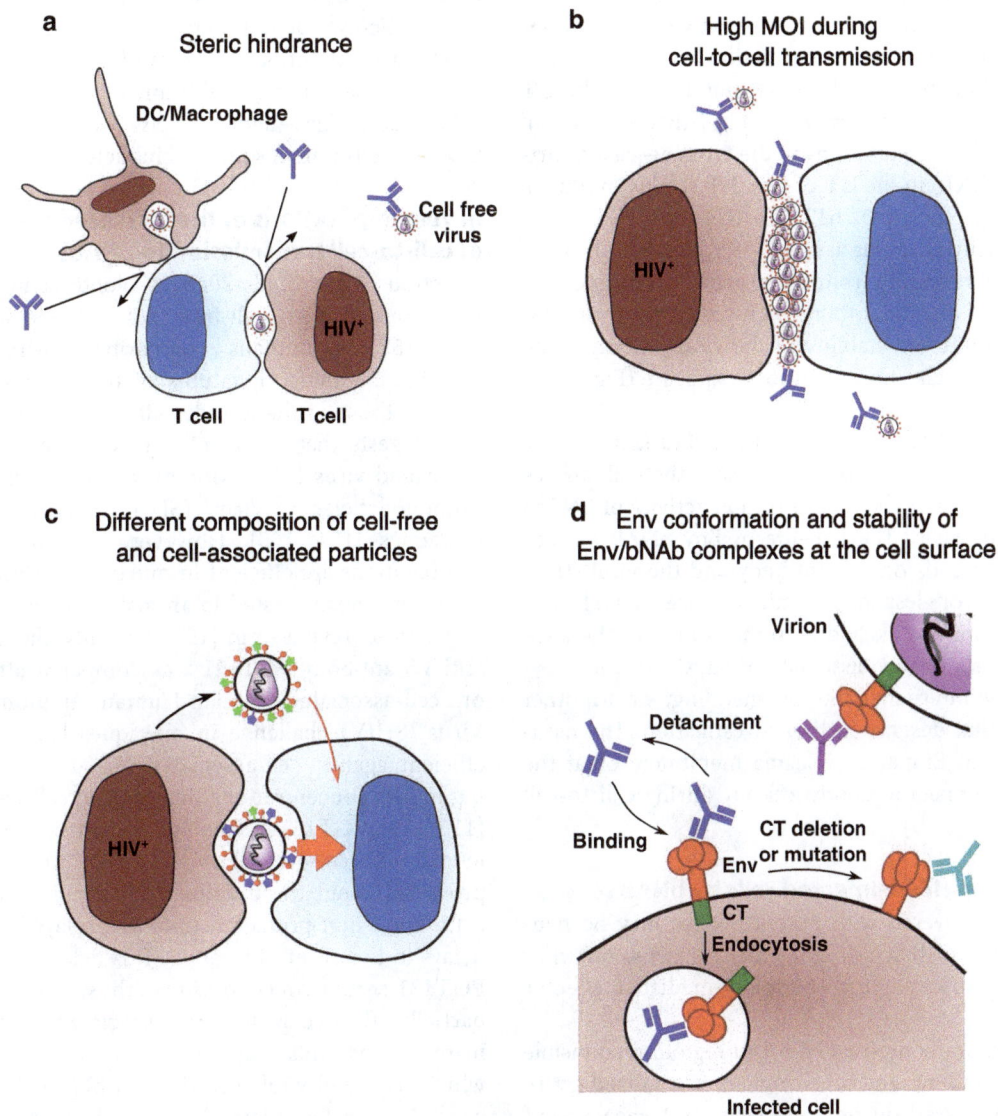

Fig. 3 Potential mechanisms explaining the increased resistance of cell-associated HIV-1 to bNAbs-mediated neutralization. **a** bNAbs may poorly access virions present at the VS because of the physical proximity of donor and target cell membranes. **b** VS-mediated HIV-1 is associated with high MOIs. **c** Viruses budding at the VS may incorporate cellular proteins differently than cell-free virions, possibly leading to different susceptibilities to bNAbs. **d** Env conformation and stability of Env-bNAb complexes at the cell surface. Env conformation may be different at the surface of cell-free virus and at the plasma membrane. The stability of Env-bNAb complexes at the cell surface depends on the antibody and the viral strain. Donor cells are in brown and uninfected cells in blue

Local variations at membrane subdomains, depending on the subcellular environment or the presence of lipids and cellular proteins, may also modify Env epitope exposure. These different dynamic parameters impact the accessibility of cell-surface Env to bNAbs. For example, the engagement of Env by CD4 exposes epitopes targeted by non-neutralizing antibodies (nnAbs) [134, 135]. Since the creation of the VS involves interaction of Env with CD4, the conformation of Env at the synapse may be different from that at other regions of the membrane. We also reported that some antibodies, such as 8ANC195, which recognizes a gp120/41 bridging epitope and neutralizes cell-free virions, does not efficiently bind to infected cells [17], confirming the existence of different conformations of Env on virions and cells.

Viral proteins may also modify epitope accessibility. Nef and Vpu modify the levels of Env at the cell surface [136, 137] and Nef decreases Env susceptibility to anti-MPER antibodies [138]. The Env cytoplasmic tail (CT) also regulates the exposure of Env epitopes, through mechanisms that deserve further characterization [139, 140]. A CT truncation increases sensitivity to neutralization during cell-to-cell transmission with little effect on cell-free infection [110]. Some mutations in the CT inhibit cell-free infection more strongly than cell-to-cell transmission [141]. Mutations in the tyrosine-based sorting signal (YXXL) in the CT of two T/F strains modulate neutralization efficacy of b12, 10-1074 and PGT126 in cell-to-cell neutralization assays [119]. This YXXL motif regulates Env recycling from the plasma membrane. The engagement of Env in recycling pathways not only modulates the amount and stability of the viral protein at the surface, but may also impact epitope exposure (Fig. 3d).

Stability of Env-bNAb complexes at the cell surface

The stability of Env-bNAb complexes at the cell surface most likely regulates the neutralization activity of bNAbs against donor cells. The half-life of Env-bNAb surface complexes depends on the antibody and the viral strain [17]. It varies from less than 30 min to more than 6 h [17]. These variations are likely due to the affinity of the antibody (association and dissociation rates), to antibody-induced Env internalization or shedding, or to other parameters that deserve further investigation. The natural recycling of Env at the plasma membrane or at the VS may also impact antibody efficacy during cell-to-cell transmission.

Elimination of HIV-1-infected cells by bNAbs

Infected cells covered with potent bNAbs may be neutralized in their ability to transmit the virus, but may also become susceptible to antibody-mediated effector functions.

Antibodies are composed of a Fab region, responsible for antigen binding, and a Fc domain, recognized by Fc receptors expressed on immune cells. FcR engagement subsequently triggers various immune effector mechanisms (for a review, see [142]). For example, NK cells recruited by bNAbs kill HIV-1-infected cells through Antibody-Dependent Cellular Cytotoxicity (ADCC) [17, 143, 144]. Other Fc-dependent mechanisms include antibody–dependent cellular phagocytosis (ADCP) and activation of the complement pathway (reviewed in [142]). ADCC is mediated by bNAbs and nnAbs, depending on Env epitope accessibility at the cell surface [135, 145]. bNAbs require Fc-mediated immunity for optimal efficacy in vivo [146–148]. In humanized mice, nnAbs clear HIV-infected cells and impose selective pressure on the virus, as observed by mutation in Env [149]. However, primary strains are often poorly susceptible to nnAbs-mediated ADCC in vitro [135, 150]. HIV-1 propagation in vivo is the result of a balance between the rate of viral transmission and the clearance of infected cells. Thus,

even if bNAbs do not totally neutralize viral cell-to-cell spread, Fc-mediated functions represent an additional mechanism of action of the antibodies against infected T cells. Whether these additional functions also impact DC/Macrophages-mediated cis- or trans-infection of CD4$^+$ T cells remains poorly characterized.

In vivo implications of the increased resistance of cell-to-cell transmission to bNAbs

Infectious body fluids such as blood, semen or breast milk contain both cell-free and cell-associated HIV-1 [151, 152]. In humans, comparing cell-free and cell-associated genetic signatures of the infecting partner's virus to those of the founder virus in the recipient partner suggests that some infections are initiated by cell-associated virus [153]. Moreover, cell-associated Simian Immunodeficiency Virus (SIV) initiates infection in macaques [154, 155]. However, even though bNAbs combinations are efficient in murine and simian models, they were mostly tested in animals challenged with cell-free HIV-1 (reviewed in [19]). Recently, the effect of the anti-V3 antibody PGT121 was compared after cell-free or cell-associated Simian-Human Immunodeficiency Virus (SHIV) challenge in macaques [156]. PGT121 is efficient against cell-associated HIV-1 in vitro, requiring higher concentrations than during cell-free infection [116, 119]. PGT121 infusion protected all 6 animals challenged with cell-free SHIV. However, the antibody only protected 3 out the 6 animals challenged with infected cells. The 3 non-protected animals displayed 1- to 7-week delays in the onset of viremia. This delay correlated with PGT121 serum concentrations. Thus, PGT121 was only partially effective against cell-associated SHIV challenge in macaques. This may be due to an "occult" infection which triggered viral spread when bNAbs levels waned, or to the transfer of latently infected cell that reactivated late after the challenge. These results highlight the need for high and sustained concentrations of antibodies to confer resistance to challenge with infected cells. In this macaque model, a high dose of cell-associated SHIV was used as a challenge. Humans probably receive a lower level of infectious challenge during natural contamination. Future trials of bNAbs will be of great interest to assess their prophylactic efficacy in humans.

Noteworthy, the main issue of using single bNAbs in vivo is the rapid occurrence of escape mutations [23–26]. Mathematical modelling suggested that escape mutations to bNAbs are more likely to happen during cell-to-cell transmission than during cell-free infection [117]. Again, current and future clinical trials using combination of bNAbs will be instrumental in determining whether this immunotherapy is counteracting the different modes of HIV-1 spread in humans.

Conclusion

HIV-1 cell-to-cell transfer has been extensively characterized in cell culture systems. In vivo experiments confirmed the contribution of this mechanism during viral spread. Conventional antiretroviral drugs efficiently inhibit cell-free and cell-associated viral transmission [157] but the impact of bNAbs on intercellular viral spread may be less marked. There are important mechanistic differences depending on antibodies, viral strains, and the nature of donor and recipient cells. The most potent bNAbs, that stably bind to infected cells and impair CD4/Env interaction or viral fusion, efficiently inhibit cell-to-cell transfer. These bNAbs display transient therapeutic efficacy in humans. In addition to neutralization, bNAbs trigger the destruction of infected cells. Future basic and clinical studies will help determining whether the targeting of infected cells by combinations of bNAbs with long half-lives and increased potency are a promising approach to the prevention, treatment, and possibly cure of HIV-1 infection.

Authors' contributions
All authors contributed to the writing of the manuscript. All authors read and approved the final manuscript.

Author details
[1] Virus and Immunity Unit, Department of Virology, Institut Pasteur, Paris, France. [2] CNRS-UMR3569, Paris, France. [3] Vaccine Research Institute, Créteil, France.

Acknowledgements
The authors thank the members of the Virus and Immunity Unit for helpful discussions.

Competing interests
The authors declare they have no competing interests.

Funding
Work in the Virus & Immunity unit is funded by Institut Pasteur, ANRS, Sidaction, the Vaccine Research Institute (ANR-10-LABX-77), the Labex IBEID (ANR-10-IHUB-0002, the "TIMTAMDEN" ANR-14-CE14-0029, the "CHIKV-Viro-Immuno" ANR-14-CE14-0015-01, L'Oréal Sponsorhip and the Gilead HIV cure program.

References
1. Barre-Sinoussi F, Chermann J, Rey F, Nugeyre M, Chamaret S, Gruest J, et al. Isolation of a T-lymphotropic retrovirus from a patient at risk for acquired immune deficiency syndrome (AIDS). Science. 1983;220:868–71.
2. Schiffner T, Sattentau QJ, Duncan CJA. Cell-to-cell spread of HIV-1 and evasion of neutralizing antibodies. Vaccine. 2013;31:5789–97.
3. Casartelli N. HIV-1 cell-to-cell transmission and antiviral strategies: an overview. Curr Drug Targets. 2016;17:65–75.
4. Bracq L, Xie M, Benichou S, Bouchet J. Mechanisms for cell-to-cell transmission of HIV-1. Front Immunol. 2018. 9:260.
5. Jolly C, Kashefi K, Hollinshead M, Sattentau QJ. HIV-1 cell to cell transfer across an Env-induced, actin-dependent synapse. J Exp Med. 2004;199:283–93.
6. Monel B, Beaumont E, Vendrame D, Schwartz O, Brand D, Mammano F. HIV cell-to-cell transmission requires the production of infectious virus particles and does not proceed through Env-mediated fusion pores. J Virol. 2012;86:3924–33.
7. Tomaras GD, Yates NL, Liu P, Qin L, Fouda GG, Chavez LL, et al. Initial B-cell responses to transmitted human immunodeficiency virus type 1: virion-binding immunoglobulin M (IgM) and IgG antibodies followed by plasma anti-gp41 antibodies with ineffective control of initial viremia. J Virol. 2008;82:12449–63.
8. Frost SDW, Wrin T, Smith DM, Pond SLK, Liu Y, Paxinos E, et al. Neutralizing antibody responses drive the evolution of human immunodeficiency virus type 1 envelope during recent HIV infection. Proc Natl Acad Sci. 2005;102:18514–9.
9. Wei X, Decker JM, Wang S, Hui H, Kappes JC, Wu X, et al. Antibody neutralization and escape by HIV-1. Nature. 2003;422:307–12.
10. Deeks SG, Schweighardt B, Wrin T, Galovich J, Hoh R, Sinclair E, et al. Neutralizing antibody responses against autologous and heterologous viruses in acute versus chronic human immunodeficiency virus (HIV) infection: evidence for a constraint on the ability of HIV to completely evade neutralizing antibody responses. J Virol. 2006;80:6155–64.
11. Simek MD, Rida W, Priddy FH, Pung P, Carrow E, Laufer DS, et al. Human immunodeficiency virus type 1 elite neutralizers: individuals with broad and potent neutralizing activity identified by using a high-throughput neutralization assay together with an analytical selection algorithm. J Virol. 2009;83:7337–48.
12. McCoy LE, Burton DR. Identification and specificity of broadly neutralizing antibodies against HIV. Immunol Rev. 2017;275:11–20.
13. Mouquet H. Antibody B cell responses in HIV-1 infection. Trends Immunol. 2014;35:549–61.
14. Kong R, Xu K, Zhou T, Acharya P, Lemmin T, Liu K, et al. Fusion peptide of HIV-1 as a site of vulnerability to neutralizing antibody. Science. 2016;352:828–33.
15. van Gils MJ, van den Kerkhof TLGM, Ozorowski G, Cottrell CA, Sok D, Pauthner M, et al. An HIV-1 antibody from an elite neutralizer implicates the fusion peptide as a site of vulnerability. Nat Microbiol. 2016;2:16199.
16. Xu K, Acharya P, Kong R, Cheng C, Chuang G-Y, Liu K, et al. Epitope-based vaccine design yields fusion peptide-directed antibodies that neutralize diverse strains of HIV-1. Nat Med. 2018;24:857–67.
17. Bruel T, Guivel-Benhassine F, Amraoui S, Malbec M, Richard L, Bourdic K, et al. Elimination of HIV-1-infected cells by broadly neutralizing antibodies. Nat Commun. 2016;7:10844.
18. Shingai M, Donau OK, Plishka RJ, Buckler-White A, Mascola JR, Nabel GJ, et al. Passive transfer of modest titers of potent and broadly neutralizing anti-HIV monoclonal antibodies block SHIV infection in macaques. J Exp Med. 2014;211:2061–74.
19. Nishimura Y, Martin MA. Of mice, macaques, and men: broadly neutralizing antibody immunotherapy for HIV-1. Cell Host Microbe. 2017;22:207–16.
20. Lu C-L, Murakowski DK, Bournazos S, Schoofs T, Sarkar D, Halper-Stromberg A, et al. Enhanced clearance of HIV-1-infected cells by broadly neutralizing antibodies against HIV-1 in vivo. Science. 2016;352:1001–4.
21. Nishimura Y, Gautam R, Chun T-W, Sadjadpour R, Foulds KE, Shingai M, et al. Early antibody therapy can induce long-lasting immunity to SHIV. Nature. 2017;543:559–63.
22. Cohen YZ, Caskey M. Broadly neutralizing antibodies for treatment and prevention of HIV-1 infection. Curr Opin HIV AIDS. 2018;13:366–737.

23. Caskey M, Klein F, Lorenzi JCC, Seaman MS, West AP, Buckley N, et al. Viraemia suppressed in HIV-1-infected humans by broadly neutralizing antibody 3BNC117. Nature. 2015;522:487–91.

24. Lynch RM, Boritz E, Coates EE, DeZure A, Madden P, Costner P, et al. Virologic effects of broadly neutralizing antibody VRC01 administration during chronic HIV-1 infection. Sci Transl Med. 2015;2015:319ra206–319ra206.

25. Caskey M, Schoofs T, Gruell H, Settler A, Karagounis T, Kreider EF, et al. Antibody 10-1074 suppresses viremia in HIV-1-infected individuals. Nat Med. 2017;23:185–91.

26. Scheid JF, Horwitz JA, Bar-On Y, Kreider EF, Lu C-L, Lorenzi JCC, et al. HIV-1 antibody 3BNC117 suppresses viral rebound in humans during treatment interruption. Nature. 2016;535:556–60.

27. Schoofs T, Klein F, Braunschweig M, Kreider EF, Feldmann A, Nogueira L, et al. HIV-1 therapy with monoclonal antibody 3BNC117 elicits host immune responses against HIV-1. Science. 2016;352:997–1001.

28. Pearce-Pratt R, Phillips DM. Studies of adhesion of lymphocytic cells: implications for sexual transmission of human immunodeficiency virus1. Biol Reprod. 1993;48:431–45.

29. Pearce-Pratt R, Malamud D, Phillips DM. Role of the cytoskeleton in cell-to-cell transmission of human immunodeficiency virus. J Virol. 1994;68:2898–905.

30. Fais S, Capobianchi MR, Abbate I, Castilletti C, Gentile M, Cordiali Fei P, et al. Unidirectional budding of HIV-1 at the site of cell-to-cell contact is associated with co-polarization of intercellular adhesion molecules and HIV-1 viral matrix protein. AIDS. 1995;9:329–35.

31. Igakura T, Stinchcombe JC, Goon PKC, Taylor GP, Weber JN, Griffiths GM, et al. Spread of HTLV-I between lymphocytes by virus-induced polarization of the cytoskeleton. Science. 2003;299:1713–6.

32. Vasiliver-Shamis G, Dustin ML, Hioe CE. HIV-1 virological synapse is not simply a copycat of the immunological synapse. Viruses. 2010;2:1239–60.

33. Rudnicka D, Feldmann J, Porrot F, Wietgrefe S, Guadagnini S, Prevost M-C, et al. Simultaneous cell-to-cell transmission of human immunodeficiency virus to multiple targets through polysynapses. J Virol. 2009;83:6234–46.

34. Roy NH, Chan J, Lambele M, Thali M. Clustering and mobility of HIV-1 Env at viral assembly sites predict its propensity to induce cell-cell fusion. J Virol. 2013;87:7516–25.

35. Weng J, Krementsov DN, Khurana S, Roy NH, Thali M. Formation of syncytia is repressed by tetraspanins in human immunodeficiency virus type 1-producing cells. J Virol. 2009;83:7467–74.

36. Roy NH, Lambele M, Chan J, Symeonides M, Thali M. Ezrin is a component of the HIV-1 virological presynapse and contributes to the inhibition of cell-cell fusion. J Virol. 2014;88:7645–58.

37. Blanco J, Bosch B, Fernández-Figueras MT, Barretina J, Clotet B, Esté JA. High level of coreceptor-independent HIV transfer induced by contacts between primary CD4 T cells. J Biol Chem. 2004;279:51305–14.

38. Hubner W, McNerney GP, Chen P, Dale BM, Gordon RE, Chuang FYS, et al. Quantitative 3D video microscopy of HIV transfer across T cell virological synapses. Science. 2009;323:1743–7.

39. Jolly C, Mitar I, Sattentau QJ. Adhesion molecule interactions facilitate human immunodeficiency virus type 1-induced virological synapse formation between T cells. J Virol. 2007;81:13916–21.

40. Puigdomenech I, Massanella M, Izquierdo-Useros N, Ruiz-Hernandez R, Curriu M, Bofill M, et al. HIV transfer between CD4 T cells does not require LFA-1 binding to ICAM-1 and is governed by the interaction of HIV envelope glycoprotein with CD4. Retrovirology. 2008;5:32.

41. Jolly C, Mitar I, Sattentau QJ. Requirement for an intact T-cell actin and tubulin cytoskeleton for efficient assembly and spread of human immunodeficiency virus type 1. J Virol. 2007;81:5547–60.

42. Haller C, Tibroni N, Rudolph JM, Grosse R, Fackler OT. Nef does not inhibit F-actin remodelling and HIV-1 cell–cell transmission at the T lymphocyte virological synapse. Eur J Cell Biol. 2011;90:913–21.

43. Sol-Foulon N, Sourisseau M, Porrot F, Thoulouze M-I, Trouillet C, Nobile C, et al. ZAP-70 kinase regulates HIV cell-to-cell spread and virological synapse formation. EMBO J. 2007;26:516–26.

44. Jolly C, Welsch S, Michor S, Sattentau QJ. The regulated secretory pathway in CD4+T cells contributes to human immunodeficiency virus type-1 cell-to-cell spread at the virological synapse. PLoS Pathog. 2011;7:e1002226.

45. Jolly C, Sattentau QJ. Human immunodeficiency virus type 1 virological synapse formation in T cells requires lipid raft integrity. J Virol. 2005;79:12088–94.

46. Malbec M, Sourisseau M, Guivel-Benhassine F, Porrot F, Blanchet F, Schwartz O, et al. HIV-1 Nef promotes the localization of Gag to the cell membrane and facilitates viral cell-to-cell transfer. Retrovirology. 2013;10:80.

47. Casartelli N, Sourisseau M, Feldmann J, Guivel-Benhassine F, Mallet A, Marcelin A-G, et al. Tetherin restricts productive HIV-1 cell-to-cell transmission. PLoS Pathog. 2010;6:e1000955.

48. Kuhl BD, Sloan RD, Donahue DA, Bar-Magen T, Liang C, Wainberg MA. Tetherin restricts direct cell-to-cell infection of HIV-1. Retrovirology. 2010;7:115.

49. Jolly C, Booth NJ, Neil SJD. Cell-cell spread of human immunodeficiency virus type 1 overcomes tetherin/BST-2-mediated restriction in T cells. J Virol. 2010;84:12185–99.

50. Compton AA, Bruel T, Porrot F, Mallet A, Sachse M, Euvrard M, et al. IFITM proteins incorporated into HIV-1 virions impair viral fusion and spread. Cell Host Microbe. 2014;16:736–47.

51. Tartour K, Appourchaux R, Gaillard J, Nguyen X-N, Durand S, Turpin J, et al. IFITM proteins are incorporated onto HIV-1 virion particles and negatively imprint their infectivity. Retrovirology. 2014;11:103.

52. Bosch B, Grigorov B, Senserrich J, Clotet B, Darlix J, Muriaux D, et al. A clathrin–dynamin-dependent endocytic pathway for the uptake of HIV-1 by direct T cell–T cell transmission. Antiviral Res. 2008;80:185–93.

53. Sloan RD, Kuhl BD, Mesplede T, Munch J, Donahue DA, Wainberg MA. Productive entry of HIV-1 during cell-to-cell transmission via dynamin-dependent endocytosis. J Virol. 2013;87:8110–23.

54. Dale BM, McNerney GP, Thompson DL, Hubner W, de los Reyes K, Chuang FYS, et al. Cell-to-cell transfer of HIV-1 via virological synapses leads to endosomal viral entry maturation that activates viral membrane fusion. Cell Host Microbe. 2011;10:551–62.

55. Herold N, Anders-Osswein M, Glass B, Eckhardt M, Muller B, Krausslich H-G. HIV-1 entry in SupT1-R5, CEM-ss, and primary CD4+T cells occurs at the plasma membrane and does not require endocytosis. J Virol. 2014;88:13956–70.

56. Sourisseau M, Sol-Foulon N, Porrot F, Blanchet F, Schwartz O. Inefficient human immunodeficiency virus replication in mobile lymphocytes. J Virol. 2007;81:1000–12.

57. Chen P, Hubner W, Spinelli MA, Chen BK. Predominant mode of human immunodeficiency virus transfer between T cells is mediated by sustained Env-dependent neutralization-resistant virological synapses. J Virol. 2007;81:12582–95.

58. Del Portillo A, Tripodi J, Najfeld V, Wodarz D, Levy DN, Chen BK. Multiploid inheritance of HIV-1 during cell-to-cell infection. J Virol. 2011;85:7169–76.

59. Russell RA, Martin N, Mitar I, Jones E, Sattentau QJ. Multiple proviral integration events after virological synapse-mediated HIV-1 spread. Virology. 2013;443:143–9.

60. Boullé M, Müller TG, Dähling S, Ganga Y, Jackson L, Mahamed D, et al. HIV cell-to-cell spread results in earlier onset of viral gene expression by multiple infections per cell. PLoS Pathog. 2016;12:e1005964.

61. Sewald X, Gonzalez DG, Haberman AM, Mothes W. In vivo imaging of virological synapses. Nat Commun. 2012;3:1320.

62. Murooka TT, Deruaz M, Marangoni F, Vrbanac VD, Seung E, von Andrian UH, et al. HIV-infected T cells are migratory vehicles for viral dissemination. Nature. 2012;490:283–7.

63. Compton AA, Schwartz O. They might be giants: does syncytium formation sink or spread HIV infection? PLoS Pathog. 2017;13:e1006099.

64. Ladinsky MS, Kieffer C, Olson G, Deruaz M, Vrbanac V, Tager AM, et al. Electron tomography of HIV-1 infection in gut-associated lymphoid tissue. PLoS Pathog. 2014;10:e1003899.

65. Law KM, Komarova NL, Yewdall AW, Lee RK, Herrera OL, Wodarz D, et al. In vivo HIV-1 cell-to-cell transmission promotes multicopy micro-compartmentalized infection. Cell Rep. 2016;15:2771–83.

66. Gousset K, Ablan SD, Coren LV, Ono A, Soheilian F, Nagashima K, et al. Real-time visualization of HIV-1 GAG trafficking in infected macrophages. PLoS Pathog. 2008;4:e1000015.

67. Groot F, Welsch S, Sattentau QJ. Efficient HIV-1 transmission from macrophages to T cells across transient virological synapses. Blood. 2008;111:4660–3.

68. Duncan CJA, Williams JP, Schiffner T, Gartner K, Ochsenbauer C, Kappes J, et al. High-multiplicity HIV-1 infection and neutralizing antibody evasion mediated by the macrophage-T cell virological synapse. J Virol. 2014;88:2025–34.

69. Wu L, KewalRamani VN. Dendritic-cell interactions with HIV: infection and viral dissemination. Nat Rev Immunol. 2006;6:859–68.

70. Laguette N, Sobhian B, Casartelli N, Ringeard M, Chable-Bessia C, Ségéral E, et al. SAMHD1 is the dendritic- and myeloid-cell-specific HIV-1 restriction factor counteracted by Vpx. Nature. 2011;474:654–7.

71. Goldstone DC, Ennis-Adeniran V, Hedden JJ, Groom HCT, Rice GI, Christodoulou E, et al. HIV-1 restriction factor SAMHD1 is a deoxynucleoside triphosphate triphosphohydrolase. Nature. 2011;480:379–82.

72. St Gelais C, de Silva S, Amie SM, Coleman CM, Hoy H, Hollenbaugh JA, et al. SAMHD1 restricts HIV-1 infection in dendritic cells (DCs) by dNTP depletion, but its expression in DCs and primary CD4 + T-lymphocytes cannot be upregulated by interferons. Retrovirology. 2012;9:105.

73. Manel N, Hogstad B, Wang Y, Levy DE, Unutmaz D, Littman DR. A cryptic sensor for HIV-1 activates antiviral innate immunity in dendritic cells. Nature. 2010;467:214–7.

74. Luban J. Innate immune sensing of HIV by dendritic cells. Cell Host Microbe. 2012;12:408–18.

75. Ayinde D, Bruel T, Cardinaud S, Porrot F, Prado JG, Moris A, et al. SAMHD1 limits HIV-1 antigen presentation by monocyte-derived dendritic cells. J Virol. 2015;89:6994–7006.

76. Lee B, Sharron M, Montaner LJ, Weissman D, Doms RW. Quantification of CD4, CCR5, and CXCR4 levels on lymphocyte subsets, dendritic cells, and differentially conditioned monocyte-derived macrophages. Proc Natl Acad Sci. 1999;96:5215–20.

77. Chauveau L, Donahue DA, Monel B, Porrot F, Bruel T, Richard L, et al. HIV fusion in dendritic cells occurs mainly at the surface and is limited by low CD4 levels. J Virol. 2017;91:e01248–17.

78. Pelchen-Matthews A, Kramer B, Marsh M. Infectious HIV-1 assembles in late endosomes in primary macrophages. J Cell Biol. 2003;162:443–55.

79. Deneka M, Pelchen-Matthews A, Byland R, Ruiz-Mateos E, Marsh M. In macrophages, HIV-1 assembles into an intracellular plasma membrane domain containing the tetraspanins CD81, CD9, and CD53. J Cell Biol. 2007;177:329–41.

80. Gaudin R, Berre S, Cunha de Alencar B, Decalf J, Schindler M, Gobert F-X, et al. Dynamics of HIV-containing compartments in macrophages reveal sequestration of virions and transient surface connections. PLoS ONE. 2013;8:e69450.

81. Cameron PU, Freudenthal PS, Barker JM, Gezelter S, Inaba K, Steinman RM. Dendritic cells exposed to human immunodeficiency virus type-1 transmit a vigorous cytopathic infection to CD4 + T cells. Science. 1992;257:383–7.

82. Hladik F, McElrath MJ. Setting the stage: host invasion by HIV. Nat Rev Immunol. 2008;8:447–57.

83. Geijtenbeek TB, Kwon DS, Torensma R, van Vliet SJ, van Duijnhoven GC, Middel J, et al. DC-SIGN, a dendritic cell-specific HIV-1-binding protein that enhances trans-infection of T cells. Cell. 2000;100:587–94.

84. Arrighi J-F, Pion M, Garcia E, Escola J-M, van Kooyk Y, Geijtenbeek TB, et al. DC-SIGN–mediated infectious synapse formation enhances X4 HIV-1 transmission from dendritic cells to T cells. J Exp Med. 2004;200:1279–88.

85. Garcia E, Pion M, Pelchen-Matthews A, Collinson L, Arrighi J-F, Blot G, et al. HIV-1 trafficking to the dendritic cell-T-cell infectious synapse uses a pathway of tetraspanin sorting to the immunological synapse: HIV-1 localization in human dendritic cells. Traffic. 2005;6:488–501.

86. Nobile C, Petit C, Moris A, Skrabal K, Abastado J-P, Mammano F, et al. Covert human immunodeficiency virus replication in dendritic cells and in DC-SIGN-expressing cells promotes long-term transmission to lymphocytes. J Virol. 2005;79:5386–99.

87. Izquierdo-Useros N, Lorizate M, Puertas MC, Rodriguez-Plata MT, Zangger N, Erikson E, et al. Siglec-1 is a novel dendritic cell receptor that mediates HIV-1 trans-infection through recognition of viral membrane gangliosides. PLoS Biol. 2012;10:e1001448.

88. Puryear WB, Akiyama H, Geer SD, Ramirez NP, Yu X, Reinhard BM, et al. Interferon-inducible mechanism of dendritic cell-mediated HIV-1 dissemination is dependent on siglec-1/CD169. PLoS Pathog. 2013;9:e1003291.

89. Akiyama H, Ramirez N-GP, Gudheti MV, Gummuluru S. CD169-mediated trafficking of HIV to plasma membrane invaginations in dendritic cells attenuates efficacy of anti-gp120 broadly neutralizing antibodies. PLoS Pathog. 2015;11:e1004751.

90. Hammonds JE, Beeman N, Ding L, Takushi S, Francis AC, Wang J-J, et al. Siglec-1 initiates formation of the virus-containing compartment and enhances macrophage-to-T cell transmission of HIV-1. PLoS Pathog. 2017;13:e1006181.

91. Rodriguez-Plata MT, Puigdomènech I, Izquierdo-Useros N, Puertas MC, Carrillo J, Erkizia I, et al. The infectious synapse formed between mature dendritic cells and CD4 + T cells is independent of the presence of the HIV-1 envelope glycoprotein. Retrovirology. 2013;10:42.

92. McDonald D, Wu L, Bohks SM, KewalRamani VN, Unutmaz D, Hope TJ. Recruitment of HIV and its receptors to dendritic cell-T cell junctions. Science. 2003;300:1295–7.

93. Ménager MM, Littman DR. Actin Dynamics regulates dendritic cell-mediated transfer of HIV-1 to T cells. Cell. 2016;164:695–709.

94. Wiley RD, Gummuluru S. Immature dendritic cell-derived exosomes can mediate HIV-1 trans infection. Proc Natl Acad Sci. 2006;103:738–43.

95. Villani A-C, Satija R, Reynolds G, Sarkizova S, Shekhar K, Fletcher J, et al. Single-cell RNA-seq reveals new types of human blood dendritic cells, monocytes, and progenitors. Science. 2017;356:eaah4573.

96. See P, Dutertre C-A, Chen J, Günther P, McGovern N, Irac SE, et al. Mapping the human DC lineage through the integration of high-dimensional techniques. Science. 2017;356:eaag3009.

97. Silvin A, Yu CI, Lahaye X, Imperatore F, Brault J-B, Cardinaud S, et al. Constitutive resistance to viral infection in human CD141+ dendritic cells. Sci Immunol. 2017;2:eaai8071.

98. Sowinski S, Jolly C, Berninghausen O, Purbhoo MA, Chauveau A, Köhler K, et al. Membrane nanotubes physically connect T cells over long distances presenting a novel route for HIV-1 transmission. Nat Cell Biol. 2008;10:211–9.

99. Eugenin EA, Gaskill PJ, Berman JW. Tunneling nanotubes (TNT) are induced by HIV-infection of macrophages: a potential mechanism for intercellular HIV trafficking. Cell Immunol. 2009;254:142–8.

100. Hashimoto M, Bhuyan F, Hiyoshi M, Noyori O, Nasser H, Miyazaki M, et al. Potential role of the formation of tunneling nanotubes in HIV-1 spread in macrophages. J Immunol. 2016;196:1832–41.

101. Kadiu I, Gendelman HE. Macrophage bridging conduit trafficking of HIV-1 through the endoplasmic reticulum and Golgi network. J Proteome Res. 2011;10:3225–38.

102. Kadiu I, Gendelman HE. Human immunodeficiency virus type 1 endocytic trafficking through macrophage bridging conduits facilitates spread of infection. J Neuroimmune Pharmacol. 2011;6:658–75.

103. Nikolic DS, Lehmann M, Felts R, Garcia E, Blanchet FP, Subramaniam S, et al. HIV-1 activates Cdc42 and induces membrane extensions in immature dendritic cells to facilitate cell-to-cell virus propagation. Blood. 2011;118:4841–52.

104. Aggarwal A, Iemma TL, Shih I, Newsome TP, McAllery S, Cunningham AL, et al. Mobilization of HIV spread by diaphanous 2 dependent filopodia in infected dendritic cells. PLoS Pathog. 2012;8:e1002762.

105. Baxter AE, Russell RA, Duncan CJA, Moore MD, Willberg CB, Pablos JL, et al. Macrophage infection via selective capture of HIV-1-infected CD4 + T cells. Cell Host Microbe. 2014;16:711–21.

106. Bracq L, Xie M, Lambelé M, Vu L-T, Matz J, Schmitt A, et al. T cell-macrophage fusion triggers multinucleated giant cell formation for HIV-1 spreading. J Virol. 2017;91:e01237–17.

107. Alfsen A, Yu H, Magérus-Chatinet A, Schmitt A, Bomsel M. HIV-1-infected blood mononuclear cells form an integrin- and agrin-dependent viral synapse to induce efficient HIV-1 transcytosis across epithelial cell monolayer. MBoC. 2005;16:4267–79.

108. Real F, Sennepin A, Ganor Y, Schmitt A, Bomsel M. Live imaging of HIV-1 transfer across T cell virological synapse to epithelial cells that promotes stromal macrophage infection. Cell Rep. 2018;23:1794–805.

109. Gupta P, Balachandran R, Ho M, Enrico A, Rinaldo C. Cell-to-cell transmission of human immunodeficiency virus type 1 in the presence of azidothymidine and neutralizing antibody. J Virol. 1989;63:2361–5.

110. Durham ND, Yewdall AW, Chen P, Lee R, Zony C, Robinson JE, et al. Neutralization resistance of virological synapse-mediated HIV-1 infection is regulated by the gp41 cytoplasmic tail. J Virol. 2012;86:7484–95.

111. Sánchez-Palomino S, Massanella M, Carrillo J, García A, García F, González N, et al. A cell-to-cell HIV transfer assay identifies humoral responses with broad neutralization activity. Vaccine. 2011;29:5250–9.

112. Purtscher M, Trkola A, Gruber G, Buchacher A, Predl R, Steindl F, et al. A broadly neutralizing human monoclonal antibody against gp41 of human immunodeficiency virus type 1. AIDS Res Hum Retroviruses. 1994;10:1651–8.

113. Pantaleo G, Demarest JF, Vaccarezza M, Graziosi C, Bansal GP, Koenig S, et al. Effect of anti-V3 antibodies on cell-free and cell-to-cell human immunodeficiency virus transmission. Eur J Immunol. 1995;25:226–31.

114. Massanella M, Puigdomènech I, Cabrera C, Fernandez-Figueras MT, Aucher A, Gaibelet G, et al. Antigp41 antibodies fail to block early events of virological synapses but inhibit HIV spread between T cells. AIDS. 2009;23:183–8.

115. Abela IA, Berlinger L, Schanz M, Reynell L, Günthard HF, Rusert P, et al. Cell-cell transmission enables HIV-1 to evade inhibition by potent CD4bs directed antibodies. PLoS Pathog. 2012;8:e1002634.

116. Malbec M, Porrot F, Rua R, Horwitz J, Klein F, Halper-Stromberg A, et al. Broadly neutralizing antibodies that inhibit HIV-1 cell to cell transmission. J Exp Med. 2013;210:2813–21.

117. Reh L, Magnus C, Schanz M, Weber J, Uhr T, Rusert P, et al. Capacity of broadly neutralizing antibodies to inhibit HIV-1 cell-cell transmission is strain- and epitope-dependent. PLoS Pathog. 2015;11:e1004966.

118. Gombos RB, Kolodkin-Gal D, Eslamizar L, Owuor JO, Mazzola E, Gonzalez AM, et al. Inhibitory effect of individual or combinations of broadly neutralizing antibodies and antiviral reagents against cell-free and cell-to-cell HIV-1 transmission. J Virol. 2015;89:7813–28.

119. Li H, Zony C, Chen P, Chen BK. Reduced potency and incomplete neutralization of broadly neutralizing antibodies against cell-to-cell transmission of HIV-1 with transmitted founder Envs. J Virol. 2017;91:e02425–16.

120. Martin N, Welsch S, Jolly C, Briggs JAG, Vaux D, Sattentau QJ. Virological synapse-mediated spread of human immunodeficiency virus type 1 between T cells is sensitive to entry inhibition. J Virol. 2010;84:3516–27.

121. Frankel SS, Steinman RM, Michael NL, Kim SR, Bhardwaj N, Pope M, et al. Neutralizing monoclonal antibodies block human immunodeficiency virus type 1 infection of dendritic cells and transmission to T cells. J Virol. 1998;72:9788–94.

122. Ganesh L, Leung K, Lore K, Levin R, Panet A, Schwartz O, et al. Infection of specific dendritic cells by CCR5-tropic human immunodeficiency virus type 1 promotes cell-mediated transmission of virus resistant to broadly neutralizing antibodies. J Virol. 2004;78:11980–7.

123. van Montfort T, Nabatov AA, Geijtenbeek TBH, Pollakis G, Paxton WA. Efficient capture of antibody neutralized HIV-1 by cells expressing DC-SIGN and transfer to CD4 + T lymphocytes. J Immunol. 2007;178:3177–85.

124. Su B, Xu K, Lederle A, Peressin M, Biedma ME, Laumond G, et al. Neutralizing antibodies inhibit HIV-1 transfer from primary dendritic cells to autologous CD4 T lymphocytes. Blood. 2012;120:3708–17.

125. Su B, Lederle A, Laumond G, Ducloy C, Schmidt S, Decoville T, et al. Broadly neutralizing antibody VRC01 prevents HIV-1 transmission from plasmacytoid dendritic cells to CD4 T lymphocytes. J Virol. 2014;88:10975–81.

126. Sagar M, Akiyama H, Etemad B, Ramirez N, Freitas I, Gummuluru S. Transmembrane domain membrane proximal external region but not surface unit-directed broadly neutralizing HIV-1 antibodies can restrict dendritic cell-mediated HIV-1 trans-infection. J Infect Dis. 2012;205:1248–57.

127. McCoy LE, Groppelli E, Blanchetot C, de Haard H, Verrips T, Rutten L, et al. Neutralisation of HIV-1 cell-cell spread by human and llama antibodies. Retrovirology. 2014;11:83.

128. Koppensteiner H, Banning C, Schneider C, Hohenberg H, Schindler M. Macrophage internal HIV-1 is protected from neutralizing antibodies. J Virol. 2012;86:2826–36.

129. Cohen YZ, Lorenzi JCC, Seaman MS, Nogueira L, Schoofs T, Krassnig L, et al. Neutralizing activity of broadly neutralizing anti-HIV-1 antibodies against clade B clinical isolates produced in peripheral blood mononuclear cells. J Virol. 2017;92:e01883–17.

130. Fortin JF, Cantin R, Lamontagne G, Tremblay M. Host-derived ICAM-1 glycoproteins incorporated on human immunodeficiency virus type 1 are biologically active and enhance viral infectivity. J Virol. 1997;71:3588–96.

131. Fortin J-F, Cantin R, Tremblay MJ. T cells expressing activated LFA-1 are more susceptible to infection with human immunodeficiency virus type 1 particles bearing host-encoded ICAM-1. J Virol. 1998;72:2105–12.

132. Fortin J-F, Cantin R, Bergeron MG, Tremblay MJ. Interaction between virion-bound host intercellular adhesion molecule-1 and the high-affinity state of lymphocyte function-associated antigen-1 on target cells renders R5 and X4 isolates of human immunodeficiency virus type 1 more refractory to neutralization. Virology. 2000;268:493–503.

133. Chojnacki J, Staudt T, Glass B, Bingen P, Engelhardt J, Anders M, et al. Maturation-dependent HIV-1 surface protein redistribution revealed by fluorescence nanoscopy. Science. 2012;338:524–8.

134. Veillette M, Desormeaux A, Medjahed H, Gharsallah N-E, Coutu M, Baalwa J, et al. Interaction with cellular CD4 exposes HIV-1 envelope epitopes targeted by antibody-dependent cell-mediated cytotoxicity. J Virol. 2014;88:2633–44.

135. Bruel T, Guivel-Benhassine F, Lorin V, Lortat-Jacob H, Baleux F, Bourdic K, et al. Lack of ADCC breadth of human nonneutralizing anti-HIV-1 antibodies. J Virol. 2017;91:e02440–16.

136. Schwartz O, Maréchal V, Danos O, Heard JM. Human immunodeficiency virus type 1 Nef increases the efficiency of reverse transcription in the infected cell. J Virol. 1995;69:4053–9.

137. Neil SJD, Zang T, Bieniasz PD. Tetherin inhibits retrovirus release and is antagonized by HIV-1 Vpu. Nature. 2008;451:425–30.

138. Lai RPJ, Yan J, Heeney J, McClure MO, Göttlinger H, Luban J, et al. Nef decreases HIV-1 sensitivity to neutralizing antibodies that target the membrane-proximal external region of TMgp41. PLoS Pathog. 2011;7:e1002442.

139. Joyner AS, Willis JR, Crowe JE, Aiken C. Maturation-induced cloaking of neutralization epitopes on HIV-1 particles. PLoS Pathog. 2011;7:e1002234.

140. Chen J, Kovacs JM, Peng H, Rits-Volloch S, Lu J, Park D, et al. Effect of the cytoplasmic domain on antigenic characteristics of HIV-1 envelope glycoprotein. Science. 2015;349:191–5.

141. Durham ND, Chen BK. HIV-1 cell-free and cell-to-cell infections are differentially regulated by distinct determinants in the Env gp41 cytoplasmic tail. J Virol. 2015;89:9324–37.

142. Lu LL, Suscovich TJ, Fortune SM, Alter G. Beyond binding: antibody effector functions in infectious diseases. Nat Rev Immunol. 2017;18:46–61.

143. von Bredow B, Arias JF, Heyer LN, Moldt B, Le K, Robinson JE, et al. Comparison of antibody-dependent cell-mediated cytotoxicity and virus neutralization by HIV-1 Env-specific monoclonal antibodies. J Virol. 2016;90:6127–39.

144. Lee WS, Kent SJ. Anti-HIV-1 antibody-dependent cellular cytotoxicity: is there more to antibodies than neutralization? Curr Opin HIV AIDS. 2018;13:160–6.

145. Richard J, Prévost J, Alsahafi N, Ding S, Finzi A. Impact of HIV-1 envelope conformation on ADCC responses. Trends Microbiol. 2018;26(4):253–65.

146. Hessell AJ, Hangartner L, Hunter M, Havenith CEG, Beurskens FJ, Bakker JM, et al. Fc receptor but not complement binding is important in antibody protection against HIV. Nature. 2007;449:101–4.

147. Bournazos S, Klein F, Pietzsch J, Seaman MS, Nussenzweig MC, Ravetch JV. Broadly neutralizing anti-HIV-1 antibodies require fc effector functions for in vivo activity. Cell. 2014;158:1243–53.

148. Horwitz JA, Halper-Stromberg A, Mouquet H, Gitlin AD, Tretiakova A, Eisenreich TR, et al. HIV-1 suppression and durable control by combining single broadly neutralizing antibodies and antiretroviral drugs in humanized mice. Proc Natl Acad Sci. 2013;110:16538–43.

149. Horwitz JA, Bar-On Y, Lu C-L, Fera D, Lockhart AAK, Lorenzi JCC, et al. Non-neutralizing antibodies alter the course of HIV-1 infection in vivo. Cell. 2017;170(637–648):e10.

150. Prévost J, Richard J, Ding S, Pacheco B, Charlebois R, Hahn BH, et al. Envelope glycoproteins sampling states 2/3 are susceptible to ADCC by sera from HIV-1-infected individuals. Virology. 2018;515:38–45.

151. Ndirangu J, Viljoen J, Bland RM, Danaviah S, Thorne C, Van de Perre P, et al. Cell-free (RNA) and cell-associated (DNA) HIV-1 and postnatal transmission through breastfeeding. PLoS ONE. 2012;7:e51493.

152. Bernard-Stoecklin S, Gommet C, Corneau AB, Guenounou S, Torres C, Dejucq-Rainsford N, et al. Semen CD4 + T cells and macrophages are productively infected at all stages of SIV infection in Macaques. PLoS Pathog. 2013;9:e1003810.

153. Zhu T, Wang N, Carr A, Nam DS, Moor-Jankowski R, Cooper DA, et al. Genetic characterization of human immunodeficiency virus type 1 in blood and genital secretions: evidence for viral compartmentalization and selection during sexual transmission. J Virol. 1996;70:3098–107.

154. Sallé B, Brochard P, Bourry O, Mannioui A, Andrieu T, Prevot S, et al. Infection of Macaques after vaginal exposure to cell-associated simian immunodeficiency virus. J Infect Dis. 2010;202:337–44.

155. Kolodkin-Gal D, Hulot SL, Korioth-Schmitz B, Gombos RB, Zheng Y, Owuor J, et al. Efficiency of cell-free and cell-associated virus in mucosal transmission of human immunodeficiency virus type 1 and simian immunodeficiency virus. J Virol. 2013;87:13589–97.

156. Parsons MS, Lloyd SB, Lee WS, Kristensen AB, Amarasena T, Center RJ, et al. Partial efficacy of a broadly neutralizing antibody against cell-associated SHIV infection. Sci Transl Med. 2017;9:eaaf1483.

157. Titanji BK, Pillay D, Jolly C. Combination antiretroviral therapy and cell–cell spread of wild-type and drug-resistant human immunodeficiency virus-1. J Gen Virol. 2017;98:821–34.

10

Non-coding RNAs and retroviruses

Xu Zhang[1,2,3], Xiancai Ma[1,2,3], Shuliang Jing[1,2,3], Hui Zhang[1,2,3*] and Yijun Zhang[4*] ⓘ

Abstract

Retroviruses can cause severe diseases such as cancer and acquired immunodeficiency syndrome. A unique feature in the life cycle of retroviruses is that their RNA genome is reverse transcribed into double-stranded DNA, which then integrates into the host genome to exploit the host machinery for their benefits. The metazoan genome encodes numerous non-coding RNAs (ncRNA), which act as key regulators in essential cellular processes such as antiviral response. The development of next-generation sequencing technology has greatly accelerated the detection of ncRNAs from viruses and their hosts. ncRNAs have been shown to play important roles in the retroviral life cycle and virus–host interactions. Here, we review recent advances in ncRNA studies with special focus on those have changed our understanding of retroviruses or provided novel strategies to treat retrovirus-related diseases. Many ncRNAs such as microRNAs (miRNAs) and long non-coding RNAs (lncRNAs) are involved in the late phase of the retroviral life cycle. However, their roles in the early phase of viral replication merit further investigations.

Keywords: Non-coding RNA, Retroviruses, Viral life cycle, Virus latency, MicroRNA, Long non-coding RNA

Background

The classification and life cycle of retroviruses

Retroviruses represent a large and diverse family of enveloped RNA viruses defined by common taxonomic denominators that include structure, composition, and replicative properties [1]. A key feature of the retroviral life cycle is that the RNA genome is reverse-transcribed to double-stranded DNA, which is subsequently integrated into the host genome and turns to a provirus. The viral genes are transcribed from the integrated proviral DNA to produce proteins and genomic RNA required to assemble the progeny viral particles. Retroviruses are further subdivided into seven groups (genus) defined by their evolutionary relatedness [2]. Retroviruses in five of these groups have oncogenic potential (formerly referred to as oncoviruses), and the other two groups are lentiviruses and spumaviruses. The representative of the lentivirus family is the human immunodeficiency virus type 1 (HIV-1), the causative agent of acquired immunodeficiency syndrome (AIDS). There are over 36 million

people living with HIV-1 worldwide, with approximately 2.1 million new infections being reported in 2015. To date, there is no cure for AIDS because of the existence of the HIV reservoir. The latent reservoir is a group of HIV-infected cells (mainly resting CD4[+] T cells) that do not actively produce new HIV-1, but could produce virus again upon stimulation [3].

The life cycle of retroviruses can be simply divided into the early and late phases. The early phase refers to the steps from cell binding to integration of the viral cDNA in the host genome, whereas the late phase begins with the expression of viral genes and is followed by the assembly, release, and maturation of progeny virions [4]. For HIV-1, the lifecycle can be briefly divided into seven steps: (1) attachment and binding, (2) fusion and uncoating, (3) reverse transcription, (4) integration, (5) transcription, (6) assembly, and (7) budding (Fig. 1A–G). Steps 1–4 represent the early phase, and steps 5–7 represent the late phase of a typical retrovirus life cycle. In addition, there is a special state of the retrovirus life cycle called latent infection. Under such conditions, the proviral DNA is transcriptionally inactive without producing infectious viral particles. As the host CD4[+] T cells are activated, the phase of latent HIV infection can be reversed to productive infection [3, 5]. Numerous host factors are involved

*Correspondence: zhangh92@mail.sysu.edu.cn; yi-jun.zhang@yale.edu
[1] Institute of Human Virology, Zhongshan School of Medicine, Sun Yat-Sen University, Guangzhou 510080, China
[4] Section of Infectious Diseases, Department of Internal Medicine, Yale University School of Medicine, New Haven, CT 06520, USA
Full list of author information is available at the end of the article

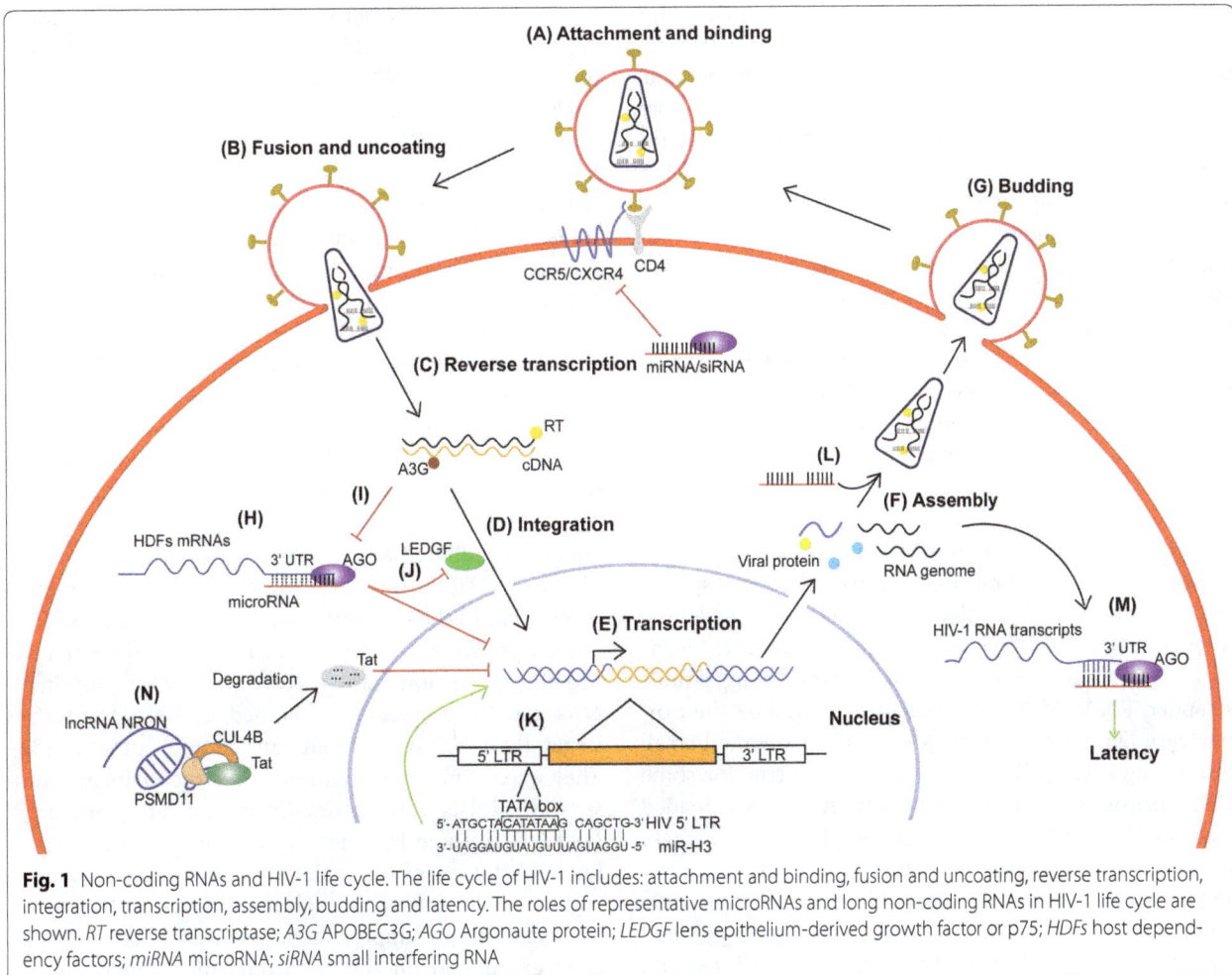

Fig. 1 Non-coding RNAs and HIV-1 life cycle. The life cycle of HIV-1 includes: attachment and binding, fusion and uncoating, reverse transcription, integration, transcription, assembly, budding and latency. The roles of representative microRNAs and long non-coding RNAs in HIV-1 life cycle are shown. *RT* reverse transcriptase; *A3G* APOBEC3G; *AGO* Argonaute protein; *LEDGF* lens epithelium-derived growth factor or p75; *HDFs* host dependency factors; *miRNA* microRNA; *siRNA* small interfering RNA

in the life cycle of retroviruses, being either indispensable or restrictive [6].

Virology and RNA biology have reciprocally influenced each other for decades [7]. The capping of eukaryotic mRNA was first discovered in reovirus and vaccinia virus [8]. Splicing and then alternative splicing were first demonstrated by analysis of adenoviral transcription [9, 10]. Analysis of viral systems, in particular picornaviruses, led to the first description of an internal ribosome entry site (IRES) [7]. Retroviruses have also played an important role in understanding the export of mRNAs from the nucleus to the cytoplasm. For host transcripts, only fully spliced mRNAs can be exported to the cytoplasm. However, for some retroviruses such as HIV-1, both spliced and unspliced transcripts need to be exported to the cytoplasm to produce viral proteins or serve as genomic RNA. HIV-1 encodes a special protein called Rev that exports its unspliced mRNA transcripts containing the Rev Response Element (RRE) to the cytoplasm [11]. To accomplish this function, Rev harbors a nuclear export

signal (NES), which was the first NES described, and still remains the prototype of the most common class of NESs [12]. Compatible with such significant progress in virus research, the recent advances in non-coding RNA (ncRNA) research have greatly extended our understanding of viruses.

The classification and functions of non-coding RNAs
Genomic studies have demonstrated that only two percent of the human genome codes for proteins, whereas the majority codes for numerous non-protein coding RNAs (or non-coding RNA, ncRNA) [13]. Based on their function, non-coding RNAs can be divided into two major groups: (1) housekeeping non-coding RNA such as ribosomal RNA (rRNA), transfer RNA (tRNA), small nuclear RNA (snRNA), and small nucleolar RNA (snoRNA); and (2) regulatory non-coding RNA such as microRNA (miRNA), long non-coding RNA (lncRNA), and piwi-interacting RNA (piRNA) [14]. The housekeeping non-coding RNAs are mainly involved in the

basic biological processes in cells, such as snRNA for pre-mRNA splicing, rRNA and tRNA for mRNA translation, snoRNA for rRNA methylation/pseudouridylation. However, the regulatory non-coding RNAs exert more diverse and sophisticated functions such as miRNA for regulating gene transcription and translation, lncRNA for modifying epigenetic signatures of chromatin, and piRNA for silencing transposons [14]. Unlike housekeeping ncRNAs, the expression of regulatory ncRNAs is usually tissue-specific and their regulation is gene-specific, which is mostly enabled by sequence-specific interactions between the ncRNA and its target(s) [15]. During viral infection, the regulatory ncRNAs exhibit more profound changes in expression and sophisticated functions compared to the housekeeping ncRNAs [16].

RNA interference and microRNA

RNA interference (RNAi) was proposed to initially evolve in plants and invertebrates as a native immune response against viruses [17]. In plant and invertebrate cells, the infection of all RNA viruses, except retroviruses, leads to the generation of perfectly base-paired long double stranded RNAs (dsRNA), which are cleaved by the exonuclease Dicer into ~ 22 bp short dsRNAs named small interfering RNA (siRNA) [17]. This is also true for some DNA viruses. One strand of the siRNA duplex is loaded into the RNA-induced silencing complex (RISC), where it guides RISC to mRNA containing complementary sequence [18]. Since these virus-derived siRNAs are fully complementary to viral mRNAs, the RISC binding guided by these siRNAs will silence their cognate viral RNAs and inhibit virus replication. In plants and nematodes, this antiviral response can be further amplified by generating a secondary wave of siRNAs through a mechanism involving RNA-dependent RNA polymerases (RdRPs) [19, 20]. In mammalian cells, RNAi mediated by siRNA is no longer a major form of the antiviral response. Instead, interferon (IFN) response and it-induced systematic antiviral state play a key role (reviewed in Ref. [21]). However, the RNAi mechanism was retained to generate endogenous microRNA (miRNA) and regulate the expression of a significant amount of genes. MicroRNAs represent an important class of regulators in many crucial biological processes in animals, plants, fungi, and viruses [22, 23]. In the nucleus, primary miRNAs (pri-miRNAs) are transcribed and processed by Drosha and its cofactor DGCR8 (also known as Pasha, located in the DiGeorge syndrome chromosomal region) to generate precursor miRNAs (pre-miRNAs) [24], which are then exported to the cytoplasm [25] and further sliced by Dicer to generate ~ 22 nt mature miRNAs [26]. Like siRNAs, one strand of mature miRNAs is bound by Argonaute (AGO) proteins and loaded into the RISC [27] for guiding the RISC to

the 3′ UTR of mRNAs to suppress translation or induce degradation. Unlike siRNAs, which fully complement to their target mRNA, most miRNAs bind to the target mRNA mainly through the "seed sequence", residues 2–8 of the guide miRNAs (Fig. 1H). The regulatory target sequences of miRNA have been extended to the 5′ UTR [28] and the coding region [29] of mRNAs to suppress translation. Moreover, miRNAs could switch from suppressor to activator of translation by targeting the 5′ UTR [30] or 3′ UTR [31] of certain mRNAs. In addition to regulating mRNA translation in the cytoplasm, mounting evidence reveals that the small RNA-Ago pathway can also positively regulate gene expression by targeting gene promoters in the nucleus, a phenomenon termed as RNA activation (RNAa), which is evolutionarily conserved from *Caenorhabditis elegans* to human [32–35].

Long non-coding RNAs

The ENCODE (The Encyclopedia of DNA Elements) Project led to the discovery of a large proportion of long transcripts from the human genome that do not code proteins (long non-coding RNAs, lncRNAs) [36]. lncRNAs can be operationally defined as RNA transcripts larger than 200 bp without any coding potential [37]. They appear in the genome in three major forms: antisense lncRNAs, intronic lncRNAs, and intergenic lncRNAs (also termed large intervening noncoding RNAs or lincRNAs). One of the major functions of lncRNA is to regulate gene activity through interactions with chromatin, especially to suppress gene expression. For instance, gene expression on the X-chromosome can be inactivated by the lncRNA Xsit [38]. Although the mechanisms of lncRNA-mediated gene regulation are diverse, three main mechanistic themes have been drawn from dozens of examples (see review by Rinn and Chang [37]). These include decoys, scaffolds, and guides. Notably, when an lncRNA guide protein complex to the target site on chromatin, how does the lncRNA recognize and interact with the target DNA is still unclear. In addition to using DNA-binding protein(s) as adapter, the RNA–DNA direct interaction through RNA:DNA hybrid or RNA:DNA:DNA triplex are also possible forms requiring further investigation [39]. Increasing attention has been given to lncRNAs due to their strong connection with the development of various diseases, especially cancers. The elevated expression of the lncRNA Hox transcript antisense intergenic RNA (HOTAIR) has been observed in human breast, colon, and liver cancers, and facilitates cancer metastasis in vivo [40–42]. Extensive studies on the role of lncRNA in cancers may provide useful insights for the study of lncRNAs in the retrovirus system.

In this review, we discuss recent advances in the study of non-coding RNAs that play important roles in the life cycle of retroviruses, with special focus on miRNAs and lncRNAs (Tables 1, 2). Moreover, the treatment of retrovirus-related diseases can also benefit from the study of non-coding RNAs.

Non-coding RNAs and the early phase of the retrovirus life cycle

The early phase of retrovirus life cycle includes binding and fusion of virions to host cells, reverse transcription of viral genomic RNA into cDNA, and its integration in the host chromosome (Fig. 1A–D). During the binding and fusion steps, viral Env proteins play a leading role. The HIV-1 Env trimer first binds to the cell surface CD4 receptor and induces conformational changes that allows

binding to the CCR5 or CXCR4 co-receptor, which mediates the fusion of viral and cell membranes. The study on how non-coding RNAs are involved in these steps is missing. In general, RNA is quite unstable in the extracellular environment and ready to be degraded by RNase. However, several reports showed that some ncRNAs, e.g. miRNAs or lncRNAs, are circulating in the blood, which can serve as biomarkers of various diseases [43, 44]. The improved stability of these ncRNAs could be due to their small size or special secondary structures [37]. An implication from the existence of these extracellular RNAs is that the non-coding RNAs can be involved in the early steps of retroviral infection, such as the binding and fusion of virions to the host cells. A possibility

Table 1 Retroviral and host microRNA

	Virus	Name	Viral target(s)	Cellular target(s)	Function	References
Viral microRNA	HIV-1	miR-H3	HIV-1 5′ LTR TATA box		Enhance HIV-1 5′ LTR transcription	[77]
		TAR-derived miRNA		ERCC1, IER3, Caspase 8, Aiolos, Ikaros, Nucleophosmin (NPM)/B23	Protect the infected cells from apoptosis, maintain balance between apoptosis and cell survival	[70, 71, 75, 76]
		miR-N367	Nef		Block HIV-1 Nef expression	[72]
		vmiRNA#1-5		Predicted	Unknown	[68]
	BLV	B1-5		Bovine HBP1, PXDN	Mimic host miR-29, tumorigenesis	[66]
	BFV	miR-BF2-5p miR-BF1-5p miR-BF1-3p			Unknown	[85]
	ALV-J	E (XSR) miRNA			Unknown, possible roles in myeloid leukosis associated with ALV-J	[86]
Host microRNA		miR-29a miR-29b miR-149 miR-378 miR-324-5p	HIV-1 Nef, Vpr, Env, Vif transcripts		Downregulate the expression of Nef protein and interfere with HIV-1 replication	[119–121]
		miR-326	Nef ORF located in the 3′ U3 of HIV-1 transcripts		Moderate HIV-1 replication in human cells	[122]
		miR-423 miR-301a miR-155	HIV-1 genome		Repress viral gene expression	[123]
		miR-28 miR-125b miR-150 miR-223 miR-382	HIV-1 mRNA 3′ ends		Contribute to HIV-1 latency	[46]
		miR-146		CXCR4	Inhibit HIV-1 infection	[47, 48]
		miR-155		ADAM10, TNPO3, Nup153, LEDGF/p75	Inhibit HIV-1 infection	[60]
		miR-198		Cyclin T1 mRNA	Restrict HIV-1 replication in monocytes	[102]
		Let-7i		IL-2 promoter TATA box	Activate IL-2 transcription, involved in HIV-1 infection-induced CD4+ T cell depletion	[78, 137]

Table 2 Retroviral and host LncRNA

	Virus	Name	Viral targets	Cellular targets	Function	References
Viral lncRNA	HIV-1	HIV-1-encoded antisense RNA	HIV-1 5′ LTR		Alter the epigenetic landscape and silence the HIV-1 promoter	[84]
	HERV-H	HERVH RNA		p300, OCT4	Activate neighboring genes and in turn regulating pluripotency-related genes	[93]
	HTLV-1	HBZ		E2F1	Promote T cell proliferation	[97, 98]
Host lncRNA		NRON	Tat	NFAT	Induce the degradation of Tat and contribute to HIV-1 latency; suppress NFAT-mediated viral gene activation	[132, 135]
		NEAT1	HIV-1 unspliced RNAs	p54nrb, PSF, Matrin3, RBM14	Inhibit nucleus-to-cytoplasm export of Rev-dependent instability element (INS)-containing HIV-1 mRNAs	[104, 106, 108–110]
		7SK snRNA		P-TEFb	Negatively regulate HIV-1 Tat transcriptional activation by specifically sequestering P-TEFb	[111, 112]
		7SL RNA	HIV-1 Gag	APOBEC3G	Enable efficient packaging of APOBEC3G into virions	[128]

is that these extracellular ncRNAs could enter the target cells along with the viruses and affect viral infectivity. The virion-associated ncRNAs might also play certain roles in these steps. A small subset of host miRNAs are shown to be concentrated in the HIV-1 virions by up to 115 folds [45]. Notably, three of the packaged miRNAs: miRNA-382, miRNA-223, and miRNA-150, were able to interact with the 3′ UTR of HIV-1 mRNA as well as contribute to HIV-1 latency [46] (see discussion in the non-coding RNAs and retrovirus assembly section below). However, their functions within the virions remain to be determined. It is interesting to investigate whether the noncoding RNAs packaged in virions are involved in viral fusion and uncoating steps, considering they have been protected by the viral particle from the damage caused by the extracellular environment. As mentioned above, these virion-enriched ncRNAs could also affect the expression of entry- or uncoating-related proteins.

As the co-receptor is important for HIV-1 entrance, the dysregulation of CCR5 or CXCR4 significantly affects HIV-1 infection. It has been shown that CXCR4 is a direct target of miR-146a in human hematopoietic normal and leukemic cells; and the transcription factor PLZF (promyelocytic leukemia zinc finger) has been identified as a repressor of miR-146a expression in megakaryocytic (Mk) cells [47]. These authors further reported that the miR-146a upregulation by AMD3100 treatment or PLZF

silencing decreases CXCR4 protein expression and prevents HIV-1 infection in monocytic cell line and CD4$^+$ T lymphocytes [48]. However, the suppression of CXCR4 by miR-146 was not confirmed at least in MT2 cells [49]. At present, there is no solid evidence for CCR5 to be regulated by any cellular or viral microRNA and the HIV-1 infection is therefore affected.

For HIV-1, the initiation of reverse transcription is coupled with the uncoating of the viral core [50]. It is well known that tRNA$_{Lys3}$ serves as the primer for reverse transcription of viral genomic RNA. In addition to primer tRNA, the reverse transcription complex (RTC) contains multiple proteins, including viral proteins MA (matrix protein, p17), CA (capsid protein, p24), NC (nucleocapsid protein, p7), IN (integrase), and Vpr [51]. The mature CA protein most likely provides the overall structure of the RTC [52, 53]. Only a few host proteins have been identified from the RTC. The cellular protein cyclophilin A (CypA) was shown to play a critical role in the correct disassembly of the HIV-1 core early after infection [54]. The APOBEC3 family is involved in the restriction of retrovirus reverse-transcription, functioning as cytosine deaminases that introduce hyper G to A mutations to the sense strand of proviral cDNA [55]. While no report shows the expression of these host factors is directly regulated by miRNA or other ncRNAs, our studies have shown that APOBEC3G and its family members cause derepression of miRNA-mediated protein translation inhibition [56], which is through interfering with the interaction between Argonaute-2 and MOV10 [57] (Fig. 1I). These findings imply that there could be a complex regulation network involving retroviruses, APOBEC3 proteins and the host miRNA pathway. It will be interesting to investigate the roles of lncRNAs during the assembly of the RTC, e.g. as a scaffold for the complex assembly. It is also intriguing to explore the roles of virion-associated miRNAs during reverse transcription, given that these miRNAs could potentially bind to the 3′ UTR of viral genomic RNA and be packaged into the virions.

At the late stage of the reverse transcription, the RTC transitions into a pre-integration complex (PIC), which is subsequently transported into the nucleus. Similarly, the integration of viral DNA into the host chromosome involves many host factors, such as proteins that help the transfer of viral DNA to nucleus and the integration of viral DNA into the host chromosome. For example, the cellular transcriptional coactivator lens epithelium-derived growth factor (LEDGF)/p75 is an essential HIV integration cofactor, which forms stable tetramers and associates with HIV-1 integrase [58, 59]. The stimulation of polyinosinic-polycytidylic acid [poly (I:C)] and bacterial lipopolysaccharide (LPS), the ligands for toll-like receptor 3 (TLR3) and TLR4, respectively, are known to decrease HIV-1 infection in monocyte-derived macrophages (MDMs), but the mechanism was unclear. It has been shown that stimulation with poly (I:C) upon TLR3 in MDMs leads to the upregulation of miR-155 expression, and consequently the downregulation of its target proteins including ADAM10, TNPO3, Nup153, and LEDGF/p75. This study indicates that a TLR3-induced miRNA exerts an anti-HIV-1 effect by targeting several HIV-1 dependency factors to inhibit HIV-1 infection [60] (Fig. 1J).

Compared to the late phase, less is known about the early steps of retrovirus life cycle, as reviewed by Nisole and Saib [4]. Accordingly, the roles of non-coding RNAs played during the early phase of retrovirus life cycle are still largely unknown.

Non-coding RNAs and the late phase of the retrovirus life cycle

Retrovirus-encoded non-coding RNAs

After integration, the provirus starts to transcribe viral genes. The transcription of the proviral genome leads to generation of diverse products including genomic RNA, spliced mRNAs, structural proteins, accessory proteins, and some non-coding RNAs [61]. These viral parts play various roles in the late stage of retroviral life cycle, and some of them are essential parts of the progeny viruses.

Below we describe the roles played by virus-encoded and cellular non-coding RNAs in the late stage of the retroviral life cycle.

HIV-1-encoded non-coding RNAs

Virus-encoded miRNAs were initially identified from Epstein–Barr viruses (EBV) [62]. Since then, an increasing number of virus-encoded miRNAs have been identified [17, 63]. Most of these miRNAs were reported in DNA viruses such as Herpes and Polyoma viruses, but rarely in RNA viruses [17]. Because of the rapid developments of next-generation sequencing (NGS, or deep-sequencing) technology, which is much more sensitive and quantitative than the conventional cDNA clone sequencing method, more RNA virus-derived miRNAs have been discovered, especially from HIV-1, West Nile Virus (WNV), and Bovine Leukemia Virus (BLV) [64–67].

It has been reported that HIV-1 encodes miRNAs and other small RNAs. Bennasser et al. first performed a computational prediction of HIV-1-encoded miRNAs and found five pre-miRNA candidates [68]. Subsequently, several groups identified miRNAs from the HIV-1 negative regulatory factor (Nef) and trans-activation response (TAR) element [69–72]. Through the NGS method, a number of HIV-1-encoded small RNAs were discovered, some of which exhibit features of miRNA siRNA [73–75]. HIV-1-derived small RNAs have been shown to modulate cellular and/or viral gene expression. The TAR-derived miRNA protects the infected cells from apoptosis by downregulating cellular genes involved in apoptosis [71, 76]. A Nef-derived miRNA-miR-N367 blocks HIV-1 Nef expression in vitro [72].

The low abundance of HIV-1-derived small RNAs has fueled the debate about the existence and function of HIV-1-encoded miRNAs [17]. A possible explanation of the low abundance of HIV-1-derived miRNAs is that the virus has been evolving to escape from or counteract the RNAi-mediated immune surveillance. HIV-1 has developed special ways to manipulate the host RNAi, such as using a non-processed transcript to produce miRNAs and targeting viral promoter DNA for the regulation of gene expression. Harwig et al. revealed that non-processive transcription from the HIV-1 LTR promoter results in the production of TAR-encoded miRNA-like small RNA [75]. Dicer cleaves these TAR RNAs and the viral transactivating regulatory protein (Tat) stimulates this processing. Through this special biogenesis pathway, HIV-1 produces the TAR-derived miRNA without cleavage of its RNA genome. Through a strategy combining in silico prediction and NGS, our group identified a novel HIV-1-encoded miRNA, miR-H3 [77]. miR-H3 is located in the mRNA region encoding the active center of reverse transcriptase (RT), and exhibits high sequence conservation among HIV-1 subtypes. The overexpression of miR-H3 increases viral production, while mutations in the miR-H3 sequence significantly impair the replication of HIV-1$_{NL43}$, suggesting that it is a viral replication-enhancing miRNA. Interestingly, miR-H3 targets the HIV-1 5′ LTR TATA box and sequence-specifically activates the viral promoter transcription. This is the first report of the promoter TATA box-targeting miRNAs that activate gene transcription [77]. These miRNAs might directly interact with the TATA box in the RNA Polymerase II pre-initiation complexes (PICs) and facilitate transcription initiation [78]. In contrast to cytoplasmic miRNAs that need a quite high expression level to bind and regulate their massive mRNA targets, the abundance of the TATA box-targeting miRNAs required for regulating promoter activity is significantly reduced, given that the copy number of their targets in the nucleus is very limited (Fig. 1K).

The secondary structure of the entire HIV-1 RNA genome is quite complicated [79]. Several groups recently found that HIV-1 transcribes not only full-length genomic RNA and multiple spliced mRNAs, but also some antisense RNAs [65, 80–82]. Some of the HIV-1-encoded antisense RNAs can suppress HIV-1 expression [83]. Particularly, one of these suppressive HIV-1-encoded antisense RNAs is a lncRNA [84]. Further experiments showed that this lncRNA could alter the epigenetic landscape of the HIV-1 promoter by recruiting DNA methyltransferase 3A (DNMT3A), enhancer of zeste homolog 2 (EZH2), histone deacetylase 1 (HDAC1), and euchromatic histone-lysine N-methyltransferase 2 (EHMT2, also known as G9a) to the HIV-1 5′ LTR. These proteins recruited by the antisense lncRNA lead to an epigenetically silenced state of the viral promoter, which is characterized by multiple suppressive epigenetic markers including histone deacetylation, H3K9 dimethylation, and H3K27 trimethylation [84].

Other retrovirus-derived non-coding RNAs
Interestingly, to prevent the cleavage of their RNA genome, some retroviruses use an alternative RNA source as miRNA precursor. A deltaretrovirus bovine leukemia virus (BLV) uses RNA Pol III transcripts to produce five miRNAs in a Drosha-independent manner [66]. Whisnant et al. identified three miRNAs from bovine foamy virus (BFV), a member of the spumavirus subfamily of retroviruses, in both BFV-infected cultured cells and BFV-infected cattle. All three viral miRNAs are generated from an ~ 122-nucleotide (nt) pri-miRNA encoded within the BFV long terminal repeat U3 region. This BFV pri-miRNA is also transcribed by

RNA polymerase III [85]. In the avian leukosis virus subgroup J (ALV-J), an alpharetrovirus, a miRNA encoded by the exogenous virus-specific (E or XSR) region has been described. Unlike the above reported miRNAs, this miRNA is generated by the canonical miRNA biogenesis pathway. The pri-miRNA is transcribed by RNA Pol II and requires Drosha and Dicer for processing [86]. This finding raises the debate on whether retroviruses can use the canonical miRNA pathway to produce miRNA again.

Besides miRNAs, retroviruses also encode lncRNAs to regulate viral or host genes expression [87]. In recent years, transposable elements (TEs) have been identified as a major lncRNA repertoire, and are treated as functional domains of lncRNAs due to their multiple RNA-, DNA-, and protein-binding properties [88]. Nearly two thirds of the mature lncRNAs are originated from transposable elements (TEs). Among them, ten percent are transcribed from endogenous retrovirus (ERV) [89]. HERV-H is one of the primate-specific endogenous retroviruses that is preferentially expressed in human embryonic stem cells (hESCs) and induced pluripotent stem cells (hiPSCs) [90, 91]. Nearly ten percent of the HERV-H transcripts are lncRNAs [92]. One of the HERV-H-driven lncRNAs was found to interact with the transcriptional coactivator p300 and pluripotency factor OCT4 and enriched in the HERV-H LTR7 regions, resulting in the activation of neighboring genes and in turn regulating pluripotency-related genes [93]. In addition to the regulation of hESCs, another ERV-derived lncRNA named Endogenous retroViral-associated ADenocarcinoma RNA (EVADR) was found to be expressed specifically in human adenocarcinoma but not in non-glandular origin tumors [94]. Human T cell leukemia virus type 1 (HTLV-1), a retrovirus of the human T-lymphotropic virus (HTLV) family, is the etiologic agent of adult T-cell leukemia (ATL) [95]. An HTLV-1-encoded protein named HTLV-1 bZIP factor (HBZ) was previously found to suppress the viral *Tax* expression [96]. Recently, researchers found that the mRNA of *HBZ* is retained in the nucleus and functions as an lncRNA to promote T cell proliferation [97, 98].

Taken together, some special features of retrovirus-derived miRNAs have emerged: (1) biogenesis—retroviruses use both canonical and non-canonical biogenesis pathways to generate miRNA; and (2) mode of action—retrovirus-encoded miRNA target can the promoter TATA box to upregulate gene transcription instead of targeting the mRNA 3′ UTR to suppress translation. These findings extend our understanding of the RNAi pathway in mammalian cells. Although the small size of retroviral RNA genomes has limited their coding ability for ncRNAs, the extraordinary diversity of viral transcripts and the enormous host gene regulation network enable the viral ncRNAs unlimited functional potentials.

Cellular non-coding RNAs and retroviral gene expression

During productive infection, plenty of host factors are involved in the transcriptional regulation of viral genes such as the P-TEFb complex and NFκ-B [99, 100]. In addition, massive interactions between viral products and host proteins or ncRNAs occur at different levels. Therefore, viral gene expression might be the most regulated step in the retroviral life cycle.

Host non-coding RNAs regulate viral transcription and RNA transport

The efficient replication of HIV-1 is dependent on many cellular transcription factors, which could also be the targets of host RNAi. As a subunit of RNA polymerase II elongation factor P-TEFb, Cyclin T1 is required for Tat transactivation of HIV-1 LTR-directed gene expression [101]. MiR-198 is relatively highly expressed in human monocytes compared to macrophages, which are more permissive for HIV-1 replication. By targeting the 3′ UTR of Cyclin T1 mRNA and suppressing its translation, miR-198 functions to restrict HIV-1 replication in monocytes [102]. Many other host miRNA-mediated indirect effects on HIV-1 transcription through targeting the host dependency factors (HDFs) have been summarized by Barichievy et al. [103] (Fig. 1H).

Cellular lncRNAs also participate in the transcriptional regulation as well as the transportation of HIV-1 RNAs. A group identified six lncRNAs that were dysregulated by HIV-1 infection in both Jurkat and MT4 cells, one of which is NEAT1 (Nuclear Paraspeckle Assembly Transcripts 1) [104]. NEAT1 contributes to the formation of paraspeckles through sequestering multiple component proteins [105–107]. Some of the NEAT1-sequestered proteins are pivotal co-factors for efficient HIV-1 gene expression, including p54nrb, PSF, Matrin3, and RBM14 [108–110]. Besides canonical lncRNAs, some non-canonical lncRNAs were also involved in HIV-1 replication [46, 111, 112]. P-TEFb, which is composed of CDK9 and Cyclin T1, is indispensable for efficient HIV-1 transcription [113]. Two independent groups identified that lncRNA 7SK small nuclear RNA (snRNA) can negatively regulate HIV-1 Tat transcriptional activation by specifically sequestering P-TEFb [111, 112]. In addition, HIV-1 unspliced RNAs can be hijacked in NEAT1-supported nuclear paraspeckles and subjected to RNA editing. Knockdown of NEAT1 significantly enhanced HIV-1 production by increasing nucleus-to-cytoplasm export of Rev-dependent HIV-1 mRNAs containing an instability element (INS) [104].

Host non-coding RNAs directly target HIV-1 RNAs for post-transcriptional suppression

HIV-1 infection suppresses the RNA interfering pathway of host cells [114]. HIV-1 infection also causes global dysregulation of host miRNA expression profiles [115, 116]. HIV-1 Tat protein is shown to be a suppressor of RNA silencing (SRS), which abrogates the host cells RNA-silencing defense by subverting the ability of Dicer to process precursor double-stranded RNAs into siRNAs [117]. The HIV-1 TAR element was also reported to inhibit the host RNAi pathway by competitively binding to TAR RNA binding protein (TRBP), a cofactor of the key RNAi component Dicer [118]. These findings suggest that HIV-1 is escaping from the restriction imposed by the host RNAi mechanism. In fact, many host miRNAs have been shown to affect HIV-1 replication in direct or indirect ways.

Since HIV-1 is a RNA virus, its genomic RNA is a potential target for host miRNAs. Using in silico approaches, a number of miRNA binding sites in HIV-1 genomic RNA or mRNA transcripts were predicted and subsequently experimentally validated. Hariharan et al. reported that miR-29a and miR-29b were predicted to target HIV-1 Nef transcripts, whereas miR-149, miR-378, and miR-324-5p were predicted to target Vpr, Env, and Vif transcripts, respectively. However, these targeting sites were not located in the HIV-1 3′ LTR [119]. These authors then showed that the cellular miRNA miR-29a downregulates the expression of Nef protein and interferes with HIV-1 replication in HEK293T and Jurkat T cells [120, 121]. Similarly, Houzet et al. predicted the target sites of 22 human miRNAs in the HIV-1 genome, five of which were capable of inhibiting HIV-1 replication in 42CD4 cells derived from HEK293 cells stably expressing CD4 and CXCR4 [122]. Houzet et al. further demonstrated that the degree of complementarity between the predicted viral sequence and cellular miR-326 correlates with the potency of miRNA-mediated inhibition of viral replication. This finding indicates the selection pressure imposed on HIV-1 by the host RNAi pathway, which may drive the evolution of HIV-1. Using the photoactivatable ribonucleoside-induced cross-linking and immunoprecipitation (PAR-CLIP) technique, Whisnant et al. discovered several binding sites in the HIV-1 genome for cellular miRNAs, a subset of which were capable of repressing viral gene expression, including miR-423, miR-301a, and miR-155 [123]. They also argued that HIV-1 transcripts have evolved to avoid inhibition by host miRNAs by adopting extensive RNA secondary structures that occlude most potential miRNA binding sites.

Collectively, the current data show that cellular non-coding RNAs directly or indirectly modulate viral transcription, RNA transportation, and translation.

Meanwhile, the viruses have been evolving to evade inhibition by the RNAi pathway, which is enabled by their hyper mutation rate as well as the complicated folding of viral RNAs.

Non-coding RNAs and retrovirus assembly: the packaging of non-coding RNAs into retroviral particles

It was noticed several decades ago that host RNAs could be packaged into retroviral particles [124, 125]. Over 30% of the RNA in retroviral particles consist of host RNAs. These host RNAs include mRNA, tRNA, and small non-coding RNAs transcribed by Pol III. The most well-known host RNA packaged into HIV-1 virions is $tRNA_{Lys3}$, which serves as the primer to initiate HIV-1 reverse transcription [126]. The non-coding RNA 7SL is another highly enriched host RNA identified in HIV-1 virions [127], which is important for the efficient packaging of APOBEC3G into virions [128]. Numerous subsets of endogenous retroelement RNAs expressed in virus-producing cells are also preferentially packaged. For example, intact endogenous retroviral transcripts like the murine VL30 elements are packaged by murine leukemia virus (MLV); and fragments of non-long terminal repeats (LTR) retroelements such as the transcripts of divergent and truncated Long INterspersed Elements (LINEs) are packaged into virions by HIV-1 [129, 130].

Through the NGS technology, a pile of host miRNAs was found to be selectively packaged into HIV-1 virions and affect viral infectivity (Fig. 1L). Using the SOLiD sequencing platform, Schopman et al. examined the miRNA profiling in a T cell line and several primary cell subsets before and after HIV-1 infection. They also examined the miRNAs in HIV-1 particles, and found that a small subset of the host miRNAs is dramatically concentrated in the virions by up to 115 folds [45]. Notably, three of the packaged miRNAs: miRNA-382, miRNA-223, and miRNA-150, are shown to contribute to HIV-1 latency [46]. Later, Bogerd et al. used the Illumina Hiseq 2000 system to investigate the packaging of cellular miRNAs into HIV-1 virions produced from CEM-SS T cells. However, they just found a 2- to 4-fold enrichment of five host miRNAs in virions. Among them, miR-155 and miR-92a were reported previously to weakly bind HIV-1 transcripts [123]. Interestingly, an artificial miRNA target site introduced into the viral genome resulted in 10- to 40-fold increase in the packaging of the cognate miRNAs into virions, which significantly inhibited HIV-1 virion infectivity [131]. Nevertheless, it remains to be clarified how these virion-enriched miRNAs exert their functions during the early phase of the HIV-1 life cycle. It is possible that these virion-enriched miRNAs can inhibit viral reverse transcription or regulate the genes needed for viral entry or uncoating, as we discussed above regarding the roles of ncRNAs in the early phase of retroviral life cycle.

Non-coding RNAs and retroviral latency

Given the inhibitory effect on gene expression mediated by miRNAs, it is intriguing to investigate the roles of host miRNAs in HIV-1 latency. Our group reported that cellular miRNAs potently inhibit HIV-1 production in resting primary CD4$^+$ T cells and contribute to HIV-1 latency [46]. We showed that the 3' ends of HIV-1 messenger RNAs are targeted by several cellular miRNAs including miR-28, miR-125b, miR-150, miR-223, and miR-382, which are enriched in resting CD4$^+$ T cells compared to activated CD4$^+$ T cells. Specific inhibitors of these miRNAs activate HIV-1 protein translation in resting CD4$^+$ T cells transfected with HIV-1 infectious clones as well as viral production from resting CD4$^+$ T cells isolated from HIV-1-infected individuals on suppressive combined antiretroviral therapy (cART) [46]. This is the first report showing that cellular miRNAs contribute to HIV-1 latency, which adds a new layer to the mechanisms of the establishment of HIV-1 latency (Fig. 1M).

In addition to miRNAs, lncRNAs have also been found to be involved in the regulation of HIV-1 latency. Recently, we found a cellular lncRNA-noncoding repressor of NFAT (NRON), which is highly expressed in resting CD4$^+$ T lymphocytes, contributes to HIV-1 latency [132]. Knockdown of NRON in latently infected resting CD4$^+$ T cells significantly enhanced HIV-1 expression without activating the cells. Early studies showed that NRON acts as a negative regulator of transcription factor NFAT, which promotes HIV-1 expression by binding to the downstream of TAR [133, 134]. NRON hijacks NFAT in the cytoplasm to suppress NFAT-mediated viral gene activation. Another group also suggested that the NRON levels were reduced by the early viral accessory protein Nef and increased by the late protein Vpu [135]. However, we found that the expression of NFAT in HIV-1 latently-infected resting CD4$^+$ T cells is quite low. The mutation of NFAT binding sites in the HIV-1 5' LTR did not abolish NRON-mediated suppression of HIV-1 transcription. These findings indicate that the suppression of HIV-1 activation by NORN is independent of NFAT in resting CD4$^+$ T cells. Intriguingly, the expression of the HIV-1 transactivator Tat decreased significantly upon NRON overexpression. Further investigations showed that NRON directly links Tat to the ubiquitin/proteasome components including CUL4B and PSMD11 to specifically induce Tat degradation, thus facilitating HIV-1 latency (Fig. 1N). Collectively, these data suggest that NRON modulates HIV-1 latency in both NFAT-dependent and -independent manners. In addition, another group reported that an HIV-1 antisense transcript called ASP interacts with polycomb repressor complex 2 (PRC2) and recruits PRC2 to the HIV-1 5' LTR. This induces the accumulation of suppressive H3K27 trimethylation and reduces viral transcription, which facilitates the establishment of HIV-1 latency [136].

Non-coding RNAs and retrovirus pathogenesis

Retrovirus infection causes severe diseases such as cancers and AIDS. As key regulators of cellular processes, non-coding RNAs are involved in the progression of diseases caused by retroviruses. We showed that HIV-1 infection decreases the expression of a cellular miRNA let-7i in CD4+ T cells by attenuating the transcription of its precursor [137]. Let-7i activates the transcription of cytokine interleukin-2 (IL-2) through targeting its promoter TATA box region [78]. It has been observed for a long time that HIV-1 infection causes a decrease in IL-2 levels, which is one of the causes of CD4+ T cell depletion, but the mechanism was not clear. Our findings reveal a novel pathway that the HIV-1 infection-induced suppression of the let-7i/IL-2 axis contributes to CD4+ T cell death [137]. Another interesting study showed that the BLV-miR-B4 shares an identical seed sequence with the cellular pro-oncogene miR-29, and both downregulate a similar set of mRNA targets [138]. Given that miR-29 overexpression is associated with B-cell neoplasms that resemble BLV-associated tumors, these findings suggest a possible miRNA-mediated mechanism contributing to BLV-induced tumorigenesis [66]. Other support for their roles in tumor onset and progression is that these miRNAs are highly expressed in preleukemic and malignant cells in which viral structural and regulatory gene expression was repressed [138]. The increasing ncRNA expression profiling data during viral infection are very helpful to identify those ncRNAs that are involved in retroviral pathogenesis.

Application of non-coding RNA approaches in the specific treatment of retrovirus-related diseases

Since non-coding RNAs can sequence-specifically block retrovirus or host factors required for viral replication, non-coding RNAs are ideal candidates for the treatment of retrovirus infection. HIV-1 latency in resting CD4+ T cells is a major obstacle for the eradication of viruses from HIV-1-infected patients receiving combination antiretroviral therapy (cART) [3, 5]. The "shock and kill" strategy aims to activate the latently-infected viruses and induce the killing of the infected cells by specific cytotoxic effects [139]. Several approaches have been developed to activate latent virus transcription for killing, including by activating T lymphocytes with IL-2 or IL-2 plus anti-CD3/anti-CD28 antibody [140, 141], protein kinase C (PKC) activators (e.g. prostatin [142]), or

activating transcription with histone deacetylases inhibitors (HDACi) without inducing host cell activation (such as valproic acid [VPA], suberoylanilide hydroxamic acid [SAHA]) [143–145]. However, the first approach has been shown to cause serious cytotoxic effects, while PKC agonists and HDACi are speculated to cause global gene expression activation with unpredictable side effects. Thus, an HIV-1 provirus-specific activating reagent is ideal for purging the latent reservoir. Our study demonstrated that the HIV-1-encoded miRNA miR-H3 could activate HIV-1 transcription in a sequence-specific manner [77] (Fig. 1K). Together with our previous findings that some cellular miRNAs contribute to the latency of HIV-1 by inhibiting HIV-1 production [46], a combination of the HIV-1 TATA box-targeting small RNA(s) and the inhibitors of these cellular miRNAs could provide an HIV-1-specific and much safer approach for activating and eradicating the HIV-1 latent reservoir [146]. In addition, lncRNAs could also be good candidates for activating HIV-1 latency. The depletion of NRON, especially in combination with a histone deacetylase (HDAC) inhibitor, significantly reactivates viral production from HIV-1-latently infected primary CD4+ T lymphocytes [132]. Collectively, our data demonstrate that non-coding RNAs could be used for the development of more effective and virus-specific latency-reversing agents [146]. Considering the significant sequence variations among different strains of retrovirus, such as HIV-1, even within a single infected individual [147], the efficacy of single small ncRNA, e.g. siRNA or miRNA, targeting the viral transcripts must vary as well. A combination of small ncRNAs that target multiple conservative sites of the viral sequence will prevent the rise of escape mutants. Moreover, the delivery efficiency of ncRNAs to infected cells needs to be further improved in the future.

Conclusion and future perspectives

Recent advances in the study of ncRNAs have greatly improved our understanding of retroviral replication, pathogenesis, and evasion from the host immune surveillance. The advent of next-generation sequencing technology, in particular, has completely changed the field of non-coding RNA research. The NGS has two main advantages compared to the classic Sanger sequencing: (1) depth, the NGS is also called deep-sequencing due to its capability to capture extreme low profiling RNA transcripts; (2) accuracy, NGS can provide both quantitative expression data (reads) and the sequence of individual RNA molecules. The successful applications of NGS in retrovirus ncRNA research have been proven by the identification of retrovirus-derived small ncRNAs [129, 130] and host small RNAs packaged into viral particles [45]. Moreover, NGS-based novel technologies such as ChIP-Seq (Chromatin ImmunoPrecipitation-sequencing) and CLIP-Seq (CrossLinking Immuno-Precipitation-sequencing) are powerful for functional analysis of non-coding RNAs [148, 149]. However, when NGS is used to study ncRNAs in a retrovirus system, some precautions need to be taken: (1) it is important to distinguish "noise" and "signal", as many low- or even high-abundant RNAs are random degradation products instead of functional molecules. In such cases, functional assays must be conducted carefully with a variety of independent approaches [77]. (2) The usage of different cell types, different protocols of viral infection such as viral titer, infection time etc., will result in differing NGS data. Therefore, the comparison of NGS data from heterogeneous sample preparations is a reliable way to identify retrovirus-derived ncRNAs and infer their roles in viral infection [123].

The study of non-coding RNAs in the retrovirus system has revealed a whole new layer of viral replication and virus–host interactions. The reports cited in this review have shown that ncRNAs are involved in the key steps of the retroviral life cycle, especially during the late phase of infection: viral transcription, translation, and assembly, as well as latency and pathogenesis (Fig. 1, Tables 1, 2). In contrast, much less is known about the roles of ncRNAs in the early phase of the retrovirus life cycle, which deserve further investigation. The increasing understanding of ncRNAs and their interactions with retroviruses will eventually benefit the therapy of retrovirus-related diseases.

Authors' contributions
YZ and HZ conceived the paper. XZ, XM, SJ and YZ wrote the manuscript, under the guidance of HZ. YZ prepared the figure. All authors read and approved the final manuscript.

Author details
[1] Institute of Human Virology, Zhongshan School of Medicine, Sun Yat-Sen University, Guangzhou 510080, China. [2] Key Laboratory of Tropical Disease Control of Ministry of Education, Zhongshan School of Medicine, Sun Yat-Sen University, Guangzhou 510080, China. [3] Guangdong Engineering Research Center for Antimicrobial Agent and Immunotechnology, Zhongshan School of Medicine, Sun Yat-Sen University, Guangzhou 510080, China. [4] Section of Infectious Diseases, Department of Internal Medicine, Yale University School of Medicine, New Haven, CT 06520, USA.

Competing interests
The authors declare that they have no competing interests.

Funding
This work was funded by Natural Science Foundation of China (NSFC)-NIH of US Project (No. 81561128007), Key Project of NSFC (No. 81730060), Guangdong Innovative Research Team Program (No. 2009010058), and the Joint-innovation Program in Healthcare for Special Scientific Research Projects of Guangzhou, China (201508020256) to HZ.

References
1. Coffin JM. Genetic diversity and evolution of retroviruses. Curr Top Microbiol Immunol. 1992;176:143–64.
2. Coffin JM, Hughes SH, Varmus HE, editors. Retroviruses. Cold Spring Harbor: Cold Spring Harbor Laboratory Press; 1997.
3. Chun TW, Stuyver L, Mizell SB, Ehler LA, Mican JA, Baseler M, Lloyd AL, Nowak MA, Fauci AS. Presence of an inducible HIV-1 latent reservoir during highly active antiretroviral therapy. Proc Natl Acad Sci USA. 1997;94:13193–7.
4. Nisole S, Saib A. Early steps of retrovirus replicative cycle. Retrovirology. 2004;1:9.
5. Siliciano RF, Greene WC. HIV latency. Cold Spring Harb Perspect Med. 2011;1:a007096.
6. Goff SP. Host factors exploited by retroviruses. Nat Rev Microbiol. 2007;5:253–63.
7. Cullen BR. The virology-RNA biology connection. RNA. 2015;21:592–4.
8. Miura K, Watanabe K, Sugiura M, Shatkin AJ. The 5'-terminal nucleotide sequences of the double-stranded RNA of human reovirus. Proc Natl Acad Sci USA. 1974;71:3979–83.
9. Berget SM, Moore C, Sharp PA. Spliced segments at the 5' terminus of adenovirus 2 late mRNA. Proc Natl Acad Sci USA. 1977;74:3171–5.
10. Schmitt P, Gattoni R, Keohavong P, Stevenin J. Alternative splicing of E1A transcripts of adenovirus requires appropriate ionic conditions in vitro. Cell. 1987;50:31–9.
11. Malim MH, Hauber J, Le SY, Maizel JV, Cullen BR. The HIV-1 rev trans-activator acts through a structured target sequence to activate nuclear export of unspliced viral mRNA. Nature. 1989;338:254–7.
12. Fischer U, Huber J, Boelens WC, Mattaj IW, Luhrmann R. The HIV-1 Rev activation domain is a nuclear export signal that accesses an export pathway used by specific cellular RNAs. Cell. 1995;82:475–83.
13. Consortium EP. An integrated encyclopedia of DNA elements in the human genome. Nature. 2012;489:57–74.
14. Eddy SR. Non-coding RNA genes and the modern RNA world. Nat Rev Genet. 2001;2:919–29.
15. Mattick JS, Makunin IV. Non-coding RNA. Hum Mol Genet. 2006;15(Spec No 1):R17–29.
16. Voinnet O. Induction and suppression of RNA silencing: insights from viral infections. Nat Rev Genet. 2005;6:206–20.
17. Umbach JL, Cullen BR. The role of RNAi and microRNAs in animal virus replication and antiviral immunity. Genes Dev. 2009;23:1151–64.
18. Rand TA, Petersen S, Du F, Wang X. Argonaute2 cleaves the anti-guide strand of siRNA during RISC activation. Cell. 2005;123:621–9.
19. Aoki K, Moriguchi H, Yoshioka T, Okawa K, Tabara H. In vitro analyses of the production and activity of secondary small interfering RNAs in C. elegans. EMBO J. 2007;26:5007–19.
20. Diaz-Pendon JA, Li F, Li WX, Ding SW. Suppression of antiviral silencing by cucumber mosaic virus 2b protein in Arabidopsis is associated with drastically reduced accumulation of three classes of viral small interfering RNAs. Plant Cell. 2007;19:2053–63.
21. Sen GC. Viruses and interferons. Annu Rev Microbiol. 2001;55:255–81.
22. Bartel DP. MicroRNAs: genomics, biogenesis, mechanism, and function. Cell. 2004;116:281–97.
23. Bushati N, Cohen SM. microRNA functions. Annu Rev Cell Dev Biol. 2007;23:175–205.
24. Lee Y, Ahn C, Han J, Choi H, Kim J, Yim J, Lee J, Provost P, Radmark O, Kim S, Kim VN. The nuclear RNase III Drosha initiates microRNA processing. Nature. 2003;425:415–9.

25. Yi R, Qin Y, Macara IG, Cullen BR. Exportin-5 mediates the nuclear export of pre-microRNAs and short hairpin RNAs. Genes Dev. 2003;17:3011–6.

26. Hutvagner G, McLachlan J, Pasquinelli AE, Balint E, Tuschl T, Zamore PD. A cellular function for the RNA-interference enzyme Dicer in the maturation of the let-7 small temporal RNA. Science. 2001;293:834–8.

27. Gregory RI, Chendrimada TP, Cooch N, Shiekhattar R. Human RISC couples microRNA biogenesis and posttranscriptional gene silencing. Cell. 2005;123:631–40.

28. Lytle JR, Yario TA, Steitz JA. Target mRNAs are repressed as efficiently by microRNA-binding sites in the 5′ UTR as in the 3′ UTR. Proc Natl Acad Sci USA. 2007;104:9667–72.

29. Tay Y, Zhang J, Thomson AM, Lim B, Rigoutsos I. MicroRNAs to Nanog, Oct4 and Sox2 coding regions modulate embryonic stem cell differentiation. Nature. 2008;455:1124–8.

30. Orom UA, Nielsen FC, Lund AH. MicroRNA-10a binds the 5′ UTR of ribosomal protein mRNAs and enhances their translation. Mol Cell. 2008;30:460–71.

31. Vasudevan S, Tong Y, Steitz JA. Switching from repression to activation: microRNAs can up-regulate translation. Science. 2007;318:1931–4.

32. Zhang Y, Zhang H. RNAa induced by TATA box-targeting MicroRNAs. Adv Exp Med Biol. 2017;983:91–111.

33. Gagnon KT, Corey DR. Argonaute and the nuclear RNAs: new pathways for RNA-mediated control of gene expression. Nucleic Acid Ther. 2012;22:3–16.

34. Portnoy V, Huang V, Place RF, Li LC. Small RNA and transcriptional upregulation. Wiley Interdiscip Rev RNA. 2011;2:748–60.

35. Li LC. Small RNA-guided transcriptional gene activation (RNAa) in mammalian cells. Adv Exp Med Biol. 2017;983:1–20.

36. Harrow J, Frankish A, Gonzalez JM, Tapanari E, Diekhans M, Kokocinski F, Aken BL, Barrell D, Zadissa A, Searle S, et al. GENCODE: the reference human genome annotation for The ENCODE Project. Genome Res. 2012;22:1760–74.

37. Rinn JL, Chang HY. Genome regulation by long noncoding RNAs. Annu Rev Biochem. 2012;81:145–66.

38. Wutz A. Gene silencing in X-chromosome inactivation: advances in understanding facultative heterochromatin formation. Nat Rev Genet. 2011;12:542–53.

39. Li Y, Syed J, Sugiyama H. RNA-DNA triplex formation by long noncoding RNAs. Cell Chem Biol. 2016;23:1325–33.

40. Yang Z, Zhou L, Wu LM, Lai MC, Xie HY, Zhang F, Zheng SS. Overexpression of long non-coding RNA HOTAIR predicts tumor recurrence in hepatocellular carcinoma patients following liver transplantation. Ann Surg Oncol. 2011;18:1243–50.

41. Kogo R, Shimamura T, Mimori K, Kawahara K, Imoto S, Sudo T, Tanaka F, Shibata K, Suzuki A, Komune S, et al. Long noncoding RNA HOTAIR regulates polycomb-dependent chromatin modification and is associated with poor prognosis in colorectal cancers. Cancer Res. 2011;71:6320–6.

42. Gupta RA, Shah N, Wang KC, Kim J, Horlings HM, Wong DJ, Tsai MC, Hung T, Argani P, Rinn JL, et al. Long non-coding RNA HOTAIR reprograms chromatin state to promote cancer metastasis. Nature. 2010;464:1071–6.

43. Turchinovich A, Weiz L, Langheinz A, Burwinkel B. Characterization of extracellular circulating microRNA. Nucleic Acids Res. 2011;39:7223–33.

44. Prensner JR, Iyer MK, Balbin OA, Dhanasekaran SM, Cao Q, Brenner JC, Laxman B, Asangani IA, Grasso CS, Kominsky HD, et al. Transcriptome sequencing across a prostate cancer cohort identifies PCAT-1, an unannotated lincRNA implicated in disease progression. Nat Biotechnol. 2011;29:742–9.

45. Schopman NC, van Montfort T, Willemsen M, Knoepfel SA, Pollakis G, van Kampen A, Sanders RW, Haasnoot J, Berkhout B. Selective packaging of cellular miRNAs in HIV-1 particles. Virus Res. 2012;169:438–47.

46. Huang J, Wang F, Argyris E, Chen K, Liang Z, Tian H, Huang W, Squires K, Verlinghieri G, Zhang H. Cellular microRNAs contribute to HIV-1 latency in resting primary CD4+ T lymphocytes. Nat Med. 2007;13:1241–7.

47. Labbaye C, Spinello I, Quaranta MT, Pelosi E, Pasquini L, Petrucci E, Biffoni M, Nuzzolo ER, Billi M, Foa R, et al. A three-step pathway comprising PLZF/miR-146a/CXCR4 controls megakaryopoiesis. Nat Cell Biol. 2008;10:788–801.

48. Quaranta MT, Olivetta E, Sanchez M, Spinello I, Paolillo R, Arenaccio C, Federico M, Labbaye C. miR-146a controls CXCR4 expression in a pathway that involves PLZF and can be used to inhibit HIV-1 infection of CD4(+) T lymphocytes. Virology. 2015;478:27–38.

49. Reynoso R, Laufer N, Hackl M, Skalicky S, Monteforte R, Turk G, Carobene M, Quarleri J, Cahn P, Werner R, et al. MicroRNAs differentially present in the plasma of HIV elite controllers reduce HIV infection in vitro. Sci Rep. 2014;4:5915.

50. Zhang H, Dornadula G, Orenstein J, Pomerantz RJ. Morphologic changes in human immunodeficiency virus type 1 virions secondary to intravirion reverse transcription: evidence indicating that reverse transcription may not take place within the intact viral core. J Hum Virol. 2000;3:165–72.

51. Hu WS, Hughes SH. HIV-1 reverse transcription. Cold Spring Harb Perspect Med. 2012;2:a006882.

52. Qi M, Yang R, Aiken C. Cyclophilin A-dependent restriction of human immunodeficiency virus type 1 capsid mutants for infection of nondividing cells. J Virol. 2008;82:12001–8.

53. Yamashita M, Emerman M. Capsid is a dominant determinant of retrovirus infectivity in nondividing cells. J Virol. 2004;78:5670–8.

54. Braaten D, Franke EK, Luban J. Cyclophilin A is required for an early step in the life cycle of human immunodeficiency virus type 1 before the initiation of reverse transcription. J Virol. 1996;70:3551–60.

55. Zhang H, Yang B, Pomerantz RJ, Zhang C, Arunachalam SC, Gao L. The cytidine deaminase CEM15 induces hypermutation in newly synthesized HIV-1 DNA. Nature. 2003;424:94–8.

56. Huang J, Liang Z, Yang B, Tian H, Ma J, Zhang H. Derepression of microRNA-mediated protein translation inhibition by apolipoprotein B mRNA-editing enzyme catalytic polypeptide-like 3G (APOBEC3G) and its family members. J Biol Chem. 2007;282:33632–40.

57. Liu C, Zhang X, Huang F, Yang B, Li J, Liu B, Luo H, Zhang P, Zhang H. APOBEC3G inhibits microRNA-mediated repression of translation by interfering with the interaction between Argonaute-2 and MOV10. J Biol Chem. 2012;287:29373–83.

58. Llano M, Saenz DT, Meehan A, Wongthida P, Peretz M, Walker WH, Teo W, Poeschla EM. An essential role for LEDGF/p75 in HIV integration. Science. 2006;314:461–4.

59. Cherepanov P, Maertens G, Proost P, Devreese B, Van Beeumen J, Engelborghs Y, De Clercq E, Debyser Z. HIV-1 integrase forms stable tetramers and associates with LEDGF/p75 protein in human cells. J Biol Chem. 2003;278:372–81.

60. Swaminathan G, Rossi F, Sierra LJ, Gupta A, Navas-Martin S, Martin-Garcia J. A role for microRNA-155 modulation in the anti-HIV-1 effects of Toll-like receptor 3 stimulation in macrophages. PLoS Pathog. 2012;8:e1002937.

61. Ocwieja KE, Sherrill-Mix S, Mukherjee R, Custers-Allen R, David P, Brown M, Wang S, Link DR, Olson J, Travers K, et al. Dynamic regulation of HIV-1 mRNA populations analyzed by single-molecule enrichment and long-read sequencing. Nucleic Acids Res. 2012;40:10345–55.

62. Pfeffer S, Zavolan M, Grasser FA, Chien M, Russo JJ, Ju J, John B, Enright AJ, Marks D, Sander C, Tuschl T. Identification of virus-encoded microRNAs. Science. 2004;304:734–6.

63. Pfeffer S, Sewer A, Lagos-Quintana M, Sheridan R, Sander C, Grasser FA, van Dyk LF, Ho CK, Shuman S, Chien M, et al. Identification of microRNAs of the herpesvirus family. Nat Methods. 2005;2:269–76.

64. Klase ZA, Sampey GC, Kashanchi F. Retrovirus infected cells contain viral microRNAs. Retrovirology. 2013;10:15.

65. Schopman NC, Willemsen M, Liu YP, Bradley T, van Kampen A, Baas F, Berkhout B, Haasnoot J. Deep sequencing of virus-infected cells reveals HIV-encoded small RNAs. Nucleic Acids Res. 2012;40:414–27.

66. Kincaid RP, Burke JM, Sullivan CS. RNA virus microRNA that mimics a B-cell oncomiR. Proc Natl Acad Sci USA. 2012;109:3077–82.

67. Hussain M, Torres S, Schnettler E, Funk A, Grundhoff A, Pijlman GP, Khromykh AA, Asgari S. West Nile virus encodes a microRNA-like small RNA in the 3′ untranslated region which up-regulates GATA4 mRNA and facilitates virus replication in mosquito cells. Nucleic Acids Res. 2012;40:2210–23.

68. Bennasser Y, Le SY, Yeung ML, Jeang KT. HIV-1 encoded candidate micro-RNAs and their cellular targets. Retrovirology. 2004;1:43.

69. Klase Z, Kale P, Winograd R, Gupta MV, Heydarian M, Berro R, McCaffrey T, Kashanchi F. HIV-1 TAR element is processed by Dicer to yield a viral micro-RNA involved in chromatin remodeling of the viral LTR. BMC Mol Biol. 2007;8:63.

70. Ouellet DL, Plante I, Landry P, Barat C, Janelle ME, Flamand L, Tremblay MJ, Provost P. Identification of functional microRNAs released through asymmetrical processing of HIV-1 TAR element. Nucleic Acids Res. 2008;36:2353–65.

71. Klase Z, Winograd R, Davis J, Carpio L, Hildreth R, Heydarian M, Fu S, McCaffrey T, Meiri E, Ayash-Rashkovsky M, et al. HIV-1 TAR miRNA protects against apoptosis by altering cellular gene expression. Retrovirology. 2009;6:18.

72. Omoto S, Ito M, Tsutsumi Y, Ichikawa Y, Okuyama H, Brisibe EA, Saksena NK, Fujii YR. HIV-1 nef suppression by virally encoded microRNA. Retrovirology. 2004;1:44.

73. Schopman NC, Willemsen M, Liu YP, Bradley T, van Kampen A, Baas F, Berkhout B, Haasnoot J. Deep sequencing of virus-infected cells reveals HIV-encoded small RNAs. Nucleic Acids Res. 2011;40:414–27.

74. Yeung ML, Bennasser Y, Watashi K, Le SY, Houzet L, Jeang KT. Pyrosequencing of small non-coding RNAs in HIV-1 infected cells: evidence for the processing of a viral-cellular double-stranded RNA hybrid. Nucleic Acids Res. 2009;37:6575–86.

75. Harwig A, Jongejan A, van Kampen AH, Berkhout B, Das AT. Tat-dependent production of an HIV-1 TAR-encoded miRNA-like small RNA. Nucleic Acids Res. 2016;44(9):4340–53.

76. Ouellet DL, Vigneault-Edwards J, Letourneau K, Gobeil LA, Plante I, Burnett JC, Rossi JJ, Provost P. Regulation of host gene expression by HIV-1 TAR microRNAs. Retrovirology. 2013;10:86.

77. Zhang Y, Fan M, Geng G, Liu B, Huang Z, Luo H, Zhou J, Guo X, Cai W, Zhang H. A novel HIV-1-encoded microRNA enhances its viral replication by targeting the TATA box region. Retrovirology. 2014;11:23.

78. Zhang Y, Fan M, Zhang X, Huang F, Wu K, Zhang J, Liu J, Huang Z, Luo H, Tao L, Zhang H. Cellular microRNAs up-regulate transcription via interaction with promoter TATA-box motifs. RNA. 2014;20:1878–89.

79. Watts JM, Dang KK, Gorelick RJ, Leonard CW, Bess JW Jr, Swanstrom R, Burch CL, Weeks KM. Architecture and secondary structure of an entire HIV-1 RNA genome. Nature. 2009;460:711–6.

80. Harwig A, Das AT, Berkhout B. HIV-1 RNAs: sense and antisense, large mRNAs and small siRNAs and miRNAs. Curr Opin HIV AIDS. 2015;10:103–9.

81. Ludwig LB, Ambrus JL Jr, Krawczyk KA, Sharma S, Brooks S, Hsiao CB, Schwartz SA. Human immunodeficiency virus-type 1 LTR DNA contains an intrinsic gene producing antisense RNA and protein products. Retrovirology. 2006;3:80.

82. Landry S, Halin M, Lefort S, Audet B, Vaquero C, Mesnard JM, Barbeau B. Detection, characterization and regulation of antisense transcripts in HIV-1. Retrovirology. 2007;4:71.

83. Kobayashi-Ishihara M, Yamagishi M, Hara T, Matsuda Y, Takahashi R, Miyake A, Nakano K, Yamochi T, Ishida T, Watanabe T. HIV-1-encoded antisense RNA suppresses viral replication for a prolonged period. Retrovirology. 2012;9:38.

84. Saayman S, Ackley A, Turner A-MW, Famiglietti M, Bosque A, Clemson M, Planelles V, Morris KV. An HIV-encoded antisense long noncoding RNA epigenetically regulates viral transcription. Mol Ther. 2014;22:1164–75.

85. Whisnant AW, Kehl T, Bao Q, Materniak M, Kuzmak J, Lochelt M, Cullen BR. Identification of novel, highly expressed retroviral microRNAs in cells infected by bovine foamy virus. J Virol. 2014;88:4679–86.

86. Yao Y, Smith LP, Nair V, Watson M. An avian retrovirus uses canonical expression and processing mechanisms to generate viral microRNA. J Virol. 2014;88:2–9.

87. Kapusta A, Feschotte C. Volatile evolution of long noncoding RNA repertoires: mechanisms and biological implications. Trends Genet. 2014;30:439–52.

88. Johnson R, Guigo R. The RIDL hypothesis: transposable elements as functional domains of long noncoding RNAs. RNA. 2014;20:959–76.

89. Kapusta A, Kronenberg Z, Lynch VJ, Zhuo X, Ramsay L, Bourque G, Yandell M, Feschotte C. Transposable elements are major contributors to the origin, diversification, and regulation of vertebrate long noncoding RNAs. PLoS Genet. 2013;9:e1003470.

90. Santoni FA, Guerra J, Luban J. HERV-H RNA is abundant in human embryonic stem cells and a precise marker for pluripotency. Retrovirology. 2012;9:111.

91. Wang J, Xie G, Singh M, Ghanbarian AT, Rasko T, Szvetnik A, Cai H, Besser D, Prigione A, Fuchs NV, et al. Primate-specific endogenous

92. retrovirus-driven transcription defines naive-like stem cells. Nature. 2014;516:405–9.

92. Kelley D, Rinn J. Transposable elements reveal a stem cell-specific class of long noncoding RNAs. Genome Biol. 2012;13:R107.

93. Lu X, Sachs F, Ramsay L, Jacques PE, Goke J, Bourque G, Ng HH. The retrovirus HERVH is a long noncoding RNA required for human embryonic stem cell identity. Nat Struct Mol Biol. 2014;21:423–5.

94. Gibb EA, Warren RL, Wilson GW, Brown SD, Robertson GA, Morin GB, Holt RA. Activation of an endogenous retrovirus-associated long noncoding RNA in human adenocarcinoma. Genome Med. 2015;7(1):22.

95. Poiesz BJ, Ruscetti FW, Gazdar AF, Bunn PA, Minna JD, Gallo RC. Detection and isolation of type C retrovirus particles from fresh and cultured lymphocytes of a patient with cutaneous T-cell lymphoma. Proc Natl Acad Sci USA. 1980;77:7415–9.

96. Mesnard JM, Barbeau B, Devaux C. HBZ, a new important player in the mystery of adult T-cell leukemia. Blood. 2006;108:3979–82.

97. Satou Y, Yasunaga J, Yoshida M, Matsuoka M. HTLV-I basic leucine zipper factor gene mRNA supports proliferation of adult T cell leukemia cells. Proc Natl Acad Sci USA. 2006;103:720–5.

98. Rende F, Cavallari I, Corradin A, Silic-Benussi M, Toulza F, Toffolo GM, Tanaka Y, Jacobson S, Taylor GP, D'Agostino DM, et al. Kinetics and intracellular compartmentalization of HTLV-1 gene expression: nuclear retention of HBZ mRNAs. Blood. 2011;117:4855–9.

99. Zhou H, Xu M, Huang Q, Gates AT, Zhang XD, Castle JC, Stec E, Ferrer M, Strulovici B, Hazuda DJ, Espeseth AS. Genome-scale RNAi screen for host factors required for HIV replication. Cell Host Microbe. 2008;4:495–504.

100. Brass AL, Dykxhoorn DM, Benita Y, Yan N, Engelman A, Xavier RJ, Lieberman J, Elledge SJ. Identification of host proteins required for HIV infection through a functional genomic screen. Science. 2008;319:921–6.

101. Wei P, Garber ME, Fang SM, Fischer WH, Jones KA. A novel CDK9-associated C-type cyclin interacts directly with HIV-1 Tat and mediates its high-affinity, loop-specific binding to TAR RNA. Cell. 1998;92:451–62.

102. Sung TL, Rice AP. miR-198 inhibits HIV-1 gene expression and replication in monocytes and its mechanism of action appears to involve repression of cyclin T1. PLoS Pathog. 2009;5:e1000263.

103. Barichievy S, Naidoo J, Mhlanga MM. Non-coding RNAs and HIV: viral manipulation of host dark matter to shape the cellular environment. Front Genet. 2015;6:108.

104. Zhang Q, Chen CY, Yedavalli VS, Jeang KT. NEAT1 long noncoding RNA and paraspeckle bodies modulate HIV-1 posttranscriptional expression. MBio. 2013;4:e00596-00512.

105. Hutchinson JN, Ensminger AW, Clemson CM, Lynch CR, Lawrence JB, Chess A. A screen for nuclear transcripts identifies two linked noncoding RNAs associated with SC35 splicing domains. BMC Genom. 2007;8:39.

106. Clemson CM, Hutchinson JN, Sara SA, Ensminger AW, Fox AH, Chess A, Lawrence JB. An architectural role for a nuclear noncoding RNA: NEAT1 RNA is essential for the structure of paraspeckles. Mol Cell. 2009;33:717–26.

107. Hirose T, Virnicchi G, Tanigawa A, Naganuma T, Li R, Kimura H, Yokoi T, Nakagawa S, Benard M, Fox AH, Pierron G. NEAT1 long noncoding RNA regulates transcription via protein sequestration within subnuclear bodies. Mol Biol Cell. 2014;25:169–83.

108. Zolotukhin AS, Michalowski D, Bear J, Smulevitch SV, Traish AM, Peng R, Patton J, Shatsky IN, Felber BK. PSF acts through the human immunodeficiency virus type 1 mRNA instability elements to regulate virus expression. Mol Cell Biol. 2003;23:6618–30.

109. Yedavalli VS, Jeang KT. Matrin 3 is a co-factor for HIV-1 Rev in regulating post-transcriptional viral gene expression. Retrovirology. 2011;8:61.

110. Budhiraja S, Liu H, Couturier J, Malovannaya A, Qin J, Lewis DE, Rice AP. Mining the human complexome database identifies RBM14 as an XPO1-associated protein involved in HIV-1 Rev function. J Virol. 2015;89:3557–67.

111. Nguyen VT, Kiss T, Michels AA, Bensaude O. 7SK small nuclear RNA binds to and inhibits the activity of CDK9/cyclin T complexes. Nature. 2001;414:322–5.

112. Yang S, Sun Y, Zhang H. The multimerization of human immunodeficiency virus type I Vif protein: a requirement for Vif function in the viral life cycle. J Biol Chem. 2001;276:4889–93.

113. Mancebo HS, Lee G, Flygare J, Tomassini J, Luu P, Zhu Y, Peng J, Blau C, Hazuda D, Price D, Flores O. P-TEFb kinase is required for HIV Tat transcriptional activation in vivo and in vitro. Genes Dev. 1997;11:2633–44.

114. Triboulet R, Mari B, Lin YL, Chable-Bessia C, Bennasser Y, Lebrigand K, Cardinaud B, Maurin T, Barbry P, Baillat V, et al. Suppression of microRNA-silencing pathway by HIV-1 during virus replication. Science. 2007;315:1579–82.

115. Yeung ML, Bennasser Y, Myers TG, Jiang G, Benkirane M, Jeang KT. Changes in microRNA expression profiles in HIV-1-transfected human cells. Retrovirology. 2005;2:81.

116. Houzet L, Yeung ML, de Lame V, Desai D, Smith SM, Jeang KT. MicroRNA profile changes in human immunodeficiency virus type 1 (HIV-1) seropositive individuals. Retrovirology. 2008;5:118.

117. Bennasser Y, Le SY, Benkirane M, Jeang KT. Evidence that HIV-1 encodes an siRNA and a suppressor of RNA silencing. Immunity. 2005;22:607–19.

118. Chendrimada TP, Gregory RI, Kumaraswamy E, Norman J, Cooch N, Nishikura K, Shiekhattar R. TRBP recruits the Dicer complex to Ago2 for microRNA processing and gene silencing. Nature. 2005;436:740–4.

119. Hariharan M, Scaria V, Pillai B, Brahmachari SK. Targets for human encoded microRNAs in HIV genes. Biochem Biophys Res Commun. 2005;337:1214–8.

120. Ahluwalia JK, Khan SZ, Soni K, Rawat P, Gupta A, Hariharan M, Scaria V, Lalwani M, Pillai B, Mitra D, Brahmachari SK. Human cellular microRNA hsa-miR-29a interferes with viral nef protein expression and HIV-1 replication. Retrovirology. 2008;5:117.

121. Sun G, Li H, Wu X, Covarrubias M, Scherer L, Meinking K, Luk B, Chomchan P, Alluin J, Gombart AF, Rossi JJ. Interplay between HIV-1 infection and host microRNAs. Nucleic Acids Res. 2012;40:2181–96.

122. Houzet L, Klase Z, Yeung ML, Wu A, Le SY, Quinones M, Jeang KT. The extent of sequence complementarity correlates with the potency of cellular miRNA-mediated restriction of HIV-1. Nucleic Acids Res. 2012;40:11684–96.

123. Whisnant AW, Bogerd HP, Flores O, Ho P, Powers JG, Sharova N, Stevenson M, Chen CH, Cullen BR. In-depth analysis of the interaction of HIV-1 with cellular microRNA biogenesis and effector mechanisms. MBio. 2013;4:e000193.

124. Bishop JM, Levinson WE, Quintrell N, Sullivan D, Fanshier L, Jackson J. The low molecular weight RNAs of Rous sarcoma virus. I. The 4 S RNA. Virology. 1970;42:182–95.

125. Telesnitsky A, Wolin SL. The host RNAs in retroviral particles. Viruses. 2016;8:235.

126. Huang Y, Mak J, Cao Q, Li Z, Wainberg MA, Kleiman L. Incorporation of excess wild-type and mutant tRNA(3Lys) into human immunodeficiency virus type 1. J Virol. 1994;68:7676–83.

127. Onafuwa-Nuga AA, Telesnitsky A, King SR. 7SL RNA, but not the 54-kd signal recognition particle protein, is an abundant component of both infectious HIV-1 and minimal virus-like particles. RNA. 2006;12:542–6.

128. Wang T, Tian C, Zhang W, Luo K, Sarkis PT, Yu L, Liu B, Yu Y, Yu XF. 7SL RNA mediates virion packaging of the antiviral cytidine deaminase APOBEC3G. J Virol. 2007;81:13112–24.

129. Eckwahl MJ, Arnion H, Kharytonchyk S, Zang T, Bieniasz PD, Telesnitsky A, Wolin SL. Analysis of the human immunodeficiency virus-1 RNA packageome. RNA. 2016;22:1228–38.

130. Eckwahl MJ, Sim S, Smith D, Telesnitsky A, Wolin SL. A retrovirus packages nascent host noncoding RNAs from a novel surveillance pathway. Genes Dev. 2015;29:646–57.

131. Bogerd HP, Kennedy EM, Whisnant AW, Cullen BR. Induced packaging of cellular MicroRNAs into HIV-1 virions can inhibit infectivity. MBio. 2017;8(1):e02125–16.

132. Li J, Chen C, Ma X, Geng G, Liu B, Zhang Y, Zhang S, Zhong F, Liu C, Yin Y, et al. Long noncoding RNA NRON contributes to HIV-1 latency by specifically inducing tat protein degradation. Nat Commun. 2016;7:11730.

133. Romanchikova N, Ivanova V, Scheller C, Jankevics E, Jassoy C, Serfling E. NFAT transcription factors control HIV-1 expression through a binding site downstream of TAR region. Immunobiology. 2003;208:361–5.

134. Willingham AT, Orth AP, Batalov S, Peters EC, Wen BG, Aza-Blanc P, Hogenesch JB, Schultz PG. A strategy for probing the function of noncoding RNAs finds a repressor of NFAT. Science. 2005;309:1570–3.

135. Imam H, Bano AS, Patel P, Holla P, Jameel S. The lncRNA NRON modulates HIV-1 replication in a NFAT-dependent manner and is differentially regulated by early and late viral proteins. Sci Rep. 2015;5:8639.

136. Zapata JC, Campilongo F, Barclay RA, DeMarino C, Iglesias-Ussel MD, Kashanchi F, Romerio F. The human immunodeficiency virus 1 ASP RNA promotes viral latency by recruiting the Polycomb Repressor Complex 2 and promoting nucleosome assembly. Virology. 2017;506:34–44.

137. Zhang Y, Yin Y, Zhang S, Luo H, Zhang H. HIV-1 infection-induced suppression of the Let-7i/IL-2 axis contributes to CD4+ T cell death. Sci Rep. 2016;6:25341.

138. Rosewick N, Momont M, Durkin K, Takeda H, Caiment F, Cleuter Y, Vernin C, Mortreux F, Wattel E, Burny A, et al. Deep sequencing reveals abundant noncanonical retroviral microRNAs in B-cell leukemia/lymphoma. Proc Natl Acad Sci USA. 2013;110:2306–11.

139. Deeks SG. HIV: shock and kill. Nature. 2012;487:439–40.

140. Manninen A, Renkema GH, Saksela K. Synergistic activation of NFAT by HIV-1 nef and the Ras/MAPK pathway. J Biol Chem. 2000;275:16513–7.

141. Chun TW, Engel D, Mizell SB, Hallahan CW, Fischette M, Park S, Davey RT Jr, Dybul M, Kovacs JA, Metcalf JA, et al. Effect of interleukin-2 on the pool of latently infected, resting CD4+ T cells in HIV-1-infected patients receiving highly active anti-retroviral therapy. Nat Med. 1999;5:651–5.

142. Kulkosky J, Culnan DM, Roman J, Dornadula G, Schnell M, Boyd MR, Pomerantz RJ. Prostratin: activation of latent HIV-1 expression suggests a potential inductive adjuvant therapy for HAART. Blood. 2001;98:3006–15.

143. Ylisastigui L, Archin NM, Lehrman G, Bosch RJ, Margolis DM. Coaxing HIV-1 from resting CD4 T cells: histone deacetylase inhibition allows latent viral expression. AIDS. 2004;18:1101–8.

144. Archin NM, Espeseth A, Parker D, Cheema M, Hazuda D, Margolis DM. Expression of latent HIV induced by the potent HDAC inhibitor suberoylanilide hydroxamic acid. AIDS Res Hum Retrovir. 2009;25:207–12.

145. Contreras X, Schweneker M, Chen CS, McCune JM, Deeks SG, Martin J, Peterlin BM. Suberoylanilide hydroxamic acid reactivates HIV from latently infected cells. J Biol Chem. 2009;284:6782–9.

146. Zhang H. Reversal of HIV-1 latency with anti-microRNA inhibitors. Int J Biochem Cell Biol. 2009;41:451–4.

147. Bandaranayake RM, Kolli M, King NM, Nalivaika EA, Heroux A, Kakizawa J, Sugiura W, Schiffer CA. The effect of clade-specific sequence polymorphisms on HIV-1 protease activity and inhibitor resistance pathways. J Virol. 2010;84:9995–10003.

148. Yang JH, Li JH, Shao P, Zhou H, Chen YQ, Qu LH. starBase: a database for exploring microRNA–mRNA interaction maps from Argonaute CLIP-Seq and Degradome-Seq data. Nucleic Acids Res. 2011;39:D202–9.

149. van Dijk EL, Auger H, Jaszczyszyn Y, Thermes C. Ten years of next-generation sequencing technology. Trends Genet. 2014;30:418–26.

11

Inhibitors of the integrase–transportin-SR2 interaction block HIV nuclear import

Jonas Demeulemeester[1,4†] ⓘ, Jolien Blokken[1†], Stéphanie De Houwer[1], Lieve Dirix[1], Hugo Klaassen[2], Arnaud Marchand[2], Patrick Chaltin[2,3], Frauke Christ[1] and Zeger Debyser[1*] ⓘ

Abstract

Background: Combination antiretroviral therapy efficiently suppresses HIV replication in infected patients, transforming HIV/AIDS into a chronic disease. Viral resistance does develop however, especially under suboptimal treatment conditions such as poor adherence. As a consequence, continued exploration of novel targets is paramount to identify novel antivirals that do not suffer from cross-resistance with existing drugs. One new promising class of targets are HIV protein–cofactor interactions. Transportin-SR2 (TRN-SR2) is a β-karyopherin that was recently identified as an HIV-1 cofactor. It has been implicated in nuclear import of the viral pre-integration complex and was confirmed as a direct binding partner of HIV-1 integrase (IN). Nevertheless, consensus on its mechanism of action is yet to be reached.

Results: Here we describe the development and use of an AlphaScreen-based high-throughput screening cascade for small molecule inhibitors of the HIV-1 IN–TRN-SR2 interaction. False positives and nonspecific protein–protein interaction inhibitors were eliminated through different counterscreens. We identified and confirmed 2 active compound series from an initial screen of 25,608 small molecules. These compounds significantly reduced nuclear import of fluorescently labeled HIV particles.

Conclusions: Alphascreen-based high-throughput screening can allow the identification of compounds representing a novel class of HIV inhibitors. These results corroborate the role of the IN–TRN-SR2 interaction in nuclear import. These compounds represent the first in class small molecule inhibitors of HIV-1 nuclear import.

Keywords: Drug discovery, Integrase, Transportin-SR2, HIV, Nuclear import

Background

Control of human immunodeficiency virus type 1 (HIV-1) infection still poses considerable challenges. Viral resistance selection under suboptimal treatment conditions together with long-term adverse effects of chronic combination antiretroviral therapy (cART), highlight the need for novel antivirals with (1) a higher barrier towards resistance development, (2) pharmacokinetic properties allowing once-daily dosing and (3) less adverse effects. Novel targets, both viral and cellular, therefore need to be evaluated for their potential to be targeted with a small molecule in order to develop new classes of antivirals. HIV is characterized by its ability to stably integrate into the host cell genome and to infect both dividing and non-dividing cells [1]. As a result, the pre-integration complex (PIC) needs to be actively transported across the nuclear envelope. Integration into host cell chromatin is a complex process catalyzed by the viral integrase (IN). Once integration has been achieved, the fate of virus and host cell are irreversibly linked, highlighting this step as the point-of-no-return in the viral replication cycle.

*Correspondence: zeger.debyser@kuleuven.be

†Jonas Demeulemeester and Jolien Blokken shared first author

[1] Laboratory for Molecular Virology and Gene Therapy, Department of Pharmaceutical and Pharmacological Sciences, KU Leuven, Kapucijnenvoer 33, VCTB +5, Bus 7001, 3000 Leuven, Flanders, Belgium

Full list of author information is available at the end of the article

Due to technical issues such as poor in vitro solubility, IN was last of the three HIV enzymes to be targeted by cART. To date, three IN inhibitors have been approved for clinical use (raltegravir, elvitegravir and dolutegravir), all belonging to a class of catalytic site inhibitors known as integrase strand transfer inhibitors (INSTIs, see [2] for a recent review). As a consequence of their common mechanism of action these inhibitors suffer a significant degree of cross-resistance. Allosteric inhibitors potently blocking IN indirectly can circumvent cross-resistance in analogy to non-nucleoside reverse transcriptase inhibitors (NNRTIs) [3]. Of note, successful integration and completion of the viral replication cycle in general, are dependent on more than just the catalytic activity of IN but also on its multimerization dynamics and interplay with cellular cofactors such as LEDGF/p75 [4–8]. Screening for inhibitors of either the LEDGF/p75-IN interaction or the integrase 3'-processing reaction independently led to the discovery of a second class of IN inhibitors, LEDGINs (also referred to as non-catalytic site integrase inhibitors, NCINIs) [9, 10]. By binding the LEDGF/p75 binding site across the IN dimerization interface, LEDGINs not only block LEDGF/p75 binding but also perturb IN multimerization, which in turn leads to inhibited catalytic activity (both 3'processing and strand transfer) and aberrant viral maturation [4–7, 11, 12].

In 2008, another IN cofactor was identified, Transportin-SR2 (TRN-SR2, Tnpo3), encoded by the *TNPO3* gene. TRN-SR2 was picked up as a cellular cofactor of HIV-1 in two genome-wide siRNA screens [13, 14] and as a binding partner of HIV IN in a yeast two-hybrid screen [15]. Through q-PCR analysis and the use of a cellular nuclear import assay [16], Christ et al. [15] showed a clear reduction in HIV nuclear import after depletion of TRN-SR2, supporting a role of TRN-SR2 in this process. Transportin-SR2 belongs to the β-karyopherin family. It has been shown to import splicing factors to the nucleus, most of which contain an RS (arginine–serine) repeat region and/or an RNA recognition motif (RRM) domain [17–19]. Its overall toroid structure, composed of stacked HEAT repeats, provides flexibility to accommodate a variety of cellular cargoes [19–21]. Charged residues on and around an Arg-rich helix in TRN-SR2 are critical for recognition of the phosphorylated RS region of cargo and hence its nuclear import [19]. Until now, crystal structures of TRN-SR2 alone [19], in complex with RanGTP [21] and in complex with the cellular cargo ASF/SF2 [19] have been described. A crystal structure of TRN-SR2 in complex with IN is not available.

A variety of viral components have been linked to nuclear import of the HIV pre-integration complex

(PIC): capsid (CA), the central polypurine tract (cPPT), IN, matrix and viral protein R [22–24]. Also for the host cell, a plethora of import factors have been implicated, most notably importin-α/β [25, 26], importin-α3 [27] and importin-7 [28]. Despite the general agreement on the importance of TRN-SR2 for HIV nuclear import, the exact mechanism of action remains a matter of debate. The TRN-SR2–CA interaction has been reported to play a role in nuclear import by some groups [29, 30], while others published evidence for a direct interaction with HIV IN [15, 31–33]. Moreover, IN was shown to be displaced from TRN-SR2 upon addition of RanGTP, as is the case with normal cargoes [20]. An IN R263A/K264A mutant is partially deficient for the interaction with TRN-SR2 [33, 34] and the corresponding virus was affected at the nuclear import step, supporting the notion that the IN–TRN-SR2 interaction is responsible for this process [34].

As evidenced by the discovery and development of LEDGINs, targeting protein–protein interactions between IN and cellular cofactors can yield new classes of viral replication inhibitors [35, 36]. Since nuclear import represents a bottleneck during HIV replication [15] we reasoned that inhibitors of this interaction might have the potential to become potent antivirals and we embarked on a drug discovery campaign targeting the interaction between HIV-1 IN and TRN-SR2. Small molecules disrupting the interaction and blocking nuclear import would additionally be valuable to study HIV nuclear import and therefore increase our understanding of this crucial step in its replication cycle.

At the time this study was initiated, the interface between TRN-SR2 and IN had not been defined and no crystal structure of TRN-SR2 was available. Therefore, we opted for a high-throughput screening (HTS) approach. Here, we describe the development and use of an amplified luminescent proximity homogenous assay (AlphaScreen)-based screening cascade to identify small-molecule inhibitors of the HIV-1 IN–TRN-SR2 interaction from a library of 25,608 compounds. We eliminated false positives and nonspecific protein–protein interaction inhibitors through the implementation of appropriate counterscreens. Five compound classes provided modest protection against HIV-1 during multiple round replication. Finally, four representative compounds were tested in a cellular fluorescent HIV nuclear import assay. Two compounds significantly reduced the number of nuclear PICs, suggesting these molecules represent a novel class of inhibitors targeting HIV nuclear import. These novel inhibitors validate the IN–TRN-SR2 interaction as an antiviral target and warrant further exploration.

Methods

Recombinant protein purification

Recombinant proteins were expressed in *E. coli* strain BL21-CodonPlus2 (DE3). N-terminally His_6-tagged and untagged IN, His_6-tagged glutathione-S-transferase (GST-His_6), maltose-binding protein (MBP)-tagged JPO2 (Cell division cycle-associated 7-like protein, CDCA7L), 3xflag-tagged LEDGF/p75 and GST-TRN-SR2 were purified as described previously [20, 37–39].

High-throughput screening

Compound stocks were dissolved at approximately 5 mM in dimethylsulfoxide (DMSO) in 96-well plates. Stocks were first diluted to 125 µM in assay buffer (150 mM NaCl, 25 mM Tris–HCl pH 7.4, 1 mM $MgCl_2$, 0.1% (v/v) Tween-20 and 0.1% (w/v) bovine serum albumin (BSA)) supplemented with 2.5% (v/v) DMSO before 10 µl was transferred to a dry 384-well PS 384-OptiPlate (Perkin Elmer) on a Freedom EVO200 liquid handling robot (Tecan). Untagged TRN-SR2 at 2.5 µM and assay buffer containing 5% DMSO were transferred from a separate 96-well plate to the assay plates and represented the positive and negative controls, respectively. Next, 5 µl each of 5× working dilutions of GST-TRN-SR2 and His_6-IN were added using an XRD-384 automated reagent dispenser (FluidX). The plate was left to incubate for 1 h at 7 °C before 5 µl of a glutathione donor and Ni^{2+}-chelate acceptor AlphaScreen bead mixture (Perkin Elmer) was added. This brought the final assay volume to 25 µl and established final concentrations of 50 µM for the compounds, 10 nM GST-TRN-SR2, 40 nM His_6-IN, 10 µg/ml donor and acceptor beads and 2% DMSO.

Hit validation and counterscreens

Both the hit validation assay and the two counterscreens (GST-His_6 and LEDGF/p75–JPO2) were performed in duplicate. Compounds were first diluted to 125 µM as during the main screen but now two doses were transferred to a dry assay plate. From this point on, the hit validation assay was performed identically to the main screen.

For the GST-His_6 counterscreen, 10 µl of a 2.5× working dilution of the recombinant GST-His_6 protein (10 nM final assay concentration) was added to the plate instead of the GST-TRN-SR2 and His_6-IN. In this case, 50 µM bromophenol blue and buffer containing the appropriate amount of DMSO represented the positive and negative controls, respectively.

The LEDGF/p75–JPO2 specificity counterscreen was performed similarly, but instead of GST-TRN-SR2 and His_6-IN, maltose-binding protein (MBP)-tagged JPO2 and 3xflag-tagged LEDGF/p75 were employed at final concentrations of 5 nM. The AlphaScreen bead mixture was modified accordingly to anti-flag acceptor beads and streptavidin donor beads coated with anti-MBP antibody according to the manufacturer's protocol (Perkin Elmer). Untagged LEDGF/p75 at a final concentration of 1 µM and buffer containing the appropriate amount of DMSO were used as positive and negative controls, respectively.

Multiple round antiviral activity assay

The inhibitory effect of antiviral compounds on the HIV-induced cytopathic effect (CPE) in MT-4 cell culture was determined by the MTT-assay [40]. The assay is based on the reduction of the yellow colored 3-(4,5-dimethyl-thiazol-2-yl)-2,5- diphenyltetrazolium bromide (MTT) by mitochondrial dehydrogenase of metabolically active cells to a blue formazan derivative, which can be measured spectrophotometrically. The 50% cell culture infective dose of the HIV strain was determined by titration of the virus stock on MT-4 cells. For the antiviral activity assays, MT-4 cells were infected with 100–300× 50% cell culture infective doses in the presence of five-fold serial dilutions of the compounds. The concentration achieving 50% protection against the HIV CPE (the 50% effective concentration, EC_{50}), was determined as well as the concentration killing 50% of the MT-4 cells (the 50% cytotoxic concentration, CC_{50}).

Single round antiviral activity assay

20,000 HeLaP4 cells were seeded into 96-well plates on the day prior to infection. Cells were infected in triplicate with 3 dilutions (typically 1×10^5, 3.3×10^4 and 1.1×10^4 pg p24) of VSV-G pseudotyped single-round HIV-1 supplemented with one of the compounds in a total volume of 200 µl per well. The virus was produced as described previously [31]. The final compound concentration in the assay was 100 µM. p24 measurements were performed with the Innotest HIV Antigen mAb kit (Fujirebio). 24 h after infection the supernatant was replaced by fresh medium. 72 h post infection cells were lysed in 50 µl of lysis buffer (50 mM Tris/HCl, pH 7.3, 200 mM NaCl, 0.2% NP40, 5% glycerol) and analyzed for firefly luciferase activity (ONE-Glo™, Promega, Belgium) according to the manufacturer's protocol. Chemiluminescence was measured with a Glomax luminometer (Promega, Belgium). The signals were normalized for protein content as determined by a BCA protein assay (Thermo Scientific Pierce).

PIC nuclear import assay

The PIC nuclear import assay was performed as previously described [34]. Briefly, to produce the fluorescent HIV particles, 293T cells were transfected with 15 µg pVpr-IN-eGFP, 15 µg pNL4-3.Luc.R-.E- (obtained from the NIH AIDS Reference and Reagent Program), and 5 µg of the pMD.G plasmid encoding the vesicular stomatitis virus glycoprotein (VSV-G) [41]. Supernatant was collected after 48 h, filtered and concentrated by ultracentrifugation. p24 was measured with the Innotest HIV Antigen mAb kit (Fujirebio). A viral inoculum of 3.10^6 pg p24 was used to infect 30,000 HeLaP4 cells in the presence of 100 µM of hit compound. PF-3450074 (PF74, Sigma-Aldrich) was tested at 2 µM and 10 µM. Five hours after infection, cells were fixed and the nuclear lamina was visualized with a monoclonal anti-lamin A/C antibody (Santa Cruz, sc-7292) followed by a secondary goat anti-mouse IgG Alexa-Fluor 633. Three-dimensional image stacks were acquired on a Zeiss LSM510 multiphoton confocal microscope (Cell Imaging Core CIC, University of Leuven) equipped with a Plan-Apochromat 63×/1.4 Oil DIC objective. The Z-step size was 0.3 µm. The quantification of PICs was performed using a homemade MatLab routine (The MathWorks, Inc.). A fluorescent spot was assigned as a PIC if at least two adjacent pixels were above the threshold and if the signal was present in at least two consecutive Z-planes. PICs were classified as cytoplasmic or nuclear based on the nuclear lamin staining.

Results

Optimization of the IN–TRN-SR2 AlphaScreen

Development of robust high-throughput assays requires optimal buffer conditions in which both proteins and the detection method are stable and reproducible. Initial conditions for an AlphaScreen assay measuring the direct protein–protein interaction between HIV-1 IN and TRN-SR2 were previously reported by our group [31]. This experience allowed us to readily adapt an assay buffer to meet the requirements for a high-throughput screen (HTS) for inhibitors of the interaction. Two modifications were made to the previously reported assay buffer: First, measurements were done in the presence of 1 mM dithiothreitol (DTT) to maintain a sufficiently reducing environment and prevent aggregation of glutathione-S-transferase (GST)-tagged protein on the surface of the glutathione donor beads [39]. Second, since protein–protein interactions can be difficult to disrupt by small molecules, we aimed to screen at a relatively high compound concentration of 50 µM. To aid compound solubility at these concentrations, aside from the already present 0.1% (v/v) Tween-20 and 0.1% (w/v) bovine serum albumin (BSA), we increased the final concentration of dimethylsulfoxide (DMSO). To assess the tolerance of the assay for DMSO, we titrated it out in a two-fold dilution series between 20 and 0.16% (v/v). The AlphaScreen signal was normalized to the 0% DMSO condition and the background signal (100 and 0%, respectively). Figure 1 shows that despite a high tolerance of the assay for DMSO the variability increases to unacceptable levels when more

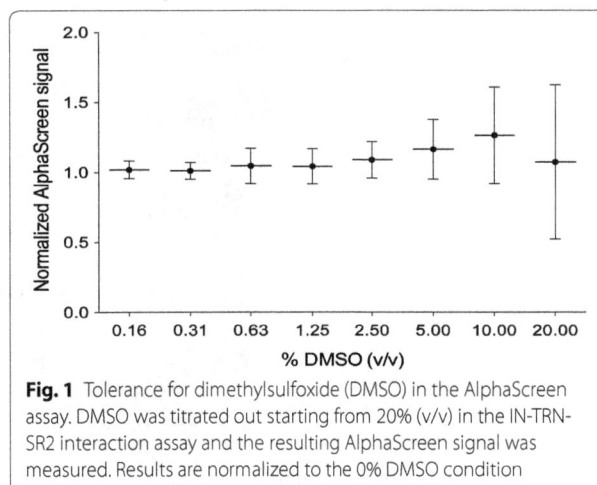

Fig. 1 Tolerance for dimethylsulfoxide (DMSO) in the AlphaScreen assay. DMSO was titrated out starting from 20% (v/v) in the IN-TRN-SR2 interaction assay and the resulting AlphaScreen signal was measured. Results are normalized to the 0% DMSO condition

than 2.5% DMSO is present. Based on these results, we opted for a final DMSO concentration in the assay buffer of 2%.

HTS assay optimization is a fine balance between identifying robust assay conditions with minimal variability and keeping costs acceptable. In the present case, costs were mainly driven by the amount of AlphaScreen beads used. However, reducing the bead concentration leads to a roughly linear decrease of the signal-to-background (S/B) ratio, and hence of the assay quality as well [39]. As a compromise, we decided to lower the final bead concentrations only two-fold to 10 µg/ml.

Next, optimal protein concentrations were determined through cross-titration of the binding partners (Fig. 2a). Concentrations of 10 nM GST-TRN-SR2 and 40 nM His_6-IN provided a good S/B ratio (> 25) with minimal protein consumption and remained well below the AlphaScreen hooking range. Hooking can be seen to occur at concentrations of 300 nM His_6-IN. Under these conditions, the Ni^{2+}-chelate acceptor beads are expected to be fully saturated and the excess of free IN protein will compete with IN on the bead surface for binding to TRN-SR2, effectively inhibiting the signal.

To monitor per plate quality, each 384-well plate contained a total of 64 control wells arranged in 2 columns of 8 positive and 8 negative wells on either side. As a positive control, we evaluated both untagged TRN-SR2 and IN to corroborate the ability of our assay to pick up inhibitors. However, untagged IN proved unable to inhibit the AlphaScreen signal to background levels (Fig. 2b), most likely due to the proneness of the enzyme to form multimers at higher concentrations [42, 43] which could still bring both beads together. Untagged TRN-SR2 did inhibit the signal (Fig. 2b) and was chosen as the positive control at a final concentration of 1 µM.

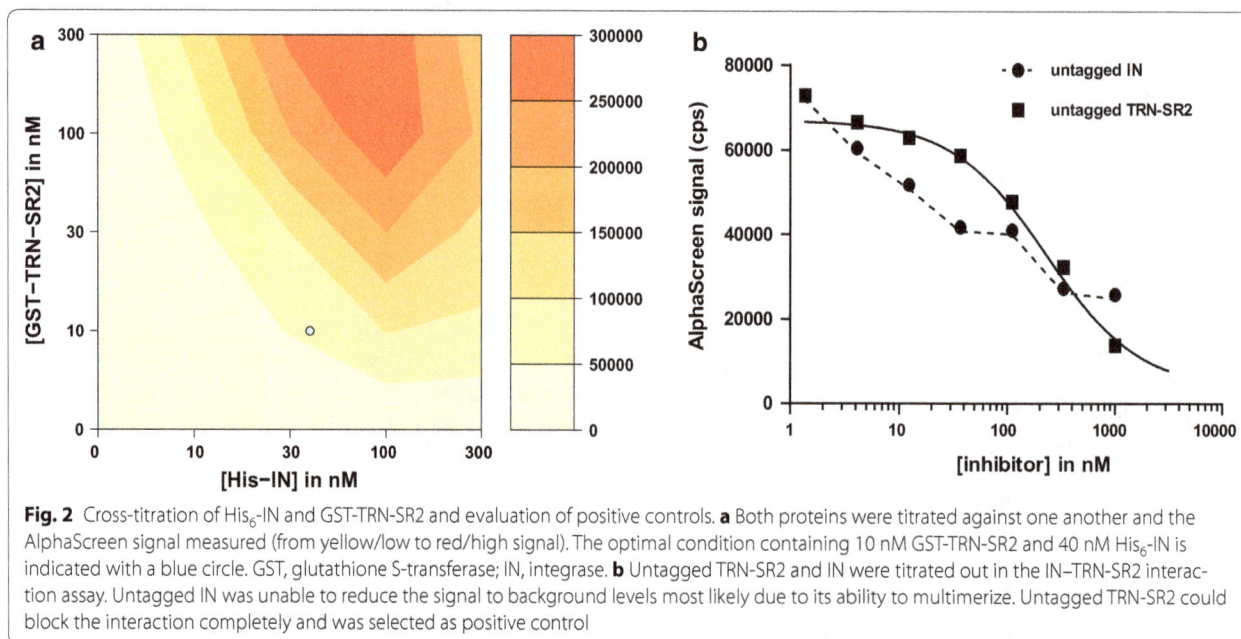

Fig. 2 Cross-titration of His$_6$-IN and GST-TRN-SR2 and evaluation of positive controls. **a** Both proteins were titrated against one another and the AlphaScreen signal measured (from yellow/low to red/high signal). The optimal condition containing 10 nM GST-TRN-SR2 and 40 nM His$_6$-IN is indicated with a blue circle. GST, glutathione S-transferase; IN, integrase. **b** Untagged TRN-SR2 and IN were titrated out in the IN–TRN-SR2 interaction assay. Untagged IN was unable to reduce the signal to background levels most likely due to its ability to multimerize. Untagged TRN-SR2 could block the interaction completely and was selected as positive control

High-throughput screening, false positives and negatives

The optimized assay was used to screen a part of the CD3 (Center for Drug Design and Discovery) library. The set of test compounds consisted of 25,608 small molecules which were selected based on (1) chemical diversity, (2) druglike properties (Lipinski rule of five compliant), (3) exclusion of known toxicophores and purchased from multiple commercial suppliers. Assay performance was evaluated on a plate-by-plate basis and remained robust throughout the entire screening campaign (Fig. 3). A median Z′-factor of 0.76 was obtained and no plates failed during screening. Considering a cut-off of 50% inhibition (percentage of inhibition (PIN) of 50%), we identified a total of 409 initial hits from the collection.

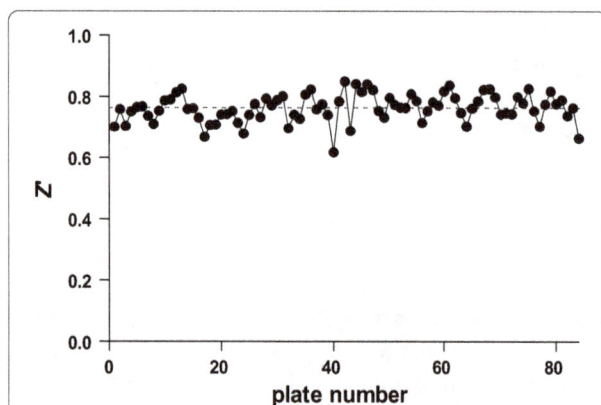

Fig. 3 Assay performance throughout the screening campaign. Assay performance per plate was monitored throughout the screening campaign. A median Z′-factor of 0.76 was determined. No plates had to be repeated

False positives often dominate initial hit lists obtained from HTS campaigns. True false positives were weeded out from the cherry-picked hit compounds by a confirmation screen in which the 409 hits were retested in duplicate in the IN–TRN-SR2 interaction assay. Figure 4a shows percentages of inhibition (PIN) of the duplicates of each compound normalized to the positive (100%) and negative (0%) controls. Linear regression results in a slope of 1.000 ± 0.004 and an R^2 of 0.9675, indicating the robustness of the platform.

AlphaScreen technology is not insensitive to interference [44]. To rid our hit lists of AlphaScreen-specific false positives including inner filter effect, $^1\Delta O_2$ quenchers, and Ni^{2+} chelators, we included in our cascade a GST-His$_6$ counterscreen described previously [39]. Figure 4b shows PIN values for the duplicates of each compound in this counterscreen normalized to the positive (bromophenol blue, inner filter effect, 100%) and negative (0%) controls. Here as well, the slope of 0.9892 ± 0.006 and R^2 of 0.9640 confirm the platform's robustness.

Combining both results by plotting the average PIN in the GST-His$_6$ counterscreen against that from the confirmation screen allowed us to confidently select positive hits (Fig. 4c). First, we opted for compounds that met the cut-off of 50% inhibition of the IN–TRN-SR2 interaction, eliminating 126 false positives. Second, compounds should preferentially be devoid of quenching at the active concentrations. Specifically, the percentage of inhibition in the GST-His$_6$ counterscreen should be below 20% or the activity observed against the IN–TRN-SR2 interaction should be > 50% stronger than the quenching. These

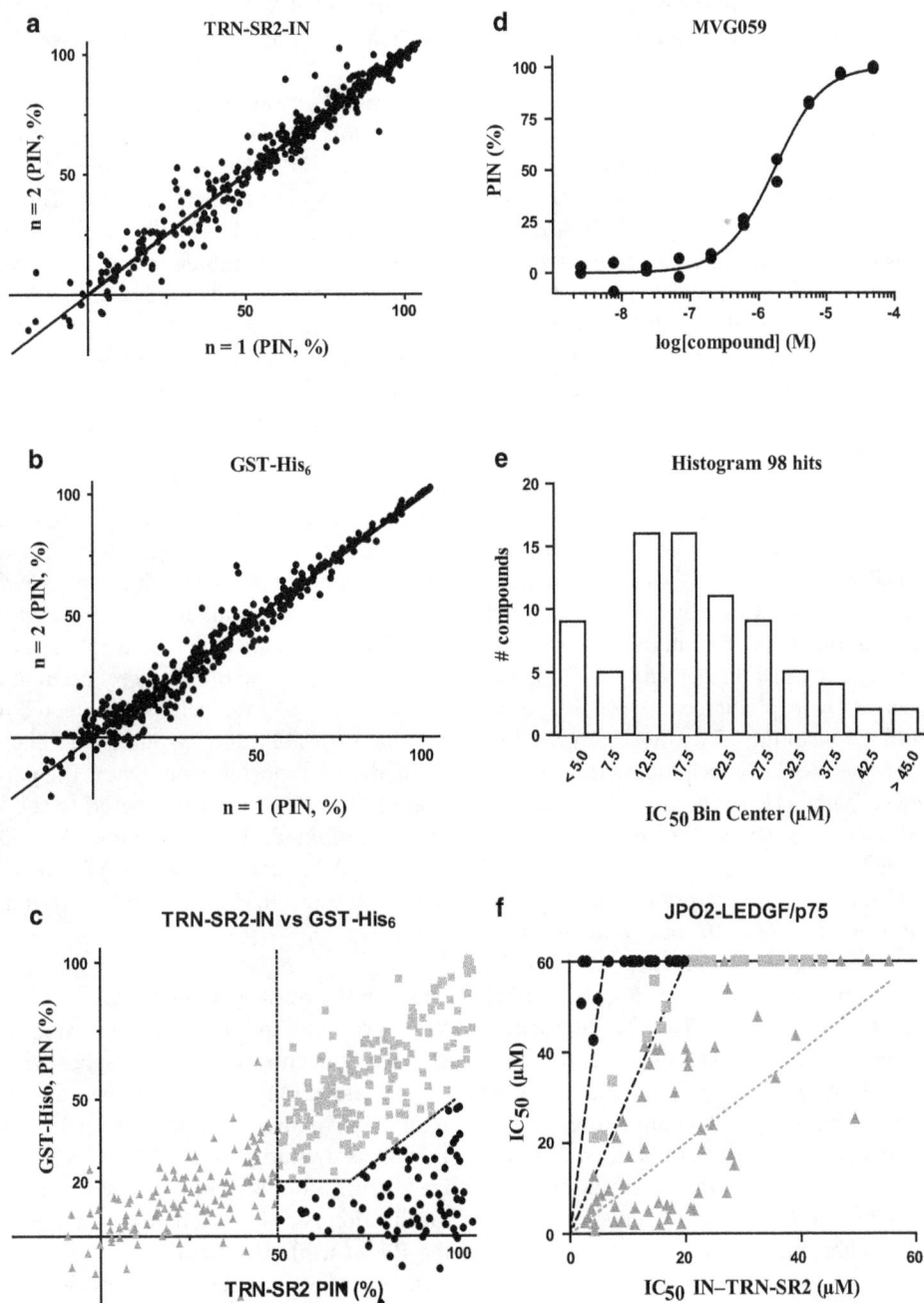

Fig. 4 AlphaScreen screening strategy (**a, b**). Normalized percentage inhibition (PIN) of duplicates of each of the 409 primary hits in (**a**) a confirmatory repeat of the IN–TRN-SR2 AlphaScreen or (**b**) the GST-His$_6$ false positive counterscreen. In both cases, the linear regression fit to the data is shown: slopes are not significantly different from 1 and R^2 values are 0.9675 and 0.9640 for (**a**) and (**b**), respectively. **c** Average percentage inhibition in the GST-His$_6$ counterscreen plotted against that observed in the IN–TRN-SR2 assay. Hits of interest show > 50% inhibition of the IN–TRN-SR2 interaction and are devoid of quenching at the active concentration (< 20% inhibition of the GST-His$_6$ signal or 50% stronger inhibition of the IN–TRN-SR2 interaction). Primary hits occupying the different areas of the result space are plotted as dark grey triangles (false positives), light grey squares (quenchers) and black circles (hits of interest). **d** Titration results and dose–response curve fit obtained for compound MVG059. Duplicates are plotted. **e** Histogram of the obtained IC$_{50}$ values for all 98 hits sorted into 5 μM bins. **f** Hit compound specificity. IC$_{50}$ values obtained against the IN–TRN-SR2 and LEDGF/p75–JPO2 interactions were plotted against one another. Compounds having an IC$_{50}$ < 20 μM against the IN–TRN-SR2 interaction and being tenfold less active or having an IC$_{50}$ > 60 μM against LEDGF/p75–JPO2 are preferred (black circles). Hits that were only between 10 and 3 times more active in the IN–TRN-SR2 assay are less promising (light grey squares). Those that were less potent (IC$_{50}$ ≥ 20 μM) but did not inhibit the LEDGF/p75–JPO2 interaction (IC$_{50}$ > 60 μM) were looked at case-by-case. Compounds falling outside of these regions were considered non-specific and not investigated further (dark grey triangles)

requirements delineated an area of the results space containing 98 clean and confirmed hit compounds (Fig. 4c, black circles).

Determination of potency and specificity

The 98 confirmed hits were next subjected to IC_{50} determination in the IN–TRN-SR2 AlphaScreen interaction assay. Compounds were titrated in duplicate in a threefold dilution series starting at 50 μM and dose–response curves were fit to the resulting data. Figure 4d shows a representative titration result while Fig. 4e provides a histogram of the obtained IC_{50} data. In total, 14 out of the 98 hits had an IC_{50} value in the single digit micromolar range.

Since the IN–TRN-SR2 protein–protein interface is believed to be relatively flat and featureless, we decided to perform a specificity counterscreen. Compounds were assayed for their inhibition of an unrelated protein–protein interaction (LEDGF/p75–JPO2) [45, 46] and their IC_{50} values were determined. Compounds were titrated as before and the inhibition of the interaction between full-length 3xflag-tagged LEDGF/p75 and MBP-tagged JPO2 was measured by AlphaScreen. Dose–response curves were fit and the resulting IC_{50} values compared to those obtained for the IN–TRN-SR2 interaction. Compounds that showed high activity ($IC_{50} < 20$ μM) in the IN–TRN-SR2 interaction assay and were tenfold less active or completely inactive ($IC_{50} > 60$ μM) against the LEDGF/p75–JPO2 interaction were prioritized (Fig. 4f). Compounds that were between 10 and 3 times more active in the IN–TRN-SR2 assay were kept as back-up compounds. Those that were less potent ($IC_{50} \geq 20$ μM) but did not inhibit the LEDGF/p75–JPO2 interaction ($IC_{50} > 60$ μM) were looked at case-by-case and evaluated as potential back-up compounds based on their PIN at the highest concentration used. All compounds falling outside these regions of the results space were considered nonspecific protein–protein interaction inhibitors and discarded from the hit list. In the end, this resulted in 23 first priority and 25 fallback compounds.

Analogues

The 23 first priority compounds were clustered into 12 classes based on their structure and the hit compounds of each cluster were repurchased. Unfortunately, the IN–TRN-SR2 activity could not be confirmed for 5 hits which left us with 7 hit compounds for which commercially available analogues were selected and ordered. These analogues were funneled through the same screening cascade consisting of the IN–TRN-SR2 interaction assay and both counterscreens (GST-His$_6$ for quenching and LEDGF/p75–JPO2 for specificity) leading to a selection of compounds which were further evaluated for

inhibition of HIV-1 replication and cellular toxicity in the MTT/MT-4 viral replication assay (see Table 1).

Antiviral activity in cell culture

A selection of active compounds was then evaluated for inhibition of HIV-1 replication and cellular toxicity in the MTT/MT-4 viral replication assay. The percentage protection against the HIV CPE was measured. Modest (up to 46% at 100 μM) protection was observed for a limited number of compounds in classes 3, 7 and 9 but no 50% effective concentration (EC_{50}) was reached at concentrations lower than the observed 50% cytotoxic concentration (CC_{50}) (Table 1).

Rapid growth (and frequent cell divisions) of the MT-4 cells during the viral replication assay however, may mask viral nuclear import defects, in particular with low potency compounds. This could imply that the MTT/MT-4 assay is not well suited to detect a block in viral nuclear import. We hence decided to evaluate four representative compounds from the most promising classes 6, 7, 9 and 10 in a single round antiviral activity assay on HeLaP4 cells. Compounds were tested at a final concentration of 100 μM and cells were infected with a threefold dilution series of a single-round virus expressing the firefly luciferase reporter gene (Fluc). The percentage inhibition of HIV replication compared to the DMSO control was determined. For compound MVG036 no inhibition could be detected while MVG010, MVG044 and MVG030 showed 34.2, 16.3 and 23.3% inhibition, respectively (Fig. 5).

Effect on HIV nuclear import

We next analyzed the selected compounds, again at 100 μM concentration, in a low throughput PIC nuclear import assay [34] to test whether the decrease in viral replication is due to inhibition of PIC nuclear import. In this assay fluorescently labeled viral PICs are visualized using confocal microscopy and their subcellular localization is evaluated based on a nuclear lamina staining (Fig. 6a, b). The ratio of nuclear PICs over the total number of PICs (percentage nuclear PICs) was then calculated as a measure of nuclear import. DMSO and Raltegravir (RAL) were used as negative controls in two independent experiments as they should not affect HIV nuclear import. The capsid-binder PF74 was used as a positive control. This compound is known to inhibit nuclear import at low concentrations (2 μM) whereas it also inhibits reverse transcription at higher concentrations (10 μM) (Fig. 6c) [47, 48]. MVG044 and MVG030 significantly reduced the number of nuclear PICs compared to both DMSO and RAL ($p < 0.05$) while MVG036 only showed significance compared to DMSO (Fig. 6d; Table 2).

Table 1 Antiviral activity and toxicity of selected hits in multiple round MTT assay

Class	Compound ID	IN–TRN-SR2 Pin at 50 μM (%)[a]	EC_{50} (μM)[b]		CC_{50} (μM)[c]		Protection (%)[d]
3	MVG001	65.3	<	8	<	8	2
	MVG002	43.4	>	13	=	13	5
	MVG003	47.2	>	80	=	80	13
	MVG004	82.6	>	21	=	21	4
	MVG005	39.7	>	57	=	57	6
	MVG006	50.5	>	63	=	63	6
	MVG007	64.8	>	74	=	74	6
	MVG008	30.1	>	99	=	99	23
	MVG009	32.0	>	51	=	51	4
6	MVG010	37.1	>	100	=	100	6
	MVG011	41.7	>	102	=	102	1
	MVG012	107.1	>	74	=	74	10
	MVG013	51.9	>	95	=	95	3
	MVG014	63.8	>	87	=	87	4
	MVG015	48.1	>	87	=	87	5
	MVG016	46.9	>	244	>	244	20
	MVG017	< 10	=	195	=	229	52
	MVG018	< 10	>	137	>	137	7
	MVG019	< 10	>	250	>	250	6
	MVG020	< 10	>	250	>	250	18
	MVG021	< 10	>	250	>	250	34
	MVG022	44.9	=	67	>	136	53
	MVG023	< 10	>	110	>	110	0
	MVG024	< 10	>	36	>	45	49
7	MVG025	72.9	>	34	=	34	4
	MVG026	45.7	>	35	=	48	4
	MVG027	43.2	>	57	=	57	6
	MVG028	58.7	>	56	=	80	13
	MVG029	48.8	>	57	=	57	3
	MVG030	71.6	>	97	=	97	25
	MVG031	62.3	>	53	=	53	4
	MVG032	46.5	>	48	=	48	5
	MVG033	49.5	>	59	=	59	20
	MVG034	43.0	>	73	=	73	16
9	MVG035	43.8	>	36	=	36	1
	MVG036	105.6	>	55	=	65	46
	MVG037	43.1	>	85	=	85	22
	MVG038	47.2	>	59	=	59	0
	MVG039	40.1	>	17	=	17	1
	MVG040	43.6	>	25	=	25	25
	MVG041	54.0	>	35	=	35	2
10	MVG042	89.6	>	55	=	55	10
	MVG043	102.0	>	67	=	67	4
	MVG044	75.9	>	250	>	250	22
	MVG045	11.4	>	203	=	203	21
	MVG046	10.3	>	207	=	207	32
	MVG047	< 10	>	250	>	250	7
	MVG048	< 10	>	87	=	87	0
	MVG049	< 10	=	165	>	231	55
	MVG050	44.1	>	250	>	250	0

Table 1 continued

Class	Compound ID	IN–TRN-SR2 Pin at 50 µM (%)[a]	EC$_{50}$ (µM)[b]		CC$_{50}$ (µM)[c]		Protection (%)[d]
	MVG051	< 10	>	250	>	250	22
	MVG052	20.1	>	66	=	66	8
	MVG053	< 10	>	167	>	167	39
	MVG054	18.0	>	225	=	225	0
	MVG055	< 10	>	167	>	167	21
	MVG056	71.1	>	250	>	250	24
	MVG057	23.3	>	250	>	250	16
	MVG058	53.7	=	170	>	250	24

[a] Compounds were tested in AlphaScreen at 50 µM for their ability to inhibit the IN-TRN-SR2 interaction. Percentage inhibition (PIN), relative to the DMSO control

[b,c] MT-4 cells were infected with HIV at 100 to 300× the 50% cell culture infective doses in the presence of 100 µM of the antiviral drugs. The compound concentration achieving 50% protection against the cytopathic effect of HIV, the 50% effective concentration (EC$_{50}$), was determined. The concentration of the compound killing 50% of the MT-4 cells, the 50% cytotoxic concentration (CC$_{50}$), was determined as well

[d] The percentage of protection against the cytopathic effect of HIV was measured in MT-4 cells as well. Values below 20% were not considered as real activities. Data are averages of triplicate measurements

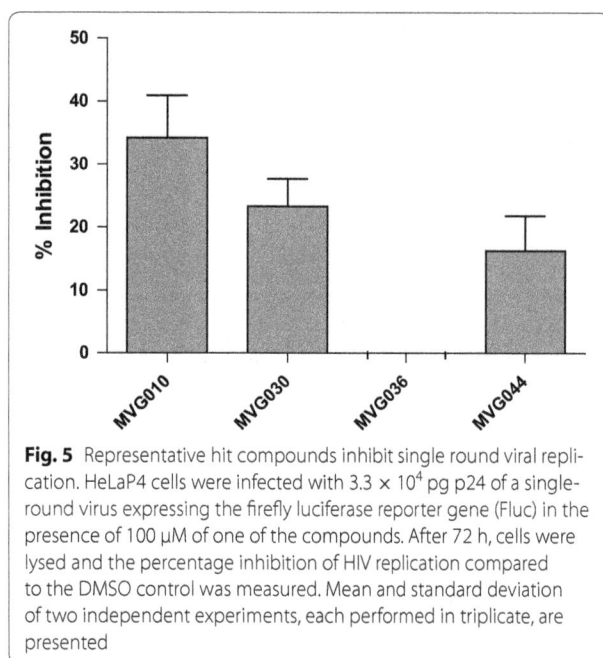

Fig. 5 Representative hit compounds inhibit single round viral replication. HeLaP4 cells were infected with 3.3 × 10^4 pg p24 of a single-round virus expressing the firefly luciferase reporter gene (Fluc) in the presence of 100 µM of one of the compounds. After 72 h, cells were lysed and the percentage inhibition of HIV replication compared to the DMSO control was measured. Mean and standard deviation of two independent experiments, each performed in triplicate, are presented

to the modest activity of our compounds. In addition, these compounds are products of commercially available libraries and have not been optimized yet for activity. The experiments on the potency determination in MT4 cells as well as the inhibition of viral infectivity in a single round viral replication assay in HeLaP4 cells, were experiments lasting for 5 and 3 days, respectively. Chemical (in)stability of the compounds might lead to a more pronounced effect when early time points are analyzed (PIC assay) in contrast to analysis after incubation over several days.

Discussion

Here we present the discovery of small HIV-1 nuclear import inhibitors targeting the interaction of HIV-1 IN and its cellular co-factor, the karyopherin TRN-SR2. We developed an AlphaScreen-based HTS assay to screen for inhibitors of the HIV IN–TRN-SR2 interaction (Figs. 1, 2, 3). We screened a diverse library of 25,608 compounds, yielding a total of 409 hits (Fig. 4). A confirmation assay on the cherry-picked hits in combination with a GST-His$_6$ counterscreen to remove AlphaScreen technology-interfering false positives narrowed down the hit list to 98 inhibitors (Fig. 4c). Of these 98 hits, 14 were found to have an IC$_{50}$ value in the single-digit micromolar range as determined in the TRN-SR2–HIV IN AlphaScreen assay (Fig. 4e). Because we anticipated the IN–TRN-SR2 interface to be relatively flat and featureless, we performed an additional specificity counterscreen for an unrelated protein–protein interaction (LEDGF/p75–JPO2). Selecting compounds that did not inhibit the LEDGF/p75–JPO2 interaction or were 10 times more potent against the IN–TRN-SR2 interaction resulted in a list of 23 first priority compounds (Fig. 4f). After clustering, hit confirmation with a new "fresh" sample, and analogs selection, the

MVG044 from compound family 10 induced the most pronounced block to nuclear import: the mean % nuclear PICs was 4.8% for DMSO (95% confidence interval [3.8; 5.9%]), 4.5% for Ral [3.4; 5.6%] and 2.1% [0.9; 3.2%] and 2.0% [1.5; 2.7%] for the two MVG044 conditions (DMSO, n = 49 cells; MVG044, n = 50 cells; p = 0.00001, Mann–Whitney U test and Ral, n = 35 cells; MVG044, n = 31 cells; p = 0.0002, Mann–Whitney U test) (Table 2).

In Table 3 we present an overview of the data for the four representative compounds. At first sight, there does not seem to be a strong correlation between the different read outs. This is not entirely unexpected, mainly due

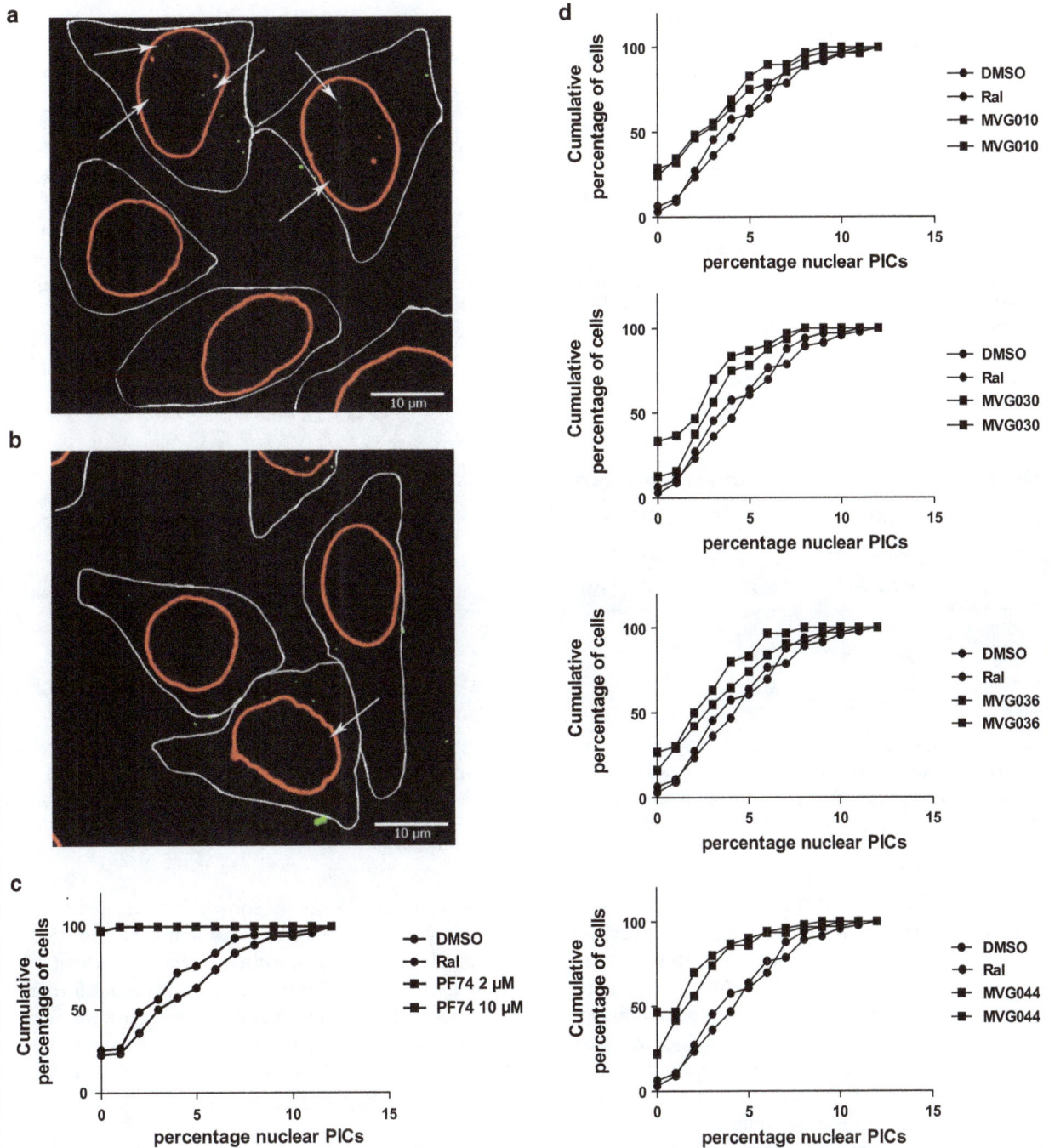

Fig. 6 Representative hit compounds reduce nuclear import of HIV. Five hours after infection with IN-eGFP labeled virus in the presence of one of four representative hit compounds (MVG010, MVG044, MVG030 or MVG036), PF74 and DMSO or RAL as controls, HeLaP4 cells were fixed and analyzed by laser-scanning confocal microscopy. The ratio of nuclear/total amount of PICs was quantified (percentage nuclear PICs). **a, b** Representative slice of a stack of cells infected with eGFP-IN labeled virus in the presence of DMSO (**a**) or MVG044 (**b**). The nuclear lamina was immunostained with anti-lamin a/c (red). PICs are identified as green dots and nuclear PICs are highlighted by white arrows. **c, d** Presented are the cumulative distributions of the percentage of cells containing the indicated percentage nuclear PICs for the positive control PF74 (**c**) and four representative hit compounds (MVG010, MVG044, MVG030 or MVG036) or DMSO and Ral as controls (**d**). Two independent experiments, with distinct virus productions, are presented for each compound

Table 2 PIC assay statistics

	Compared to DMSO				Compared to Raltegravir			
	n^a	p value[b]	% nuclear PICs[c]	95% CI[d]	n^a	p value[b]	% nuclear PICs[c]	95% CI[d]
DMSO		–	–	–	49	0.8099	4.8	[3.8; 5.9]
Ral	35	0.8099	4.5	[3.4; 5.6]		–	–	–
MVG010	32	0.1209	3.8	[2.3; 5.4]	29	0.1152	4.2	[2.2; 6.3]
MVG044	31	0.00001	2.1	[1.5; 2.7]	50	0.0002	2.0	[0.9; 3.2]
MVG030	30	0.0411	3.3	[2.3; 4.2]	33	0.0019	2.2	[1.4; 3.0]
MVG036	31	0.0011	2.3	[1.6; 3.1]	30	0.0700	3.2	[2.2; 4.2]

Summary of two independent PIC assays comparing the four representative hit compounds to the DMSO and Ral control. HeLaP4 cells were fixed and analyzed by confocal microscopy 5 h after infection with an eGFP-labeled IN virus. PICs were assigned as cytoplasmic or nuclear based on nuclear lamina staining

[a] Number of HeLaP4 cells counted in each condition

[b] p values (Mann–Whitney U test) compared to DMSO or RAL control

[c] Mean percentage of nuclear PICs in each cell calculated using a homemade MatLab routine (The MathWorks, Inc.)

[d] 95% confidence interval (CI) for the percentage of nuclear PICs

Table 3 Overview of the data for four representative compounds

	In vitro		MT4 cells			HeLaP4 cells	
	AlphaScreen[a]		MTT[b]			Fluc[c]	PIC assay[d]
	IC$_{50}$ (µM)	PIN (%)	EC$_{50}$ (µM)	CC$_{50}$ (µM)	% Protection	PIN (%)	p value
MVG010	54.6	37.1	> 100	100	6	34.2	0.1209
MVG030	33.6	71.6	> 97	97	25	23.3	0.0411
MVG036	37.6	105.6	> 55	65	46	–	0.0011
MVG044	17.1	75.9	> 250	> 250	22	16.3	0.00001

[a] HIV-1 IN–TRN-SR2 AlphaScreen IC$_{50}$ values and percentage inhibition (PIN) are presented. All compounds were tested at 50 µM

[b] EC$_{50}$ and CC$_{50}$ values in MT4 cells are given as well as the percentage of protection against the cytopathic effect of HIV

[c] HeLaP4 cells were infected with a single-round virus expressing the firefly luciferase reporter gene (Fluc) in the presence of one of the compounds (100 µM) and the results are expressed as a percentage inhibition relative to the DMSO control

[d] For the PIC assay in HeLaP4 cells, p values (Mann–Whitney U test), compared to the DMSO control, are given

best compounds selected from 6 series were evaluated for their ability to block HIV replication in infected cells. For five of the classes we were able to detect modest protection against the HIV CPE in an MTT/MT-4 antiviral activity assay (Table 1). In a next step, compounds from the most promising classes 6, 7, 9 and 10 were tested in a single-round antiviral activity assay and a HIV nuclear import assay on HeLaP4 cells. Although only modest inhibition of viral replication could be detected (Fig. 5), two of the compounds significantly reduced the number of nuclear PICs while the other two showed a trend towards less nuclear import (Fig. 6; Table 3).

As previously mentioned, no information on the structure and interface of the TRN-SR2–HIV IN complex was available at the start of our screening campaign. In 2012, De Houwer et al. identified the interaction hot spots in IN for the IN–TRN-SR2 interaction [32]. Amino acids R262/R263/K264 and K266/R269 in the C-terminal domain of IN were found to be the main determinants of the interaction. These results were independently confirmed by

Larue et al. [33]. More recently, the structures of TRN-SR2 alone and its complexes with Ran-GTP and ASF/SF2 were published [19, 21]. Although the structure of TRN-SR2–IN has not yet been solved, structural information together with the mutagenesis data point towards a large, charged and relatively flat interaction interface. Targeting the TRN-SR2–IN interaction with high affinity may therefore require design of completely new chemotypes [49].

Conclusions

Our efforts evidenced that an Alphascreen-based HTS can allow the identification of compounds representing a novel class of HIV inhibitors. Their activity in the PIC nuclear import assay confirms that nuclear import of HIV can be targeted by small molecules. While the effects are clear-cut in the PIC assay, the activities of the compounds in the MTT/MT-4 and the single round antiviral activity assay are only modest (Table 3). Several reasons may be conceived to explain this discrepancy. First, rapid growth (and frequent cell divisions) of the cell culture-adapted MT-4 cells during the viral replication assay may relieve the bottleneck of nuclear import. Disassembly and reassembly of the nuclear membrane during the frequent mitoses could give incoming viral PICs periodic access to the condensed, LEDGF/p75-decorated chromatin, masking nuclear import defects. Second, while the single round antiviral activity assay gives a global view of viral replication after 72 h, the PIC assay is a kinetic assay, providing a snapshot of the population of cytoplasmic and nuclear PICs at 5 h after infection. As nuclear import is a bottleneck process [15], PICs accumulating at the nuclear periphery may remain there for some time before being bound and imported by TRN-SR2 (or being degraded). Depending on its affinity and kinetics, an inhibitor of the IN–TRN-SR2 interaction could delay the import process and shift PICs towards degradation in the cytoplasm. Our compounds may not induce sufficient delay in import and a few PICs may make it into the cell's nucleus masking the inhibition.

One of the caveats of targeting pathogen-host protein–protein interactions is the risk of inducing cellular toxicity due to inhibition of the host protein function. Notably, none of the active classes exhibited prominent toxicity in the MTT/MT-4 assay.

Recently, De Houwer et al. [34] reported an IN mutant virus that is partially defective for interaction with TRN-SR2 and nuclear import. Together with these findings, the identification of molecules inhibiting HIV-1 PIC nuclear import from a HTS campaign against the IN–TRN-SR2 interaction underscores the importance of the interaction for HIV-1 nuclear import.

Authors' contributions

JD, JB, SDH and LD performed the experiments; JD, JB, SDH and LD analysed the data; JD, JB and SDH have written the manuscript with help from FC, AM and ZD. HK, AM and PC contributed with compounds, reagents, materials and analysis tools. All authors read and approved the final manuscript.

Author details

[1] Laboratory for Molecular Virology and Gene Therapy, Department of Pharmaceutical and Pharmacological Sciences, KU Leuven, Kapucijnenvoer 33, VCTB +5, Bus 7001, 3000 Leuven, Flanders, Belgium. [2] Center for Innovation and Stimulation of Drug Discovery (CISTIM), Leuven, Belgium. [3] Center for Drug Design and Development (CD3), KU Leuven R&D, Leuven, Belgium. [4] Present Address: The Francis Crick Institute, London, UK.

Acknowledgements

We thank Barbara Van Remoortel and Nam Joo Van der Veken for excellent technical support and Dr. Woan-Yuh Tarn (Inst. of Biomedical Sciences, Taiwan) for the pGEX-TRN-SR2 expression plasmid.

Competing interests

The authors declare that they have no competing interests.
availability of these data due to ongoing chemical optimization. Data on some compounds are however available from the authors upon reasonable request and with permission of CISTIM.

Consent for publication

Not applicable.

Funding

This work was supported by grants from the FWO (G.0487.10 N), (G.0A53.16 N), the IAP BelVir, FP7 CHAARM, hiveranet EURECA and the KU Leuven BOF. JD and LD were doctoral fellows of the Research Foundation Flanders (FWO) and SDH was a doctoral fellow of the agency for Innovation by Science and Technology (IWT). JB is part of the academic and teaching staff of KU Leuven. FC is an Industrial Research Fund (IOF) fellow.

References

1. Weinberg JB, Matthews TJ, Cullen BR, Malim MH. Productive human immunodeficiency virus type 1 (HIV-1) infection of nonproliferating human monocytes. J Exp Med. 1991;174(6):1477–82 **(Epub 1991/12/01)**.
2. Podany AT, Scarsi KK, Fletcher CV. Comparative clinical pharmacokinetics and pharmacodynamics of HIV-1 integrase strand transfer inhibitors. Clin Pharmacokinet. 2017;56(1):25–40 **(Epub 2016/06/19)**.
3. Christ F, Debyser Z. The LEDGF/p75 integrase interaction, a novel target for anti-HIV therapy. Virology. 2013;435(1):102–9 **(Epub 2012/12/12)**.
4. Desimmie BA, Schrijvers R, Demeulemeester J, Borrenberghs D, Weydert C, Thys W, et al. LEDGINs inhibit late stage HIV-1 replication by modulating integrase multimerization in the virions. Retrovirology. 2013;10:57 **(Epub 2013/06/01)**.
5. Christ F, Shaw S, Demeulemeester J, Desimmie BA, Marchand A, Butler S, et al. Small-molecule inhibitors of the LEDGF/p75 binding site of integrase block HIV replication and modulate integrase multimerization. Antimicrob Agents Chemother. 2012;56(8):4365–74 **(Epub 2012/06/06)**.
6. Balakrishnan M, Yant SR, Tsai L, O'Sullivan C, Bam RA, Tsai A, et al. Non-catalytic site HIV-1 integrase inhibitors disrupt core maturation and induce a reverse transcription block in target cells. PLoS ONE. 2013;8(9):e74163 **(Epub 2013/09/17)**.
7. Jurado KA, Engelman A. Multimodal mechanism of action of allosteric HIV-1 integrase inhibitors. Expert Rev Mol Med. 2013;15:e14 **(Epub 2013/11/28)**.
8. Cherepanov P, Maertens G, Proost P, Devreese B, Van Beeumen J, Engelborghs Y, et al. HIV-1 integrase forms stable tetramers and associates with LEDGF/p75 protein in human cells. J Biol Chem. 2003;278(1):372–81 **(Epub 2002/10/31)**.
9. Fader LD, Malenfant E, Parisien M, Carson R, Bilodeau F, Landry S, et al. Discovery of BI 224436, a noncatalytic site integrase inhibitor (NCINI) of HIV-1. ACS Med Chem Lett. 2014;5(4):422–7 **(Epub 2014/06/06)**.
10. Christ F, Voet A, Marchand A, Nicolet S, Desimmie BA, Marchand D, et al. Rational design of small-molecule inhibitors of the LEDGF/p75-integrase interaction and HIV replication. Nat Chem Biol. 2010;6(6):442–8 **(Epub 2010/05/18)**.
11. Kessl JJ, Jena N, Koh Y, Taskent-Sezgin H, Slaughter A, Feng L, et al. Multimode, cooperative mechanism of action of allosteric HIV-1 integrase inhibitors. J Biol Chem. 2012;287(20):16801–11 **(Epub 2012/03/23)**.
12. Tsiang M, Jones GS, Niedziela-Majka A, Kan E, Lansdon EB, Huang W, et al. New class of HIV-1 integrase (IN) inhibitors with a dual mode of action. J Biol Chem. 2012;287(25):21189–203 **(Epub 2012/04/27)**.

13. Brass AL, Dykxhoorn DM, Benita Y, Yan N, Engelman A, Xavier RJ, et al. Identification of host proteins required for HIV infection through a functional genomic screen. Science. 2008;319(5865):921–6 **(Epub 2008/01/12)**.

14. Konig R, Zhou Y, Elleder D, Diamond TL, Bonamy GM, Irelan JT, et al. Global analysis of host-pathogen interactions that regulate early-stage HIV-1 replication. Cell. 2008;135(1):49–60 **(Epub 2008/10/16)**.

15. Christ F, Thys W, De Rijck J, Gijsbers R, Albanese A, Arosio D, et al. Transportin-SR2 imports HIV into the nucleus. Curr Biol CB. 2008;18(16):1192–202 **(Epub 2008/08/30)**.

16. Albanese A, Arosio D, Terreni M, Cereseto A. HIV-1 pre-integration complexes selectively target decondensed chromatin in the nuclear periphery. PLoS ONE. 2008;3(6):e2413 **(Epub 2008/06/12)**.

17. Lai MC, Lin RI, Huang SY, Tsai CW, Tarn WY. A human importin-beta family protein, transportin-SR2, interacts with the phosphorylated RS domain of SR proteins. J Biol Chem. 2000;275(11):7950–7 **(Epub 2000/03/14)**.

18. Lai MC, Kuo HW, Chang WC, Tarn WY. A novel splicing regulator shares a nuclear import pathway with SR proteins. EMBO J. 2003;22(6):1359–69 **(Epub 2003/03/12)**.

19. Maertens GN, Cook NJ, Wang W, Hare S, Gupta SS, Oztop I, et al. Structural basis for nuclear import of splicing factors by human transportin 3. Proc Natl Acad Sci USA. 2014;111(7):2728–33 **(Epub 2014/01/23)**.

20. Taltynov O, Demeulemeester J, Christ F, De Houwer S, Tsirkone VG, Gerard M, et al. Interaction of transportin-SR2 with Ras-related nuclear protein (Ran) GTPase. J Biol Chem. 2013;288(35):25603–13 **(Epub 2013/07/24)**.

21. Tsirkone VG, Beutels KG, Demeulemeester J, Debyser Z, Christ F, Strelkov SV. Structure of transportin SR2, a karyopherin involved in human disease, in complex with Ran. Acta Crystallogr Sect F Struct Biol Commun. 2014;70(Pt 6):723–9 **(Epub 2014/06/11)**.

22. Yamashita M, Emerman M. The cell cycle independence of HIV infections is not determined by known karyophilic viral elements. PLoS Pathog. 2005;1(3):e18 **(Epub 2005/11/18)**.

23. De Rijck J, Vandekerckhove L, Christ F, Debyser Z. Lentiviral nuclear import: a complex interplay between virus and host. BioEssays News Rev Mol Cell Dev Biol. 2007;29(5):441–51 **(Epub 2007/04/24)**.

24. Suzuki Y, Craigie R. The road to chromatin—nuclear entry of retroviruses. Nat Rev Microbiol. 2007;5(3):187–96 **(Epub 2007/02/17)**.

25. Gallay P, Hope T, Chin D, Trono D. HIV-1 infection of nondividing cells through the recognition of integrase by the importin/karyopherin pathway. Proc Natl Acad Sci USA. 1997;94(18):9825–30 **(Epub 1997/09/02)**.

26. Kamata M, Nitahara-Kasahara Y, Miyamoto Y, Yoneda Y, Aida Y. Importin-alpha promotes passage through the nuclear pore complex of human immunodeficiency virus type 1 Vpr. J Virol. 2005;79(6):3557–64 **(Epub 2005/02/26)**.

27. Ao Z, Danappa Jayappa K, Wang B, Zheng Y, Kung S, Rassart E, et al. Importin alpha3 interacts with HIV-1 integrase and contributes to HIV-1 nuclear import and replication. J Virol. 2010;84(17):8650–63 **(Epub 2010/06/18)**.

28. Fassati A, Gorlich D, Harrison I, Zaytseva L, Mingot JM. Nuclear import of HIV-1 intracellular reverse transcription complexes is mediated by importin 7. EMBO J. 2003;22(14):3675–85 **(Epub 2003/07/11)**.

29. Krishnan L, Matreyek KA, Oztop I, Lee K, Tipper CH, Li X, et al. The requirement for cellular transportin 3 (TNPO3 or TRN-SR2) during infection maps to human immunodeficiency virus type 1 capsid and not integrase. J Virol. 2010;84(1):397–406 **(Epub 2009/10/23)**.

30. De Iaco A, Luban J. Inhibition of HIV-1 infection by TNPO3 depletion is determined by capsid and detectable after viral cDNA enters the nucleus. Retrovirology. 2011;8:98 **(Epub 2011/12/08)**.

31. Thys W, De Houwer S, Demeulemeester J, Taltynov O, Vancraenenbroeck R, Gerard M, et al. Interplay between HIV entry and transportin-SR2 dependency. Retrovirology. 2011;8:7 **(Epub 2011/02/01)**.

32. De Houwer S, Demeulemeester J, Thys W, Taltynov O, Zmajkovicova K, Christ F, et al. Identification of residues in the C-terminal domain of HIV-1 integrase that mediate binding to the transportin-SR2 protein. J Biol Chem. 2012;287(41):34059–68 **(Epub 2012/08/09)**.

33. Larue R, Gupta K, Wuensch C, Shkriabai N, Kessl JJ, Danhart E, et al. Interaction of the HIV-1 intasome with transportin 3 protein (TNPO3 or TRN-SR2). J Biol Chem. 2012;287(41):34044–58 **(Epub 2012/08/09)**.

34. De Houwer S, Demeulemeester J, Thys W, Rocha S, Dirix L, Gijsbers R, et al. The HIV-1 integrase mutant R263A/K264A is 2-fold defective for TRN-SR2 binding and viral nuclear import. J Biol Chem. 2014;289(36):25351–61 **(Epub 2014/07/27)**.

35. Debyser Z, Christ F, De Rijck J, Gijsbers R. Host factors for retroviral integration site selection. Trends Biochem Sci. 2015;40(2):108–16 **(Epub 2015/01/04)**.

36. Demeulemeester J, Chaltin P, Marchand A, De Maeyer M, Debyser Z, Christ F. LEDGINs, non-catalytic site inhibitors of HIV-1 integrase: a patent review (2006–2014). Expert Opin Ther Pat. 2014;24(6):609–32 **(Epub 2014/03/29)**.

37. Maertens G, Cherepanov P, Pluymers W, Busschots K, De Clercq E, Debyser Z, et al. LEDGF/p75 is essential for nuclear and chromosomal targeting of HIV-1 integrase in human cells. J Biol Chem. 2003;278(35):33528–39 **(Epub 2003/06/11)**.

38. Busschots K, Vercammen J, Emiliani S, Benarous R, Engelborghs Y, Christ F, et al. The interaction of LEDGF/p75 with integrase is lentivirus-specific and promotes DNA binding. J Biol Chem. 2005;280(18):17841–7 **(Epub 2005/03/08)**.

39. Demeulemeester J, Tintori C, Botta M, Debyser Z, Christ F. Development of an AlphaScreen-based HIV-1 integrase dimerization assay for discovery of novel allosteric inhibitors. J Biomol Screen. 2012;17(5):618–28 **(Epub 2012/02/18)**.

40. Pauwels R, Balzarini J, Baba M, Snoeck R, Schols D, Herdewijn P, et al. Rapid and automated tetrazolium-based colorimetric assay for the detection of anti-HIV compounds. J Virol Methods. 1988;20(4):309–21 **(Epub 1988/08/01)**.

41. Naldini L, Blomer U, Gallay P, Ory D, Mulligan R, Gage FH, et al. In vivo gene delivery and stable transduction of nondividing cells by a lentiviral vector. Science. 1996;272(5259):263–7 **(Epub 1996/04/12)**.

42. Guiot E, Carayon K, Delelis O, Simon F, Tauc P, Zubin E, et al. Relationship between the oligomeric status of HIV-1 integrase on DNA and enzymatic activity. J Biol Chem. 2006;281(32):22707–19 **(Epub 2006/06/16)**.

43. Deprez E, Tauc P, Leh H, Mouscadet JF, Auclair C, Brochon JC. Oligomeric states of the HIV-1 integrase as measured by time-resolved fluorescence anisotropy. Biochemistry. 2000;39(31):9275–84 **(Epub 2000/08/05)**.

44. Baell JB, Holloway GA. New substructure filters for removal of pan assay interference compounds (PAINS) from screening libraries and for their exclusion in bioassays. J Med Chem. 2010;53(7):2719–40 **(Epub 2010/02/06)**.

45. Maertens GN, Cherepanov P, Engelman A. Transcriptional co-activator p75 binds and tethers the Myc-interacting protein JPO2 to chromatin. J Cell Sci. 2006;119(Pt 12):2563–71 **(Epub 2006/06/01)**.

46. Bartholomeeusen K, Christ F, Hendrix J, Rain JC, Emiliani S, Benarous R, et al. Lens epithelium-derived growth factor/p75 interacts with the transposase-derived DDE domain of PogZ. J Biol Chem. 2009;284(17):11467–77 **(Epub 2009/02/27)**.

47. Shi J, Zhou J, Shah VB, Aiken C, Whitby K. Small-molecule inhibition of human immunodeficiency virus type 1 infection by virus capsid destabilization. J Virol. 2011;85(1):542–9 **(Epub 2010/10/22)**.

48. Peng K, Muranyi W, Glass B, Laketa V, Yant SR, Tsai L, et al. Quantitative microscopy of functional HIV post-entry complexes reveals association of replication with the viral capsid. ELife. 2014;3:e04114 **(Epub 2014/12/18)**.

49. Wells JA, McClendon CL. Reaching for high-hanging fruit in drug discovery at protein–protein interfaces. Nature. 2007;450(7172):1001–9 **(Epub 2007/12/14)**.

12

Stabilizing HIV-1 envelope glycoprotein trimers to induce neutralizing antibodies

Alba Torrents de la Peña[1] and Rogier W. Sanders[1,2]*

Abstract

An effective HIV-1 vaccine probably will need to be able to induce broadly neutralizing HIV-1 antibodies (bNAbs) in order to be efficacious. The many bNAbs that have been isolated from HIV-1 infected patients illustrate that the human immune system is able to elicit this type of antibodies. The elucidation of the structure of the HIV-1 envelope glycoprotein (Env) trimer has further fueled the search for Env immunogens that induce bNAbs, but while native Env trimer mimetics are often capable of inducing strain-specific neutralizing antibodies (NAbs) against the parental virus, they have not yet induced potent bNAb responses. To improve the performance of Env trimer immunogens, researchers have studied the immune responses that Env trimers have induced in animals; they have evaluated how to best use Env trimers in various immunization regimens; and they have engineered increasingly stabilized Env trimer variants. Here, we review the different approaches that have been used to increase the stability of HIV-1 Env trimer immunogens with the aim of improving the induction of NAbs. In particular, we draw parallels between the various approaches to stabilize Env trimers and ones that have been used by nature in extremophile microorganisms in order to survive in extreme environmental conditions.

Background

The development of an effective and safe vaccine against HIV-1 requires a detailed understanding of the virological and immunological characteristics of HIV-1 infection. The virus has the ability to mutate very quickly, resulting in great viral diversity and making the development of an effective vaccine very challenging. Therefore, many research groups in the HIV-1 vaccine field pursue the development of a vaccine that can induce broadly neutralizing antibodies (bNAbs), i.e. antibodies that can target the functional envelope glycoprotein (Env) on many different virus isolates.

A focus of vaccine design is the generation of soluble Env trimer mimetics that can induce such antibodies and much progress has been made over the last few years in generating recombinant Env trimers that resemble the native Env spike. This required negating the inherent instability and flexibility of the native Env trimer and was accomplished by molecular design, resulting in

soluble stable Env trimers, of which SOSIP.664 trimers were the prototype [1–4]. The clade A BG505 SOSIP.664 trimer, now the gold standard in HIV native-like trimer immunogen design, allowed the determination of the high-resolution structure of the Env trimer [5–7]. A recent structure of the membrane-derived JR-FL trimer confirmed that the soluble and stabilized BG505 trimer resembled the native Env trimer present on the viral membrane [8]. Moreover, the SOSIP.664 design could be extrapolated to HIV-1 isolates other than BG505, thereby expanding the toolkit for HIV-1 vaccine design [9–14]. When used as immunogens in animal trials, SOSIP.664 proteins from various strains elicited autologous (strain-specific) Tier-2 neutralizing antibodies (NAbs); however, these immunogens failed to elicit potent bNAbs in most animals [15–18].

Here, we describe several approaches that have been pursued in order to increase the performance of soluble Env trimer mimetics as immunogens to induce NAbs. First, we review different methods that have been used to improve the stability of HIV-1 Env trimers, including forced viral evolution, structure-based design, high throughput screening of mutant trimers and selection

*Correspondence: r.w.sanders@amc.uva.nl
[1] Department of Medical Microbiology, Academic Medical Center, University of Amsterdam, 1105 AZ Amsterdam, The Netherlands
Full list of author information is available at the end of the article

of improved trimers by mammalian cell display. We also review which epitopes on Env trimer mimetics are targeted by the immune system, and we assess different immunization strategies in which Env trimer immunogens can be employed, including cocktail and sequential vaccination regimens.

Generating and validating mimetics of the native Env spike

The native Env trimer is unstable and flexible (conformationally heterogeneous), and the same applies to early generation soluble Env trimer derivates. As a consequence it took many years to elucidate its high-resolution structure by X-ray crystallography and cryo-electron microscopy (EM) techniques [19–21]. Initial low resolution cryo-electron tomography reconstructions of membrane-bound and soluble trimers provided new insights [22, 23], but high-resolution structures of the trimer were solved by using BG505 SOSIP.664 and the wide assortment of potent bNAbs that became available over the last decade [5, 24, 25]. Large gains in resolution were obtained with the first Env trimer crystal structure (4.7 Å resolution), which included a complex of the BG505 SOSIP.664 trimer with the V3-glycan bNAb PGT122 [20], and the first cryo-EM derived model of the same trimer in complex with the CD4 binding site bNAb PGV04 at a resolution of 5.8 Å [19]. In addition to providing lattice contacts to facilitate crystallization and 3D features to facilitate EM reconstruction, these bNAbs also provided validation of the structures, as the respective bNAb epitopes were clearly present.

The next step was to improve the resolution of the trimer structure by complexing the trimer with a combination of several new bNAbs. The use of the 35O22 bNAb directed to the gp120-gp41 interface and antibodies of the PGT121-family increased the resolution to ~ 3.5 Å and then 3.0 Å, and provided new details of the prefusion conformation of gp41, especially in HR1, a partially disordered region [6, 7, 26]. The SOSIP platform has been applied to trimers from different HIV-1 clades and their structures in complex with diverse bNAbs have also been elucidated, providing valuable new information for structure-based vaccine design [12, 21, 27–30]. Overall, the structures of all SOSIP trimers showed a highly similar trimer core, but revealed some differences in the variable loops that emanate from the core [21].

Another breakthrough came with the elucidation of the cryo-EM structure of a membrane-derived JR-FL trimer that was stabilized by the bNAb PGT151, but not by SOSIP mutations [8]. The overall structural features of the membrane-derived trimer as well as bNAb epitopes agree well to those of the soluble SOSIP trimers. However, subtle differences were observed in the

HR1 region of gp41, where the I559P substitution in the soluble trimer breaks a helix that is present in the full-length Env structure, exactly as it was meant to do [1, 8]. The high similarity of the membrane-derived and the soluble version of the Env confirm the value of the SOSIP design for generating soluble Env spike mimetics. A modification of the SOSIP design involves the introduction of a flexible Gly-Ser linker between gp120 and gp41 to replace the furin cleavage site, sometimes with additional modifications, effectively resulting in single chains trimers that do not require furin cleavage [31–33].

Designing next-generation Env trimers: learning from HIV-1 itself

A strategy to stabilize the Env trimers is by understanding and exploiting stability on the virus. To protect Env from NAbs, the virus evolves in a Darwinian way by selecting mutations in Env, in particular its variable loops, and by masking the protein surface with a shifting glycan shield. Virus evolution can also be exploited in the lab to obtain valuable information about mutations that can stabilize the Env trimer while retaining its functionality [34–37]. Such mutations can then be used to stabilize recombinant Env vaccine candidates.

By culturing HIV-1 virus under harsh conditions such as unphysiological temperatures (45–55 °C) or incremental concentrations of denaturant (GuHCl), Leaman and colleagues identified a more stable Env mutant that contained seven mutations compared to its wild-type counterpart. Most of the mutations were located in the gp120-gp41 interface, including positions 535 and 543 (Fig. 1, Table 1) [34]. These substitutions were also identified by an earlier study in which the sequence of the early generation but relatively stable KNH1144 SOSIP protein was compared to that of the unstable JR-FL SOSIP [38]. De Taeye et al. introduced, when not present, the 535M and 543N mutations into distinct clade B (AMC008 and B41) and clade C trimers (ZM197M) in order to increase their trimerization and stability [10].

Other substitutions that can improve native-like trimers were selected based on studies on how the virus becomes dependent on the entry inhibitor VIR165, and how HIV-1 can adapt to cold [39, 40]. These substitutions are located in C1 domain of gp120 (E64K, H66R and H66A; Fig. 1, Table 1) and likely keep the virus in the prefusion conformation by impeding steps towards the CD4-bound conformation by interacting with the HR1 region in gp41 [10, 41]. Thus, mutations that increase the stability of the native Env spike on virions can also be useful for the development of stable soluble native-like Env immunogens.

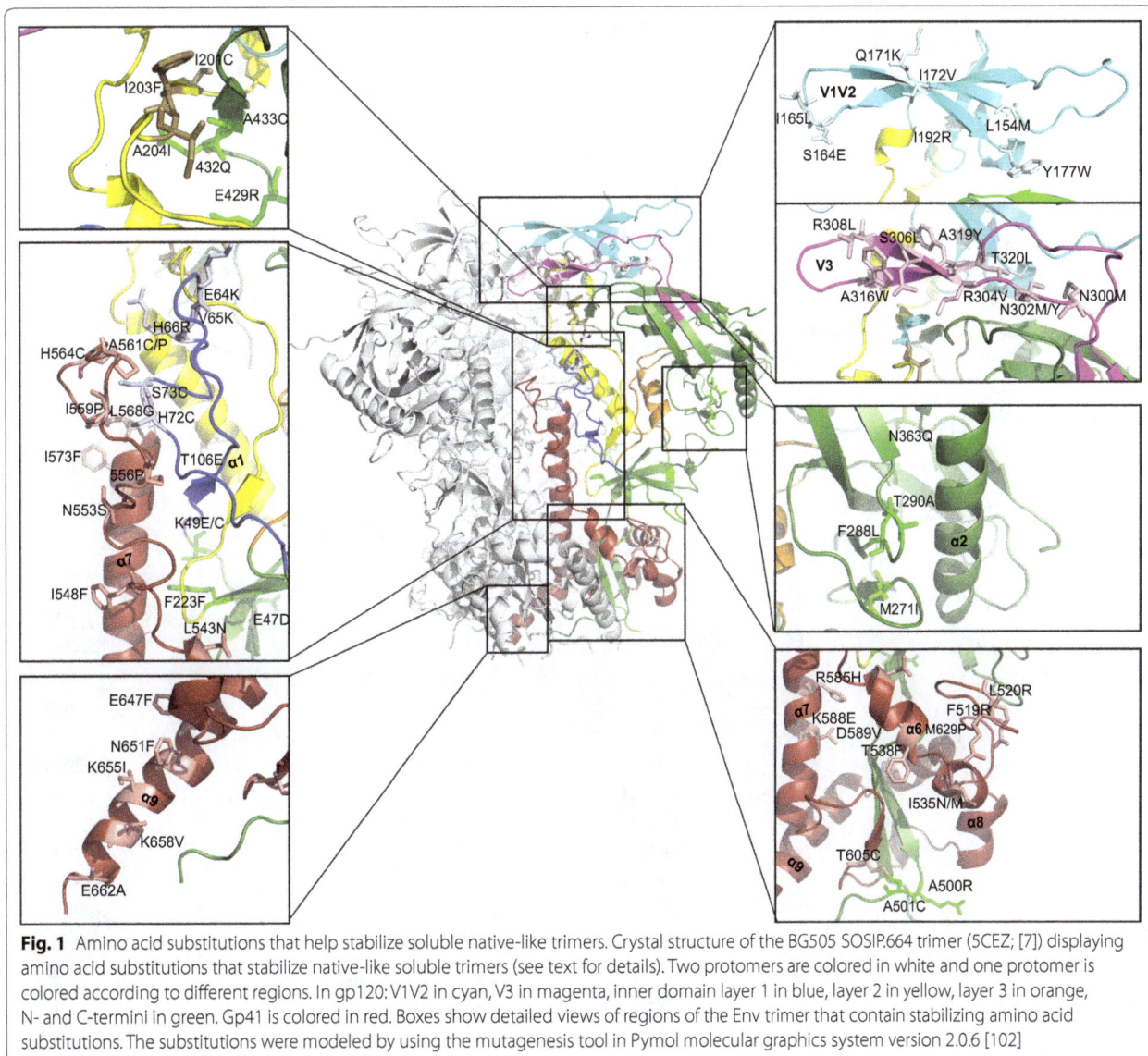

Fig. 1 Amino acid substitutions that help stabilize soluble native-like trimers. Crystal structure of the BG505 SOSIP.664 trimer (5CEZ; [7]) displaying amino acid substitutions that stabilize native-like soluble trimers (see text for details). Two protomers are colored in white and one protomer is colored according to different regions. In gp120: V1V2 in cyan, V3 in magenta, inner domain layer 1 in blue, layer 2 in yellow, layer 3 in orange, N- and C-termini in green. Gp41 is colored in red. Boxes show detailed views of regions of the Env trimer that contain stabilizing amino acid substitutions. The substitutions were modeled by using the mutagenesis tool in Pymol molecular graphics system version 2.0.6 [102]

Designing next-generation Env trimers: learning from extremophile organisms

SOSIP trimers based on most virus isolates other than BG505 initially did not form stable native-like trimers efficiently. However, the available trimer structures provided sufficient structural details to design modifications that improve the structure and stability of Env trimers, and that allowed generating stable trimers from many different isolates and clades.

When considering how to stabilize vaccine antigens, much can be learnt from nature. Extremophile bacteria and archea, which thrive in extreme environmental conditions such as high and low temperatures (between 45–122 °C and below − 15 °C, respectively) or alkaline and acidic conditions (pH > 11 and pH < 1, respectively)

[42–44], have evolved highly stable proteins compared to their mesophilic homologues [43, 45]. In extremophile organisms, natural evolution has applied six methods of protein stabilization. Several of these methods have been applied, either intentionally or not, to HIV-1 Env trimer vaccine design.

First, thermophilic proteins often have an increased number of hydrophobic residues at domain and oligomer interfaces, facilitating tighter packing of protein domains [46, 47]. A similar strategy was applied to HIV-1 Env trimers to stabilize the trimer and prevent the exposure of non-NAbs [48–53]. For example, de Taeye et al. avoided the spontaneous exposure of the V3 loop by increasing the hydrophobic interactions within the V3 domain and between the V3 and V1V2 domains, by

Table 1 Amino acid substitutions that stabilize soluble native-like trimers

	Hydrophobic	Aromatic	Proline/glycine	Disulfide bonds	Charged	Other
C1				E49C-L555C[a]	E47D[b]	E106T[b]
				H72C-H564C[a]	K49E[b]	
				A73C-A561C[a]	E64K[c]	
					V65K[b]	
					H66R[c]	
					T106E[d]	
V1	L154M[e]	Y177W[e]			S164E[b]	
V2	I165L[b]				Q171K[f]	
	I172V[f]				I192R[f]	
C2	A204I[g]	I203F[h]		I201C-A433C[m,n]		
	M271I[d]	F223W[d]				
	F288L[d]					
	T290A[d]					
V3	N300M[e]	N302Y/F[j]			H308R[b]	
	N302M[e]	A316W[c]				
	R304V[d]	A319Y[d]				
	S306L[i]					
	R308L[i]					
	T320L[e]					
C3						N363Q[d]
C4	Y420M[e]			I201C-A433C[m,n]	E429R[b]	R432Q[b]
C5				A501C-T605C[k]	A500R[b]	
FP[p]					F519R[j]	F516S[d]
					L520R[j]	
HR1[q]	D589V[g]	T538F[h]	L556P[g]	E49C-L555C[a]	L568D[d]	I535N/M[c,g,o]
		I548F[h]	I559G/P[l]	H72C-H564C[a]	K588E[g]	L543N[b,c]
		I573F[g]	A561P[d]	A73C-A561C[a]	G588R[b]	N553S[b]
			L568G[j]			V570H[d]
			T569G/P[j,l]			R585H[d]
						K588Q[g]
DSL[r]				A501C-T605C[k]		
	K655I[g]	E647F[g]	M629P[h]			
HR2[s]	K658V[g]	N651F[g]	S636G[j]			
	E662A[b]					

[a] Torrents de la Pena et al. Cell Rep. 2017

[b] Guenaga et al. J Virol. 2015

[c] de Taeye et al. Cell. 2015

[d] Steichen et al., Immunity. 2016

[e] Chuang et al. J Virol. 2017

[f] Ringe et al. J Virol. 2017

[g] Rutten et al. Cell Rep. 2018

[h] Sullivan et al. J Virol. 2017

[i] de Taeye et al. J Biol Chem. 2017

[j] Guenaga et al. Immunity. 2017

[k] Binley et al. J Virol. 2000

[l] Sanders et al. J Virol. 2002

[m] Guenaga et al. Plos Path. 2015

[n] Do Kwon et al., Nat. Struct. Mol. Biol. 2015

[o] Dey et al., Virol. 2007

[p] Fusion peptide

[q] Heptad repeat 1

[r] Disulfide loop

[s] Heptad repeat 2

introducing two Leu residues (S306L, R308L) in the V3 loop (Fig. 1, Table 1) [53]. Similarly, Chuang et al., Kulp et al., Steichen et al. and Rutten et al., introduced hydrophobic mutations in the trimer core (A204I, T320L, E381M, Q422L) or the trimer stem (D589V, K655I, K658V, E662A) using structure-based design and mammalian cell display, which resulted in increased Env packing and reduced flexibility (Fig. 1, Table 1) [49–51, 54].

Second, extremophile proteins contain a higher number of aromatic amino acids, which can enhance protein thermostability through ring stacking interactions as well as hydrophobic packing [55–57]. In structure-based HIV-1 immunogen design, several groups used the same principle and introduced aromatic residues to reduce V3 exposure (A316W, A319Y), and to increase stability of the trimer apex (Y177W, N302Y, N302F), the trimer base (E647F, N651F) and the trimer interface (gp120-gp41 interface: A223W, T538F and I548F; gp41-gp41 interface: I573F) (Fig. 1, Table 1) [10, 48–51, 54]. Overall, the introduction of hydrophobic and aromatic residues accounts for ~ 45% of the total number of mutations that are described in the literature to increase Env trimer stability.

Third, proteins from thermophilic organisms tend to have an increased number of charged residues involved in internal ion pairing and hydrogen bonding, as well as an increased number of positively charged residues at the solvent-exposed surface to provide stability at the surface [57]. For HIV-1 Env trimers the introduction of charged amino acids at the gp120 and gp41 interface also contributed to formation of well-ordered native-like trimers from different clades with enhanced thermostability (A500R, A558R) (Fig. 1, Table 1) [13, 58].

Fourth, proteins from thermophilic organisms usually contain many more predicted disulfide bonds than mesophilic organisms, which increases protein stability dramatically [45, 59, 60]. In mesophiles, proteins with many disulfide bonds are rare. As a consequence, there is a strong positive correlation between the number of disulfide bonds in proteins and the maximum growth temperature of thermophilic organisms [45, 59, 60]. Some viruses, such as influenza and vaccinia viruses, contain a disulfide bond that links the two Env subunits together, but HIV-1 Env naturally does not have such a disulfide bond, resulting in shedding of the gp120 subunit. The first step of generating stable native-like trimers was therefore the introduction of a disulfide bond between the gp120 and gp41 subunits (A501C-T605C) (Fig. 1, Table 1) [2]. To stabilize the flexible trimer interface, additional disulfide bonds have been introduced in the Env trimer: an intersubunit disulfide bond (A73C-A561C) and an interprotomer disulfide bond (E49C-L555C) (Fig. 1,

Table 1) [7, 61]. Furthermore, an intrasubunit disulfide bond (I201C-A433C) described by Kwon et al. and Guenaga et al. also stabilized the trimer in its prefusion state (Fig. 1, Table 1) [62, 63]. Combining three non-native disulfide bonds (A501C-T605C + A73C-A561C + I201C-A433C or A501C-T605C + A73C-A561C + E49C-L555C) resulted in hyperstable trimers that reached melting temperatures of up to 81 °C and 92 °C, respectively [61].

Fifth, thermophilic organisms increase the number of proline and glycine residues in loops to provide conformational rigidity to the protein [43]. In the HIV field, similar approaches have been used to generate soluble Env trimers. Since the HR1 region forms a helix in the post-fusion state and it adopts a partially disordered conformation in the pre-fusion state, we introduced the I559P mutation in the loop of HR1 to destabilize the post-fusion state of gp41 and stabilize the pre-fusion state [1]. Similarly, the introduction of glycine or proline residues in the HR1 and HR2 (N554G, L556P, A558P, I559G, T569P, T569G and S636G) further stabilized soluble HIV-1 Env trimers (Fig. 1, Table 1) [1, 54, 58]. Kong et al. computationally modeled HR1 loops with low Gibbs free energy that resulted in increased numbers of proline residues and rigidification of the HR1 loop [64].

A last mechanism that thermophilic organisms apply to survive at high temperatures is the reduction of asparagine and glutamine residues to prevent deamidation. This strategy has not been (intentionally) used for HIV vaccine design yet.

Thus, strategies to stabilize Env trimers from BG505 and other isolates using high throughput screening, selection by mammalian display, and structure-based design, in many ways mirror what extremophiles have achieved in nature to survive under extreme conditions. The resulting improvements in stability of soluble Env trimers allow us to use these immunogens in immunogenicity studies by facilitating the generation of a toolkit of trimers from different clades. Several of these trimers have been evaluated as immunogens and some studies have suggested that in some cases increased thermostability translates into increased immunogenicity [61, 65]. Furthermore, by increasing the trimer shelf life and avoiding cold chain transportation and storage will help to eventually produce a vaccine that is globally available.

Evaluating Env trimers in vivo: learning from immunization experiments

Native-like Env trimers have been tested as immunogens in small animals, mostly rabbits, and nonhuman primates. These studies indicated that native-like trimers consistently induced, for the first time, NAb responses against hard-to-neutralize (Tier 2) primary HIV-1 isolates. However, heterologous primary isolates were not, or only weakly and sporadically neutralized. Highly stable native-like trimers have been designed to improve the immunogenicity of the trimer by increasing its half-life in vivo and thus the presentation of bNAb epitopes. Immunogenicity studies with the highly stable trimers did not increase the generation of autologous NAb responses, but they induced weak heterologous Tier 2 responses in some cases. While trimer thermostability in vitro is a useful parameter that can be linked to in vivo observations [61, 65], it will also be important to investigate additional stability parameters such as trimer stability in serum at 37 °C.

Immunization with SOSIP trimers also induced strong non-neutralizing antibody (non-NAb) responses against V3 epitopes and neo-epitopes at the bottom of the trimer [10, 15, 16, 66]. Heterologous primary isolates were not, or only weakly and sporadically neutralized, pointing to possible directions of further research to improve native-like trimer immunogens.

First, it has recently been shown that the NAb responses in animals immunized with BG505 SOSIP trimers are dominated by specificities targeting a hole in the glycan shield, specifically the peptidic surface surrounding amino acids at positions 241 and 289, where most virus isolates have N-linked glycans [17, 67]. While autologous NAb responses might in some cases be a starting point for generating bNAb responses [7, 68], they could also distract or compete for such responses. If the latter scenario were true, one might want to dampen immunodominant isolate-specific, glycan-hole directed NAb responses. One strategy to counteract the immunogenicity of the BG505 specific glycan hole would be to immunize with trimers that contain glycans at positions N241 and N289. Previous studies have shown that immunizations with trimers based on isolates with a denser glycan shield (AMC008 and ZM197M) induced a broader heterologous NAb response compared to trimers from isolates with large holes in the glycan shield (BG505 and B41), which supports the pursuit of this strategy [69].

Second, immunization with BG505 SOSIP.664 trimers induced a strong response against non-NAb V3 epitopes [10, 50, 53, 70], leading to the hypothesis that this immunodominant V3-response interfered with the generation of bNAb responses. When rabbits were immunized with an improved version of the trimer, the BG505 SOSIP. v4 trimer, which contained the A316W mutation that sequestered the V3 epitope, these SOSIP trimers induced weaker anti-V3 responses and V3-directed Tier 1A virus NAb responses, without affecting the autologous NAb response [10, 16]. In a next iteration of trimer design, two additional hydrophobic residues were incorporated in the V3 loop of the BG505 SOSIP.v4 trimer (R306L and

R308L) to completely abolish the responses against the V3 loop [53]. Although these modifications reduced V3 immunogenicity, they did not improve the autologous NAb responses, nor did they result in a broadening of the NAb response. Similar results were recently obtained by Kulp et al. using different V3 designs [16, 50].

Third, the generation of soluble Env trimers resulted in the exposure of neo-epitopes at the bottom of the trimer, which is occluded by the viral membrane when the Env trimer is presented on virions. It has been suggested that the bottom of the trimer presents another immunodominant non-NAb epitope that could interfere with NAb responses [66, 70]; M. J. van Gils, C. A. Cottrell, A. B. Ward, R. W. Sanders unpublished data). To prevent the exposure of this epitope one could hide it, for example by placing the trimer on a nanoparticle.

Although interference by V3 and trimer bottom non-NAb responses is an attractive hypothesis, there is no formal proof yet that these non-NAb responses interfere with more desirable NAb and bNAb reponses. However, the V3 and trimer bottom non-NAb epitopes are usually solely of peptidic nature. B cells recognizing such epitopes are much more frequent in the naïve B cell repertoire and probably have higher affinity than naïve B cells recognizing composite peptide-glycan bNAb epitopes [70]. Higher affinity B cells might have a selective advantage over the lower affinity B cells targeting bNAb epitopes, because they might bind and process more antigen and, as a consequence, receive more T cell help. This will make it unlikely that B cells with the intrinsic capacity to mature into bNAbs will thrive in an environment that favors B cells targeting non-NAb or strain-specific glycan hole NAb epitopes. However, these arguments are somewhat theoretical in the HIV-1 context and the immune responses raised against Env trimers in animal and human vaccination experiments should be dissected in more detail to address these concerns.

To improve our understanding of the fate of Env trimers in vivo a number of studies focused on the germinal center responses against Env trimers. Macaques were immunized with stable Env trimers and germinal center cells from the lymph nodes were collected over time using fine needle aspirates (FNA), thereby avoiding the need to take lymph node biopsies and thereby blunting the response in that lymph node [18, 70]. While all the macaques generated immune responses against the trimer, the NAb responses correlated quantitatively with GC B cell frequencies. These studies provide a frame-of-reference for further studies on germinal center B cells and Tfh cells and their roles in epitope immunodominance and subdominance. Furthermore, insights in the amount of Env that enters the lymph nodes and the half-life of the Env protein in circulation would help efforts to study how the immunogen is delivered to B cells and how this can be improved. Previous work on other immunogens, including on gp120, suggest that it is worthwhile to exploit fluorescently tagged native-like trimers and to answer some of these questions, especially whether highly stable trimers show longer trimer half life in the presence of serum and proteases [71–73].

Evaluating Env trimers in vivo: learning from different immunization regimens

Until now, monovalent immunization with soluble HIV-1 Env trimers has only induced strong NAb responses against autologous viruses, and only weak and sporadic heterologous Tier 2 NAb responses. One strategy to increase neutralization breadth involves exploring different vaccine regimens such as cocktails of different immunogens. HIV-1 is a highly diverse pathogen, as is influenza virus. For influenza virus we use annually updated vaccines composed of a trivalent or tetravalent cocktail of different inactivated influenza viruses. However, annual influenza vaccination only protects against viral variants that are closely related to the vaccine strains, which exemplifies how difficult it is to induce a bNAb response against highly diverse viruses. The search for a universal flu vaccine shares similarities with the search for a bNAb-inducing HIV-1 vaccine.

To increase neutralization breadth, we have explored the use of cocktail and sequential regimens [17, 69]. We observed that immunization with a combination of immunogens in a cocktail formulation or in sequence did not induce bNAbs, but merely autologous NAb responses. Furthermore, the autologous NAb responses were prominent against the most immundominant trimer of the cocktail [69]. Thus, the immune response shows narrow specificity, similar to what has been reported for influenza vaccines [74]. These results indicate that an HIV-1 Env vaccine based on a cocktail or sequence of randomly chosen trimers is unlikely to induce bNAbs.

An alternative to the cocktail and sequential formulations could be to guide naïve B cell lineages towards bNAb activity by rational design. Since in natural infection the bNAbs develop through the co-evolution of the virus and the antibodies, one strategy that is being pursued is immunization with longitudinal Env sequences from patients that developed a bNAb response [75–80]. This strategy aims to recapitulate the evolutionary path of the virus and assumes that the development of the bNAb response largely depends on viral characteristics. Another, but somewhat related strategy, termed germline-targeting, focuses on the activation of rare subsets of naïve B cell that express B cell receptors (germline precursors) that have the intrinsic capacity to develop into bNAbs. SOSIP trimers generally do not bind inferred germline versions of bNAbs and several groups are designing immunogens that bind specifically to germline antibodies to guide the B cell responses towards the development of broadly neutralizing antibodies [51, 81–87].

Trimers can also be used to boost responses that are primed by epitope-specific immunogens. For example, Xu et al. applied trimers in an immunization regimen aimed at focusing immune responses to the fusion peptide. They immunized guinea pigs and macaques with a fusion peptide coupled to the carrier protein KLH, and boosted the responses with stabilized BG505 SOSIP trimers. This immunization strategy induced autologous NAb responses in all the animals and substantial NAb responses against heterologous Tier-2 viruses in some animals [88]. When they isolated the antibodies that were responsible for the broad neutralization they could confirm that these antibodies targeted the fusion peptide on both autologous and heterologous viruses [88].

Another strategy to overcome the low affinity of the immunogens to the desired but rare germline precursors of bNAbs is to multimerize the antigen, thereby increasing the potency of the Ab response by cross-linking the B cell receptors. The use of liposomes and ferritin nanocages that present Env trimers on their surface indeed improve the NAb response [89–91]. The flexibility of the nanoparticle system would allow the incorporation of trimers from different clades or lineages to enhance NAb responses against conserved B cell epitopes.

Applying the lessons learnt to other viral pathogens

We described how to make stable HIV-1 Env trimers for structural and immunological studies and how to use them in the quest for an HIV-1 vaccine. However, the lessons learnt in the HIV-1 field can also be applied to other viruses and *vice versa*. Similar to HIV-1 Env, other viral fusion proteins, such as the respiratory syncytial virus (RSV) F protein, are intrinsically metastable and easily switch from the pre-fusion to the post-fusion form. While a lot of efforts had to be invested to produce a stable soluble HIV-1 Env trimer, the influenza HA protein is comparatively stable and can be easily expressed. In contrast, the RSV F protein is, similarly to HIV Env, quite unstable and it adopts the post-fusion conformation when purified as soluble protein. While McLellan and colleagues introduced a disulfide bond and hydrophobic residues to keep the RSV glycoprotein in the pre-fusion state [92], Krarup et al. prevented the transition of this protein to the post-fusion state by introducing helix-breaking prolines in the refolding region 1, quite similar to what has been done for HIV-1 Env [93].

Recently, high-resolution structures of other viral glycoproteins were solved, including those of human parainfluenza virus 5, ebola virus, lassa virus, human betacoronavirus HKS1, lymphocytic choriomeningitis virus, herpes simplex virus 1 and severe fever with thrombocytopenia syndrome virus [92, 94–100]. The above-mentioned strategies that worked for HIV-1 Env have also benefited the stabilization and native-like pre-fusion forms of several of these glycoproteins. To keep the Middle East respiratory syndrome coronavirus (MERS-CoV) glycoprotein in the pre-fusion state, Pallesen et al. introduced two prolines at the start of the central helix of the protein, similarly to the I559P substitution introduced in the HIV-1 Env trimer [1, 96]. Similarly, to retain the lassa virus glycoprotein in the pre-fusion conformation, Hastie and colleagues incorporated a proline in the HR1 domain [98]. To further improve the stability the authors introduced a disulfide bond between the two subunits and improved the cleavage site as previously done for the HIV-1 Env trimer. Thus, the general strategy is to retain the viral glycoprotein in the pre-fusion conformation by structure-based design [2, 92, 96].

To further improve the immunogenicity of Env trimers, we can also learn from the recombinant vaccines against viral pathogens that are currently available. Hepatitis B virus, hepatitis E virus and human papillomavirus use recombinant virus-like particles as the immunogen [101]. These vaccines are self-assembling nanoparticles that mimic the native virions and expose neutralizing epitopes on their surface. As previously discussed, improvement of the nanoparticle design in the HIV-1 vaccine field is being pursued by several groups including us. In short, the strategies used to improve HIV-1 immunogen design provide a template to design vaccine candidates for other viruses and *vice versa*.

Conclusion
Here, we reviewed the latest design strategies to stabilize the soluble HIV-1 Env trimers as well as different immunization strategies maximize their value. The development of native-like trimers as immunogens, the availability of high-resolution structures, the design of different immunization strategies, the promise of germline-targeting and nanoparticle presentation, combined with an increased understanding of the host immunological responses against Env trimers, should advance the field of HIV-1 trimer vaccinology. These efforts should advance

the HIV-1 field and provide lessons for subunit vaccines against other viruses for which diversity is an issue, such as, but not limited to, influenza virus, dengue virus and hepatitis C virus.

Abbreviations
bNAbs: Broadly neutralizing antibodies; Env: Envelope glycoprotein; NAbs: Neutralizing antibodies; EM: Electron microscopy; non-NAb: Non-neutralizing antibody; FNA: Fine needle aspirates; RSV: Respiratory syncytial virus; MERS-CoV: Middle East respiratory syndrome coronavirus.

Authors' contributions
ATdIP and RWS wrote the review. Both authors read and approved the final manuscript.

Author details
[1] Department of Medical Microbiology, Academic Medical Center, University of Amsterdam, 1105 AZ Amsterdam, The Netherlands. [2] Department of Microbiology and Immunology, Weill Medical College of Cornell University, New York, NY 10021, USA.

Competing interests
RWS is listed on patents and patent applications related to stabilized HIV-1 Env trimers.

Funding
This work was supported by National Institutes of Health Grants P01 AI110657, the Bill and Melinda Gates Foundation, Grant #OPP1132237 and the Aids fonds Netherlands, Grant #2012041. RWS is a recipient of a Vidi grant from the Netherlands Organization for Scientific Research (NWO) and a Starting Investigator Grant from the European Research Council (ERC-StG-2011–280829-SHEV).

References
1. Sanders RW, Vesanen M, Schuelke N, Master A, Schiffner L, Kalyanaraman R, et al. Stabilization of the soluble, cleaved, trimeric form of the envelope glycoprotein complex of human immunodeficiency virus type 1. J Virol. 2002;76:8875–89.
2. Binley JM, Sanders RW, Clas B, Schuelke N, Master A, Guo Y, et al. A recombinant human immunodeficiency virus type 1 envelope glycoprotein complex stabilized by an intermolecular disulfide bond between the gp120 and gp41 subunits is an antigenic mimic of the trimeric virion-associated structure. J Virol. 2000;74:627–43.
3. Khayat R, Lee JH, Julien J-P, Cupo A, Klasse PJ, Sanders RW, et al. Structural characterization of cleaved, soluble HIV-1 envelope glycoprotein trimers. J Virol. 2013;87:9865–72.
4. Klasse PJ, Depetris RS, Pejchal R, Julien J-P, Khayat R, Lee JH, et al. Influences on trimerization and aggregation of soluble, cleaved HIV-1 SOSIP envelope glycoprotein. J Virol. 2013;87:9873–85.
5. Sanders RW, Derking R, Cupo A, Julien JP, Yasmeen A, de Val N, et al. A next-generation cleaved, soluble HIV-1 Env trimer, BG505 SOSIP.664 gp140, expresses multiple epitopes for broadly neutralizing but not non-neutralizing antibodies. PLoS Pathog. 2013;9:e1003618.
6. Pancera M, Zhou T, Druz A, Georgiev IS, Soto C, Gorman J, et al. Structure and immune recognition of trimeric pre-fusion HIV-1 Env. Nature. 2014;514:455–61.

7. Garces F, Lee JHH, de Val N, Torrents de la Peña A, Kong L, Puchades C, et al. Affinity maturation of a potent family of HIV antibodies is primarily focused on accommodating or avoiding glycans. Immunity. 2015;43:1053–63.

8. Lee JH, Ozorowski G, Ward AB. Cryo-EM structure of a native, fully glycosylated, cleaved HIV-1 envelope trimer. Science. 2016;351:1043–8.

9. Pugach P, Ozorowski G, Cupo A, Ringe R, Yasmeen A, de Val N, et al. A native-like SOSIP.664 trimer based on an hiv-1 subtype B env gene. J Virol. 2015;89:3380–95.

10. de Taeye SW, Ozorowski G, Torrents de la Peña A, Guttman M, Julien JP, van den Kerkhof TLGM, et al. Immunogenicity of stabilized HIV-1 envelope trimers with reduced exposure of non-neutralizing epitopes. Cell. 2015;163:1702–15.

11. Julien J, Lee JH, Ozorowski G, Hua Y, Torrents de la Peña A, de Taeye SW, et al. Design and structure of two HIV-1 clade C SOSIP.664 trimers that increase the arsenal of native-like Env immunogens. Proc Natl Acad Sci USA. 2015;112:1–6.

12. Stewart-Jones GBE, Soto C, Lemmin T, Chuang GY, Druz A, Kong R, et al. Trimeric HIV-1-Env structures define glycan shields from clades A, B, and G. Cell. 2016;165:813–26.

13. Guenaga J, de Val N, Tran K, Feng Y, Satchwell K, Ward AB, et al. Well-ordered trimeric HIV-1 subtype B and C soluble spike mimetics generated by negative selection display native-like properties. PLoS Pathog. 2015;11:e1004570.

14. Ringe RP, Yasmeen A, Ozorowski G, Go EP, Pritchard LK, Guttman M, et al. Influences on the design and purification of soluble, recombinant native-like HIV-1 envelope glycoprotein trimers. J Virol. 2015;89:12189–210.

15. Sanders RW, van Gils MJ, Derking R, Sok D, Ketas TJ, Burger JA, et al. HIV-1 neutralizing antibodies induced by native-like envelope trimers. Science. 2015;349:aac4223.

16. Pauthner M, Havenar-Daughton C, Sok D, Nkolola JP, Bastidas R, Boopathy AV, et al. elicitation of robust Tier 2 neutralizing antibody responses in nonhuman primates by HIV envelope trimer immunization using optimized approaches. Immunity. 2017;46:1073–88.

17. Klasse PJ, LaBranche CC, Ketas TJ, Ozorowski G, Cupo A, Pugach P, et al. Sequential and simultaneous immunization of rabbits with HIV-1 envelope glycoprotein SOSIP.664 trimers from clades A, B and C. PLoS Pathog. 2016;12:1–31.

18. Havenar-Daughton C, Reiss SM, Carnathan DG, Wu JE, Kendric K, Torrents de la Peña A, et al. Cytokine-independent detection of antigen-specific germinal center T follicular helper cells in immunized nonhuman primates using a live cell activation-induced marker technique. J Immunol. 2016;197:994–1002.

19. Lyumkis D, Julien J-P, de Val N, Cupo A, Potter CS, Klasse P-J, et al. Cryo-EM structure of a fully glycosylated soluble cleaved HIV-1 envelope trimer. Science. 2013;342:1484–90.

20. Julien J-P, Cupo A, Sok D, Stanfield RL, Lyumkis D, Deller MC, et al. Crystal structure of a soluble cleaved HIV-1 envelope trimer. Science. 2013;342:1477–83.

21. Ward AB, Wilson IA. The HIV-1 envelope glycoprotein structure: nailing down a moving target. Immunol Rev. 2017;275:21–32.

22. Harris A, Borgnia MJ, Shi D, Bartesaghi A, He H, Pejchal R, et al. Trimeric HIV-1 glycoprotein gp140 immunogens and native HIV-1 envelope glycoproteins display the same closed and open quaternary molecular architectures. Proc Natl Acad Sci USA. 2011;108:11440–5.

23. Liu J, Bartesaghi A, Borgnia MJ, Sapiro G, Subramaniam S. Molecular architecture of native HIV-1 gp120 trimers. Nature. 2008;455:109–13.

24. Wu X, Parast AB, Richardson BA, Nduati R, John-stewart G, Mbori-ngacha D, et al. Neutralization escape variants of human immunodeficiency virus type 1 are transmitted from mother to infant. J Virol. 2006;80:835–44.

25. McCoy LE, Burton DR. Identification and specificity of broadly neutralizing antibodies against HIV. Immunol Rev. 2017;275:11–20.

26. Doria-Rose N, Schramm C, Gorman J, Moore PL, Bhiman JN, DeKosky BJ, et al. Developmental pathway for potent V1V2-directed HIV-neutralizing antibodies. Nature. 2014;509:55–62.

27. Jardine JG, Sok D, Julien JP, Briney B, Sarkar A, Liang CH, et al. Minimally mutated HIV-1 broadly neutralizing antibodies to guide reductionist vaccine design. PLoS Pathog. 2016;12:1–33.

28. Kong L, Torrents De La Peña A, Deller MC, Garces F, Sliepen K, Hua Y, et al. Complete epitopes for vaccine design derived from a crystal structure of the broadly neutralizing antibodies PGT128 and 8ANC195 in complex with an HIV-1 Env trimer. Acta Crystallogr Sect D: Biol Crystallogr. 2015;71:2099–108.

29. Scharf L, Wang H, Gao H, Chen S, McDowall AW, Bjorkman PJ. Broadly neutralizing antibody 8ANC195 recognizes closed and open states of HIV-1 Env. Cell. 2015;162:1379–90.

30. Lee JH, Andrabi R, Su CY, Yasmeen A, Julien JP, Kong L, et al. A broadly neutralizing antibody targets the dynamic HIV envelope trimer apex via a long, rigidified, and anionic β-hairpin structure. Immunity. 2017;46:690–702.

31. Georgiev IS, Joyce MG, Yang Y, Sastry M, Zhang B, Baxa U, et al. Single-chain soluble BG505.SOSIP gp140 trimers as structural and antigenic mimics of mature closed HIV-1 Env. J Virol. 2015;89:5318–29.

32. Sharma SK, deVal N, Bale S, Guenaga J, Tran K, Feng Y, et al. Cleavage-independent HIV-1 Env trimers engineered as soluble native spike mimetics for vaccine design. Cell Rep. 2015;11:539–50.

33. Kong L, He L, De Val N, Vora N, Morris CD, Azadnia P, et al. Uncleaved prefusion-optimized gp140 trimers derived from analysis of HIV-1 envelope metastability. Nat Commun. 2016;7:1–15.

34. Leaman DP, Zwick MB. Increased functional stability and homogeneity of viral envelope spikes through directed evolution. PLoS Pathog. 2013;9:e1003184.

35. Agrawal N, Leaman DP, Rowcliffe E, Kinkead H, Nohria R, Akagi J, et al. Functional stability of unliganded envelope glycoprotein spikes among isolates of human immunodeficiency virus type 1 (HIV-1). PLoS ONE. 2011;6:e21339.

36. Bontjer I, Land A, Eggink D, Verkade E, Tuin K, Baldwin C, et al. Optimization of human immunodeficiency virus type 1 envelope glycoproteins with V1/V2 deleted, using virus evolution. J Virol. 2009;83:368–83.

37. Bontjer I, Melchers M, Eggink D, David K, Moore JP, Berkhout B, et al. Stabilized HIV-1 envelope glycoprotein trimers lacking the V1V2 domain, obtained by virus evolution. J Biol Chem. 2010;285:36456–70.

38. Dey AK, David KB, Klasse PJ, Moore JP. Specific amino acids in the N-terminus of the gp41 ectodomain contribute to the stabilization of a soluble, cleaved gp140 envelope glycoprotein from human immunodeficiency virus type 1. Virology. 2007;360:199–208.

39. Eggink D, de Taeye SW, Bontjer I, Klasse PJ, Langedijk JPM, Berkhout B, et al. HIV-1 escape from a peptidic anchor inhibitor by envelope glycoprotein spike stabilization. J Virol. 2016;90:10587–99.

40. Kassa A, Finzi A, Pancera M, Courter JR, Smith AB, Sodroski J. Identification of a human immunodeficiency virus type 1 envelope glycoprotein variant resistant to cold inactivation. J Virol. 2009;83:4476–88.

41. Finzi A, Xiang SH, Pacheco B, Wang L, Haight J, Kassa A, et al. Topological layers in the HIV-1 gp120 inner domain regulate gp41 interaction and CD4-triggered conformational transitions. Mol Cell. 2010;37:656–67.

42. D'Amico S, Gerday C, Feller G. structural determinants of cold adaptation and stability in a large protein. J Biol Chem. 2001;276:25791–6.

43. Redd JC, Lewis H, Trejo E, Winston V, Evilia C. Protein adaptations in archael extremophiles. Archaea. 2013;2013:1–14.

44. del Vecchio P, Elias M, Merone L, Graziano G, Dupuy J, Mandrich L, et al. Structural determinants of the high thermal stability of SsoPox from the hyperthermophilic archaeon Sulfolobus solfataricus. Extremophiles. 2009;13:461–70.

45. Liszka MJ, Clark ME, Schneider E, Clark DS. Nature versus nurture: developing enzymes that function under extreme conditions. Annu Rev Chem Biomol Eng. 2012;3:77–102.

46. Melchionna S, Sinibaldi R, Briganti G. Explanation of the stability of thermophilic proteins based on unique micromorphology. Biophys J. 2006;90:4204–12.

47. Razvi A, Scholtz JM. Lessons in stability from thermophilic proteins. Protein Sci. 2006;15:1569–78.

48. Sullivan JT, Sulli C, Nilo A, Yasmeen A, Ozorowski G, Sanders RW, et al. High-throughput protein engineering improves the antigenicity and stability of soluble HIV-1 envelope glycoprotein SOSIP trimers. J Virol. 2017;91:e00862.

49. Chuang G-Y, Gneg H, Pancera M, Xu K, Cheng C, Acharya P, et al. Structure-based design of a soluble prefusion-closed HIV-1 Env trimer with reduced CD4 affinity and improved immunogenicity. J Virol. 2017;91:1–18.

50. Kulp DW, Steichen JM, Pauthner M, Hu X, Schiffner T, Liguori A, et al. Structure-based design of native-like HIV-1 envelope trimers to silence non-neutralizing epitopes and eliminate CD4 binding. Nat Commun. 2017;8:1655.

51. Steichen JM, Kulp DW, Tokatlian T, Escolano A, Dosenovic P, Stanfield RL, et al. HIV vaccine design to target germline precursors of glycan-dependent broadly neutralizing antibodies. Immunity. 2016;45:483–96.

52. de Taeye SW, Moore JP, Sanders RW. HIV-1 Envelope trimer design and immunization strategies to induce broadly neutralizing antibodies. Trends Immunol. 2016;37:221–32.

53. de Taeye SW, Torrents de la Peña A, Vecchione A, Scutigliani E, Sliepen K, Burger JA, et al. Stabilization of the gp120 V3 loop through hydrophobic interactions reduces the immunodominant V3-directed non-neutralizing response to HIV-1 envelope trimers. J Biol Chem. 2017;120:1688–701.

54. Rutten L, Lai YT, Blokland S, Truan D, Bisschop IJM, Strokappe NM, et al. A universal approach to optimize the folding and stability of prefusion-closed HIV-1 envelope trimers. Cell Rep. 2018;23:584–95.

55. Goldstein RA. Amino-acid interactions in psychrophiles, mesophiles, thermophiles, and hyperthermophiles: insights from the quasi-chemical approximation. Protein Sci. 2007;16:1887–95.

56. Makwana KM, Mahalakshmi R. Implications of aromatic-aromatic interactions: from protein structures to peptide models. Protein Sci. 2015;24:1920–33.

57. Zhou XX, Wang YB, Pan YJ, Li WF. Differences in amino acids composition and coupling patterns between mesophilic and thermophilic proteins. Amino Acids. 2008;34:25–33.

58. Guenaga J, Garces F, De Val N, Ward AB, Wilson IA, Wyatt RT, et al. Glycine substitution at helix-to-coil transitions facilitates the structural determination of a stabilized subtype c hiv envelope glycoprotein. Immunity. 2017;46:792–803.

59. Beeby M, O'Connor BD, Ryttersgaard C, Boutz DR, Perry LJ, Yeates TO. The genomics of disulfide bonding and protein stabilization in thermophiles. PLoS Biol. 2005;3:1549–58.

60. Ladenstein R, Ren B. Reconsideration of an early dogma, saying "there is no evidence for disulfide bonds in proteins from archaea". Extremophiles. 2008;12:29–38.

61. Torrents de la Peña A, Julien J-P, De Taeye SW, Ward AB, Wilson IA, Sanders RW. Improving the immunogenicity of native-like HIV-1 envelope trimers by hyperstabilization. Cell Rep. 2017;20:1805–17.

62. Do Kwon Y, Pancera M, Acharya P, Georgiev IS, Crooks ET, Gorman J, et al. Crystal structure, conformational fixation and entry-related interactions of mature ligand-free HIV-1 Env. Nat Struct Mol Biol. 2015;22:522–31.

63. Guenaga J, Dubrovskaya V, de Val N, Sharma SK, Carrette B, Ward AB, et al. Structure-guided redesign increases the propensity of HIV Env to generate highly stable soluble trimers. J Virol. 2016;90:2806–17.

64. Kong L, He L, De Val N, Vora N, Morris CD, Azadnia P, et al. Uncleaved prefusion-optimized gp140 trimers derived from analysis of HIV-1 envelope metastability. Nat Commun. 2016;7:1–15.

65. Feng Y, Tran K, Bale S, Kumar S, Guenaga J, Wilson R, et al. Thermostability of well-ordered HIV spikes correlates with the elicitation of autologous Tier 2 neutralizing antibodies. PLoS Pathog. 2016;12:1–26.

66. Hu JK, Crampton JC, Cupo A, Ketas T, van Gils MJ, Sliepen K, et al. Murine antibody responses to cleaved soluble HIV-1 envelope trimers are highly restricted in specificity. J Virol. 2015;89:10383–98.

67. McCoy LE, van Gils MJ, Ozorowski G, Messmer T, Briney B, Voss JE, et al. Holes in the glycan shield of the native hiv envelope are a target of trimer-elicited neutralizing antibodies. Cell Rep. 2016;16:2327–38.

68. Lynch RM, Wong P, Tran L, O'Dell S, Nason MC, Li Y, et al. HIV-1 Fitness cost associated with escape from the VRC01 class of CD4 binding site neutralizing antibodies. J Virol. 2015;89:4201–13.

69. Torrents de la Peña A, de Taeye SW, Sliepen K, LaBranche C, Burger JA, Schermer EE, et al. Immunogenicity in rabbits of SOSIP trimers from clades A, B and C given individually, sequentially or in combinations. J Virol. 2018;92:e01957.

70. Havenar-Daughton C, Lee JH, Crotty S. Tfh cells and HIV bnAbs, an immunodominance model of the HIV neutralizing antibody generation problem. Immunol Rev. 2017;275:49–61.

71. Park C, Arthos J, Cicala C, Kehrl JH. The HIV-1 envelope protein gp120 is captured and displayed for B cell recognition by SIGN-R1 + lymph node macrophages. Elife. 2015;4:1–23.

72. Sliepen K, Van Montfort T, Ozorowski G, Pritchard LK, Crispin M, Ward AB, et al. Engineering and characterization of a fluorescent native-like HIV-1 envelope glycoprotein trimer. Biomolecules. 2015;5:2919–34.

73. Forthal DN, Gilbert PB, Landucci G, Phan T. Recombinant gp120 vaccine-induced antibodies inhibit clinical strains of HIV-1 in the presence of Fc receptor-bearing effector cells and correlate inversely with HIV infection rate. J Immunol. 2007;178:6596–603.

74. Gerdil C. The annual production cycle for influenza vaccine. Vaccine. 2003;21:1776–9.

75. Bonsignori M, Liao H-X, Gao F, Williams WB, Alam SM, Montefiori DC, et al. Antibody-virus co-evolution in HIV infection: paths for HIV vaccine development. Immunol Rev. 2017;275:145–60.

76. Landais E, Huang X, Havenar-Daughton C, Murrell B, Price MA, Wickramasinghe L, et al. Broadly neutralizing antibody responses in a large longitudinal sub-saharan HIV primary infection cohort. PLoS Pathog. 2016;12:1–22.

77. Landais E, Murrell B, Briney B, Murrell S, Rantalainen K, Berndsen ZT, et al. HIV Envelope glycoform heterogeneity and localized diversity govern the initiation and maturation of a V2 apex broadly neutralizing antibody lineage. Immunity. 2017;47:990–1003.

78. Moore PL, Gray ES, Wibmer CK, Bhiman JN, Nonyane M, Sheward DJ, et al. Evolution of an HIV glycan–dependent broadly neutralizing antibody epitope through immune escape. Nat Med. 2012;18:1688–92.

79. Hraber P, Korber B, Wagh K, Giorgi EE, Bhattacharya T, Gnanakaran S, et al. Longitudinal antigenic sequences and sites from intra-host evolution (LASSIE) identifies immune-selected HIV variants. Viruses. 2015;7:5443–75.

80. Tian M, Cheng C, Chen X, Duan H, Cheng HL, Dao M, et al. Induction of HIV neutralizing antibody lineages in mice with diverse precursor repertoires. Cell. 2016;166:1471–84.

81. Briney B, Sok D, Jardine JG, Kulp DW, Skog P, Menis S, et al. Tailored immunogens direct affinity maturation toward HIV neutralizing antibodies. Cell. 2016;166:1459–70.

82. Jardine J, Julien J-P, Menis S, Ota T, Kalyuzhniy O, McGuire A, et al. Rational HIV immunogen design to target specific germline B cell receptors. Science. 2013;340:711–6.

83. Jardine JG, Ota T, Sok D, Pauthner M, Kulp DW, Kalyuzhniy O, et al. Priming a broadly neutralizing antibody response to HIV-1 using a germline-targeting immunogen. Science. 2015;349:156–61.

84. Sok D, Pauthner M, Briney B, Lee JH, Saye-Francisco KL, Hsueh J, et al. A prominent site of antibody vulnerability on HIV envelope incorporates a motif associated with CCR5 binding and its camouflaging glycans. Immunity. 2016;45:1–23.

85. McGuire AT, Hoot S, Dreyer AM, Lippy A, Stuart A, Cohen KW, et al. Engineering HIV envelope protein to activate germline B cell receptors of broadly neutralizing anti-CD4 binding site antibodies. J Exp Med. 2013;210:655–63.

86. Medina-Ramírez M, Garces F, Escolano A, Skog P, de Taeye SW, del Moral-Sanchez I, et al. Design and crystal structure of a native-like HIV-1 envelope trimer that engages multiple broadly neutralizing antibody precursors in vivo. J Exp Med. 2017;214:2573–90.

87. Sliepen K, Medina-Ramírez M, Yasmeen A, Moore JP, Klasse PJ, Sanders RW. Binding of inferred germline precursors of broadly neutralizing HIV-1 antibodies to native-like envelope trimers. Virology. 2015;486:116–20.

88. Kai Xu, Acharya P, Kong R, Cheng C, Chuang G-Y, Liu K, et al. Epitope-based vaccine design yields fusion peptide-directed antibodies that neutralize diverse strains of HIV-1. Nat Med. 2018;24:857–67.

89. Ingale J, Stano A, Guenaga J, Sharma SK, Nemazee D, Zwick MB, et al. High-density array of well-ordered HIV-1 spikes on synthetic liposomal nanoparticles efficiently activate B cells. Cell Rep. 2016;15:1986–99.

90. Sliepen K, Ozorowski G, Burger JA, van Montfort T, Stunnenberg M, LaBranche C, et al. Presenting native-like HIV-1 envelope trimers on ferritin nanoparticles improves their immunogenicity. Retrovirology. 2015;12:82.

91. Georgiev IS, Joyce MG, Chen RE, Leung K, McKee K, Druz A, et al. Two-component ferritin nanoparticles for multimerization of diverse trimeric antigens. ACS Infect Dis. 2018;4:788–96.

92. McLellan JS, Chen M, Joyce MG, Sastry M, Stewart-Jones GBE, Yang Y, et al. Structure-based design of a fusion glycoprotein vaccine for respiratory syncytial virus. Science. 2013;342:592–8.

93. Krarup A, Truan D, Furmanova-Hollenstein P, Bogaert L, Bouchier P, Bisschop IJM, et al. A highly stable prefusion RSV F vaccine derived from structural analysis of the fusion mechanism. Nat Commun. 2015;6:8143.

94. Yin HS, Wen X, Paterson RG, Lamb RA, Jardetzky TS. Structure of the parainfluenza virus 5 F protein in its metastable, prefusion conformation. Nature. 2006;439:38–44.

95. Lee JE, Fusco ML, Hessell AJ, Oswald WB, Burton DR, Saphire EO. Structure of the Ebola virus glycoprotein bound to an antibody from a human survivor. Nature. 2008;454:177–82.

96. Pallesen J, Wang N, Corbett KS, Wrapp D, Kirchdoerfer RN, Turner HL, et al. Immunogenicity and structures of a rationally designed prefusion MERS-CoV spike antigen. Proc Natl Acad Sci. 2017;114:E7348–57.

97. Kong L, Giang E, Nieusma T, Kadam RU, Cogburn KE, Hua Y, et al. Hepatitis C virus E2 envelope glycoprotein core structure. Science. 2013;342:1090–4.

98. Hastie KM, Igonet S, Sullivan BM, Legrand P, Zandonatti MA, Robinson JE, et al. Crystal structure of the prefusion surface glycoprotein of the prototypic arenavirus LCMV. Nat Struct Mol Biol. 2016;23:513–21.

99. Zeev-Ben-Mordehai T, Vasishtan D, Hernández Durán A, Vollmer B, White P, Prasad Pandurangan A, et al. Two distinct trimeric conformations of natively membrane-anchored full-length herpes simplex virus 1 glycoprotein B. Proc Natl Acad Sci. 2016;113:4176–81.

100. Kirchdoerfer RN, Cottrell CA, Wang N, Pallesen J, Yassine HM, Turner HL, et al. Prefusion structure of a human coronavirus spike protein. Nature. 2016;74:27–34.

101. Zhao Q, Li S, Yu H, Xia N, Modis Y. Virus-like particle-based human vaccines: quality assessment based on structural and functional properties. Trends Biotechnol. 2013;31:654–63.

102. Schrodinger LLC. The PyMOL molecular graphics system, version 1.3r1. 2010.

13

Recent advances in retroviruses via cryo-electron microscopy

Johnson Mak[1] and Alex de Marco[2*] (ID)

Abstract

Cryo-electron microscopy has undergone a revolution in recent years and it has contributed significantly to a number of different areas in biological research. In this manuscript, we will describe some of the recent advancements in cryo-electron microscopy focussing on the advantages that this technique can bring rather than on the technology. We will then conclude discussing how the field of retrovirology has benefited from cryo-electron microscopy.

Keywords: Cryo-electron microscopy, Cryo-electron tomography, Structural biology, Single particle, Subtomogram averaging

Introduction

Biological systems are complex environments populated with millions of molecules that include structural proteins, enzymes, nucleic acids and lipids [1]. Many of these molecules interact with multiple partners in order to fulfil their role. Duration, stability and specificity of those interactions vary from one situation to the next [2] and understanding these intermolecular relationships can provide insights into their mechanisms of action. Data about a specific interaction can be used to develop computational models to predict how these molecules function [3–5], examples include the study of the interactome of YGL161G in Yeast [3]. In the case of pathogens, such structural knowledge can be used for the design of vaccines [6, 7] and novel therapeutics [8, 9]. Currently, the three major techniques commonly used for structural determination are X-ray crystallography, Nuclear Magnetic Resonance (NMR) and cryo-Electron Microscopy (cryoEM) [10]. All three of these approaches can be used to resolve the structure of a protein (or complexes) to atomic or near-atomic resolution. Through X-Ray

crystallography and NMR, it has been possible to resolve the structure of isolated proteins or complexes in isolated states. Despite the significant information provided through these methods, the result can be prone to artefacts and poor interpretation. One reason for such drawback is that these approaches do not take into account the environment where the proteins or complexes normally exist. In this review, we will share the basic principles of cryoEM and highlight some of the recent advances, we will discuss advantages and potential pitfalls of this technique. In particular, we will provide examples of how cryoEM has revealed aspects of retrovirology that were previously unknown to us.

Cryo-electron microscopy and related techniques
The electron microscope

The term CryoEM covers a broad range of methods that share the common ground of imaging, through a transmission electron microscope (TEM), a radiation sensitive sample that is kept at cryogenic temperature [11]. A TEM provides a detailed map of the electron densities distributed across the inspected sample. Similarly, a light microscope provides a map of the optical density of a sample, but the resolution that can be achieved by these two techniques differs significantly due to the diffraction limit of the wavelength in use. Accordingly, using visible light,

---

*Correspondence: alex.demarco@monash.edu
[2] Department of Biochemistry and Molecular Biology, Monash University, Clayton, VIC, Australia
Full list of author information is available at the end of the article

observable features are limited to ~ 200 nm resolution, while by using soft X-Rays the resolution limit is down to ~ 30 nm. To be noted that this limit depends on the current limitations in lens manufacturing. In contrast, electrons have a wavelength of ~ 2 pm at 300 keV and the lens system in these microscopes allow a resolution limit to the angstrom (Å) range. In this latter case, the resolution limit of the instrument is not limiting, while the structural variability within the samples together with their sensitivity to the electron beam will be the major limiting factors.

In TEMs, electrons are emitted by a source filament (that can be thermoionic or cold depending on the material and operation principle) and accelerated at voltages typically ranging between 60 and 300 keV. The electron beam is shaped and directed to the sample through an electromagnetic condenser lens system. While passing through the sample, each electron scatters differently depending on the local composition of the specimen (atomic cross-section) [12]. The scattered beam is then refocused through another set of electromagnetic lenses (objective lens) that will project a magnified image on a detector. Over the past few years, the development of new imaging detectors allowed for the capture of images with extremely low electron doses and short exposures. This is attributed to the ability to directly detect electrons (Direct Electron Detectors), having both a high quantum efficiency (up to 70% depending on energy and frequency) and fast readout speed (up to 400 frames/s). These advancements allow for collecting images with high signal-to-noise ratio at the higher frequencies (if compared to the film and CCD data). The poor signal-to-noise ratio is recognized as one of the major limiting factors in achieving high-resolution until 2012 [13, 14].

The sample preparation

CryoEM analysis consists of imaging samples maintained at cryogenic temperatures (80–120 K). Cryogenic conditions limit the effects of radiation damage on biological samples [15] and provide a means for instantaneous fixation. In fact, if the freezing process is fast enough all the water in the sample will become vitreous and any activity (down to molecular level) will stop [15]. Vitreous ice is an amorphous solid form of water, which can withstand a high vacuum environment (such as the one found inside a TEM) without displaying significant sublimation. Vitreous ice also has the same electron transparency as liquid water making cryoEM ideal to inspect proteins. In fact, an electron accelerated at 300 keV (the most commonly used energy in high-resolution cryoEM) can travel through a region up to ~ 250 nm of water and statistically undergoing a single elastic scatter event (mean free path) [16].

Vitreous ice, however, is not a condition that is easily achieved. A rapid drop in temperature throughout the whole sample (from room temperature to cryogenic temperature) must be reached within ~ 1 ms. For a thin sample that is less than 10 μm, vitreous ice can be achieved through plunge freezing the sample in liquid ethane [15]. For thicker samples, the preferred method is High-Pressure Freezing (HPF). HPF consists of a rapid cooling of biological samples (even up to 200 μm in thickness) within ~ 2 ms, while the pressure is increased to 2000 bars to prevent the formation of crystalline ice [17].

The most common method of sample preparation (including purified proteins, protein complexes and viruses) requires deposition of a water-soluble substrate onto a TEM grid support that is covered with a holey carbon foil. Once the sample has been spread throughout the grid, excess liquid is removed by blotting in order to leave the thinnest possible film. This is then plunged into liquid ethane.

Different samples require different approaches

Currently, cryoEM comprises of a multitude of applications from imaging of purified proteins to its application on intact entities. These include large macromolecular complexes, viruses, bacteria or even tissue sections. Depending on the sample and the question to be addressed, multiple potential workflows can be applied for cryoEM based structure determination. Currently, the preferred method to resolve the structure of purified proteins and protein complexes is Single Particle cryoEM (SP cryoEM). As previously mentioned, biological samples are extremely sensitive to high energy electrons, therefore images must be taken using a very low dose. Imaging at low dose lead to an extremely low signal-to-noise ratio, and since scattering is a stochastic event it can lead to incomplete sampling. Another limitation comes from the fact that molecules are three-dimensional objects, while electron micrographs are two-dimensional projections, which can, per se, only provide an incomplete description of the sample. The simplest way to overcome these problems consists of 'averaging' multiple copies of the same molecule which have been imaged from enough orientations to cover every view. This is to some extent analogous to what is done in X-ray crystallography, where the quality of the signal obtained in the diffractogram depends in part on the number of repeated unit cells present in the imaging area and the uniformity of the unit cells. By imaging multiple copies of the same molecule in random orientations, it is possible to obtain three-dimensional structural information of the complex in question. All projection images will be classified based on orientation and (if applicable) conformation. Once enough views have been identified and enough statistics are available for each of those, relevant images will be averaged and combined, through back-projection, to form a noise-free three-dimensional representation of the molecule under study. One of the major advantages of Single Particle cryoEM is that the crystallization step in X-ray crystallography may be bypassed. Furthermore, the structure can be determined while the molecule is in a state that is closer to physiological, rather than the solid form of a protein crystal that may or may not be biologically relevant. At the same time, the heterogeneity (of the structural folds in solution) resulting from the allowed flexibility can become a significant hurdle to providing high-resolution 3D reconstructions that are more readily achieved via X-ray crystallography [18]. An increasing number of algorithms are being developed to overcome this problem of heterogeneity and hopefully obtain a model describing all the states that a molecule can adopt in solution. As of today, this type of comprehensive description of state has been only possible for a restricted set of molecules [19].

Complexes that are organised following a defined high order symmetry (such as actin filaments, microtubules or enveloped viruses), can be extremely unlikely to crystallize. For those, a similar approach as described for single particle cryoEM can be used to determine the high-resolution structure of the complex. In this case, the high-order symmetry is advantageous since the symmetry helps to initiate the alignment by often providing strong low-resolution information. Furthermore, the symmetry provides multiple views of the same protein in each particle and the orientation between each monomer is defined by the symmetry. The two techniques that are mostly used to resolve the structure of the monomers for these type of symmetrical assemblies are helical and icosahedral reconstruction [18]. Owing to the fact that the sample flexibility is limited by the molecular packing and considering that each individual particle contains multiple views of the same object (inherent in the symmetry), both techniques demonstrated their potential leading to resolutions below 3Å even in times when cryoEM was a very niche field and automated microscopes and direct detectors were not available [20–26].

If one is interested in understanding the structural organization of complexes in their native biological context, these appear as the convolution of molecules that are located across multiple layers, the relative position of each molecule does not necessarily follow any high order symmetry nor any relationship. This type of arrangement is valid also for purified large macromolecular complexes such as viral capsids or vesicles that can be pleomorphic but still display local symmetry or order. Consequently, the determination of these structures cannot be achieved through single particle cryoEM. One potential way to overcome this conundrum is to produce a 3D representation of the sample by performing a tomographic acquisition. This technique is known as cryo-Electron Tomography (cryoET) and consists of imaging the same area from multiple different angles, which is then followed by a back-projection step. CryoET can be used to analyse the landscape of a cellular region or to resolve structures of proteins or protein complexes: the process required for these two different types of data collection changes significantly between these two applications.

Since tomographic acquisition is slow (40'—1 h/tomogram), regardless of whether the objective is to obtain a detailed description of the cellular landscape or determine the structure of the complex to high resolution, the magnification will be lowered to the minimum allowable level that would still resolve the structure of interest by maximising the field of view. For example, if the goal is to obtain landscape information at a resolution of ~ 3 to 5 nm, the electron dose will be maximised to the limit allowed by the sample (more than 100 $e^-/Å^2$) to provide the best possible contrast. Alternatively, should the goal be to obtain molecular structural information in details, the electron dose needs to be minimised to prevent damage (between 50 and 100 $e^-/Å^2$) during data acquisition, and the magnification can be increased in order to boost the signal to noise ratio at high-resolution. In fact, the camera response or efficiency in digitizing the image (Detector Quantum Efficiency or DQE) is higher in the middle and low-frequency range.

The ability to describe a sample in three dimensions through tomography depends on the ability to image it from different angles. A major limitation of cryoET is linked to the impossibility of tilting the sample up to 90°, as past 60°–70° the grid becomes too thick to image. Typically the resolution achievable from a single tomogram is comprised between 3 and 5 nm in XY (resolution here is limited by the maximum electron dose a sample can sustain) and lower in Z (depending on the completeness of the tilt range). This is the effect of the so-called missing wedge of information [27]. In order to eliminate the anisotropy derivations from the incomplete tilt range as well as boosting the signal (and therefore the resolution), one can apply an averaging for structural determination. This approach, called "subtomogram averaging", is the equivalent of single particle analyses but performed on three-dimensional data instead of the projection data. Typically small subregions that are expected to contain the complex of interest are extracted from the tomograms (subtomograms), those are iteratively aligned and averaged. It has been shown that this approach is capable of providing near-atomic resolution, similarly to cryoEM Single Particle Analyses [28, 29].

Hybrid techniques and correlative light and electron microscopy

Finding multiple copies of samples within an EM grid for imaging in nanometre resolution is like finding a needle in a haystack. A typical problem arising upon the inspection of a tomogram collected on a cell is that it appears as a constellation of densities, and only a small fraction of those densities can be unequivocally recognised through their shape and/or location from the sample grid for imaging. Over the past few years, the use of Correlative Light and Electron Microscopy (CLEM) has been extended toward cryopreserved samples, making it much easier to identify rare events (or protein complexes in this case) for structural determination [30–32]. Current developments in cryo-CLEM showed that it is possible to predict the position of a molecule in three dimensions with a precision within 200 nm [33,34], and it is possible (where needed) to thin a sample using cryo-focused ion beam (cryo-FIB) so that it would become compatible with cryoET [35, 36].

Where did cryoEM help in understanding retroviral biology?

Analyses of glycoproteins of SIV and HIV-1 enveloped viruses

For a long time, viral proteins have been among the most studied by structural biologists, not only for the high pathological relevance but also because a significant portion of the viruses studied over the years has a capsid which is organised following a strict icosahedral symmetry [37]. Glycoproteins in icosahedral viruses are generally distributed following the symmetry of the capsid. The structure in those cases can be obtained together with the capsid structure through cryoEM and icosahedral reconstruction [38]. With the implementation of sub-tomogram averaging, it is now possible to resolve the structure of viral glycoproteins located on the membrane of irregular enveloped viruses. Even without knowing the exact location of the target proteins, the typical workflow consists of the indiscriminate extraction of observed density located on the membrane surface followed by an iterative alignment. This methods works based on the idea that the most abundant feature will predominate in the final average, while all densities that do not match will be excluded based on correlation threshold when compared to the average. A few densities are manually picked based on the expected shape and size, which are then used to provide a reference model. The classification can be done by applying a threshold to the cross-correlation value calculated during the alignment with the reference or with the sum of the densities after alignment.

Subtomogram averaging was used to successfully determine the structure of the gp120 trimer on the surface of SIV and HIV-1 virions at a resolution close to 2 nm [39, 40] (Fig. 1a). The analysis, in this case, allowed an understanding of the binding dynamics and conformational changes induced by the broadly neutralising antibodies (bNAb). Broadly neutralising antibodies have been a subject of intense research, and understanding how bNAbs can be elicited in human hosts would be vital for the development of HIV vaccine candidate. Generally speaking, there are five target sites for bNAbs against HIV envelope: the V2 site, the N332 supersite, the CD4 binding site, the gp120-41 interface, and the membrane proximal external region (MPER) (for review see Wibmer et al. [41]). The structural arrangement of the interaction between env and the antibody have been resolved through cryoEM [42–49].

Over the years there have been multiple attempts to resolve the structure of the envelope gp120 trimer for both SIV and HIV-1 [39,50–54] (Fig. 1b, d). In addition to an increase of the resolution limit as the technology

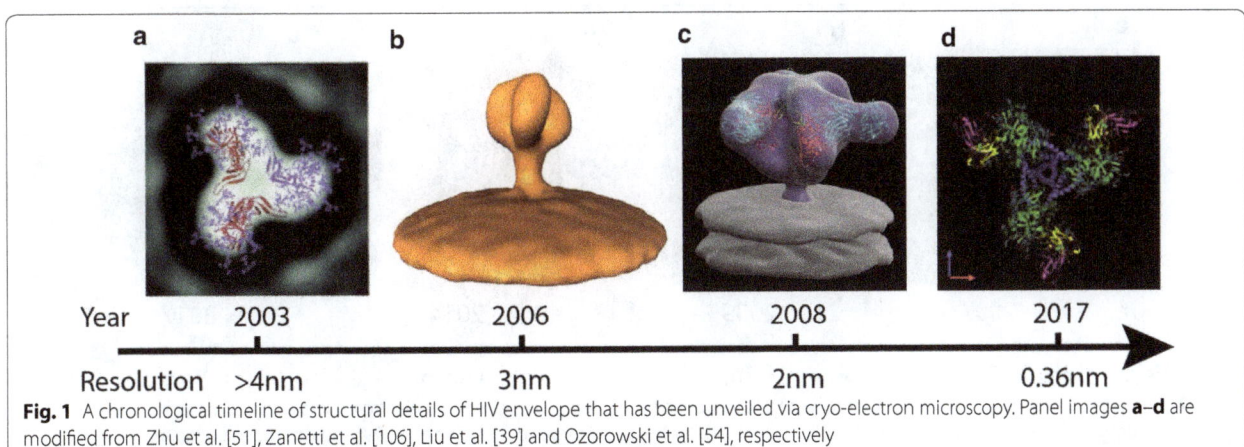

Fig. 1 A chronological timeline of structural details of HIV envelope that has been unveiled via cryo-electron microscopy. Panel images **a–d** are modified from Zhu et al. [51], Zanetti et al. [106], Liu et al. [39] and Ozorowski et al. [54], respectively

improves, there are also visible differences between individual cryoEM structures that depend on the preparation of the envelope protein trimeric structure, such as a fully glycosylated cleaved version of the protein [44], a complex that involves binding with CD4 receptor, co-receptor or receptor mimic antibody [42, 45, 47, 49, 55–57]. The bindings between HIV envelope trimer with antibody, CD4 receptor or co-receptor generally leads to structural reorganization (review see [41, 49]). The combination of super-resolution microscopy and cryoEM has also suggested that the virion particle also undergoes a size expansion upon CD4 receptor engagement [58], which might be important to facilitate the subsequent biological process of HIV infection.

As previously discussed in [59], there have been evident differences in the processing methods used and the type of controls applied. This learning curve has helped to define a procedure to validate any structure that is computed through cryoEM or cryoET. Nonetheless, it is still important to be conscious that cryoEM is still a developing field, therefore there are still potential pitfalls that a novice can run into [60, 61], and incorporation of validation standards is currently considered a high priority for experts and developers in this field [62–64].

Analyses of the retroviral capsid during viral assembly and maturation

It has long been known that retroviruses assemble an immature virion through the accumulation of multiple copies of its structural polyprotein Gag. This assembly process occurs underneath the plasma membrane of the host cells (with the exception of the spumaviruses and betaretroviruses where the assembly phase takes place in the cytoplasm). Immediately after budding, a set of proteolytic cleavages induce a dramatic change in the structural organisation. The macroscopic differences between

mature and immature forms of the virus are striking enough that these are visible through conventional TEM analyses, but the real breakthrough in understanding the re-arrangement of Gag's domains throughout this process came from the application of cryoET [65]. In fact, the inherent pleomorphism present across all retroviruses made it impossible to obtain a detailed model of the virions through other methods such as X-ray crystallography.

The early studies on immature virions were conducted on lentiviruses, specifically on HIV-1. It was shown that Gag assembles underneath the membrane and this layer can adopt multiple curvatures and some patches appeared disordered [66]. Later it was shown that the Gag layer is organised to form a hexagonal lattice, with an 8 nm spacing (Fig. 2), and that the changes in curvature are accommodated through the introduction of imperfections in the lattice [67]. Thanks to the recent improvements in both hardware and image processing tools, over the past years the resolution at which the organisation of the immature Gag lattice was resolved went from multiple nanometers to near atomic [28] (Fig. 2). The immature Gag lattice has been studied and its structure has also been resolved for alpha and betaretroviruses (respectively for Rous Sarcoma Virus—RSV—[68] and Mason-Pfizer Monkey Virus—M-PMV—[69]). For all these studies, the advancements in cryoET have been critical, in fact, early-low resolution–reconstructions performed on all those viruses suggested a high level of conservation throughout CA [70]. Recently it has been possible to reconstruct the lattice of immature virions for all these three viruses at significantly higher resolutions [68, 71], those structures showed that the arrangement of CA in the C-terminal domain (CTD) is well conserved across the family, while the N-terminal domain (NTD) appear to differ significantly. For example, the NTD in

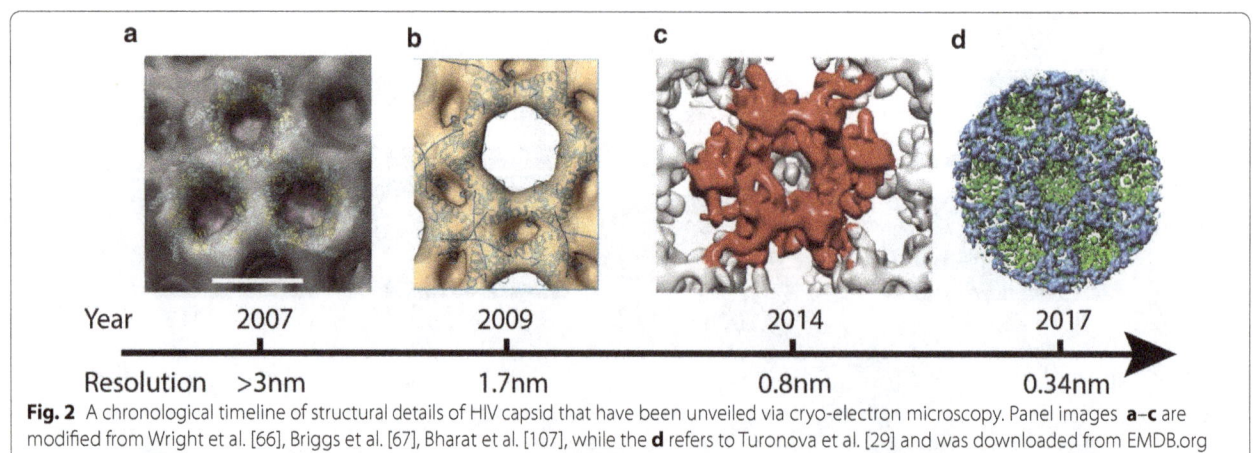

Fig. 2 A chronological timeline of structural details of HIV capsid that have been unveiled via cryo-electron microscopy. Panel images **a–c** are modified from Wright et al. [66], Briggs et al. [67], Bharat et al. [107], while the **d** refers to Turonova et al. [29] and was downloaded from EMDB.org

alpha retroviruses (RSV) have large contacts to ensure a tight interaction between neighbouring hexamers along the lattice. In addition, it appears that RSV stabilises the lattice through the interactions of the p10 domain [72].

It is well known that a common step for retroviruses is the maturation. The virion buds out from the infected cell in immature and non-infectious form. Upon the activation of the viral protease, the polyprotein Gag is cleaved in multiple positions, and these induce a dramatic rearrangement of the virion core, leading to the formation of an infectious particle [73]. HIV-1, because of its pathological importance, is the virus whose maturation process has been studied the most. Macroscopically the changes include the rearrangement of the lattice from an incomplete sphere to a fullerene cone and the increase of the spacing in the CA lattice from 8 to 10 nm [73]. The maturation process in HIV-1 occurs through 5 sequential proteolytic cleavages whose order and rate have been measured [74] and their roles in the maturation have been analysed through infectivity and morphological studies [75, 76]. Although the cleavage order in nature is probably not as strict as in vitro, and cleavages on different molecules might happen on different sites at the same time, the data available as of today [74] suggest that the cleavage between SP1 and NC is the first proteolytic processing event to occur, and it leads to the detachment of the capsid-based lattice from the NC proteins (therefore the RNA genomes) [76]. The second step is the detachment of the C-terminus p6 domain from the NC domains, this is required for a proper reorganisation of the RNA genome and it is needed for the infectivity of HIV [75]. (3) The third proteolytic cleavage event occurs between MA and CA, and this event induces the most dramatic change in the virion. Consequently, the CA lattice is reorganised completely, and it no longer displays the 8 nm hexameric arrangement upon MA-CA cleavage [76–78]. The fourth proteolytic cleavage event separates NC from SP2, which leads to genome condensation, although this cleavage appears not to be strictly required neither for infectivity nor proper genome condensation [75]. The final cleavage event is critical for the infectivity and to allow re-assembly of the core in the mature form [76, 79]. The last cleavage event, which has been intensely studied, is the site where novel anti-retroviral maturation inhibitor Bevirimat acts, which prevents the formation of an infectious virion. Through cryoET studies, it is now appreciated that Bevirimat suppresses HIV maturation by stabilising the immature CA lattice intermediate to prevent further maturation by denying viral protease access to the cleavage site [28, 77]. Thanks to the use of cryoET, it has been possible to identify the effects of allosteric integrase inhibitors (ALLINIs), which impair

the maturation displaying electron-dense aggregates located next to a malformed mature capsid [80].

In general, the structure of immature, mature and "maturing" virions, could not have been determined without the application of cryoET because retroviruses are pleomorphic. If every virion is different, then classical structural biology techniques, which are based on averaging multiple identical objects are inapplicable. As of today, the only way to obtain a good description of viruses that lack symmetry—and more generally any object composed of multiple layers that are oriented independently from each other—is to perform a tomographic acquisition. An example of this need comes from the evidence that in multiple cases the mature core of HIV-1 is not always a fullerene cone. The models obtained previously showed that the mature core in HIV-1 follows the geometry of the fullerene, based on information obtained mostly from projection images [81–84] and fitting the structure of hexamer and pentamer CA assembly that had been crystallised [82, 85]. The first sub-nanometre 3D reconstruction of a mature like lattice on a tubular assembly showed that a three-helix bundle is critical for the lattice assembly, as it provides a strong set of hydrophobic interactions [86]. Recently the mature CA lattice has been solved at 8 Å directly in the virus [87]. To highlight the importance of conducting structural studies with minimal purifications and if possible directly in situ, the comparison between the existing crystal structures [82, 85] and the EM structure showed a most evident crystallisation artefact around the structure of the CA pentamer [87]. While it is known that the most common form of the mature CA core is a fullerene cone, it has been frequently reported that other conformations such as cylindrical cores, spherical as well as non-closed or incomplete shells, are possible [84, 87, 88]. Currently, there are two models proposed for the mature core formation: a de novo assembly which was proposed through computational models [85] and is currently supported by the available high-resolution reconstructions obtained from multiple mature virions and [87, 89]. An alternative model proposes the phase transition as non-diffusional but as the result of a gradual conversion which would roll on itself to form a mature core [90]. Frank et al. also produced for the first time evidence of a possible trimeric arrangement of the MA layer [90].

The HIV-1 intasome

Another aspect of HIV biology that has benefited a great deal from cryo-EM is our understanding of the integration process. Upon infection, retroviruses integrate their genome into the host cell chromosomes. This integration process results in a permanent presence of the retroviral genome within the host cell [91]. Retroviral integration is carried out by the viral integrase, which oligomerises and complexes with the viral DNA to form the stable synaptic complex (SSC). The stable synaptic complex (also known as intasome) will subsequently transport into the nucleus and facilitate the insertion of the viral genome into the host [91, 92].

Structural studies of the intasome have been attempted for many years because of its relevance as a potential antiretroviral target, including the refinement of integrase inhibitors. The main challenge in studying intasome is the tendency of the intasomes to aggregate, making the crystallisation process extremely complicated. As of today, the intasome of RSV [93] and PFV [94] have been successfully crystalised, however, thanks to the simpler requirements for cryoEM in structural determination, the structures of four additional intasomes have been resolved. The structure of the PFV intasome/nucleosome complex has been resolved at 0.78 nm resolution [95] providing the bases for understanding the mechanism behind the nucleosome capture by the retroviral integration machinery. In addition, the structure of the intasome from two more genera have now been resolved, including the Betaretroviruses (on MMTV) [96] and Lentiviruses (on HIV-1) [97]. Lately, the structure of the lentiviral intasome nucleoprotein complex (obtained from the Maedi-visna virus (MVV)) was obtained at 0.49 nm resolution [98]. This structure has been proposed as a platform for drug design of HIV-1 IN inhibitors.

Correlative microscopy: a help to find the needle in the haystack

As mentioned in the introduction, despite the great resolution that cryoEM can deliver, biological samples are extremely complex and only a subset of the molecules imaged in a cryoEM micrograph can be unequivocally identified. Moreover, most of the biological samples are pleomorphic, meaning that it is impossible to predict with high certainty the location of a molecule or a complex. A major consequence of this incomplete understanding of the sample is that locating objects and/or events that are rare and smaller than 1 μm can be an extremely challenging and time-consuming activity. Moreover, there will be numerous cases where the complex might not be unequivocally identifiable. Here the aid provided by the combination of light microscopy with electron microscopy is invaluable and typically is referred as correlative microscopy. A number of different combination of correlative microscopy approaches have been described based on the objectives of the research questions [31, 35, 99].

This technique has been successfully used to image rare events linked to the retroviral replication cycle such as viral budding and entry. Early studies using correlative light and scanning electron microscopy showed that it was possible to identify with micrometric precision the location of a bud on an infected cell [100]. Other cases displayed a simplified approach where the focus was on the identification of cells that had been infected, in order to speed up the screening [101] and allow the identification of locations presenting viral buds for further structural analyses. Another rare and isolated event in the replication cycle is the viral entry. Here free virions have been identified through live cell imaging, their movements have been followed and the cells after plunge freezing have been inspected first through cryo-fluorescence microscopy and then through cryoEM [34, 99].

Final notes

The objective of this review was to provide an overview of the emerging capabilities available for structural studies through cryo-electron microscopy that can be of aid in the field of retrovirology. The impact that Cryo-EM and related techniques can be seen throughout all fields related to cellular biology. While electron microscopy was temporarily "out of fashion" as a research tool near the end of the 20th century; the recent technological advances, together with the wider spread of cryoEM have already shown how the structural determination of large protein complexes at near atomic resolution is possible for an increasing number of molecules. Cryo-electron microscopy, more specifically, single particle cryoEM was recognised as 'Method of the year in 2015' by Nature Methods [102] and the subject of 2017 Nobel Prize in Chemistry. With the continuous advancement of the field, it is now possible to perform cryoEM on larger assemblies, such as entire pleomorphic virus particles. The recent advances in image processing for cryoET showed that it is possible to achieve near atomic resolution on isolated pleomorphic virions [28, 29], in the future, we can expect a routine combination of cryoET on cellular samples through the use cryo-Focused Ion Beam Milling. As this combination has already allowed the resolution of structures within the cell [36, 103–105] it is reasonable to expect an improvement of resolution in the coming future. It is an exciting time for cryo-electron microscopy and virology in general.

Authors' contributions
JM and AdM equally contributed to design, write and revise the manuscript. Both authors read and approved the final manuscript.

Author details
[1] Institute for Glycomics, Griffith University Gold Coast, Southport, QLD, Australia. [2] Department of Biochemistry and Molecular Biology, Monash University, Clayton, VIC, Australia.

References

1. Milo R. What is the total number of protein molecules per cell volume? A call to rethink some published values. BioEssays. 2013;35:1050–5.
2. Berendsen HJ, Hayward S. Collective protein dynamics in relation to function. Curr Opin Struct Biol. 2000;10:165–9.
3. Deng M, Zhang K, Mehta S, Chen T, Sun F. Prediction of protein function using protein-protein interaction data. J Comput Biol. 2003;10:947–60.
4. Kitao A, Go N. Investigating protein dynamics in collective coordinate space. Curr Opin Struct Biol. 1999;9:164–9.
5. Moosavi S, Rahgozar M, Rahimi A. Protein function prediction using neighbour relativity in protein-protein interaction network. Comput Biol Chem. 2013;43:11–6.
6. Xiang SH. Recent advances on the use of structural biology for the design of novel envelope immunogens of HIV-1. Curr HIV Res. 2013;11:464–72.
7. Liljeroos L, Malito E, Ferlenghi I, Bottomley MJ. Structural and computational biology in the design of immunogenic vaccine antigens. J Immunol Res. 2015;2015:156241.
8. Fan E, O'Neal CJ, Mitchell DD, Robien MA, Zhang Z, Pickens JC, Tan XJ, Korotkov K, Roach C, Krumm B, et al. Structural biology and structure-based inhibitor design of cholera toxin and heat-labile enterotoxin. Int J Med Microbiol. 2004;294:217–23.
9. Scapin G. Structural biology in drug design: selective protein kinase inhibitors. Drug Discov Today. 2002;7:601–11.
10. Campbell ID. Timeline: the March of structural biology. Nat Rev Mol Cell Biol. 2002;3:377–81.
11. Frank J. Single-particle imaging of macromolecules by cryo-electron microscopy. Annu Rev Biophys Biomol Struct. 2002;31:303–19.
12. Reimer L. Transmission electron-microscopy. Diagn Appl Thin Films 1992:1–20.
13. Bammes BE, Rochat RH, Jakana J, Chen DH, Chiu W. Direct electron detection yields cryo-EM reconstructions at resolutions beyond 3/4 Nyquist frequency. J Struct Biol. 2012;177:589–601.
14. Li X, Mooney P, Zheng S, Booth CR, Braunfeld MB, Gubbens S, Agard DA, Cheng Y. Electron counting and beam-induced motion correction enable near-atomic-resolution single-particle cryo-EM. Nat Methods. 2013;10:584–90.
15. Dubochet J, Adrian M, Chang JJ, Homo JC, Lepault J, McDowall AW, Schultz P. Cryo-electron microscopy of vitrified specimens. Q Rev Biophys. 1988;21:129–228.
16. Holtz ME, Yu YC, Gao J, Abruna HD, Muller DA. In Situ electron energy-loss spectroscopy in liquids. Microsc Microanal. 2013;19:1027–35.
17. Bachmann L, Schmitt WW. Improved cryofixation applicable to freeze etching. Proc Natl Acad Sci USA. 1971;68:2149–52.
18. Jensen GJ. Part B: 3-D reconstruction. Preface. Methods Enzymol. 2010;482:xv–xvi.
19. Dashti A, Schwander P, Langlois R, Fung R, Li W, Hosseinizadeh A, Liao HY, Pallesen J, Sharma G, Stupina VA, et al. Trajectories of the ribosome as a Brownian nanomachine. Proc Natl Acad Sci USA. 2014;111:17492–7.
20. Chen JZ, Settembre EC, Aoki ST, Zhang X, Bellamy AR, Dormitzer PR, Harrison SC, Grigorieff N. Molecular interactions in rotavirus assembly and uncoating was seen by high-resolution cryo-EM. Proc Natl Acad Sci USA. 2009;106:10644–8.
21. Jiang W, Baker ML, Jakana J, Weigele PR, King J, Chiu W. Backbone structure of the infectious epsilon15 virus capsid revealed by electron cryomicroscopy. Nature. 2008;451:1130–4.
22. Liu H, Jin L, Koh SB, Atanasov I, Schein S, Wu L, Zhou ZH. Atomic structure of human adenovirus by cryo-EM reveals interactions among protein networks. Science. 2010;329:1038–43.
23. Sachse C, Chen JZ, Coureux PD, Stroupe ME, Fandrich M, Grigorieff N. High-resolution electron microscopy of helical specimens: a fresh look at tobacco mosaic virus. J Mol Biol. 2007;371:812–35.
24. Zhang X, Jin L, Fang Q, Hui WH, Zhou ZH. 3.3 A cryo-EM structure of a nonenveloped virus reveals a priming mechanism for cell entry. Cell. 2010;141:472–82.
25. Zhang X, Settembre E, Xu C, Dormitzer PR, Bellamy R, Harrison SC, Grigorieff N. Near-atomic resolution using electron cryomicroscopy and single-particle reconstruction. Proc Natl Acad Sci USA. 2008;105:1867–72.
26. Zhou ZH. Towards atomic resolution structural determination by single-particle cryo-electron microscopy. Curr Opin Struct Biol. 2008;18:218–28.
27. Crowther RA, Amos LA, Finch JT, De Rosier DJ, Klug A. Three-dimensional reconstructions of spherical viruses by Fourier synthesis from electron micrographs. Nature. 1970;226:421–5.
28. Schur FK, Obr M, Hagen WJ, Wan W, Jakobi AJ, Kirkpatrick JM, Sachse C, Krausslich HG, Briggs JA. An atomic model of HIV-1 capsid-SP1 reveals structures regulating assembly and maturation. Science. 2016;353(6298):506–8. https://doi.org/10.1126/science.aaf9620.
29. Turonova B, Schur FKM, Wan W, Briggs JAG. Efficient 3D-CTF correction for cryo-electron tomography using NovaCTF improves subtomogram averaging resolution to 3.4A. J Struct Biol. 2017;199(3):187–95. https://doi.org/10.1016/j.jsb.2017.07.007.
30. Sartori A, Gatz R, Beck F, Rigort A, Baumeister W, Plitzko JM. Correlative microscopy: bridging the gap between fluorescence light microscopy and cryo-electron tomography. J Struct Biol. 2007;160:135–45.
31. Schorb M, Briggs JAG. Correlated cryo-fluorescence and cryo-electron microscopy with high spatial precision and improved sensitivity. Ultramicroscopy. 2014;143:24–32.
32. Jasnin M, Ecke M, Baumeister W, Gerisch G. Actin organization in cells responding to a perforated surface, revealed by live imaging and cryo-electron tomography. Structure. 2016;24:1031–43.
33. Hampton CM, Strauss JD, Ke Z, Dillard RS, Hammonds JE, Alonas E, Desai TM, Marin M, Storms RE, Leon F, et al. Correlated fluorescence microscopy and cryo-electron tomography of virus-infected or transfected mammalian cells. Nat Protoc. 2017;12:150–67.
34. Jun S, Ke D, Debiec K, Zhao G, Meng X, Ambrose Z, Gibson GA, Watkins SC, Zhang P. Direct visualization of HIV-1 with correlative live-cell microscopy and cryo-electron tomography. Structure. 2011;19:1573–81.
35. Arnold J, Mahamid J, Lucic V, de Marco A, Fernandez J-J, Laugks T, Mayer T, Hyman AA, Baumeister W, Plitzko JM. Site-specific cryo-focused ion beam sample preparation guided by 3D correlative microscopy. Biophys J. 2016;110:860.
36. Mahamid J, Pfeffer S, Schaffer M, Villa E, Danev R, Cuellar LK, Forster F, Hyman AA, Plitzko JM, Baumeister W. Visualizing the molecular sociology at the HeLa cell nuclear periphery. Science. 2016;351:969–72.
37. Prasad BV, Schmid MF. Principles of virus structural organization. Adv Exp Med Biol. 2012;726:17–47.
38. Mancini EJ, de Haas F, Fuller SD. High-resolution icosahedral reconstruction: fulfilling the promise of cryo-electron microscopy. Structure. 1997;5:741–50.
39. Liu J, Bartesaghi A, Borgnia MJ, Sapiro G, Subramaniam S. Molecular architecture of native HIV-1 gp120 trimers. Nature. 2008;455:109–13.
40. White TA, Bartesaghi A, Borgnia MJ, Meyerson JR, de la Cruz MJ, Bess JW, Nandwani R, Hoxie JA, Lifson JD, Milne JL, Subramaniam S. Molecular architectures of trimeric SIV and HIV-1 envelope glycoproteins on intact viruses: strain-dependent variation in quaternary structure. PLoS Pathog. 2010;6:e1001249.
41. Wibmer CK, Moore PL, Morris L. HIV broadly neutralizing antibody targets. Curr Opin HIV AIDS. 2015;10:135–43.
42. Julien JP, Lee JH, Ozorowski G, Hua Y, de la Torrents Pena A, de Taeye SW, Nieusma T, Cupo A, Yasmeen A, Golabek M, et al. Design and structure of two HIV-1 clade C SOSIP.664 trimers that increase the arsenal of native-like Env immunogens. Proc Natl Acad Sci USA. 2015;112:11947–52.
43. Lee JH, Leaman DP, Kim AS, Torrents de la Pena A, Sliepen K, Yasmeen A, Derking R, Ramos A, de Taeye SW, Ozorowski G, et al. Antibodies to a conformational epitope on gp41 neutralize HIV-1 by destabilizing the Env spike. Nat Commun. 2015;6:8167.

44. Lyumkis D, Julien JP, de Val N, Cupo A, Potter CS, Klasse PJ, Burton DR, Sanders RW, Moore JP, Carragher B, et al. Cryo-EM structure of a fully glycosylated soluble cleaved HIV-1 envelope trimer. Science. 2013;342:1484–90.

45. Rasheed M, Bettadapura R, Bajaj C. Computational refinement and validation protocol for proteins with large variable regions applied to model HIV env spike in CD4 and 17b bound state. Structure. 2015;23:1138–49.

46. Tran K, Poulsen C, Guenaga J, de Val N, Wilson R, Sundling C, Li Y, Stanfield RL, Wilson IA, Ward AB, et al. Vaccine-elicited primate antibodies use a distinct approach to the HIV-1 primary receptor binding site informing vaccine redesign. Proc Natl Acad Sci USA. 2014;111:E738–47.

47. Wang H, Cohen AA, Galimidi RP, Gristick HB, Jensen GJ, Bjorkman PJ. Cryo-EM structure of a CD4-bound open HIV-1 envelope trimer reveals structural rearrangements of the gp120 V1V2 loop. Proc Natl Acad Sci USA. 2016;113:E7151–8.

48. Wang H, Gristick HB, Scharf L, West AP, Galimidi RP, Seaman MS, Freund NT, Nussenzweig MC, Bjorkman PJ: Asymmetric recognition of HIV-1 Envelope trimer by V1V2 loop-targeting antibodies. Elife 2017; 6

49. Ward AB, Wilson IA. The HIV-1 envelope glycoprotein structure: nailing down a moving target. Immunol Rev. 2017;275:21–32.

50. Zanetti G, Briggs JA, Grunewald K, Sattentau QJ, Fuller SD. Cryo-electron tomographic structure of an immunodeficiency virus envelope complex in situ. PLoS Pathog. 2006;2:e83.

51. Zhu P, Chertova E, Bess J Jr, Lifson JD, Arthur LO, Liu J, Taylor KA, Roux KH. Electron tomography analysis of envelope glycoprotein trimers on HIV and simian immunodeficiency virus virions. Proc Natl Acad Sci USA. 2003;100:15812–7.

52. Zhu P, Liu J, Bess J Jr, Chertova E, Lifson JD, Grise H, Ofek GA, Taylor KA, Roux KH. Distribution and three-dimensional structure of AIDS virus envelope spikes. Nature. 2006;441:847–52.

53. Zhu P, Winkler H, Chertova E, Taylor KA, Roux KH. Cryoelectron tomography of HIV-1 envelope spikes: further evidence for tripod-like legs. PLoS Pathog. 2008;4:e1000203.

54. Ozorowski G, Pallesen J, de Val N, Lyumkis D, Cottrell CA, Torres JL, Copps J, Stanfield RL, Cupo A, Pugach P, et al. Open and closed structures reveal allostery and pliability in the HIV-1 envelope spike. Nature. 2017;547:360–3.

55. Bartesaghi A, Merk A, Borgnia MJ, Milne JL, Subramaniam S. Prefusion structure of trimeric HIV-1 envelope glycoprotein determined by cryo-electron microscopy. Nat Struct Mol Biol. 2013;20:1352–7.

56. Lee JH, Ozorowski G, Ward AB. Cryo-EM structure of a native, fully glycosylated, cleaved HIV-1 envelope trimer. Science. 2016;351:1043–8.

57. Liu Q, Acharya P, Dolan MA, Zhang P, Guzzo C, Lu J, Kwon A, Gururani D, Miao H, Bylund T, et al. Quaternary contact in the initial interaction of CD4 with the HIV-1 envelope trimer. Nat Struct Mol Biol. 2017;24:370–8.

58. Pham S, Tabarin T, Garvey M, Pade C, Rossy J, Monaghan P, Hyatt A, Bocking T, Leis A, Gaus K, Mak J. Cryo-electron microscopy and single molecule fluorescent microscopy detect CD4 receptor induced HIV size expansion prior to cell entry. Virology. 2015;486:121–33.

59. Subramaniam S. The SIV surface spike imaged by electron tomography: one leg or three? PLoS Pathog. 2006;2:e91.

60. Mao Y, Wang L, Gu C, Herschhorn A, Xiang SH, Haim H, Yang X, Sodroski J. Subunit organization of the membrane-bound HIV-1 envelope glycoprotein trimer. Nat Struct Mol Biol. 2012;19:893–9.

61. Mao Y, Wang L, Gu C, Herschhorn A, Desormeaux A, Finzi A, Xiang SH, Sodroski JG. Molecular architecture of the uncleaved HIV-1 envelope glycoprotein trimer. Proc Natl Acad Sci USA. 2013;110:12438–43.

62. Henderson R. Avoiding the pitfalls of single particle cryo-electron microscopy: Einstein from noise. Proc Natl Acad Sci USA. 2013;110:18037–41.

63. Subramaniam S. Structure of trimeric HIV-1 envelope glycoproteins. Proc Natl Acad Sci USA. 2013;110:E4172–4.

64. van Heel M. Finding trimeric HIV-1 envelope glycoproteins in random noise. Proc Natl Acad Sci USA. 2013;110:E4175–7.

65. Sundquist WI, Krausslich HG. HIV-1 assembly, budding, and maturation. Cold Spring Harb Perspect Med. 2012;2:a006924.

66. Wright ER, Schooler JB, Ding HJ, Kieffer C, Fillmore C, Sundquist WI, Jensen GJ. Electron cryotomography of immature HIV-1 virions reveals the structure of the CA and SP1 Gag shells. EMBO J. 2007;26:2218–26.

67. Briggs JA, Riches JD, Glass B, Bartonova V, Zanetti G, Krausslich HG. Structure and assembly of immature HIV. Proc Natl Acad Sci USA. 2009;106:11090–5.

68. Schur FK, Dick RA, Hagen WJ, Vogt VM, Briggs JA. The structure of immature virus-like rous sarcoma virus gag particles reveals a structural Role for the p10 domain in assembly. J Virol. 2015;89:10294–302.

69. Bharat TA, Davey NE, Ulbrich P, Riches JD, de Marco A, Rumlova M, Sachse C, Ruml T, Briggs JA. Structure of the immature retroviral capsid at 8 A resolution by cryo-electron microscopy. Nature. 2012;487:385–9.

70. de Marco A, Davey NE, Ulbrich P, Phillips JM, Lux V, Riches JD, Fuzik T, Ruml T, Krausslich HG, Vogt VM, Briggs JA. Conserved and variable features of Gag structure and arrangement in immature retrovirus particles. J Virol. 2010;84:11729–36.

71. Schur FK, Hagen WJ, Rumlova M, Ruml T, Muller B, Krausslich HG, Briggs JA. Structure of the immature HIV-1 capsid in intact virus particles at 8.8 A resolution. Nature. 2015;517:505–8.

72. Phillips JM, Murray PS, Murray D, Vogt VM. A molecular switch required for retrovirus assembly participates in the hexagonal immature lattice. The EMBO journal. 2008;27:1411–20.

73. de Marco A, Kraeusslich HG, Briggs JAG: Structural biology of HIV assembly. In Advances in HIV-1 assembly and release. Springer, New York, NY; 2013: 1–22

74. Pettit SC, Moody MD, Wehbie RS, Kaplan AH, Nantermet PV, Klein CA, Swanstrom R. The p2 domain of human immunodeficiency virus type 1 Gag regulates sequential proteolytic processing and is required to produce fully infectious virions. J Virol. 1994;68:8017–27.

75. de Marco A, Heuser AM, Glass B, Krausslich HG, Muller B, Briggs JAG. Role of the SP2 domain and its proteolytic cleavage in HIV-1 structural maturation and infectivity. J Virol. 2012;86:13708–16.

76. de Marco A, Muller B, Glass B, Riches JD, Krausslich HG, Briggs JA. Structural analysis of HIV-1 maturation using cryo-electron tomography. PLoS Pathog. 2010;6:e1001215.

77. Keller PW, Adamson CS, Heymann JB, Freed EO, Steven AC. HIV-1 maturation inhibitor bevirimat stabilizes the immature Gag lattice. J Virol. 2011;85:1420–8.

78. Checkley MA, Luttge BG, Soheilian F, Nagashima K, Freed EO. The capsid-spacer peptide 1 Gag processing intermediate is a dominant-negative inhibitor of HIV-1 maturation. Virology. 2010;400:137–44.

79. Mattei S, Schur FK, Briggs JA. Retrovirus maturation-an extraordinary structural transformation. Curr Opin Virol. 2016;18:27–35.

80. Fontana J, Jurado KA, Cheng N, Ly NL, Fuchs JR, Gorelick RJ, Engelman AN, Steven AC. Distribution and redistribution of HIV-1 nucleocapsid protein in immature, mature, and integrase-inhibited virions: a role for integrase in maturation. J Virol. 2015;89:9765–80.

81. Ganser BK, Li S, Klishko VY, Finch JT, Sundquist WI. Assembly and analysis of conical models for the HIV-1 core. Science. 1999;283:80–3.

82. Pornillos O, Ganser-Pornillos BK, Yeager M. Atomic-level modelling of the HIV capsid. Nature. 2011;469:424–7.

83. Yeager M. Design of in vitro symmetric complexes and analysis by hybrid methods reveal mechanisms of HIV capsid assembly. J Mol Biol. 2011;410:534–52.

84. Briggs JA, Wilk T, Welker R, Krausslich HG, Fuller SD. Structural organization of authentic, mature HIV-1 virions and cores. EMBO J. 2003;22:1707–15.

85. Pornillos O, Ganser-Pornillos BK, Kelly BN, Hua Y, Whitby FG, Stout CD, Sundquist WI, Hill CP, Yeager M. X-ray structures of the hexameric building block of the HIV capsid. Cell. 2009;137:1282–92.

86. Zhao G, Perilla JR, Yufenyuy EL, Meng X, Chen B, Ning J, Ahn J, Gronenborn AM, Schulten K, Aiken C, Zhang P. Mature HIV-1 capsid structure by cryo-electron microscopy and all-atom molecular dynamics. Nature. 2013;497:643–6.

87. Mattei S, Glass B, Hagen WJ, Krausslich HG, Briggs JA. The structure and flexibility of conical HIV-1 capsids determined within intact virions. Science. 2016;354:1434–7.

88. Yu Z, Dobro MJ, Woodward CL, Levandovsky A, Danielson CM, Sandrin V, Shi J, Aiken C, Zandi R, Hope TJ, Jensen GJ. Unclosed HIV-1 capsids suggest a curled sheet model of assembly. J Mol Biol. 2013;425:112–23.

89. Grime JM, Dama JF, Ganser-Pornillos BK, Woodward CL, Jensen GJ, Yeager M, Voth GA. Coarse-grained simulation reveals key features of HIV-1 capsid self-assembly. Nat Commun. 2016;7:11568.

90. Frank GA, Narayan K, Bess JW Jr, Del Prete GQ, Wu X, Moran A, Hartnell LM, Earl LA, Lifson JD, Subramaniam S. Maturation of the HIV-1 core by a non-diffusional phase transition. Nat Commun. 2015;6:5854.

91. Craigie R, Bushman FD. HIV DNA integration. Cold Spring Harb Perspect Med. 2012;2:a006890.

92. Lesbats P, Engelman AN, Cherepanov P. Retroviral DNA integration. Chem Rev. 2016;116:12730–57.

93. Yin Z, Shi K, Banerjee S, Pandey KK, Bera S, Grandgenett DP, Aihara H. Crystal structure of the Rous sarcoma virus intasome. Nature. 2016;530:362–6.

94. Maertens GN, Hare S, Cherepanov P. The mechanism of retroviral integration from X-ray structures of its key intermediates. Nature. 2010;468:326–9.

95. Maskell DP, Renault L, Serrao E, Lesbats P, Matadeen R, Hare S, Lindemann D, Engelman AN, Costa A, Cherepanov P. Structural basis for retroviral integration into nucleosomes. Nature. 2015;523:366–9.

96. Ballandras-Colas A, Brown M, Cook NJ, Dewdney TG, Demeler B, Cherepanov P, Lyumkis D, Engelman AN. Cryo-EM reveals a novel octameric integrase structure for betaretroviral intasome function. Nature. 2016;530:358–61.

97. Passos DO, Li M, Yang R, Rebensburg SV, Ghirlando R, Jeon Y, Shkriabai N, Kvaratskhelia M, Craigie R, Lyumkis D. Cryo-EM structures and atomic model of the HIV-1 strand transfer complex intasome. Science. 2017;355:89–92.

98. Ballandras-Colas A, Maskell DP, Serrao E, Locke J, Swuec P, Jonsson SR, Kotecha A, Cook NJ, Pye VE, Taylor IA, et al. A supramolecular assembly mediates lentiviral DNA integration. Science. 2017;355:93–5.

99. Kukulski W, Schorb M, Welsch S, Picco A, Kaksonen M, Briggs JA. Correlated fluorescence and 3D electron microscopy with high sensitivity and spatial precision. J Cell Biol. 2011;192:111–9.

100. Larson DR, Johnson MC, Webb WW, Vogt VM. Visualization of retrovirus budding with correlated light and electron microscopy. Proc Natl Acad Sci USA. 2005;102:15453–8.

101. Carlson LA, de Marco A, Oberwinkler H, Habermann A, Briggs JAG, Kraeusslich HG, Gruenewald K: Cryo electron tomography of native HIV-1 budding sites. PLoS Pathogens 2010, 6.

102. Method of the Year 2015. Nat Methods 2016, 13:1.

103. Bykov YS, Schaffer M, Dodonova SO, Albert S, Plitzko JM, Baumeister W, Engel BD, Briggs JA. The structure of the COPI coat determined within the cell. Elife 2017; 6.

104. Asano S, Engel BD, Baumeister W. In situ cryo-electron tomography: a post-reductionist approach to structural biology. J Mol Biol. 2016;428:332–43.

105. Engel BD, Schaffer M, Albert S, Asano S, Plitzko JM, Baumeister W. In situ structural analysis of Golgi intracisternal protein arrays. Proc Natl Acad Sci USA. 2015;112:11264–9.

106. Zanetti G, Briggs JAG, Grünewald K, Sattentau QJ, Fuller SD. Cryo-electron tomographic structure of an immunodeficiency virus envelope complex in situ. PLoS Pathog. 2006;2:0790–7.

107. Bharat TA, Castillo Menendez LR, Hagen WJ, Lux V, Igonet S, Schorb M, Schur FK, Krausslich HG, Briggs JA. Cryo-electron microscopy of tubular arrays of HIV-1 Gag resolves structures essential for immature virus assembly. Proc Natl Acad Sci USA. 2014;111:8233–8.

14

HIV evolution and diversity in ART-treated patients

Gert van Zyl[1], Michael J. Bale[2] and Mary F. Kearney[2]* (iD)

Abstract

Characterizing HIV genetic diversity and evolution during antiretroviral therapy (ART) provides insights into the mechanisms that maintain the viral reservoir during ART. This review describes common methods used to obtain and analyze intra-patient HIV sequence data, the accumulation of diversity prior to ART and how it is affected by suppressive ART, the debate on viral replication and evolution in the presence of ART, HIV compartmentalization across various tissues, and mechanisms for the emergence of drug resistance. It also describes how CD4+ T cells that were likely infected with latent proviruses prior to initiating treatment can proliferate before and during ART, providing a renewable source of infected cells despite therapy. Some expanded cell clones carry intact and replication-competent proviruses with a small fraction of the clonal siblings being transcriptionally active and a source for residual viremia on ART. Such cells may also be the source for viral rebound after interrupting ART. The identical viral sequences observed for many years in both the plasma and infected cells of patients on long-term ART are likely due to the proliferation of infected cells both prior to and during treatment. Studies on HIV diversity may reveal targets that can be exploited in efforts to eradicate or control the infection without ART.

Keywords: HIV diversity, Antiretroviral therapy (ART), HIV genetics, HIV replication, HIV reservoir, HIV persistence, Expanded clones

Background

A signature of HIV infection is its vast genetic diversity and rapid evolution within and between infected individuals. HIV diversity results primarily from the lack of a proofreading mechanism by its reverse transcriptase (RT) enzyme that copies its RNA genome into DNA prior to integration into the host genome where it either remains latent or is expressed using the host cell machinery. HIV diversity is also influenced by a large population size and high recombination rate [1–4]. Other factors that contribute to the high genetic diversity of HIV are host APOBEC-mediated substitutions [5, 6] and changes in the population of susceptible cells over the duration of infection [7, 8] and across different anatomical compartments, such as the brain [9–11]. HIV evolution is driven, in large part, by the selection of expressed variants that carry mutations allowing escape from cell killing or virus neutralization by host immune responses [12–15]. Immune escape is also one mechanism that allows the virus to persist within the host, with another mechanism being proliferation of latently-infected cells [16, 17]. The latter mechanism is not affected by ART and is an important reservoir for the virus during suppressive treatment [18–20]. The interplay of all these factors explains why HIV sequences within an infected individual can differ by 5% or more [12, 21]. The major implications of viral diversity are the persistence of HIV despite strong immune responses, the selection of drug resistant mutations on ART, and the difficulties it imposes on the development of vaccines and curative strategies. In this review article, we will discuss some methods used to measure and view HIV diversity, the accumulation of HIV diversity in untreated individuals, the influence that ART imposes on HIV diversity, the relationship between HIV diversity and the reservoir on ART, and how HIV diversity can lead to the emergence of drug resistant variants and virologic failure.

*Correspondence: kearneym@ncifcrf.gov; kearneym@mail.nih.gov
[2] HIV Dynamic and Replication Program, Center for Cancer Research, National Cancer Institute at Frederick, 1050 Boyles Street, Building 535, Room 109, Frederick, MD 21702-1201, USA
Full list of author information is available at the end of the article

Methods to investigate HIV diversity in vivo

Single-genome amplification and sequencing

The methods by which we measure and analyze intra-patient viral populations are paramount to our understanding of HIV diversity and evolution. Early studies utilized bulk PCR amplification and cloning to measure HIV diversity and to detect the emergence of drug resistance mutations [22–25]. However, a letter by Liu et al. discussed the issues with this type of sequence analysis, especially in the context of low viral burden, showing that the resampling probability is inversely proportional to sample size—i.e. viral burden—and thus, bulk PCR and cloning can give erroneous estimates of intra-patient diversity [26]. This skewed quantitation of intra-patient sequence diversity resulted in detection of only the majority variants present in the HIV population [26–30].

In 2005, Palmer et al. [30] showed that the standard genotyping methods missed drug resistance mutations including mutations that were linked on the same viral genomes. In order to better understand intra-patient HIV populations, Palmer et al. developed an approach, based on similar approaches by Simmonds et al. [31], by utilizing limiting-dilution PCR to amplify from single HIV RNA or DNA templates [30]. Single-genome amplification or single-genome sequencing (SGA and SGS respectively) has been shown to have a low error rate of 0.003%, and a very small assay recombination rate of less than one crossover event in 66,000 bp [30]. Salazar-Gonzales et al. later showed that, in a side-by-side comparison of bulk methods to SGS, that sequences derived by bulk methods had a noticeable error rate that contributed to a statistically significant difference between the two sets of paired sequences [13]. Jordan et al. further showed that neither bulk PCR/cloning nor SGS provided more bias than the other but noted that SGS could provide a deeper look at those sequences which would be missed by bulk PCR/cloning methods [27].

Next-generation sequencing

Although SGS has become the gold-standard assay for studying HIV populations, it can only provide a limited look—without a herculean effort—at the intra-patient population. To address the issue of finding minority variants, and generating the maximum amount of data, various platforms of next-generation sequencing have been applied to HIV. High-throughput sequencing techniques have recently become popular and provide a deeper look at the HIV populations within patients and to search for variants that might be missed with lower throughput methods, such as rare drug resistance mutations. 454 pyrosequencing by Roche Diagnostics/454 Life Sciences has been the most prevalent deep sequencing method by which intra-host populations have been analyzed. It

has been used to look at HIV populations with multiple alleles at single sites as well as searching for minority variants that may contribute to virological failure on ART [32–35]. However, in contrast to SGS, the requirement of a bulk PCR step in 454 and other deep sequencing methods can introduce artifactual recombination creating variants that are not present in the original population. PCR recombination rates have been reported to range from 5.4% recombinants to up to 37% recombinants [28, 36]. To combat these recombination rates, which hinder the search for linked minority mutations in HIV populations, Boltz and Rausch et al. [36] developed an ultrasensitive SGS (uSGS) assay, performed on the Illumina Miseq platform, that reduces PCR recombination to about 0.1%. uSGS works by incorporating primer-IDs onto cDNA molecules at the RT-PCR step [37] and then ligates adaptors which limits PCR bias and recombination by avoiding PCR with lengthy primers [36] used in other deep sequencing approaches. When applied to clinical samples, uSGS gave between 30- and 80-fold more sequences than standard SGS. However, in its current version, it is limited by the fragment length that can be analyzed, about 500 base pairs. Other advancements in deep sequencing approaches have allowed for the generation of whole- or near full-length genome sequences for rapid genotyping, SNP frequency calculations, and phylogenetic analyses [38–42]. In addition, more recent advances such as the Oxford Nanopore Technologies MinION and Pacific Biosciences SMRT sequencing are rapidly gaining traction as third generation technologies for HIV analyses [43].

Analysis of intra-patient HIV sequence data

Methods used to analyze HIV sequence data are equally important to those used to generate them. Average pairwise distance (APD) is the most common sequence-based statistic used in SGS studies as it can inform estimations of the within-host genetic diversity of the HIV populations. The traditional way to visualize the diversity of HIV populations is by phylogenetic trees. The most basic approach to phylogenetic analyses of intra-patient HIV sequence data are neighbor joining methods. Neighbor joining trees generate branch lengths solely from the absolute genetic distance between sequences and (generally) make no assumptions on either a temporal structure or rates between transitions or transversions. However, maximum-likelihood methods and Bayesian methods of phylogeny, which have also been applied to intra-patient HIV sequence sets [44–47], apply evolutionary models that account for frequencies of transitions and transversions and may consider the time of sample collection in generating the trees. Using the branch lengths on trees as surrogates for evolutionary change can provide insight into the relative levels of polymorphism between sequences and into changes in the population structure over time. Studies investigating compartmentalization or divergence over time utilize different hypothesis-testing methods, such as the test for panmixia [48, 49] or the Slatkin–Maddison test [50], to show the presence, or lack thereof, of different population structures either between anatomical compartments or at different timepoints. Analyses of intra-patient HIV sequence data have led to a better understanding of HIV transmission [12, 51], the accumulation of viral diversity prior to ART initiation [4, 12, 52], the HIV population size [3, 4], the sources of persistent viremia on ART [46, 53, 54], and the mechanisms that maintain the HIV reservoir on ART [16, 17].

HIV genetic diversity and divergence in vivo
Accumulation of diversity in early and chronic HIV infection

HIV transmission is a relatively inefficient process with less than 1% of heterosexual exposures resulting in transmission and most associated with a single founder virus [12, 51]. During sexual transmission, mucosal infection of the new host results in a bottleneck which selects for viruses with higher overall fitness [55]. However, in men who have sex with men (MSM) or intravenous drug users (IVDU), when the exposure risk is high, selection for fit variants is less stringent. Moreover, the transmission of a first variant statistically increases the chance that another would transmit (transmissions do not follow a Poisson distribution). Thus, multiple founding viruses are not uncommon among MSM and IVDU, but their frequency varies across studies in accordance with the variable exposure risk [55–57]. Similar to heterosexual transmission, mother to child transmission is usually associated with one variant only, suggesting a stringent bottleneck [58]. Founding viruses are more likely CCR5 tropic, although, in some studies, up to 20% may be CXCR4 tropic [51, 59, 60]. As the initial infected target cells are activated CD4+ T cells, founding viruses require a high CD4 receptor density and may be underglycosylated compared to strains from chronic infection [61].

When only one founding virus is transmitted, the viral population is initially homogenous (Fig. 1a) but diversifies as it adapts to a new host to levels of about 1–2.5% in the viral enzymes [12] and to 5% or more in the structural genes (Fig. 1b) [12, 13, 52]. This finding was more recently demonstrated in Zanini et al. [40, 42] through whole-genome analysis of untreated patients followed longitudinally. The authors showed that the HIV genome does not evolve uniformly, with the viral enzymes having a lower

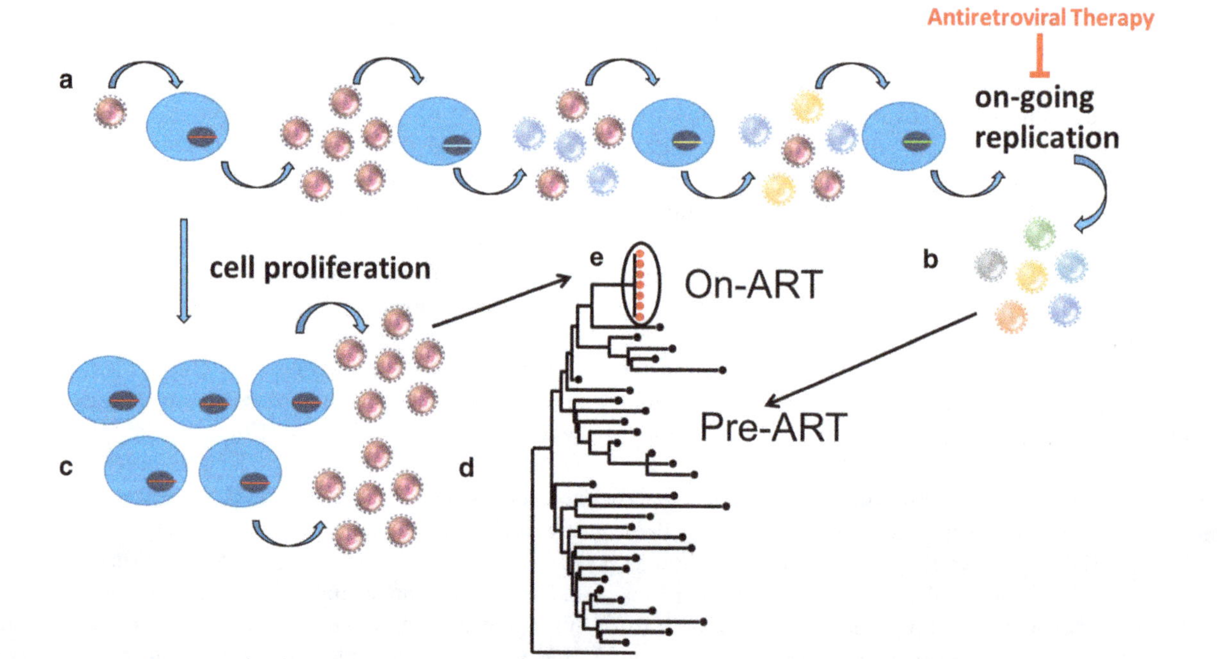

Fig. 1 Without ART, about 10^6–10^9 CD4+ T cells are infected daily by HIV-1 [141] (**a**). The HIV-1 population accumulates genetic diversity with each round of viral replication at a rate of about 1 mutation in 10^5 nucleotides copied [142] (**b**). An unknown fraction of the infected CD4+ T cells persist despite infection and undergoes cellular proliferation [16, 17] (**c**). Some clonally expanded populations of HIV-1 infected cells carry proviruses that can generate virus particles [77] (**d**). It has been shown that the identical sequences observed in persistent viremia on ART can originate from expanded clones [77] (**e**)

rate of divergence compared to gp120 and nef. In cases with multiple founding viruses, viral populations evolve through recombination in addition to mutation [12, 56, 57, 62–64]. In non-controlling patients, HIV diversifies rapidly as variants that escape dominant cytotoxic T lymphocyte (CTL) responses are selected [12, 13, 40, 65]. However, when the HLA class I haplotype of the transmitting donor corresponds to the recipient, the transmitted variant may be a pre-adapted escape variant. Such transmission of escape variants as well as higher multiplicities of infection have been associated with a higher viral load and a more rapid disease progression in the new host [66]. In contrast, natural controllers are characterized by a greater magnitude, polyfunctionality, and breadth of CTL responses and the targeting of epitopes are conserved due to the high fitness cost of escape [67, 68]. Similar to CTL escape, escape from neutralizing antibodies through evolution of *env*, encoding the surface glycoprotein, occur as early as in the first months of infection [69]. In chronic untreated infection, viral evolution may favor the selection of strains that are less resistant to CTL killing but could infect a larger range of host cells, which may manifest as a switch from CCR5 tropic strains to dual tropic or CXCR4 tropic strains [70]. This tropism switch is associated with more rapid disease progression [71]. In untreated individuals, adaptive responses to evolving B cell epitopes and sequential antibody escape, can result in the development of broadly neutralizing antibodies. Approximately 20% of chronically infected individuals develop broadly neutralizing antibodies, usually appearing late, as they are often produced by B-cells that have evolved extensively through somatic hypermutation and B cell selection [72, 73]. As mentioned above, although HIV diversifies rapidly in patients, patients in chronic infection experience a diversification plateau independent of continued viral turnover [4].

HIV genetic diversity on ART

The dynamics of plasma HIV RNA decay after initiating ART occurs in four phases and, oftentimes, results in an associated decline in the overall HIV genetic diversity [53, 74–76]. The first phase of decay occurs from the rapid death of most infected cells within days after initiating ART. The second phase is from the clearance of infected cells with half-lives of about 2–3 weeks. The third is from longer-lived cells with half-lives of 6-44 months and the last phase has a slope that is not significantly different from zero, likely resulting from the persistence and/or proliferation of infected cells that were previously latently-infected but, some fraction of which, produce virus upon stochastic activation [74–78]. A study by Besson et al. [79] investigated the decay of HIV DNA on ART and showed that the infected cell populations

decline initially but then achieve a steady state with the persistence of about 10% of infected cells during long-term ART. The persistence of a small fraction of infected cells during ART may be achieved by maintaining a balance between cellular proliferation and cell death.

The diversity of HIV populations is influenced by the loss of the vast majority of infected cells on ART and the unveiling of identical proviruses that persist in proliferating populations of CD4+ T cells (Fig. 1c) [46, 53, 54, 80]. These monotypic sequences were first described by Bailey et al. [46] and were detected in the plasma, likely resulting from virion release from some members within clonally expanded populations (Fig. 1d, e). Maldarelli et al. [16] and Wagner et al. [17] were the first to directly show that HIV-infected cells can clonally expand and persist despite ART, and that the proviral integration site may influence this phenomenon. In one case, a provirus in an expanded cell clone was shown to match the single viral variant present at detectable levels in the persistent viremia during ART [77]. Furthermore, the virus particles produced by the clonally expanded cells were replication competent [77]. This one example is the only case, thus far, where the source of infectious virus in blood has been traced to a clone of infected cells carrying a mostly latent provirus. However, studies by Lorenzi et al. [20], Bui et al. [18], and Hosmane et al. [81] demonstrated that expanded cell clones harboring replication-competent proviruses are not uncommon among ART treated patients.

Characterizing the genetics of the HIV reservoir may help us to elucidate the mechanisms that established it prior to ART and that maintain it during ART. It is thought that the reservoir is comprised by a small number of resting, memory CD4+ T cells carrying transcriptionally silent HIV proviruses [82, 83]. Reports showing that the virus can reemerge months to years after treatment interruption in patients hoped to have been cured by bone marrow transplantation [84] or early treatment [85] support the idea that HIV can rebound from a pool of latently infected cells. However, more recent studies suggest that it may also consist of cells with transcriptionally active proviruses during ART that match those that rebound when ART is interrupted [86]. Although there is considerable patient-to-patient variation, the frequency of resting CD4+ T cells that harbor HIV proviruses detectable by PCR has been very roughly estimated to average about 1 cell in 10^3; however, the number of latently infected cells carrying replication-competent proviruses has been reported to be much lower [5, 87]. The difference is due to the presence of a large number of defective proviruses. Ho et al. [87] described the proviruses in resting CD4+ T cells that were not induced to produce replication-competent virus after a single round of maximal T cell activation. Almost half of these proviruses had large internal deletions that preclude replication, while another third were lethally hypermutated by the host restriction factor APOBEC3G. Other defects and further analyses brought the fraction of defective proviruses up to > 98% [5]. Additionally, Ho et al. found that some of the intact proviruses were capable of producing infectious virions following a second round of activation [87], even though they had not been induced by the prior activation. Bui et al. [18] confirmed this finding and showed that sequential rounds of activation induced proliferation and expression from expanded cell clones.

Long-fragment PCR and sequencing revealed the proviral population structure in patients prior to ART and how the structure changes on long-term ART [5]. Early after infection, a large proportion of proviruses have ABOBEC-induced hypermutations and few have large internal deletions. However, as hypermutated proviruses produce and present aberrant peptides on HLA class I and are recognized by CTL, they are often eliminated whereas those with large internal deletions, and not producing antigen, may persist and continue to expand [88]. In contrast, reservoir cells harboring fully intact, replication-competent proviruses have been reported to be resistant to CTL killing, even though the viruses they release upon in vitro stimulation can be recognized by CTL [88]. This resistance to CTL killing may be due to a large fraction of the infected cells being transcriptionally silent in vivo and may explain the stability of this small pool of "true" reservoir cells [78].

Controversy of ongoing HIV replication during ART

Residual viremia per se is not evidence for ongoing replication. Current ART inhibits attachment and fusion, reverse transcription, integration, or particle maturation after release. However, it does not prevent virus production or release which requires the transcription of provirus, translation, virus assembly and exocytosis. Considering this, as long as infected cells persist and may become activated, viral release is possible, even in the absence of the infection of new cells. Although it has been shown that one mechanism that maintains the HIV reservoir is the persistence and proliferation of cells infected before the initiation of ART [16, 17, 19, 20, 38, 39, 77], there is continued debate as to whether the reservoir can also be maintained from ongoing viral replication in potential ART sanctuary sites, such as lymph nodes (LN) [44, 89–92] with subsequent trafficking of recently infected cells into the blood [44, 93]. If ongoing replication in tissues maintains the HIV reservoir, then preventing infection of new cells by developing antiretrovirals that better penetrate sanctuary sites, such as LN,

would be a high priority. Conversely, if current ART is fully effective at blocking full cycles of viral replication in both tissues and blood, then elimination of proliferating and long-lived infected cells would be the highest priority to achieve an HIV-1 cure. It is therefore critical that the efficacy of current ART be fully understood to identify the most appropriate curative strategy.

Residual viremia due to ongoing viral replication, in patients without drug resistance, would require the presence of drug sanctuaries where the drug penetration is insufficient, allowing ongoing rounds of infection. Evidence of poor drug penetration in LN and mucosa associated lymphoid tissue (MALT) exist [90] and recently an investigation using 454 sequencing and a Bayesian evolution model on samples from LN tissue and blood of 3 patients reported evidence of evolution in LN with trafficking to the blood [44]. The authors concluded that the reservoir is replenished by ongoing replication and suggest the need for better ART with improved penetration into drug sanctuaries. These findings have, however, not been reproduced by other investigators or by applying different models of evolution on the same dataset [94]. If ongoing replication is important in replenishing the reservoir, viral diversification would continue in most patients on therapy and newly emergent variants would be detectable in the periphery as infected cells migrate between compartments. However, most studies of patients on long-term suppressive antiretroviral regimens have not found evidence of sequence diversification from pre-therapy in blood or tissues [41, 45, 46, 53, 54, 95]. Also, if low level viremia was due to ongoing HIV replication as a result of inadequate suppression of replication by triple combination therapy, the addition of a fourth drug, referred to as therapy intensification, would result in a decreased viral load. However, most investigations reported no viral load reduction with treatment intensification [96–99]. Taken together there exists no conclusive evidence that modern combination ART is inadequate and contributes to viral persistence in individuals with viral loads below the detection limit of commercial assays.

Most studies addressing the question of ongoing replication on ART analyzed HIV sequence data in longitudinal samples for evidence of evolution of virion RNA or proviral DNA in adults who initiated ART in chronic infection [44, 46, 53, 54, 86, 100], in adults who initiated ART in early infection [53, 54], and in perinatally-infected infants [101, 102]. Performing SGS on individuals in early infection makes it easy to detect the mutations that accumulate with viral replication since the background genetic diversity is typically low. Using measures of diversity, divergence, and increasing branch lengths on phylogenetic trees over time, significant changes in HIV populations have not been reported in patients with sustained suppression of viremia on ART [53, 54, 102, 103] and suggest that the HIV reservoir is likely maintained largely, if not solely, by the persistence and expansion of cells that were infected prior to the initiation of treatment. However, most studies looking for evidence of HIV evolution on ART due to viral replication have been conducted on blood samples. Fewer studies have been performed on tissues collected from various anatomical sites. Results of studies on HIV evolution during ART in tissues, including those using nonhuman primate models, have been conflicting with some showing evidence of viral compartmentalization and evolution [44] while others claim the opposite conclusion [104]. The conflicting outcomes may result from differences in the methods used to perform the sequencing (deep sequencing vs. SGS), from the methods used to analyze the data (neighbor joining vs. Bayesian phylogenetics), whether the identical variants are collapsed to a single sequence or not [105], or simply from sampling error. It is obvious that more studies are needed to determine if ongoing cycles of HIV replication occur in any tissues during ART to levels that could sustain the reservoir and lead to viral rebound when ART is interrupted.

HIV compartmentalization

Viral compartmentalization describes tissues or cell types where viral replication occurred but anatomical barriers restrict both ingoing and outgoing viral gene flow [106]. As discussed earlier, one theory is that the viral reservoir is maintained by ongoing HIV replication in sanctuary sites where drug penetration is sub-optimal [90]. In addition to the LN, the gut lymphoid tissue has also been posited as another such site of compartmentalization. A study by van Marle et al. [107] analyzed samples from the esophagus, stomach, duodenum, and colorectum and found evidence of compartmentalization in the *nef* region of the HIV genome. Furthermore, a study by Yukl et al. [108] showed that the overall burden of HIV within the gut is much higher than in the blood which may suggest that ongoing replication during ART persists within this compartment. Along these lines, a later study by Rueda et al. [109] showed increased and prolonged activation of the immune system within the gut, suggesting that immune cells were being exposed to viral protein. In contrast, Imamichi et al. showed a lack of compartmentalization between the proviral sequences derived from PBMC and from the ileum and colon [110]. This result was later corroborated by Evering et al. [45] who showed no difference in proviral sequences from the blood or gut mucosa. Evering further demonstrated that there was no evidence of ongoing rounds of viral replication due to a lack of

detectable accumulation of diversity within the sequence data despite higher levels of immune activation within the gut [45]. This latter result was confirmed by Josefsson et al. [54] and, later, Simonetti et al. [77] who found minimal genetic changes over time and no evidence for compartmentalization between the periphery and the gut after long-term therapy.

Although there is some debate regarding the compartmentalization of HIV in lymphoid tissue, the central nervous system (CNS) is one such compartment in which heavy restriction of gene flow affects the population structure [9–11, 111]. The compartmentalization of the CNS has been found to be strongly associated with HIV-Associated Dementia (HAD) [112, 113]. Studies by Schnell et al. [9, 10] and later, Sturdevant et al. [11] found two distinct types of compartmentalization within the cerebrospinal fluid (CSF). The authors reported that the T cell tropic virus found in the CSF was generally clonal in nature, and associated with pleocytosis, whereas macrophage-tropic virus (CD4+ low) was generally diverse and contained variants not represented in the plasma [9, 10]. These results suggested that HIV could replicate in at least two cell types within the CNS, but the authors noted that there was no relationship between the tropism of the virus and HAD diagnosis [11]. A recent study by Stefic et al. [111] attempted to enumerate differential selective pressures between the blood and CNS in the context of neutralizing antibodies. The authors reported that variants in the CNS had no differential ability to escape autologous neutralization when compared to the blood, but that there was a general increase in resistance to broadly neutralizing antibodies that was independent of compartmentalization, suggesting that the CNS could have clinical implications for immunotherapies [111].

Multiple studies have shown that the genital and genitourinary tracts are another site of compartmentalization within an HIV-infected patient [114–116]. However, in contrast to these studies, Bull and colleagues published two studies showing that female genital tract sequences are typically monotypic in nature, most likely due to cellular clonal expansion of single variants [105, 117]. Bull and colleagues later showed that these monotypic populations do not form distinct lineages over time and are well mixed with the blood [118]. In addition, a study by Chaillon et al. [119] found evidence of compartmentalization between semen and blood, but that this structure did not persist over the timepoints analyzed. Taken together, these studies show that there is a complex interplay between the plasma and various anatomical sites throughout the body and that eradication strategies may require monitoring of both the blood and these anatomical sites.

Production of virus from clonally-expanded populations of infected cells

When HIV infected cells proliferate, proviral sequences are replicated with the high-fidelity cellular DNA polymerase, resulting in identical copies of the original provirus. Evidence for clonal proliferation as the source of persistent viremia, rather than ongoing cycles of viral replication, was first provided by finding the persistence of a large proportion of identical plasma sequences during residual viremia [46, 53]. This suggested that the identical viruses found in plasma may be produced by cells that have undergone clonal proliferation. The large majority of virus producing clones have defective proviruses, as intact *gag* alone is required for non-infectious particles to assemble [120]. Defective proviruses are the likely major contributor to persisting low level viremia. This explains the large proportion of identical sequences in residual viremia and the lack of linkage of persisting low level viremia with replication competent virus or virus rebounding after therapy interruption [46, 100]. Recently, novel assays to investigate HIV integration sites have been developed, which revealed that proviral integration in or near growth genes is associated with selective survival and expansion of infected CD4+ T cell clones [16, 17]. As described previously, it has also been shown that CD4 clones could harbor intact and replication-competent proviruses [18, 20, 77, 81] and that these clones contain members that are transcriptionally active [77, 78] and can be the source of persistent viremia [77] and of viral rebound [86]. In addition, recent studies have focused on the different T cell subsets with respect to locating clones with intact proviruses. Lee and colleagues found that identical variants were preferentially in Th1-polarized cells [38] and Hiener et al. [39] found intact proviruses in effector memory T cells. Taken together, these studies emphasize the role of cellular proliferation in maintaining of the HIV reservoir and suggest that further studies are needed to determine the association between different cell subsets and the clonal expansion of infected cells. It has been further suggested that there is an inverse relationship between the size of proviral clones and their probability of harboring replication-competent virus [20]. This may be explained by CD4 clones with large internal proviral deletions being less susceptible to CTL killing [88]. Taken together this explains why residual viremia in patients on long term ART may predominantly originate from defective proviruses and why there is an absence of correlation of residual viremia and quantitative infectious virus recovery [121].

Emergence of drug resistance

Although ART is highly effective at inhibiting viral replication, drug resistant variants can emerge if ART is taken intermittently or if resistance mutations were present in the population prior to its initiation. HIV drug resistance was first observed with zidovudine/azidothymidine (AZT) monotherapy with the selection of thymidine-associated mutations (TAMs) in the reverse transcriptase gene that were likely present at low levels prior to AZT exposure [122]. In contrast, triple combination ART, which first included either a protease inhibitor (PI) and two nucleos(t)ide reverse transcriptase inhibitors (NRTIs) or a non-nucleoside reverse transcriptase inhibitor with two NRTIs, resulted in sustained viral suppression in the majority of patients and a low prevalence of drug resistance in patients with high levels of adherence [123–125].

The remarkable success of combination ART has two main explanations. First, variants carrying multiple drug resistance mutations are unlikely to be present in the viral population prior to ART and, therefore, cannot be selected when adherence is sufficiently high enough to virtually block further ongoing cycles of viral replication. The much lower frequency of virologic failure due to drug resistance on combination ART is consistent with studies showing a lack of viral replication and evolution on therapy. Secondly, when combination therapy includes drugs with a high genetic barrier (requiring multiple mutations for resistance), such as the newer integrase strand transfer inhibitors (INSTIs), or when mutations have a high fitness cost, the probability of their existence and selection is even lower [126]. In particular, resistance to the new INSTI, dolutegravir (DTG), when used in combination ART appears to be exceedingly rare. This phenomena can be explained by its high genetic barrier and the high fitness cost of the drug resistant variants [127]. Consequently, dual treatment combinations of DTG with lamivudine or rilpivirine are currently being investigated in clinical trials [128, 129]. Nevertheless, when patients who are INSTI-experienced, have inadequate adherence or received DTG monotherapy, resistance has occurred [130–132]. Thus, even regimens with high genetic barriers could be compromised by pre-existing resistance, inadequate regimen formulations and insufficient adherence. In addition to high genetic barrier, the potency of particular drugs has been related to their ability to prevent new rounds of infection in single-cycle replication assays, referred to as the instantaneous inhibitory potential (IIP). Drugs with a high IIP may contribute to highly durable regimens by virtually halting viral replication and thereby preventing viral evolution [133, 134]. Taken together, high potency and high genetic barrier regimens have contributed to the prevention of antiviral escape and the success of combination ART to prevent disease progression.

Considering the effectiveness of modern ART, it begs the question why virologic failure due to drug resistance still occurs. A major predictor of regimen failure is significant pre-existing drug resistance resulting from previous drug exposure [35, 135, 136], transmitted drug resistance [137], or possibly, high viral population size [3, 138]. However, even without pre-existing resistance, inadequate adherence could create a favorable environment for the stochastic emergence and subsequent selection of resistant mutants. As the different components of combination regimens have different half-lives, breaks in therapy could effectively result in monotherapy of the component with the longest half-life, leading to the selection of drug resistance mutations. In particular, breaks in therapy containing NNRTIs that have long half-lives, are associated with a high risk of failure [139, 140].

Conclusions

Studies on intra-patient HIV genetic diversity on ART have contributed to our understanding of the establishment and maintenance of the reservoir that results in viral rebound when ART is interrupted [16, 17, 46, 53, 77, 86]. To date, scientific consensus has established that HIV replication is virtually halted in the peripheral blood of individuals fully suppressed on ART as most studies conclude that the viral population in PBMC does not diverge due to viral replication from pre-therapy populations for up to about 20 years on potent and adherent therapy [40, 53, 54, 102, 103]. However, whether viral replication persists in tissues, such as lymph nodes and gut, to levels that can maintain the HIV reservoir is still controversial [44, 45, 90, 104, 107, 110]. Because newly infected cells are not detected in the peripheral blood even after many years on ART, if viral replication persists in tissues, it indicates that these cells rarely migrate outside of their anatomical site of infection. Studies on proviral compartmentalization aim to investigate viral gene flow to better understand the migration patterns of infected cells and address the question of ongoing HIV replication during ART in tissues. However, such studies, thus far, have come to contradicting conclusions with some showing evidence of compartmentalization between blood and lymphoid tissues [44, 107] and others showing a lack of compartmentalization [45, 54, 110]. The conflicting findings may be due to differences in methods used to obtain the sequence data and analyze them or in differences in the region or length of the gene fragments investigated. More in depth studies on HIV populations in multiple genes are needed to resolve this controversy and to determine if ongoing cycles of viral replication contribute to maintaining the HIV reservoir on ART.

It is now well established that a small fraction of the cells that were likely infected prior to starting ART or during treatment interruptions can persist on long-term ART through cellular proliferation. It is likely through silencing of viral gene transcription (latent infection) that these cells survive and divide despite infection. Furthermore, the proliferation of infected cells is, in some instances, is driven by the interruption of the cell cycle by integration of HIV proviruses into oncogenes or genes that regulate cell growth [16, 17]. In one case, it was demonstrated that a large HIV infected cell clone was the source of persistent viremia and carried an archived, intact provirus that was capable of producing infectious virus in in vitro experiments [77]. This study was followed by others demonstrating that clones of cells carrying intact and replication-competent proviruses is not uncommon in individuals on suppressive ART [18, 20, 81]. These studies clearly show that a common reservoir for HIV infection during ART is the persistence and proliferation of cells infected with intact proviruses. More studies are needed to determine if such variants are always archival or if they can emerge from new rounds of infection in tissues during ART and to understand the distribution of cell clones across different anatomical compartments. Furthermore, single-cell studies are needed to confirm if the mechanism that allows the persistence of such clones is, indeed, HIV latency. Understanding the mechanisms that maintain the HIV reservoir will guide the design of strategies to eradicate the infection, such as the further development of agents aimed at driving infected cells out of latency, without inducing further cellular proliferation, so that HIV proteins can be targeted by, perhaps, a boosted immune system. Future studies on HIV diversity and evolution will likely guide this process and may contribute to evaluating the efficacy of curative interventions for HIV infection.

Abbreviations
ART: antiretroviral therapy; PBMC: peripheral blood mononuclear cells; LN: lymph node(s); APOBEC: apolipoprotein B mRNA editing enzyme, catalytic polypeptide-like; CNS: central nervous system; CSF: cerebral spinal fluid; IIP: instantaneous inhibitory potential; 454: 454 pyrosequencing.

Authors' contributions
GVZ, MJB, MFK wrote the article. All authors read and approved the final manuscript.

Author details
[1] Division of Medical Virology, Stellenbosch University and NHLS Tygerberg, Cape Town, South Africa. [2] HIV Dynamic and Replication Program, Center for Cancer Research, National Cancer Institute at Frederick, 1050 Boyles Street, Building 535, Room 109, Frederick, MD 21702-1201, USA.

Acknowledgements
We thank John Coffin and John Mellors for helpful advice and Connie Kinna for administrative support.

Competing interests
The authors declare that they have no competing interests.

Funding
Funding was provided by National Cancer Institute (Intramural) and National Institutes of Health (Grant No. 1U01AI116138-01).

References

1. Hu WS, Hughes SH. HIV-1 reverse transcription. Cold Spring Harb Perspect Med. 2012;2:a006882.
2. Coffin J, Swanstrom R. HIV pathogenesis: dynamics and genetics of viral populations and infected cells. Cold Spring Harb Perspect Med. 2013;3:a012526.
3. Boltz VF, Ambrose Z, Kearney MF, Shao W, Kewalramani VN, Maldarelli F, Mellors JW, Coffin JM. Ultrasensitive allele-specific PCR reveals rare preexisting drug-resistant variants and a large replicating virus population in macaques infected with a simian immunodeficiency virus containing human immunodeficiency virus reverse transcriptase. J Virol. 2012;86:12525–30.
4. Maldarelli F, Kearney M, Palmer S, Stephens R, Mican J, Polis MA, Davey RT, Kovacs J, Shao W, Rock-Kress D, et al. HIV populations are large and accumulate high genetic diversity in a nonlinear fashion. J Virol. 2013;87:10313–23.
5. Bruner KM, Murray AJ, Pollack RA, Soliman MG, Laskey SB, Capoferri AA, Lai J, Strain MC, Lada SM, Hoh R, et al. Defective proviruses rapidly accumulate during acute HIV-1 infection. Nat Med. 2016;22:1043–9.
6. Yu Q, Konig R, Pillai S, Chiles K, Kearney M, Palmer S, Richman D, Coffin JM, Landau NR. Single-strand specificity of APOBEC3G accounts for minus-strand deamination of the HIV genome. Nat Struct Mol Biol. 2004;11:435–42.
7. Zhou S, Bednar MM, Sturdevant CB, Hauser BM, Swanstrom R. Deep Sequencing of the HIV-1 env gene reveals discrete X4 lineages and linkage disequilibrium between X4 and R5 viruses in the V1/V2 and V3 variable regions. J Virol. 2016;90:7142–58.
8. Arrildt KT, LaBranche CC, Joseph SB, Dukhovlinova EN, Graham WD, Ping LH, Schnell G, Sturdevant CB, Kincer LP, Mallewa M, et al. Phenotypic correlates of HIV-1 macrophage tropism. J Virol. 2015;89:11294–311.
9. Schnell G, Joseph S, Spudich S, Price RW, Swanstrom R. HIV-1 replication in the central nervous system occurs in two distinct cell types. PLoS Pathog. 2011;7:e1002286.
10. Schnell G, Price RW, Swanstrom R, Spudich S. Compartmentalization and clonal amplification of HIV-1 variants in the cerebrospinal fluid during primary infection. J Virol. 2010;84:2395–407.
11. Sturdevant CB, Joseph SB, Schnell G, Price RW, Swanstrom R, Spudich S. Compartmentalized replication of R5 T cell-tropic HIV-1 in the central nervous system early in the course of infection. PLoS Pathog. 2015;11:e1004720.
12. Kearney M, Maldarelli F, Shao W, Margolick JB, Daar ES, Mellors JW, Rao V, Coffin JM, Palmer S. Human immunodeficiency virus type 1 population genetics and adaptation in newly infected individuals. J Virol. 2009;83:2715–27.
13. Salazar-Gonzalez JF, Bailes E, Pham KT, Salazar MG, Guffey MB, Keele BF, Derdeyn CA, Farmer P, Hunter E, Allen S, et al. Deciphering human immunodeficiency virus type 1 transmission and early envelope diversification by single-genome amplification and sequencing. J Virol. 2008;82:3952–70.

14. Phillips RE, Rowland-Jones S, Nixon DF, Gotch FM, Edwards JP, Ogunlesi AO, Elvin JG, Rothbard JA, Bangham CR, Rizza CR, et al. Human immunodeficiency virus genetic variation that can escape cytotoxic T cell recognition. Nature. 1991;354:453–9.
15. Wei X, Decker JM, Wang S, Hui H, Kappes JC, Wu X, Salazar-Gonzalez JF, Salazar MG, Kilby JM, Saag MS, et al. Antibody neutralization and escape by HIV-1. Nature. 2003;422:307–12.
16. Maldarelli F, Wu X, Su L, Simonetti FR, Shao W, Hill S, Spindler J, Ferris AL, Mellors JW, Kearney MF, et al. HIV latency. Specific HIV integration sites are linked to clonal expansion and persistence of infected cells. Science. 2014;345:179–83.
17. Wagner TA, McLaughlin S, Garg K, Cheung CY, Larsen BB, Styrchak S, Huang HC, Edlefsen PT, Mullins JI, Frenkel LM. HIV latency. Proliferation of cells with HIV integrated into cancer genes contributes to persistent infection. Science. 2014;345:570–3.
18. Bui JK, Halvas EK, Fyne E, Sobolewski MD, Koontz D, Shao W, Luke B, Hong FF, Kearney MF, Mellors JW. Ex vivo activation of CD4+ T-cells from donors on suppressive ART can lead to sustained production of infectious HIV-1 from a subset of infected cells. PLoS Pathog. 2017;13:e1006230.
19. Bui JK, Sobolewski MD, Keele BF, Spindler J, Musick A, Wiegand A, Luke BT, Shao W, Hughes SH, Coffin JM, et al. Proviruses with identical sequences comprise a large fraction of the replication-competent HIV reservoir. PLoS Pathog. 2017;13:e1006283.
20. Lorenzi JC, Cohen YZ, Cohn LB, Kreider EF, Barton JP, Learn GH, Oliveira T, Lavine CL, Horwitz JA, Settler A, et al. Paired quantitative and qualitative assessment of the replication-competent HIV-1 reservoir and comparison with integrated proviral DNA. Proc Natl Acad Sci USA. 2016;113:E7908–16.
21. Korber B, Gaschen B, Yusim K, Thakallapally R, Kesmir C, Detours V. Evolutionary and immunological implications of contemporary HIV-1 variation. Br Med Bull. 2001;58:19–42.
22. Simmonds P, Zhang LQ, McOmish F, Balfe P, Ludlam CA, Brown AJ. Discontinuous sequence change of human immunodeficiency virus (HIV) type 1 env sequences in plasma viral and lymphocyte-associated proviral populations in vivo: implications for models of HIV pathogenesis. J Virol. 1991;65:6266–76.
23. Meyerhans A, Cheynier R, Albert J, Seth M, Kwok S, Sninsky J, Morfeldt-Manson L, Asjo B, Wain-Hobson S. Temporal fluctuations in HIV quasispecies in vivo are not reflected by sequential HIV isolations. Cell. 1989;58:901–10.
24. St Clair MH, Martin JL, Tudor-Williams G, Bach MC, Vavro CL, King DM, Kellam P, Kemp SD, Larder BA. Resistance to ddI and sensitivity to AZT induced by a mutation in HIV-1 reverse transcriptase. Science. 1991;253:1557–9.
25. Leitner T, Halapi E, Scarlatti G, Rossi P, Albert J, Fenyo EM, Uhlen M. Analysis of heterogeneous viral populations by direct DNA sequencing. Biotechniques. 1993;15:120–7.
26. Liu SL, Rodrigo AG, Shankarappa R, Learn GH, Hsu L, Davidov O, Zhao LP, Mullins JI. HIV quasispecies and resampling. Science. 1996;273:415–6.
27. Jordan MR, Kearney M, Palmer S, Shao W, Maldarelli F, Coakley EP, Chappey C, Wanke C, Coffin JM. Comparison of standard PCR/cloning to single genome sequencing for analysis of HIV-1 populations. J Virol Methods. 2010;168:114–20.
28. Shao W, Boltz VF, Spindler JE, Kearney MF, Maldarelli F, Mellors JW, Stewart C, Volfovsky N, Levitsky A, Stephens RM, Coffin JM. Analysis of 454 sequencing error rate, error sources, and artifact recombination for detection of Low-frequency drug resistance mutations in HIV-1 DNA. Retrovirology. 2013;10:18.
29. Kearney M, Palmer S, Maldarelli F, Shao W, Polis MA, Mican J, Rock-Kress D, Margolick JB, Coffin JM, Mellors JW. Frequent polymorphism at drug resistance sites in HIV-1 protease and reverse transcriptase. AIDS. 2008;22:497–501.
30. Palmer S, Kearney M, Maldarelli F, Halvas EK, Bixby CJ, Bazmi H, Rock D, Falloon J, Davey RT Jr, Dewar RL, et al. Multiple, linked human immunodeficiency virus type 1 drug resistance mutations in

treatment-experienced patients are missed by standard genotype analysis. J Clin Microbiol. 2005;43:406–13.

31. Simmonds P, Balfe P, Ludlam CA, Bishop JO, Brown AJ. Analysis of sequence diversity in hypervariable regions of the external glycoprotein of human immunodeficiency virus type 1. J Virol. 1990;64:5840–50.

32. Bushman FD, Hoffmann C, Ronen K, Malani N, Minkah N, Rose HM, Tebas P, Wang GP. Massively parallel pyrosequencing in HIV research. AIDS. 2008;22:1411–5.

33. Rozera G, Abbate I, Bruselles A, Vlassi C, D'Offizi G, Narciso P, Chillemi G, Prosperi M, Ippolito G, Capobianchi MR. Massively parallel pyrosequencing highlights minority variants in the HIV-1 env quasispecies deriving from lymphomonocyte sub-populations. Retrovirology. 2009;6:15.

34. Eriksson N, Pachter L, Mitsuya Y, Rhee SY, Wang C, Gharizadeh B, Ronaghi M, Shafer RW, Beerenwinkel N. Viral population estimation using pyrosequencing. PLoS Comput Biol. 2008;4:e1000074.

35. Boltz VF, Zheng Y, Lockman S, Hong F, Halvas EK, McIntyre J, Currier JS, Chibowa MC, Kanyama C, Nair A, et al. Role of low-frequency HIV-1 variants in failure of nevirapine-containing antiviral therapy in women previously exposed to single-dose nevirapine. Proc Natl Acad Sci USA. 2011;108:9202–7.

36. Boltz VF, Rausch J, Shao W, Hattori J, Luke B, Maldarelli F, Mellors JW, Kearney MF, Coffin JM. Ultrasensitive single-genome sequencing: accurate, targeted, next generation sequencing of HIV-1 RNA. Retrovirology. 2016;13:87.

37. Jabara CB, Jones CD, Roach J, Anderson JA, Swanstrom R. Accurate sampling and deep sequencing of the HIV-1 protease gene using a Primer ID. Proc Natl Acad Sci USA. 2011;108:20166–71.

38. Lee GQ, Orlova-Fink N, Einkauf K, Chowdhury FZ, Sun X, Harrington S, Kuo HH, Hua S, Chen HR, Ouyang Z, et al. Clonal expansion of genome-intact HIV-1 in functionally polarized Th1 CD4+ T cells. J Clin Invest. 2017;127:2689–96.

39. Hiener B, Horsburgh BA, Eden JS, Barton K, Schlub TE, Lee E, von Stockenstrom S, Odevall L, Milush JM, Liegler T, et al. Identification of genetically intact HIV-1 proviruses in specific CD4(+) T cells from effectively treated participants. Cell Rep. 2017;21:813–22.

40. Zanini F, Brodin J, Thebo L, Lanz C, Bratt G, Albert J, Neher RA. Population genomics of intrapatient HIV-1 evolution. Elife. 2015;4:e11282.

41. Brodin J, Zanini F, Thebo L, Lanz C, Bratt G, Neher RA, Albert J. Establishment and stability of the latent HIV-1 DNA reservoir. Elife. 2016;5:e18889.

42. Zanini F, Brodin J, Albert J, Neher RA. Error rates, PCR recombination, and sampling depth in HIV-1 whole genome deep sequencing. Virus Res. 2017;239:106–14.

43. Dilernia DA, Chien JT, Monaco DC, Brown MP, Ende Z, Deymier MJ, Yue L, Paxinos EE, Allen S, Tirado-Ramos A, Hunter E. Multiplexed highly-accurate DNA sequencing of closely-related HIV-1 variants using continuous long reads from single molecule, real-time sequencing. Nucleic Acids Res. 2015;43:e129.

44. Lorenzo-Redondo R, Fryer HR, Bedford T, Kim EY, Archer J, Pond SLK, Chung YS, Penugonda S, Chipman J, Fletcher CV, et al. Persistent HIV-1 replication maintains the tissue reservoir during therapy. Nature. 2016;530:51–6.

45. Evering TH, Mehandru S, Racz P, Tenner-Racz K, Poles MA, Figueroa A, Mohri H, Markowitz M. Absence of HIV-1 evolution in the gut-associated lymphoid tissue from patients on combination antiviral therapy initiated during primary infection. PLoS Pathog. 2012;8:e1002506.

46. Bailey JR, Sedaghat AR, Kieffer T, Brennan T, Lee PK, Wind-Rotolo M, Haggerty CM, Kamireddi AR, Liu Y, Lee J, et al. Residual human immunodeficiency virus type 1 viremia in some patients on antiretroviral therapy is dominated by a small number of invariant clones rarely found in circulating CD4+ T cells. J Virol. 2006;80:6441–57.

47. Kieffer TL, Finucane MM, Nettles RE, Quinn TC, Broman KW, Ray SC, Persaud D, Siliciano RF. Genotypic analysis of HIV-1 drug resistance at the limit of detection: virus production without evolution in treated adults with undetectable HIV loads. J Infect Dis. 2004;189:1452–65.

48. Hudson RR, Boos DD, Kaplan NL. A statistical test for detecting geographic subdivision. Mol Biol Evol. 1992;9:138–51.

49. Achaz G, Palmer S, Kearney M, Maldarelli F, Mellors JW, Coffin JM, Wakeley J. A robust measure of HIV-1 population turnover within chronically infected individuals. Mol Biol Evol. 2004;21:1902–12.

50. Slatkin M, Maddison WP. A cladistic measure of gene flow inferred from the phylogenies of alleles. Genetics. 1989;123:603–13.

51. Keele BF, Giorgi EE, Salazar-Gonzalez JF, Decker JM, Pham KT, Salazar MG, Sun C, Grayson T, Wang S, Li H, et al. Identification and characterization of transmitted and early founder virus envelopes in primary HIV-1 infection. Proc Natl Acad Sci USA. 2008;105:7552–7.

52. Shankarappa R, Gupta P, Learn GH Jr, Rodrigo AG, Rinaldo CR Jr, Gorry MC, Mullins JI, Nara PL, Ehrlich GD. Evolution of human immunodeficiency virus type 1 envelope sequences in infected individuals with differing disease progression profiles. Virology. 1998;241:251–9.

53. Kearney MF, Spindler J, Shao W, Yu S, Anderson EM, O'Shea A, Rehm C, Poethke C, Kovacs N, Mellors JW, et al. Lack of detectable HIV-1 molecular evolution during suppressive antiretroviral therapy. PLoS Pathog. 2014;10:e1004010.

54. Josefsson L, von Stockenstrom S, Faria NR, Sinclair E, Bacchetti P, Killian M, Epling L, Tan A, Ho T, Lemey P, et al. The HIV-1 reservoir in eight patients on long-term suppressive antiretroviral therapy is stable with few genetic changes over time. Proc Natl Acad Sci USA. 2013;110:E4987–96.

55. Carlson JM, Schaefer M, Monaco DC, Batorsky R, Claiborne DT, Prince J, Deymier MJ, Ende ZS, Klatt NR, DeZiel CE, et al. Selection bias at the heterosexual HIV-1 transmission bottleneck. Science. 2014;345:1254031.

56. Bar KJ, Li H, Chamberland A, Tremblay C, Routy JP, Grayson T, Sun C, Wang S, Learn GH, Morgan CJ, et al. Wide variation in the multiplicity of HIV-1 infection among injection drug users. J Virol. 2010;84:6241–7.

57. Li H, Bar KJ, Wang S, Decker JM, Chen Y, Sun C, Salazar-Gonzalez JF, Salazar MG, Learn GH, Morgan CJ, et al. High multiplicity infection by HIV-1 in men who have sex with men. PLoS Pathog. 2010;6:e1000890.

58. Russell ES, Kwiek JJ, Keys J, Barton K, Mwapasa V, Montefiori DC, Meshnick SR, Swanstrom R. The genetic bottleneck in vertical transmission of subtype C HIV-1 is not driven by selection of especially neutralization-resistant virus from the maternal viral population. J Virol. 2011;85:8253–62.

59. Sheppard HW, Celum C, Michael NL, O'Brien S, Dean M, Carrington M, Dondero D, Buchbinder SP. HIV-1 infection in individuals with the CCR5-Delta32/Delta32 genotype: acquisition of syncytium-inducing virus at seroconversion. J Acquir Immune Defic Syndr. 1999;2002(29):307–13.

60. Chalmet K, Dauwe K, Foquet L, Baatz F, Seguin-Devaux C, Van Der Gucht B, Vogelaers D, Vandekerckhove L, Plum J, Verhofstede C. Presence of CXCR4-using HIV-1 in patients with recently diagnosed infection: correlates and evidence for transmission. J Infect Dis. 2012;205:174–84.

61. Ping LH, Joseph SB, Anderson JA, Abrahams MR, Salazar-Gonzalez JF, Kincer LP, Treurnicht FK, Arney L, Ojeda S, Zhang M, et al. Comparison of viral Env proteins from acute and chronic infections with subtype C human immunodeficiency virus type 1 identifies differences in glycosylation and CCR5 utilization and suggests a new strategy for immunogen design. J Virol. 2013;87:7218–33.

62. Abrahams M-R, Anderson JA, Giorgi EE, Seoighe C, Mlisana K, Ping L-H, Athreya GS, Treurnicht FK, Keele BF, Wood N, et al. Quantitating the multiplicity of infection with human immunodeficiency virus type 1 subtype C reveals a non-poisson distribution of transmitted variants. J Virol. 2009;83:3556–67.

63. Novitsky V, Wang R, Margolin L, Baca J, Rossenkhan R, Moyo S, van Widenfelt E, Essex M. Transmission of single and multiple viral variants in primary HIV-1 subtype C infection. PLoS ONE. 2011;6:e16714.

64. Batorsky R, Kearney MF, Palmer SE, Maldarelli F, Rouzine IM, Coffin JM. Estimate of effective recombination rate and average selection coefficient for HIV in chronic infection. Proc Natl Acad Sci USA. 2011;108:5661–6.

65. Fischer W, Ganusov VV, Giorgi EE, Hraber PT, Keele BF, Leitner T, Han CS, Gleasner CD, Green L, Lo C-C, et al. Transmission of single HIV-1 genomes and dynamics of early immune escape revealed by ultra-deep sequencing. PLoS ONE. 2010;5:e12303.

66. Carlson JM, Du VY, Pfeifer N, Bansal A, Tan VYF, Power K, Brumme CJ, Kreimer A, DeZiel CE, Fusi N, et al. Impact of pre-adapted HIV transmission. Nat Med. 2016;22:606–13.

67. Brennan CA, Ibarrondo FJ, Sugar CA, Hausner MA, Shih R, Ng HL, Detels R, Margolick JB, Rinaldo CR, Phair J, et al. Early HLA-B*57-restricted CD8+ T lymphocyte responses predict HIV-1 disease progression. J Virol. 2012;86:10505–16.

68. Shahid A, Olvera A, Anmole G, Kuang XT, Cotton LA, Plana M, Brander C, Brockman MA, Brumme ZL. Consequences of HLA-B*13-associated

escape mutations on HIV-1 replication and Nef function. J Virol. 2015;89:11557–71.

69. Bar KJ, Tsao C-Y, Iyer SS, Decker JM, Yang Y, Bonsignori M, Chen X, Hwang K-K, Montefiori DC, Liao H-X, et al. Early low-titer neutralizing antibodies impede HIV-1 replication and select for virus escape. PLoS Pathog. 2012;8:e1002721.

70. Hill AL, Rosenbloom DIS, Nowak MA. Evolutionary dynamics of HIV at multiple spatial and temporal scales. J Mol Med. 2012;90:543–61.

71. Waters L, Mandalia S, Randell P, Wildfire A, Gazzard B, Moyle G. The impact of HIV tropism on decreases in CD4 cell count, clinical progression, and subsequent response to a first antiretroviral therapy regimen. Clin Infect Dis. 2008;46:1617–23.

72. Wu X, Zhang Z, Schramm Chaim A, Joyce MG, Do Kwon Y, Zhou T, Sheng Z, Zhang B, O'Dell S, McKee K, et al. Maturation and diversity of the VRC01-antibody lineage over 15 years of chronic HIV-1 infection. Cell. 2015;161:470–85.

73. Liao H-X, Lynch R, Zhou T, Gao F, Alam SM, Boyd SD, Fire AZ, Roskin KM, Schramm CA, Zhang Z, et al. Co-evolution of a broadly neutralizing HIV-1 antibody and founder virus. Nature. 2013;496:469–76.

74. Palmer S, Maldarelli F, Wiegand A, Bernstein B, Hanna GJ, Brun SC, Kempf DJ, Mellors JW, Coffin JM, King MS. Low-level viremia persists for at least 7 years in patients on suppressive antiretroviral therapy. Proc Natl Acad Sci USA. 2008;105:3879–84.

75. Maldarelli F, Palmer S, King MS, Wiegand A, Polis MA, Mican J, Kovacs JA, Davey RT, Rock-Kress D, Dewar R, et al. ART suppresses plasma HIV-1 RNA to a stable set point predicted by pretherapy viremia. PLoS Pathog. 2007;3:e46.

76. Perelson AS, Essunger P, Cao Y, Vesanen M, Hurley A, Saksela K, Markowitz M, Ho DD. Decay characteristics of HIV-1-infected compartments during combination therapy. Nature. 1997;387:188–91.

77. Simonetti FR, Sobolewski MD, Fyne E, Shao W, Spindler J, Hattori J, Anderson EM, Watters SA, Hill S, Wu X, et al. Clonally expanded CD4+ T cells can produce infectious HIV-1 in vivo. Proc Natl Acad Sci USA. 2016;113:1883–8.

78. Wiegand A, Spindler J, Hong FF, Shao W, Cyktor JC, Cillo AR, Halvas EK, Coffin JM, Mellors JW, Kearney MF. Single-cell analysis of HIV-1 transcriptional activity reveals expression of proviruses in expanded clones during ART. Proc Natl Acad Sci USA. 2017;114:E3659–68.

79. Besson GJ, Lalama CM, Bosch RJ, Gandhi RT, Bedison MA, Aga E, Riddler SA, McMahon DK, Hong F, Mellors JW. HIV-1 DNA decay dynamics in blood during more than a decade of suppressive antiretroviral therapy. Clin Infect Dis. 2014;59:1312–21.

80. von Stockenstrom S, Odevall L, Lee E, Sinclair E, Bacchetti P, Killian M, Epling L, Shao W, Hoh R, Ho T, et al. Longitudinal genetic characterization reveals that cell proliferation maintains a persistent HIV type 1 DNA pool during effective HIV therapy. J Infect Dis. 2015;212:596–607.

81. Hosmane NN, Kwon KJ, Bruner KM, Capoferri AA, Beg S, Rosenbloom DI, Keele BF, Ho YC, Siliciano JD, Siliciano RF. Proliferation of latently infected CD4+ T cells carrying replication-competent HIV-1: potential role in latent reservoir dynamics. J Exp Med. 2017;214:959–72.

82. Chun TW, Carruth L, Finzi D, Shen X, DiGiuseppe JA, Taylor H, Hermankova M, Chadwick K, Margolick J, Quinn TC, et al. Quantification of latent tissue reservoirs and total body viral load in HIV-1 infection. Nature. 1997;387:183–8.

83. Chun TW, Finzi D, Margolick J, Chadwick K, Schwartz D, Siliciano RF. In vivo fate of HIV-1-infected T cells: quantitative analysis of the transition to stable latency. Nat Med. 1995;1:1284–90.

84. Henrich TJ, Hanhauser E, Marty FM, Sirignano MN, Keating S, Lee TH, Robles YP, Davis BT, Li JZ, Heisey A, et al. Antiretroviral-free HIV-1 remission and viral rebound after allogeneic stem cell transplantation: report of 2 cases. Ann Intern Med. 2014;161:319–27.

85. Luzuriaga K, Gay H, Ziemniak C, Sanborn KB, Somasundaran M, Rainwater-Lovett K, Mellors JW, Rosenbloom D, Persaud D. Viremic relapse after HIV-1 remission in a perinatally infected child. N Engl J Med. 2015;372:786–8.

86. Kearney MF, Wiegand A, Shao W, Coffin JM, Mellors JW, Lederman M, Gandhi RT, Keele BF, Li JZ. Origin of rebound plasma HIV includes cells with identical proviruses that are transcriptionally active before stopping of antiretroviral therapy. J Virol. 2015;90:1369–76.

87. Ho YC, Shan L, Hosmane NN, Wang J, Laskey SB, Rosenbloom DI, Lai J, Blankson JN, Siliciano JD, Siliciano RF. Replication-competent

88. Pollack RA, Jones RB, Pertea M, Bruner KM, Martin AR, Thomas AS, Capoferri AA, Beg SA, Huang S-H, Karandish S, et al. Defective HIV-1 proviruses are expressed and can be recognized by cytotoxic T lymphocytes, which shape the proviral landscape. Cell Host Microbe. 2017;21(494–506):e494.

89. Cory TJ, Schacker TW, Stevenson M, Fletcher CV. Overcoming pharmacologic sanctuaries. Curr Opin HIV AIDS. 2013;8:190–5.

90. Fletcher CV, Staskus K, Wietgrefe SW, Rothenberger M, Reilly C, Chipman JG, Beilman GJ, Khoruts A, Thorkelson A, Schmidt TE, et al. Persistent HIV-1 replication is associated with lower antiretroviral drug concentrations in lymphatic tissues. Proc Natl Acad Sci USA. 2014;111:2307–12.

91. Huang Y, Hoque MT, Jenabian MA, Vyboh K, Whyte SK, Sheehan NL, Brassard P, Belanger M, Chomont N, Fletcher CV, et al. Antiretroviral drug transporters and metabolic enzymes in human testicular tissue: potential contribution to HIV-1 sanctuary site. J Antimicrob Chemother. 2016;71:1954–65.

92. Chun TW, Nickle DC, Justement JS, Large D, Semerjian A, Curlin ME, O'Shea MA, Hallahan CW, Daucher M, Ward DJ, et al. HIV-infected individuals receiving effective antiviral therapy for extended periods of time continually replenish their viral reservoir. J Clin Invest. 2005;115:3250–5.

93. Boritz EA, Darko S, Swaszek L, Wolf G, Wells D, Wu X, Henry AR, Laboune F, Hu J, Ambrozak D, et al. Multiple origins of virus persistence during natural control of HIV infection. Cell. 2016;166:1004–15.

94. Kearney MF, Wiegand A, Shao W, McManus WR, Bale MJ, Luke B, Maldarelli F, Mellors JW, Coffin JM. Ongoing HIV replication during ART reconsidered. Open Forum Infect Dis. 2017;4:ofx173-ofx173.

95. Wagner TA, McKernan JL, Tobin NH, Tapia KA, Mullins JI, Frenkel LM. An increasing proportion of monotypic HIV-1 DNA sequences during antiretroviral treatment suggests proliferation of HIV-infected cells. J Virol. 2013;87:1770–8.

96. Dinoso JB, Kim SY, Wiegand AM, Palmer SE, Gange SJ, Cranmer L, O'Shea A, Callender M, Spivak A, Brennan T, et al. Treatment intensification does not reduce residual HIV-1 viremia in patients on highly active antiretroviral therapy. Proc Natl Acad Sci USA. 2009;106:9403–8.

97. Gandhi RT, Zheng L, Bosch RJ, Chan ES, Margolis DM, Read S, Kallungal B, Palmer S, Medvik K, Lederman MM, et al. The effect of raltegravir intensification on low-level residual viremia in HIV-infected patients on antiretroviral therapy: a randomized controlled trial. PLoS Med. 2010;7:e1000321.

98. McMahon D, Jones J, Wiegand A, Gange SJ, Kearney M, Palmer S, McNulty S, Metcalf JA, Acosta E, Rehm C, et al. Short-course raltegravir intensification does not reduce persistent low-level viremia in patients with HIV-1 suppression during receipt of combination antiretroviral therapy. Clin Infect Dis. 2010;50:912–9.

99. Wang X, Mink G, Lin D, Song X, Rong L. Influence of raltegravir intensification on viral load and 2-LTR dynamics in HIV patients on suppressive antiretroviral therapy. J Theor Biol. 2017;416:16–27.

100. Joos B, Fischer M, Kuster H, Pillai SK, Wong JK, Böni J, Hirschel B, Weber R, Trkola A, Günthard HF. Swiss HIV Cohort Study TSHC: HIV rebounds from latently infected cells, rather than from continuing low-level replication. Proc Natl Acad Sci USA. 2008;105:16725–30.

101. Persaud D, Ray SC, Kajdas J, Ahonkhai A, Siberry GK, Ferguson K, Ziemniak C, Quinn TC, Casazza JP, Zeichner S, et al. Slow human immunodeficiency virus type 1 evolution in viral reservoirs in infants treated with effective antiretroviral therapy. AIDS Res Hum Retroviruses. 2007;23:381–90.

102. Van Zyl GU, Katusiime MG, Wiegand A, McManus WR, Bale MJ, Halvas EK, Luke B, Boltz VF, Spindler J, Laughton B, et al. No evidence of HIV replication in children on antiretroviral therapy. J Clin Invest. 2017;127:3827–34.

103. Vancoillie L, Hebberecht L, Dauwe K, Demecheleer E, Dinakis S, Vaneechoutte D, Mortier V, Verhofstede C. Longitudinal sequencing of HIV-1 infected patients with low-level viremia for years while on ART shows no indications for genetic evolution of the virus. Virology. 2017;510:185–93.

104. Kearney MF, Anderson EM, Coomer C, Smith L, Shao W, Johnson N, Kline C, Spindler J, Mellors JW, Coffin JM, Ambrose Z. Well-mixed plasma and tissue viral populations in RT-SHIV-infected macaques implies a lack of

viral replication in the tissues during antiretroviral therapy. Retrovirology. 2015;12:93.

105. Bull M, Learn G, Genowati I, McKernan J, Hitti J, Lockhart D, Tapia K, Holte S, Dragavon J, Coombs R, et al. Compartmentalization of HIV-1 within the female genital tract is due to monotypic and low-diversity variants not distinct viral populations. PLoS ONE. 2009;4:e7122.

106. Nickle DC, Jensen MA, Shriner D, Brodie SJ, Frenkel LM, Mittler JE, Mullins JI. Evolutionary indicators of human immunodeficiency virus type 1 reservoirs and compartments. J Virol. 2003;77:5540–6.

107. van Marle G, Gill MJ, Kolodka D, McManus L, Grant T, Church DL. Compartmentalization of the gut viral reservoir in HIV-1 infected patients. Retrovirology. 2007;4:87.

108. Yukl SA, Gianella S, Sinclair E, Epling L, Li Q, Duan L, Choi AL, Girling V, Ho T, Li P, et al. Differences in HIV burden and immune activation within the gut of HIV-positive patients receiving suppressive antiretroviral therapy. J Infect Dis. 2010;202:1553–61.

109. Rueda CM, Velilla PA, Chougnet CA, Montoya CJ, Rugeles MT. HIV-induced T-cell activation/exhaustion in rectal mucosa is controlled only partially by antiretroviral treatment. PLoS ONE. 2012;7:e30307.

110. Imamichi H, Degray G, Dewar RL, Mannon P, Yao M, Chairez C, Sereti I, Kovacs JA. Lack of compartmentalization of HIV-1 quasispecies between the gut and peripheral blood compartments. J Infect Dis. 2011;204:309–14.

111. Stefic K, Chaillon A, Bouvin-Pley M, Moreau A, Braibant M, Bastides F, Gras G, Bernard L, Barin F. Probing the compartmentalization of HIV-1 in the central nervous system through its neutralization properties. PLoS ONE. 2017;12:e0181680.

112. Evering TH, Kamau E, St Bernard L, Farmer CB, Kong XP, Markowitz M. Single genome analysis reveals genetic characteristics of Neuroadaptation across HIV-1 envelope. Retrovirology. 2014;11:65.

113. Ritola K, Pilcher CD, Fiscus SA, Hoffman NG, Nelson JA, Kitrinos KM, Hicks CB, Eron JJ Jr, Swanstrom R. Multiple V1/V2 env variants are frequently present during primary infection with human immunodeficiency virus type 1. J Virol. 2004;78:11208–18.

114. Chomont N, Hocini H, Gresenguet G, Brochier C, Bouhlal H, Andreoletti L, Becquart P, Charpentier C, de Dieu Longo J, Si-Mohamed A, et al. Early archives of genetically-restricted proviral DNA in the female genital tract after heterosexual transmission of HIV-1. AIDS. 2007;21:153–62.

115. Chaudhary S, Noel RJ, Rodriguez N, Collado S, Munoz J, Kumar A, Yamamura Y. Correlation between CD4 T cell counts and virus compartmentalization in genital and systemic compartments of HIV-infected females. Virology. 2011;417:320–6.

116. Blasi M, Carpenter JH, Balakumaran B, Cara A, Gao F, Klotman ME. Identification of HIV-1 genitourinary tract compartmentalization by analyzing the env gene sequences in urine. AIDS. 2015;29:1651–7.

117. Bull ME, Learn GH, McElhone S, Hitti J, Lockhart D, Holte S, Dragavon J, Coombs RW, Mullins JI, Frenkel LM. Monotypic human immunodeficiency virus type 1 genotypes across the uterine cervix and in blood suggest proliferation of cells with provirus. J Virol. 2009;83:6020–8.

118. Bull ME, Heath LM, McKernan-Mullin JL, Kraft KM, Acevedo L, Hitti JE, Cohn SE, Tapia KA, Holte SE, Dragavon JA, et al. Human immunodeficiency viruses appear compartmentalized to the female genital tract in cross-sectional analyses but genital lineages do not persist over time. J Infect Dis. 2013;207:1206–15.

119. Chaillon A, Smith DM, Vanpouille C, Lisco A, Jordan P, Caballero G, Vargas M, Gianella S, Mehta SR. HIV trafficking between blood and semen during early untreated HIV infection. J Acquir Immune Defic Syndr. 2017;74:95–102.

120. Delchambre M, Gheysen D, Thines D, Thiriart C, Jacobs E, Verdin E, Horth M, Burny A, Bex F. The GAG precursor of simian immunodeficiency virus assembles into virus-like particles. EMBO J. 1989;8:2653–60.

121. Eriksson S, Graf EH, Dahl V, Strain MC, Yukl SA, Lysenko ES, Bosch RJ, Lai J, Chioma S, Emad F, et al. Comparative analysis of measures of viral reservoirs in HIV-1 eradication studies. PLoS Pathog. 2013;9:e1003174.

122. Wainberg MA, Rooke R, Tremblay M, Li X, Parniak MA, Gao Q, Yao XJ, Tsoukas C, Montaner J, Fanning M, Ruedy J. Clinical significance and characterization of AZT-resistant strains of HIV-1. Can J Infect Dis. 1991;2:5–11.

123. Collier AC, Coombs RW, Schoenfeld DA, Bassett RL, Timpone J, Baruch A, Jones M, Facey K, Whitacre C, McAuliffe VJ, et al. Treatment of human immunodeficiency virus infection with saquinavir, zidovudine, and zalcitabine. N Engl J Med. 1996;334:1011–8.

124. Montaner JS, Hogg R, Raboud J, Harrigan R, O'Shaughnessy M. Antiretroviral treatment in 1998. The Lancet. 1998;352:1919–22.

125. Montaner JS, Reiss P, Cooper D, Vella S, Harris M, Conway B, Wainberg MA, Smith D, Robinson P, Hall D, et al. A randomized, double-blind trial comparing combinations of nevirapine, didanosine, and zidovudine for HIV-infected patients: the INCAS Trial. Italy, The Netherlands, Canada and Australia Study. JAMA. 1998;279:930–7.

126. Altmann A, Beerenwinkel N, Sing T, Savenkov I, Doumer M, Kaiser R, Rhee S-Y, Fessel WJ, Shafer RW, Lengauer T. Improved prediction of response to antiretroviral combination therapy using the genetic barrier to drug resistance. Antivir Ther. 2007;12:169–78.

127. Brenner BG, Wainberg MA. Clinical benefit of dolutegravir in HIV-1 management related to the high genetic barrier to drug resistance. Virus Res. 2017;239:1–9.

128. Gantner P, Cuzin L, Allavena C, Cabie A, Pugliese P, Valantin M-A, Bani-Sadr F, Joly V, Ferry T, Poizot-Martin I, et al. Efficacy and safety of dolutegravir and rilpivirine dual therapy as a simplification strategy: a cohort study. HIV Medicine. 2017;18:704–8.

129. Maggiolo F, Gulminetti R, Pagnucco L, Digaetano M, Benatti S, Valenti D, Callegaro A, Ripamonti D, Mussini C. Lamivudine/dolutegravir dual therapy in HIV-infected, virologically suppressed patients. BMC Infect Dis. 2017;17:215.

130. Lepik KJ, Harrigan PR, Yip B, Wang L, Robbins MA, Zhang WW, Toy J, Akagi L, Lima VD, Guillemi S, et al. Emergent drug resistance with integrase strand transfer inhibitor-based regimens. AIDS. 2017;31:1425–34.

131. Naeger LK, Harrington P, Komatsu T, Deming D. Effect of dolutegravir functional monotherapy on HIV-1 virological response in integrase strand transfer inhibitor resistant patients. Antivir Ther. 2016;21:481–8.

132. Oldenbuettel C, Wolf E, Ritter A, Noe S, Heldwein S, Pascucci R, Wiese C, Von Krosigk A, Jaegel-Guedes E, Jaeger H, et al. Dolutegravir monotherapy as treatment de-escalation in HIV-infected adults with virological control: DoluMono cohort results. Antivir Ther. 2016;22:169–72.

133. Rabi SA, Laird GM, Durand CM, Laskey S, Shan L, Bailey JR, Chioma S, Moore RD, Siliciano RF. Multi-step inhibition explains HIV-1 protease inhibitor pharmacodynamics and resistance. J Clin Invest. 2013;123:3848–60.

134. Sampah MES, Shen L, Jilek BL, Siliciano RF. Dose-response curve slope is a missing dimension in the analysis of HIV-1 drug resistance. Proc Natl Acad Sci. 2011;108:7613–8.

135. Jourdain G, Ngo-Giang-Huong N, Le Coeur S, Bowonwatanuwong C, Kantipong P, Leechanachai P, Ariyadej S, Leenasirimakul P, Hammer S, Lallemant M. Intrapartum exposure to nevirapine and subsequent maternal responses to nevirapine-based antiretroviral therapy. N Engl J Med. 2004;351:229–40.

136. Boltz VF, Bao Y, Lockman S, Halvas EK, Kearney MF, McIntyre JA, Schooley RT, Hughes MD, Coffin JM, Mellors JW, Team OA. Low-frequency nevirapine (NVP)-resistant HIV-1 variants are not associated with failure of antiretroviral therapy in women without prior exposure to single-dose NVP. J Infect Dis. 2014;209:703–10.

137. Li JZ, Paredes R, Ribaudo HJ, Svarovskaia ES, Kozal MJ, Hullsiek KH, Miller MD, Bangsberg DR, Kuritzkes DR. Relationship between minority nonnucleoside reverse transcriptase inhibitor resistance mutations, adherence, and the risk of virologic failure. AIDS (London, England). 2012;26:185–92.

138. Goodman DD, Zhou Y, Margot NA, McColl DJ, Zhong L, Borroto-Esoda K, Miller MD, Svarovskaia ES. Low level of the K103N HIV-1 above a threshold is associated with virological failure in treatment-naive individuals undergoing efavirenz-containing therapy. AIDS. 2011;25:325–33.

139. Parienti JJ, Das-Douglas M, Massari V, Guzman D, Deeks SG, Verdon R, Bangsberg DR. Not all missed doses are the same: sustained NNRTI treatment interruptions predict HIV rebound at low-to-moderate adherence levels. PLoS ONE. 2008;3:e2783.

140. Hosseinipour MC, Gupta RK, Van Zyl G, Eron JJ, Nachega JB. Emergence of HIV drug resistance during first- and second-line antiretroviral therapy in resource-limited settings. J Infect Dis. 2013;207:S49–56.

141. Coffin JM. HIV population dynamics in vivo: implications for genetic variation, pathogenesis, and therapy. Science. 1995;267:483–9.

142. Mansky LM, Temin HM. Lower in vivo mutation rate of human immunodeficiency virus type 1 than that predicted from the fidelity of purified reverse transcriptase. J Virol. 1995;69:5087–94.

15

Replacement of feline foamy virus *bet* by feline immunodeficiency virus *vif* yields replicative virus with novel vaccine candidate potential

Carmen Ledesma-Feliciano[1], Sarah Hagen[2], Ryan Troyer[1,5], Xin Zheng[1], Esther Musselman[1], Dragana Slavkovic Lukic[2,7], Ann-Mareen Franke[2,8], Daniel Maeda[2,6], Jörg Zielonka[3,4], Carsten Münk[3], Guochao Wei[2,9], Sue VandeWoude[1] and Martin Löchelt[2*]

Abstract

Background: Hosts are able to restrict viral replication to contain virus spread before adaptive immunity is fully initiated. Many viruses have acquired genes directly counteracting intrinsic restriction mechanisms. This phenomenon has led to a co-evolutionary signature for both the virus and host which often provides a barrier against interspecies transmission events. Through different mechanisms of action, but with similar consequences, spumaviral feline foamy virus (FFV) Bet and lentiviral feline immunodeficiency virus (FIV) Vif counteract feline APOBEC3 (feA3) restriction factors that lead to hypermutation and degradation of retroviral DNA genomes. Here we examine the capacity of *vif* to substitute for *bet* function in a chimeric FFV to assess the transferability of anti-feA3 factors to allow viral replication.

Results: We show that *vif* can replace *bet* to yield replication-competent chimeric foamy viruses. An in vitro selection screen revealed that an engineered Bet-Vif fusion protein yields suboptimal protection against feA3. After multiple passages through feA3-expressing cells, however, variants with optimized replication competence emerged. In these variants, Vif was expressed independently from an N-terminal Bet moiety and was stably maintained. Experimental infection of immunocompetent domestic cats with one of the functional chimeras resulted in seroconversion against the FFV backbone and the heterologous FIV Vif protein, but virus could not be detected unambiguously by PCR. Inoculation with chimeric virus followed by wild-type FFV revealed that repeated administration of FVs allowed superinfections with enhanced antiviral antibody production and detection of low level viral genomes, indicating that chimeric virus did not induce protective immunity against wild-type FFV.

Conclusions: Unrelated viral antagonists of feA3 cellular restriction factors can be exchanged in FFV, resulting in replication competence in vitro that was attenuated in vivo. Bet therefore may have additional functions other than A3 antagonism that are essential for successful in vivo replication. Immune reactivity was mounted against the heterologous Vif protein. We conclude that Vif-expressing FV vaccine vectors may be an attractive tool to prevent or modulate lentivirus infections with the potential option to induce immunity against additional lentivirus antigens.

Keywords: Foamy virus, In vitro virus evolution, In vivo host factor requirement, Replicating vaccine vector, Lentivirus, Bet function, Vif function, APOBEC3, Restriction factor, Superinfection

*Correspondence: m.loechelt@dkfz.de
[2] Department of Molecular Diagnostics of Oncogenic Infections, Research Program Infection, Inflammation and Cancer, German Cancer Research Center, (Deutsches Krebsforschungszentrum Heidelberg, DKFZ), Im Neuenheimer Feld 242, 69120 Heidelberg, Germany
Full list of author information is available at the end of the article

Background

Foamy viruses (FVs) are ancient retroviruses comprising the only genus of the subfamily *Spumaretrovirinae*, which are different in many aspects from the *Orthoretrovirinae* that comprise all other known retroviruses including lentiviruses (LVs) [1–3]. Despite having a wide tissue tropism in infected animals, FVs have historically been regarded as apathogenic and are endemic in primates, bovids, felids, and other hosts. Clusters of highly related viruses have been documented in closely related hosts [4–7]. While humans do not have endemic FVs, they are susceptible to zoonotic infections from non-human primates [8, 9]. FVs and LVs such as feline immunodeficiency virus (FIV) have been used to develop vectors for vaccine antigen delivery and gene therapy in a variety of mammals [10–17]. In domestic cats (*Felis catus*), feline foamy virus (FFV) and FIV establish lifelong infections despite specific host antiviral immune responses [18–21]. In contrast to FFV infection, FIV infection leads to the development of an immunosuppressive AIDS-like syndrome in some cats [18, 20, 22–24]. Thus, FVs are an attractive alternative to LV vectors due to their apathogenicity, wide tissue tropism, and establishment of a persistent infection with ongoing virus gene expression and replication [6, 7, 12, 13, 21, 25, 26]. Other advantageous features of FV-based vectors are a safer integration profile than gammaretroviral and LV vectors [11, 27], a large packaging capacity, and the ability to introduce self-inactivating properties [17, 28–31]. Investigating FV vector candidates could thus yield potential new therapies to benefit both humans and animals [16].

Both LVs and FVs are complex retroviruses encoding the canonical Gag, Pol, and Env proteins, regulatory proteins essential for replication in all cells, and accessory proteins required only in certain cells. For instance, LV Tat and FV Tas (also designated Bel1) proteins are both transactivators for virus gene expression, however, their mode of action is completely different (for review [32]). Regardless, both regulatory genes induce a positive feedback loop to generate more transactivator protein in addition to transcription of structural genes required for infectivity [32]. FVs additionally encode Bet that is generated via splicing, consisting of N-terminal Tas sequences while the majority of the protein is encoded by another reading frame, the *bel2* gene [32]. Bet is the functional homologue of the LV Vif protein, both of which are involved in countering the host intrinsic antiviral restriction factors of the APOBEC3 (A3) family [33–38].

Like all other viruses, LVs and FVs are restricted by intrinsic cell mechanisms that impair or even suppress the different phases of virus replication, progeny production, and establishment of infection in the new host (for review see [39, 40]). Nonspecific innate immunity and

cell-based intrinsic immunity employing antiviral restriction factors are both absolutely required to control pathogen replication before adaptive immunity matures for long-term suppression of viral replication [41, 42]. Therefore, a fine-tuned crosstalk between innate, intrinsic, and adaptive immunity is needed to control and eliminate the pathogen as well as to build up immunological memory [41–43]. Pathogens have evolved a plethora of counteracting strategies in order to evade this control, often by the acquisition of counteracting proteins [39, 40]. The idea and concept of host-encoded restriction factors and the viral counter-defense have been in part established in human immunodeficiency virus (HIV) research. These initial studies analyzed the interplay between host-encoded A3 cytidine deaminases that result mainly in lethal mutagenesis (C to U/T exchanges) of the retroviral HIV genome during reverse transcription, and the counter-defense by LV Vif (or Bet in FVs) which result in A3 degradation (via Vif) or sequestration (via Bet) [33, 34, 36, 40, 44].

Analogous to human A3 function, feline A3 (feA3) proteins are produced in many cell types and introduce missense and stop mutations into nascent viral genomes, ultimately restricting viral replication through hypermutation and degradation [33, 34, 39]. Several studies on the function of FIV Vif and FFV Bet, which are of very different size and share no obvious sequence or structural homology [36, 38, 45], have revealed that they employ completely different modes of action to achieve the same end goal: preventing the packaging of feA3 proteins into the particle to avoid subsequent viral lethal mutagenesis. The FIV Vif protein (25 kDa) functions as an adapter molecule, binding to cognate or highly-related feA3 proteins and recruiting the ubiquitin proteasome degradation machinery, resulting in the removal of feA3 proteins from the virus-producing cell [44, 46–49]. This is the critical prerequisite to prevent cytidine deamination during or after reverse transcription of the genome. In contrast, FV Bet proteins (of 43 to 56 kDa) tightly bind A3 proteins of their cognate host species without leading to degradation, likely acting via sequestration or blocking of essential binding and multimerization sites [34, 36, 37, 45]. Therefore, *vif* and *bet* are essential viral genes required to allow productive replication in cells with active A3 expression [39, 50, 51].

Domestic cats produce multiple A3 proteins in one and two-domain forms. One-domain feA3 proteins include the A3Z2 (present as A3Z2a, A3Z2b, and A3Z2c) and A3Z3 isoforms, while read-through transcription leads to the production of two-domain feA3Z2-Z3 proteins (in A3Z2b-Z3 and A3Z2c-Z3 isoforms) [52]. These feA3 proteins have differential effects on FFV and FIV: A3Z2s markedly reduce titers of FFV lacking *bet*, while the A3Z3 and A3Z2-Z3 proteins inhibit FIV virions lacking *vif* with intermediate and high efficiency, respectively. Interestingly, both Bet and Vif counteract all feA3 regardless of whether the specific A3 isoforms efficiently restrict FFV or FIV [33, 34, 44, 46, 47, 52], suggesting a more complex relationship between these accessory genes and host restriction factor regulation than has yet been described.

Here we describe the generation and in vitro selection of FFV-Vif chimeras in which FIV *vif* partially or almost fully restored the replication capacity of *bet*-deficient FFV constructs in vitro. An in vitro-selected FFV-Vif variant that drives expression of the heterologous lentivirus Vif independent from any FFV protein and which is highly dependent on Vif expression in A3-producing cells, was used for infection of domestic cats to test the chimera's replication competence and immunogenicity. Replication of the FFV-Vif chimera was attenuated in cats compared to wild-type FFV. Cats infected with the FFV-Vif chimera developed persistent antibody responses towards FFV proteins and FIV Vif but proviral FFV-Vif chimeric genomes were at or below the limit of detection in peripheral blood mononuclear cells (PBMC) of infected cats. In contrast, proviral genomes were consistently detected in wild-type FFV-infected cats. Inoculation of cats in the FFV-Vif chimera cohort with wild-type FFV or re-inoculation with FFV-Vif chimeric virus boosted anti-FFV Gag antibody titer following re-infection. These results suggest that compensatory changes arising in vitro seemingly allowed FIV-Vif to substitute for FFV-Bet function, but were incapable of fully supporting FFV-Vif chimeric replication competence in vivo. These findings additionally suggest the capacity of spumaviruses to superinfect cats following prior attenuated FFV replication, indicating the potential suitability of chimeric FFV as a vaccine vector in the face of a pre-existing infection and immunity.

Results

FIV Vif and FFV Bet confer protection from feA3 restriction in vitro

Previous studies have shown that the FIV Vif accessory protein has the capacity to direct proteasomal degradation of all known feA3 cytidine deaminase restriction factors irrespective of whether they strongly or moderately restrict FIV replication [44, 46, 47, 52]. Similarly, FFV Bet binds to all feA3 isoforms and inactivates their restriction potential by a degradation-independent, different mechanism not comparable to FIV Vif [33, 34]. In addition, FIV Vif can protect the replication capacity of *bet*-deficient FFV while FFV Bet correspondingly counteracts feA3-mediated restriction of *vif*-deficient FIV [39, 44].

To confirm here that the viral defense proteins of FFV and FIV are functionally interchangeable to protect

infectivity against feA3 restriction [33, 34, 44, 46, 47, 52], transient transfection studies were conducted and representative data are shown here. First, we analyzed the susceptibility of FIV∆*vif*-luc, a *vif*-deficient FIV luciferase (luc) expression vector ("Methods", [44]) towards one-domain feA3Z3, and two-domain feA3Z2-Z3 isoforms (Additional file 1A). The efficacy of *luc* marker gene transduction was determined in the presence of co-transfection with FFV *bet*, FIV *vif*, or an empty control vector. Both FIV Vif and FFV Bet restored the FIV vector titer almost fully while different levels of feA3-mediated restriction were detectable only in the absence of any viral defense protein. Similarly, the replication competence of the *bet*-deleted and feA3-sensitive pCF7-BBtr FFV mutant (Table 1, [25]) was rescued by Bet and Vif. In the absence of Vif and Bet proteins, the expression of the feA3Z2b isoform strongly suppressed the titers of *bet*-deficient pCF7-BBtr (Additional file 1B). This antiviral restriction by feA3Z2b was partially or fully abrogated by co-expression of either FFV Bet or FIV Vif, respectively.

Substitution of FFV Bet by functional Vif confers FFV replication competence in feA3 expressing cells

To initially assess whether FFV Bet could be functionally replaced by FIV Vif, resulting in feA3-resistant FFV variants, *bet* sequences downstream of the essential *tas* transactivator gene (at Bet amino acid 117) in the full-length FFV clone pCF7-BetMCS (Table 1) [25, 50] were replaced by a codon-optimized FIV *vif* gene [44, 52] shown schematically and in detail in Fig. 1a and Additional file 2. Similar to other Bet fusion proteins engineered in the FFV proviral context [12, 25], an FFV protease (PR) cleavage site was introduced between the truncated N-terminus of Bet and the intact FIV *vif* gene start codon. Gene swapping did not affect FFV *tas*, and we have previously demonstrated that the N-terminal Bet sequence retained in the pCF7-Vif clones does not counteract feA3-mediated restriction of FFV replication [45]. Sequencing of resultant clones was conducted to confirm the genetic identity and correctness of the newly created clone pCF7-Vif-4 (Table 1). A spontaneous frame shift mutation arose in subclone pCF7-Vif-39 (Table 1), abrogating Bet[tr]Vif fusion protein expression completely, making this clone suitable for use as a negative control.

Plasmids pCF7-Vif-4, pCF7-Vif-39, and parental wild-type FFV full-length pCF-7 genome (Table 1) were transfected into human embryonic kidney (HEK) 293T cells. Supernatants were passaged twice on Crandell feline kidney (CrFK) cells (known to express feA3 [52]) to assess the ability of the chimeras to replicate in feline-origin cells. The full-length Bet[tr]Vif fusion protein and the mature Vif processing products were stably expressed by clone pCF7-Vif-4 which was, as expected, not the

Table 1 Viral clones and stocks used in this study

Clones	Viral stock name[a]	Major mutation	Effect on replication (CrFK)
pCF-7 [25]	Wild-type FFV[b]	–	–
pCF7-BBtr	FFV-BBtr	Truncation at Bet amino acid 117	Fully susceptible towards feA3-mediated restriction in vitro
pCF7-BetMCS [50]	FFV-BetMCS	Insertion and replacement of Bet residues at amino acid 117 by insertion of a multiple cloning site	Fully susceptible towards feA3-mediated restriction in vitro
pCF7-Vif-4	FFV-Vif-4	Engineered Bet-Vif fusion protein	Partially susceptible towards feA3-mediated restriction in vitro
pCF7-Vif-39	FFV-Vif-39	Spontaneous frameshift	Fully susceptible towards feA3-mediated restriction in vitro
pCF7-Vif W/*1	FFV-Vif W/*1[b]	Trp to Stop mutation (TGG to TGA), unlinked vif gene	Enhanced, compared to pCF7-Vif-4
pCF7-Vif W/*2	FFV-Vif W/*2	Trp to Stop mutation (TGGG to TAGA), unlinked vif gene	Enhanced, compared to pCF7-Vif-4
pCF7-Vif W/*1 M+	–	Optimized upstream Met codon in pCF7-Vif W/*1	Similar to pCF7-Vif W/*1
pCF7-Vif W/*2 M+	–	Optimized upstream Met codon in pCF7-Vif W/*2	Similar to pCF7-Vif W/*2
pCF7-Vif W/*1 M/T	–	Upstream Met codon mutated to Thr in pCF7-Vif W/*1	Similar to pCF7-Vif W/*1
pCF7-Vif W/*2 M/T	–	Upstream Met codon mutated to Thr in pCF7-Vif W/*2	Similar to pCF7-Vif W/*2

[a] FFV-Vif variants collectively referred to as "FFV Vif chimeras"

[b] Viral stocks used in domestic cat infection experiments

case for the frame shift mutant pCF7-Vif-39 (Fig. 1b, top panel). FFV Bet was only expressed by the wild-type pCF-7 genome upon transfection and serial passages (Fig. 1b, middle panel). Similar amounts of full-length FFV p52^{Gag} and the processed p48^{Gag} were synthesized by pCF7-Vif-4 and wild-type pCF-7 in transfected HEK 293T and infected CrFK cells while in clone pCF7-Vif-39, Gag expression was almost lost at the second CrFK cell passage (Fig. 1b, bottom panel). The loss of Gag expression of clone pCF7-Vif-39 was paralleled by a very rapid decline of infectivity (Fig. 2a). In contrast, titers of pCF-7 were higher than those of pCF7-Vif-4 and none of them showed a sharp decline of viral infectivity. These data indicate that intact FIV vif-chimeric pCF7-Vif-4 is replication-competent in feA3-positive CrFK cells, albeit at lower efficiency than wild-type FFV (Fig. 2a).

Passage through CrFK enhances FFV-Vif chimera replication efficiency

We continued passaging progeny of wild-type pCF-7 and chimeric pCF7-Vif-4 (see above, Fig. 2a) for 20 passages in order to use in vitro selection and evolution to obtain FFV-Vif variants with higher replication capacity in the presence of the feA3 proteins endogenously expressed in CrFK cells [34]. During the first seven passages, wild-type pCF-7 displayed titers between 10^6 and 10^7 focus-forming units per ml (FFU/ml) (Fig. 2a). During this phase, infectivity of the chimeric clone pCF7-Vif-4 was approximately one to two logs lower (10^4–10^6 FFU/ml). Starting at passage eight, however, titers of pCF7-Vif-4

progeny approached that of wild-type pCF-7, indicating emergence of pCF7-Vif variants with enhanced replicative ability in vitro (Fig. 2a). Selected samples harvested during CrFK passaging were analyzed for FFV Gag and Vif expression (Fig. 2b). FFV Gag expression was consistently detectable in all cell lysates using FFV reference serum from cat 8014 (Fig. 2b, middle panel). Early, during viral passages 2 and 5, the Bet^{tr}Vif fusion protein and its proteolytic cleavage products were the primary Vif-reactive proteins detectable. At passage 10, Bet^{tr}Vif became undetectable and the Vif protein of approximately 25 kDa was detected, along with additional Vif-reactive bands of higher molecular mass. At passage 15, mostly Vif proteins in the 25 kDa size range were identified (Fig. 2b, top panel).

To detect potential adaptive genetic changes in the FFV genome, DNA was prepared from FFV-Vif-4-infected CrFK cells at passage 18 and used as template for PCR to amplify and clone the complete bet^{tr}vif region. In seven of nine amplicons, a tryptophan codon (TGG, Trp) located in the bet sequence 50 codons upstream of the vif ORF had mutated to become TAG and TGA stop codons (Fig. 2c and Additional file 2). These changes were transitions of either the first or second G residue to an A (Fig. 2c, top panel) yielding two different stop codons, indicated by an asterisk (*), as either a TGA (five out of seven sequences, designated W/*1) or a TAG stop codon (two out of seven sequences, designated W/*2). In the five clones that had incorporated the TGA stop codon in the bet sequence, a G172R mutation in the overlapping

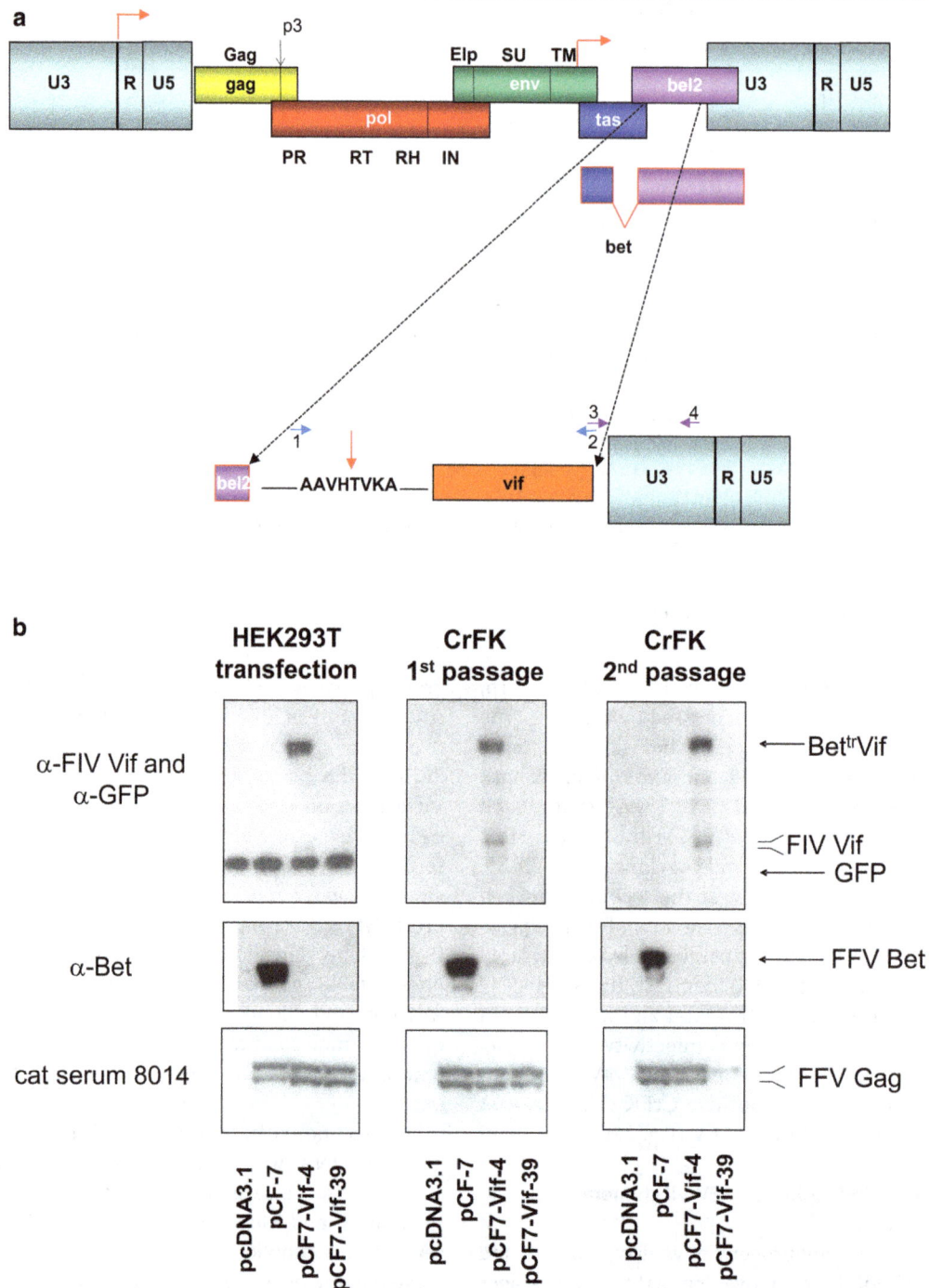

Fig. 1 Schematic presentation of the construction of FFV-Vif chimeras and their molecular features. **a** Schematic presentation of the FFV genome with its genes and protein domains as well as the LTR and internal promoters (red bent arrows, top) and presentation of the engineered Bet^trVif fusion protein (bottom). The non-functional N-terminus of *bet* (purple) was fused in-frame to the codon-optimized FIV *vif* gene including the *vif* ATG start codon. A short linker encompassing the FFV PR cleavage site (vertical red arrow, bottom) was inserted between the N-terminus of Bet and Vif. Primer pairs used to insert the *vif* gene into the FFV genome are shown in blue and violet and with numbering in the bottom panel. **b** HEK 293T were transfected with wild-type pCF-7, functional clone pCF7-Vif-4, non-functional clone pCF7-Vif-39, and pcDNA3.1 control DNA. Two days after transfection, cell culture supernatants and cells were harvested as described in the "Methods" section. Cleared supernatants were used for serial passaging in feA3-expressing CrFK cells and FFV titer determination (Fig. 2a). At 3 days p.i., infected CrFK cells and supernatants were harvested and used as above. Cell lysates from transfected HEK 293T cells and CrFK cells after the first and second passage were subjected to immunoblotting against FIV Vif and co-transfected GFP, FFV Bet, and FFV Gag (cat serum 8014). The positions and names of the detected proteins are given at the right margin

Tas-coding sequence occurred. In the two TGG to TAG mutants, a G residue following the TGG codon was also changed to A (i.e. TGGG was altered to TAGA). This resulted in a G172L exchange in Tas and a D/N change directly downstream of the new *bet* stop codon. All nucleotide exchanges correspond to C/T exchanges of the antisense strand in a sequence context PyPyC (Fig. 2c; Py = pyrimidine residue), corresponding to the canonical A3 mutation context in retroviral genomes [34, 53]. Additional genetic changes were not consistently detected in the *bet^tr vif* region.

Unlinking *vif* from *bet* by Trp/stop mutagenesis is essential for increased infectivity

The importance of the identified Trp/stop (W/*) mutations upstream of the *vif* sequence was analyzed using reverse genetics. Both W/* mutations in the *bel2* linker sequence upstream of *vif* were inserted into the original pCF7-Vif-4 to determine whether they represent adaptive mutations increasing the titer of the corresponding FFV-Vif chimera. These clones were named pCF7-Vif W/*1 (TGG/TGA) and pCF7-Vif W/*2 (TGG/TAG, Table 1).

An additional outcome of the W/* mutations was the "emergence" of an in-frame ATG codon between the new W/* stop codon and the authentic *vif* start codon (Additional file 2). To test whether this ATG codon could serve as an alternative translational initiation codon for the inserted *vif* gene, this Met ATG was replaced in the engineered pCF7-Vif W/*1 and -W/*2 clones and the parental pCF7-Vif-4 clone by a threonine (Thr) codon (suffix M/T, see Fig. 2c lower panel and Table 1). In addition, and as a complementing strategy, the surrounding nucleotide sequence of this ATG codon was converted to an optimal Kozak translational initiation context sequence (GCCA/GCCATGG, start codon underlined, [54]) as shown in Fig. 2c, lower panels. The corresponding clones are labeled by the suffix M + (Table 1). The M/T mutation resulted in a silent mutation at the *tas* C-terminus while the change to a Kozak sequence resulted in two amino acid exchanges in *tas* at the C-terminus, i.e. D206H

and A208G, and, in addition, a leucine to phenylalanine (L/F) exchange upstream, and a leucine to valine (L/V) exchange directly downstream of the potential Met start codon in the linker sequence (see Fig. 2c).

Transient co-transfection studies using a luc FFV LTR reporter construct together with either a CMV-IE promoter-driven Tas expression clone and a CMV-IE-driven β-gal plasmid or the FFV genomes pCF-7, pCF7-Vif-4, pCF7-Vif W/*1, and the different M/T and M + derivatives thereof were conducted. While the CMV-IE promoter-driven Tas expression clone yielded very high luc activities, the genomic wild-type and chimeric proviral FFV clones described above did not show significant differences in Tas transactivation, indicating that the mutations introduced do not significantly influence overall transactivation and gene expression (Additional file 3).

Clones pCF7-Vif W/*1 and -W/*2 and the different M/T and M + derivatives were transfected into HEK 293T cells and supernatants were tested for the replication competence of the FFV-Vif chimera in feA3-positive CrFK cells by serial CrFK cell passaging as described above. Serial passaging after either 60 or 84 h (Additional file 4A and 4B) showed similar outcomes: the pCF-7-encoded wild-type FFV had slightly higher titers (about fivefold) than mutants pCF7-Vif W/*1 and -W/*2 and their derivatives. For these clones and the corresponding M/T and M + clones, titers were stable during serial passages. This was not the case for the original pCF7-Vif-4 clone encoding the Bet^tr Vif fusion protein, where titers steadily and reproducibly declined upon serial passages in several independent experiments. The data show that both W/* mutations in the FFV *bet* sequence upstream of the *vif* gene cause in feA3-expressing CrFK cells a clear increase of replication competence compared to the pCF-Vif-4 encoding the Bet^tr Vif fusion protein. However, the replication competence of the pCF7-Vif W/*1 and -W/*2 clones was slightly lower than that of the wild-type FFV genome pCF-7. In addition, the FFV-encoded, in-frame ATG codon located 14 codons upstream of *vif* is probably not used as a start codon for Vif protein expression

(See figure on next page.)

Fig. 2 In vitro selection and molecular characterization of pCF7-Vif-4 variants with increased replication competence. Plasmids pCF7-Vif-4, -39, and pCF-7 were transfected into HEK 293T cells. Two days after transfection, cell-free supernatants were inoculated on CrFK cells and serially passaged twice a week on CrFK cells (every 3 or 4 days) as described above for Fig. 1b. **a** FFV titers were determined in duplicate using FeFAB reporter cells and are shown as bar diagram for selected passages over time. Error bars represent the standard deviation. **b** Selected cell extracts from the CrFK passages were subjected to immunoblotting. The immune-detection with a Vif-specific antiserum initially showed mainly the engineered Bet^tr Vif and the proteolytically released Vif, then various unidentified Vif variants, and finally (passages 10 and 15) predominantly the authentic Vif protein. FFV Gag proteins were detected in all samples as expected using cat antiserum 8014 while in the bottom panel the β-actin loading control is shown. **c** Sequence context of the in vitro-selected W/* mutations (light blue original Trp to the stop codon in red) suggests feA3 editing of the minus strand of FF7-Vif-4-derived reverse transcription intermediates in the PyPyC sequence context (top panel, Py = pyrimidine residue). Below, mutagenesis of the in-frame ATG 14 codons upstream of the *vif* gene is shown only for the sense strand (bottom panel). The ATG start codon is shown in light blue and the engineered residues and changes amino acids are in red

a

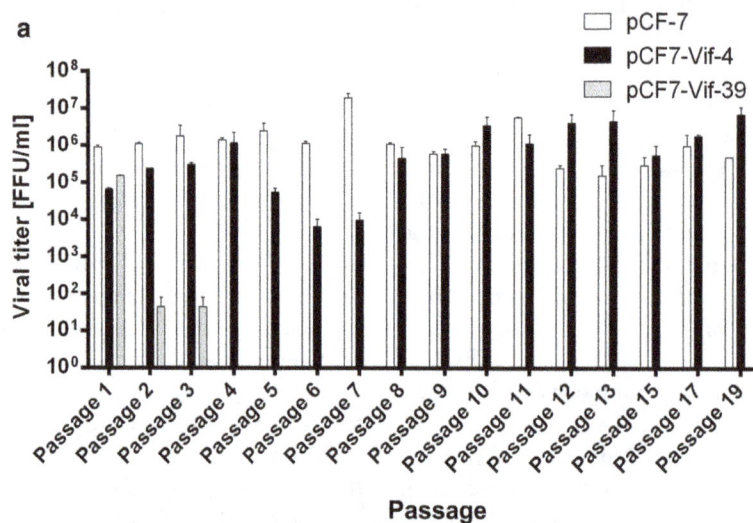

b

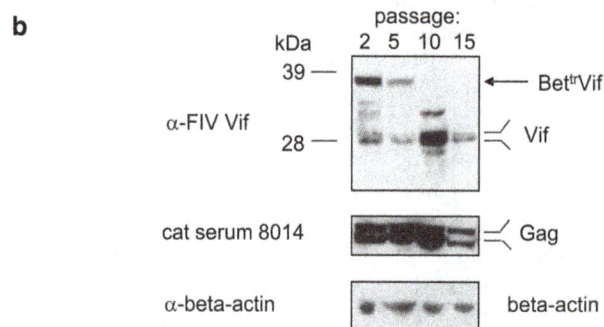

c   *in vitro* **selected FFV-Vif4 variants**

```
5'-GCT TGG GAC-3'              wild-type
3'-CGA ACC CTG-5'
   AlaTrpAsp
```

```
5'-GCT TAGAC-3'                W/*1 exchange, 5/7 clones
3'-CGA TCTC-5'
   Ala***Asp
```

```
5'-GCT A AAC-3'                W/*2 exchange, 2/7 clones
3'-CGA T TTG-5'
   Ala***Asn
```

mutagenesis of the potential upstream ATG start codon

```
5'-TTGACT ATG CTA-3'           wild-type
   LeuThrMetLeu
```

```
5'-TTGACT C CTA-3'             M-T mutation
   LeuThrThrLeu
```

```
5'-TTCACT ATG GTA-3'           M* mutation
   PheThrMetVal
```

since its replacement by a Thr codon, or the optimization of the surrounding residues towards more efficient translational initiation, did not significantly affect viral titers.

Reduced steady state levels of feA3Z2b by FFV-Vif chimeric clones pCF-Vif-4 and pCF7-Vif W/*1 and -W/*2

Co-transfection experiments were conducted to study whether the steady state levels of feA3Z2b are decreased by Bet^{tr}Vif fusion protein or the authentic Vif encoded by FFV-Vif chimeric clones pCF-Vif-4 or pCF7-Vif W/*1 and -W/*2, respectively (Table 1). As indicated in Fig. 3 (bottom panel), parental wild-type FFV full-length pCF-7 genome and FFV-Vif chimeric clones pCF-Vif-4, pCF7-Vif W/*1, and -W/*2 were transfected into HEK 293T cells together with a plasmid encoding HA-tagged feA3Z2b (the major feA3 restriction factor of Bet-deficient FFV) [33, 34]. Cells transfected with the plasmid encoding feA3Z2b and pcDNA as well as pcDNA-only-transfected HEK 293T cells served as controls. Cellular antigens were harvested two d after transfection

and subjected to immunoblotting (Fig. 3). The control blots conducted confirm proper loading of samples (anti β-actin, bottom panel) and comparable expression of FFV proteins in wild-type and chimeric FFV provirus-transfected samples and Bet^{tr}Vif fusion proteins and FIV Vif by FFV-Vif chimeric clones pCF-Vif-4 and pCF7-Vif W/*1 and -W/*2, respively (anti FFV Gag and anti FIV Vif, middle panels). As expected and previously shown [33, 34], the steady-state levels of HA-tagged feA3Z2b were not significantly affected by co-expression of wild-type FFV expressing Bet (anti HA, top panel, compare lanes 2 to 3 and 8 to 9). In stark contrast, levels of HA-tagged feA3Z2b were reproducibly and strongly reduced in cells expressing either Bet^{tr}Vif and/or authentic FIV Vif (compare lane 2 to 4, 5, and 6 and lane 8 to 10, 11, and 12 in Fig. 3, top panel). In another and independent experiment with a highly similar outcome, only co-transfection of CMV-IE promoter-based and codon-optimized FIV Vif expression plasmids reduced feA3Z2b to undetectable levels (data not shown). In summary, the data clearly

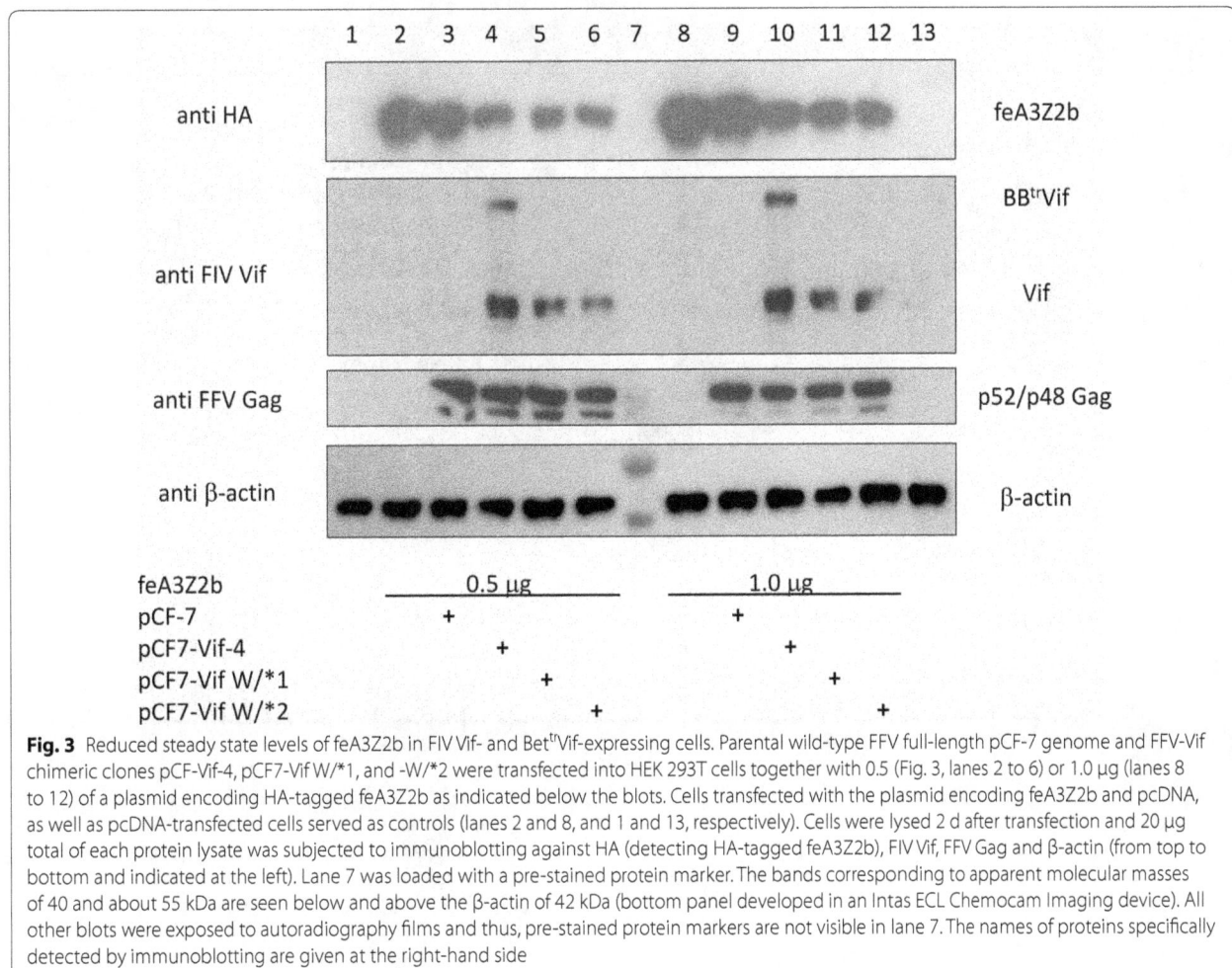

Fig. 3 Reduced steady state levels of feA3Z2b in FIV Vif- and Bet^{tr}Vif-expressing cells. Parental wild-type FFV full-length pCF-7 genome and FFV-Vif chimeric clones pCF-Vif-4, pCF7-Vif W/*1, and -W/*2 were transfected into HEK 293T cells together with 0.5 (Fig. 3, lanes 2 to 6) or 1.0 µg (lanes 8 to 12) of a plasmid encoding HA-tagged feA3Z2b as indicated below the blots. Cells transfected with the plasmid encoding feA3Z2b and pcDNA, as well as pcDNA-transfected cells served as controls (lanes 2 and 8, and 1 and 13, respectively). Cells were lysed 2 d after transfection and 20 µg total of each protein lysate was subjected to immunoblotting against HA (detecting HA-tagged feA3Z2b), FIV Vif, FFV Gag and β-actin (from top to bottom and indicated at the left). Lane 7 was loaded with a pre-stained protein marker. The bands corresponding to apparent molecular masses of 40 and about 55 kDa are seen below and above the β-actin of 42 kDa (bottom panel developed in an Intas ECL Chemocam Imaging device). All other blots were exposed to autoradiography films and thus, pre-stained protein markers are not visible in lane 7. The names of proteins specifically detected by immunoblotting are given at the right-hand side

support the conclusion that the Vif protein in the FFV-Vif chimeric clones leads to decreased steady state levels of feA3Z2b, most probably via proteasomal degradation [33, 44, 46, 47, 52].

Experimental infection of cats with chimeric virus FFV-Vif W/*1

To investigate whether the FFV-Vif chimera with the Bet-independent expression of Vif is replication-competent and immunogenic in cats, we performed inoculation experiments with FFV-Vif W/*1 (Table 1). This clone was selected for in vivo infection studies since it is the major variant detected in our in vitro experiments and is caused by only a single nucleotide exchange from the original engineered pCF7-Vif-4 chimera. Cats were separated into naïve (N), wild-type (WT), or chimeric (CH) groups based on inoculum type. The timeline of inoculations, sample collections, and final necropsy are shown in Fig. 4. None of the cats displayed signs of clinical illness or hematologic changes indicative of disease throughout the duration of the study.

Wild-type inoculated cats exhibited persistent FFV DNA proviral loads in PBMC in contrast to chimera-inoculated cats

To compare viral load and kinetics between inoculation groups, we evaluated the presence of FFV proviral DNA in PBMC over time (Figs. 4, 5). Naïve control cats remained absolutely PCR-negative at all time points tested (Additional file 5). Cats in the WT group developed a persistent PBMC proviral load as early as 21 days post-infection (p.i.) (Figs. 5a, 6), while indeterminate PCR reactions were detected earlier (Fig. 5a and Additional file 5). By day 42 p.i., all WT cats were PCR positive and positivity was consistently detected throughout the rest of the study (Fig. 5a). Cat WT3 (subsequently also referred to as "outlier") had a PBMC FFV DNA pattern that differed from the rest of the WT cohort (Fig. 6). This animal was not PCR-positive until day 42 (vs. day 21 as in its cohort-mates). Throughout the rest of the study, the outlier cat's overall viral load was however much higher (highest at 5920 viral copies/10^6 cells on day 142 p.i.) than the other WT cats (WT2 had the highest viral load at 1230 viral copies/10^6 cells on day 28 p.i.) (Fig. 6).

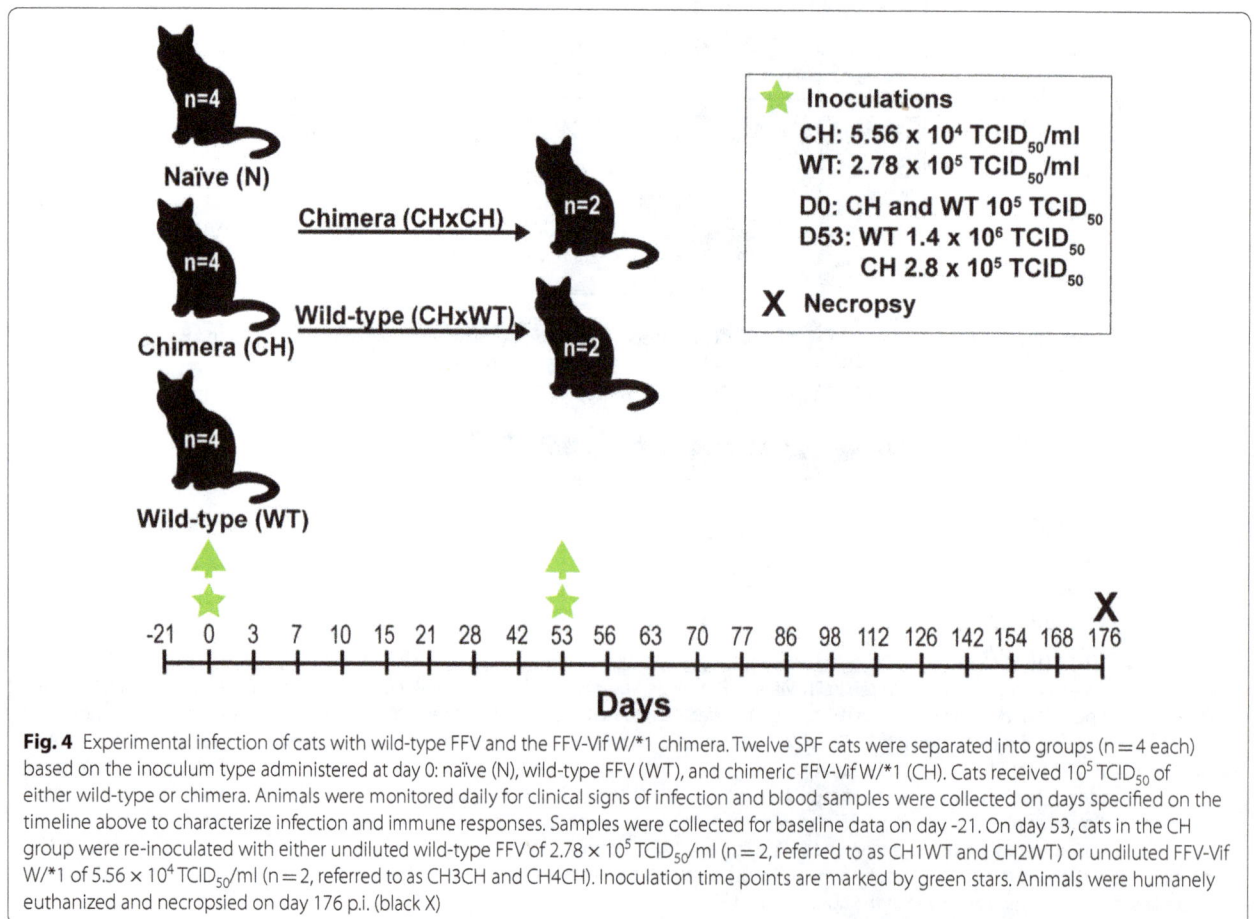

Fig. 4 Experimental infection of cats with wild-type FFV and the FFV-Vif W/*1 chimera. Twelve SPF cats were separated into groups (n=4 each) based on the inoculum type administered at day 0: naïve (N), wild-type FFV (WT), and chimeric FFV-Vif W/*1 (CH). Cats received 10^5 TCID$_{50}$ of either wild-type or chimera. Animals were monitored daily for clinical signs of infection and blood samples were collected on days specified on the timeline above to characterize infection and immune responses. Samples were collected for baseline data on day -21. On day 53, cats in the CH group were re-inoculated with either undiluted wild-type FFV of 2.78 × 10^5 TCID$_{50}$/ml (n=2, referred to as CH1WT and CH2WT) or undiluted FFV-Vif W/*1 of 5.56 × 10^4 TCID$_{50}$/ml (n=2, referred to as CH3CH and CH4CH). Inoculation time points are marked by green stars. Animals were humanely euthanized and necropsied on day 176 p.i. (black X)

a

WT	Day	-21	0	3	7	10	15	21	28	42	56	70	86	112	142	168
	PCR															
	Nested						▽○□△	▼●□▲	▼●○▲	▼●■▲				▼●■▲		
	qPCR	▽○□△	▽○□△	▽●□△	▽○□△	▽●□△	▼●■▲	▼●□▲	▼●■▲	▼●■▲	▼●■▲	▼●■▲	▼●■▲	▼●■▲	▼●■▲	▼●■▲
	ELISA															
	Gag	▽○□△					▽○□△	▼●■△	▼●■▲	▼●■▲	▼●■▲		■		■▲	▼●■▲
	Bet	▽○□△					▽○□△	▽○□△	▽●□△	▼●■▲	▼●■▲		■		■▲	▼●■▲

b

CH	Day	-21	0	3	7	10	15	21	28	42
	PCR									
	Nested						▽○□△	▽○□△	▽○□△	▽○□△
	qPCR	▽○□△	▽○□△	▽●□△	▽○□△	▽○□△	▽●□△	▽●■▲	▽●□▲	▽○■△
	ELISA									
	Gag	▽○□△					▼○□△	▼●□▲	▼●■▲	▼●■▲
	Bet	▽○□△					▽○□△	▽○□△	▽○□△	▽○□△
	Vif						▼●■△	▼●■△	▼●■△	▼●■△

Cat	Negative	Positive	Indeterminate
1	▽	▼	▾
2	○	●	◦
3	□	■	▪
4	△	▲	▴

c

CHxWT	Day	63	70	77	86	98	112	126	142	154	168
	PCR										
	Nested		▽○	▽●		▽	▽	▽		▽●	▽●
	qPCR	▽●	▽○	▼●	▽●	▼●	▽●	▽	▽●	▽●	▽●
	ELISA										
	Gag		▼●	▼●	▼●	▼●	▼●		●	●	▼●
	Bet		▽○	▽○	▽●	▼●	▼●		●	●	▼●
	Vif	▼●			▼●		▼●	▼●			▼●

d

CHxCH	Day	63	70	77	86	98	112	126	142	154	168
	PCR										
	Nested		□△	□△		□△	□△	□△		□△	□△
	qPCR	□△	□△	□△	□▲	□▲	□▲	□△	■▲	□△	□△
	ELISA										
	Gag		■▲						■		■▲
	Bet		□△						□		□△
	Vif	■▲			■△		■△	■△			■▲

Fig. 5 Results of PCR and ELISA assays over the entire study period. Summary of real time quantitative and nested PCR (qPCR and nPCR, respectively) on PBMCs and ELISAs for FFV Gag and Bet and FIV Vif performed before and following inoculation as given in the panels. The same symbols were used for cats 1–4 in WT and CH groups. Only the cats for which symbols are present (see inserted legend) were tested at the corresponding time point. Gray boxes represent time points where animals were not tested. CH-group cats were re-inoculated on day 53 (not shown) as described in "Methods". **a** WT group results (days -21 to 168 p.i.). **b** CH group results (days -21 to 42 p.i.). **c** CH×WT group results (days 63 to 168 p.i.). **d** CH×CH group results (days 63 to 168 p.i.)

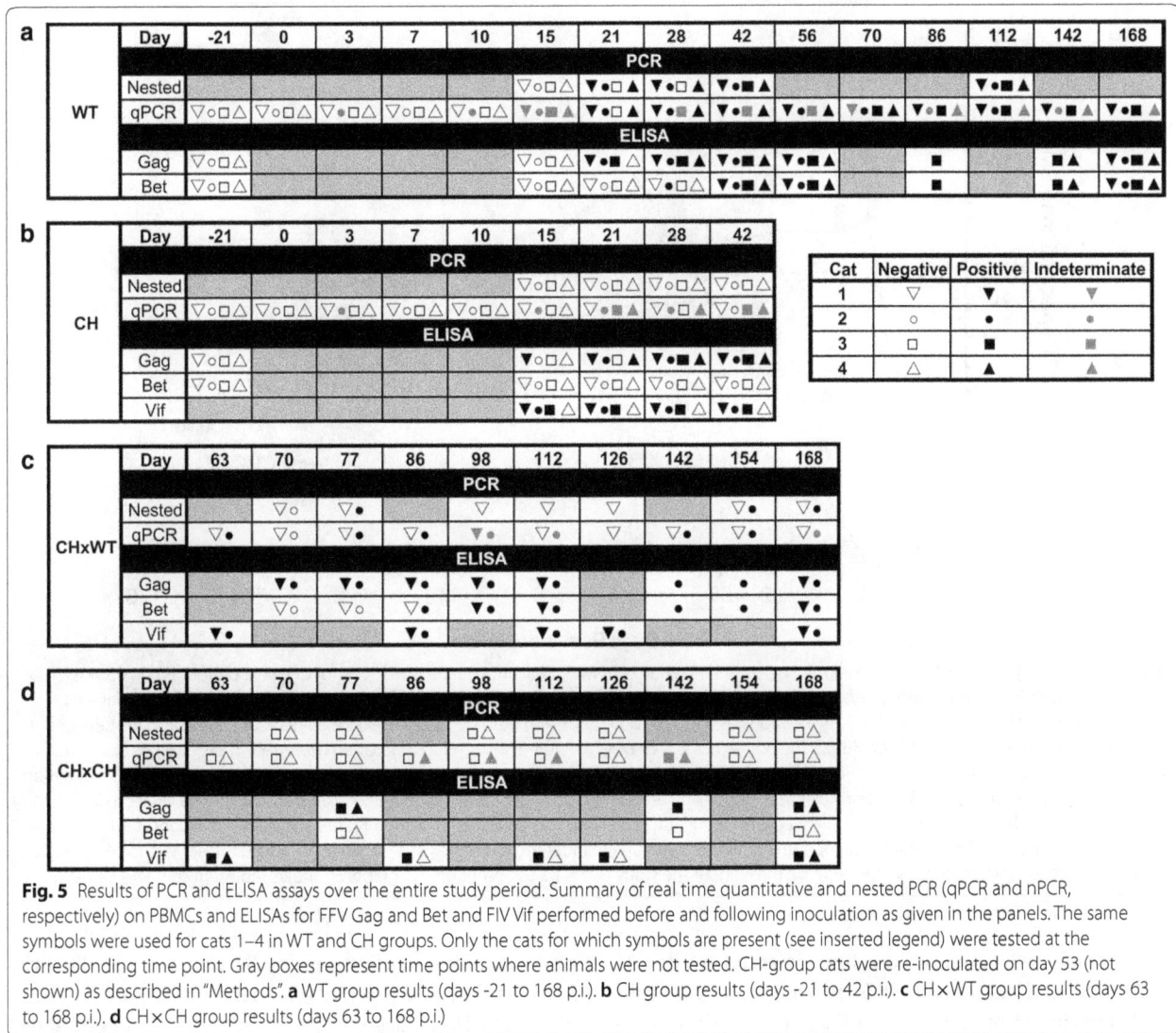

Three out of four cats inoculated with only FFV-Vif chimeric virus (CH group) showed indeterminate results for FFV PBMC provirus DNA by qPCR analysis at some of the time points tested prior to re-inoculation on day 53 p.i. (Fig. 5b and Additional file 5). One of the chimera-inoculated cats re-inoculated on day 53 with wild-type virus (cat CH2WT) demonstrated FFV proviral DNA in PBMC 24 d post re-inoculation, while the other cat in this cohort remained indeterminate or negative throughout the study (Fig. 5c). The highest viral load recorded for cat CH2WT was 656 viral copies/10^6 cells 24 days post re-inoculation (Fig. 6). Both cats re-exposed to the FFV-Vif chimera displayed repeated indeterminate PCR results in blood before and after superinfection (Fig. 5b, d).

Gag-specific immune reactivity in infected animals confirms replication competence of wild-type FFV and FFV-Vif chimera

All FFV-infected cats strongly seroconverted against Gag while all naïve control animals were negative (Additional file 6, reactivity at 1:50 dilution). In order to determine the kinetics and strength of anti-Gag reactivity, selected serum samples from wild-type FFV and FFV-Vif-infected animals were analyzed before and after superinfection (only cats in the CH group received a second inoculation, Fig. 7a, b). Wild-type FFV-infected cats had detectable specific anti-Gag antibody responses as early as 21 or 28 days p.i. (Fig. 5a and Additional file 5). Antibody levels for these cats continued to increase to final titers between 500 and 2500 (Fig. 7a). FFV Gag antibodies of

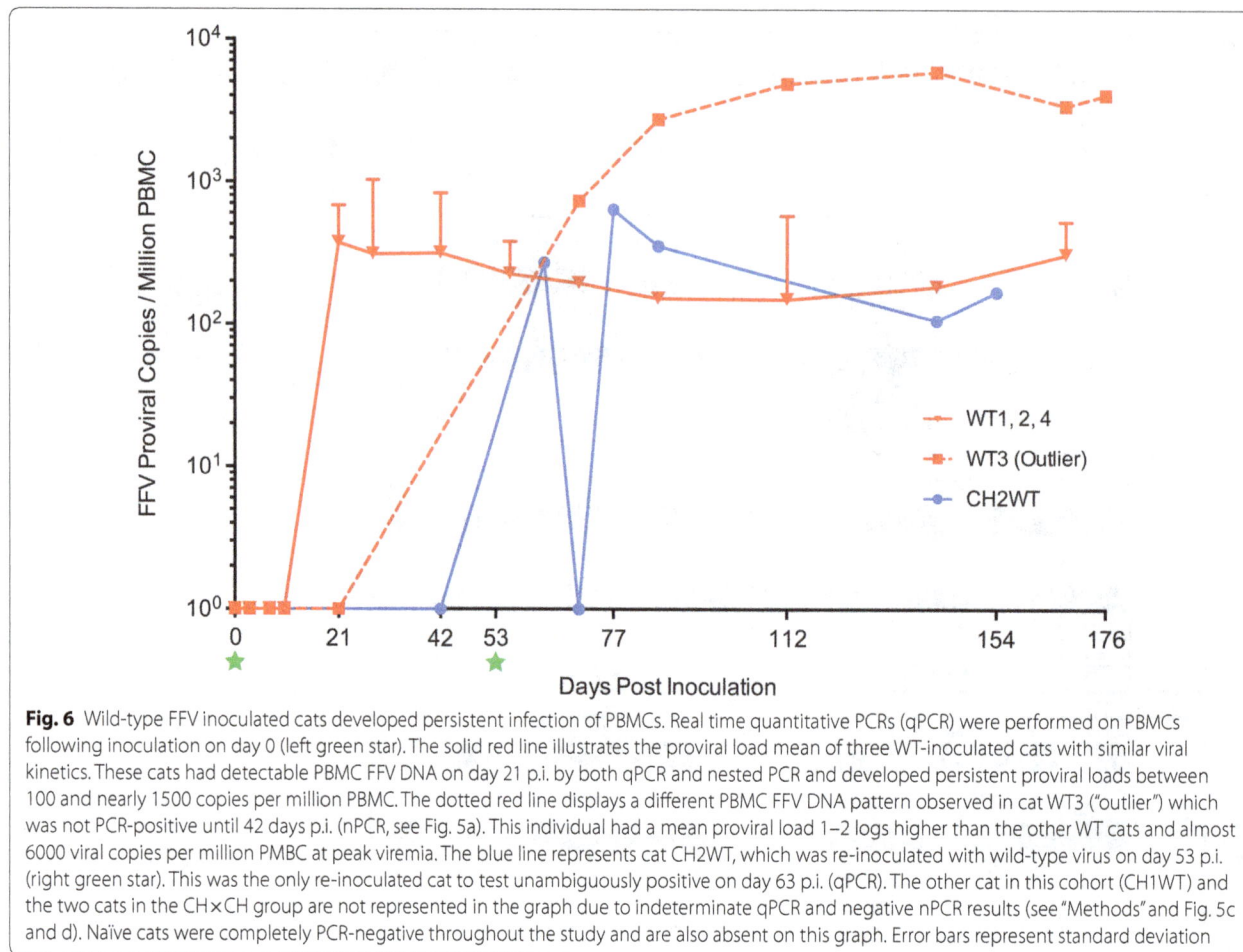

Fig. 6 Wild-type FFV inoculated cats developed persistent infection of PBMCs. Real time quantitative PCRs (qPCR) were performed on PBMCs following inoculation on day 0 (left green star). The solid red line illustrates the proviral load mean of three WT-inoculated cats with similar viral kinetics. These cats had detectable PBMC FFV DNA on day 21 p.i. by both qPCR and nested PCR and developed persistent proviral loads between 100 and nearly 1500 copies per million PBMC. The dotted red line displays a different PBMC FFV DNA pattern observed in cat WT3 ("outlier") which was not PCR-positive until 42 days p.i. (nPCR, see Fig. 5a). This individual had a mean proviral load 1–2 logs higher than the other WT cats and almost 6000 viral copies per million PMBC at peak viremia. The blue line represents cat CH2WT, which was re-inoculated with wild-type virus on day 53 p.i. (right green star). This was the only re-inoculated cat to test unambiguously positive on day 63 p.i. (qPCR). The other cat in this cohort (CH1WT) and the two cats in the CH×CH group are not represented in the graph due to indeterminate qPCR and negative nPCR results (see "Methods" and Fig. 5c and d). Naïve cats were completely PCR-negative throughout the study and are also absent on this graph. Error bars represent standard deviation

FFV-Vif-infected animals were first detected by day 15 p.i. (Fig. 5b and Additional file 5) and increased gradually until superinfection, after which Gag-specific titers were attained that were equivalent to wild-type-infected cats (Fig. 7a, b). Anti-Gag reactivity was detected in all four CH group cats at approximately the same seroconversion rate as wild-type FFV-infected cats, though titers tended to be lower prior to re-exposure in the CH group (Fig. 7b and Additional file 5).

Infected cats seroconverted against accessory FFV Bet and FIV Vif proteins

All cats infected with wild-type FFV only (WT 1–4) or FFV-Vif plus wild-type FFV (CH1WT and CH2WT) demonstrated substantial FFV Bet sero-reactivity by day 168 p.i. (Figs. 5a, c, 8a, and Additional file 5). As observed in previous studies [12, 21], Bet-specific antibodies appeared slightly later than Gag sero-reactivity (Fig. 5 and Additional file 5). Naïve controls and cats CH3CH and CH4CH were Bet-antibody negative as expected. Most importantly, Vif reactivity in three out of four FFV-Vif-infected animals was clearly positive at day 42 p.i.,

prior to superinfection on day 53 p.i. (Fig. 8b). Surprisingly, Vif-specific reactivity in these animals was detectable by day 15 p.i. despite the fact that qPCR did not detect provirus (Fig. 5b and Additional file 5). Re-inoculation of these cats with either wild-type FFV (animals CH1WT, CH2WT) or FFV-Vif chimera (CH3CH) resulted in a boost in Vif sero-reactivity at day 63 p.i. Animal CH4CH, which showed no Vif reactivity prior to superinfection, exhibited only transient FIV Vif reactivity after re-exposure (Fig. 8b).

Discussion
This study describes the generation of replication-competent variants of FFV that express FIV Vif in lieu of FFV Bet. An engineered FFV genome expressing a fusion protein of a non-functional N-terminal Bet domain fused to the full-length Vif was clearly attenuated in vitro. Second-generation FFV-Vif chimeras expressing the authentic codon-optimized *vif* gene showed much higher *vif*-dependent replication competence in feA3-expressing cells, only slightly decreased in vitro compared to wild-type FFV. In experimentally infected cats, replication of

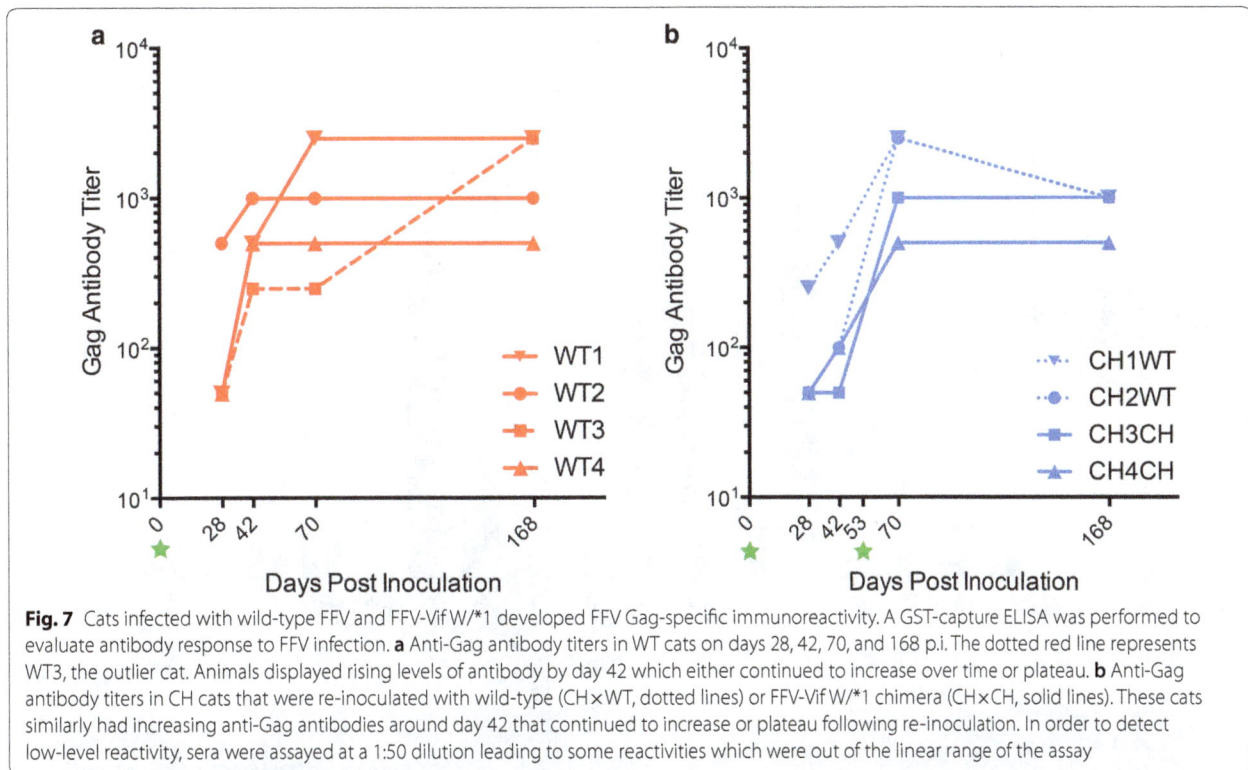

Fig. 7 Cats infected with wild-type FFV and FFV-Vif W/*1 developed FFV Gag-specific immunoreactivity. A GST-capture ELISA was performed to evaluate antibody response to FFV infection. **a** Anti-Gag antibody titers in WT cats on days 28, 42, 70, and 168 p.i. The dotted red line represents WT3, the outlier cat. Animals displayed rising levels of antibody by day 42 which either continued to increase over time or plateau. **b** Anti-Gag antibody titers in CH cats that were re-inoculated with wild-type (CH×WT, dotted lines) or FFV-Vif W/*1 chimera (CH×CH, solid lines). These cats similarly had increasing anti-Gag antibodies around day 42 that continued to increase or plateau following re-inoculation. In order to detect low-level reactivity, sera were assayed at a 1:50 dilution leading to some reactivities which were out of the linear range of the assay

the chimeric FFV-Vif variant was attenuated but led to the induction of FFV Gag-specific antibodies together with those directed against the engineered heterologous FIV Vif protein. Importantly, cats infected with the FFV-Vif chimera could be superinfected with wild-type FFV or the chimera, in both cases resulting in a strong immunological boost of sero-reactivity against FFV and FIV Vif.

The successful replacement of FFV *bet* by FIV *vif* in the context of the FFV genome may have been aided by two mechanisms. First, a codon-optimized and thus Rev-independent FIV *vif* gene was inserted, allowing for efficient translation of the Vif protein [32]. Second, LV Vif proteins function as catalytic regulators of proteasomal feA3 degradation; therefore, much lower amounts of fully functional Vif may be required to inactivate A3 activity compared to FV Bet, which acts stoichiometrically via direct binding to the feA3 protein [33]. Thus, the attenuated replication of the initially constructed pCF7-Vif-4 chimera was likely due to high expression levels of the functionally impaired Bet^{tr}Vif fusion protein.

In support of the hypothesis that Bet and Vif are differentially expressed in vivo, Bet sero-reactivity is high and has diagnostic value in infected cats and bovines [55, 56]. In contrast, while anti-Vif antibodies have been described in HIV patients [57, 58], Vif has not been shown to be a major humoral immune target of FIV infection, and

seroconversion against Vif has not been well studied in FIV infection (personal communication, Dr. Chris Grant).

Apparently, inhibitory effects of either the complete N-terminal part of Bet plus the linker sequence, or the N-terminal residues of the linker residues present downstream of the engineered FFV PR cleavage site (see Fig. 1a) favored the emergence of Trp/stop (W/*) variants. This is strongly suggested by the fact that two independent, yet highly related mutational events led to the W/* mutation in the linker sequence upstream of *vif*. The reverse genetic experiments conducted do not support translational initiation at the upstream Met residue located in the linker sequence as important for Vif protein expression. We thus assume that in the in vitro-selected clones, fully functional Vif is expressed from its authentic start codon, though the exact mechanism by which FIV Vif protein is expressed from pCF7-Vif W/*1 and pCF7-Vif W/*2 is unknown. We assume that internal re-initiation of protein biosynthesis may be involved, but other mechanisms cannot be excluded. While the mechanism of Vif expression of clones pCF7-Vif W/*1 and pCF7-Vif W/*2 is unknown, all FIV Vif proteins engineered into the FFV genome including the first-generation clone pCF7-Vif-4 encoding the Bet^{tr}Vif fusion protein lead to dramatically reduced steady state levels of

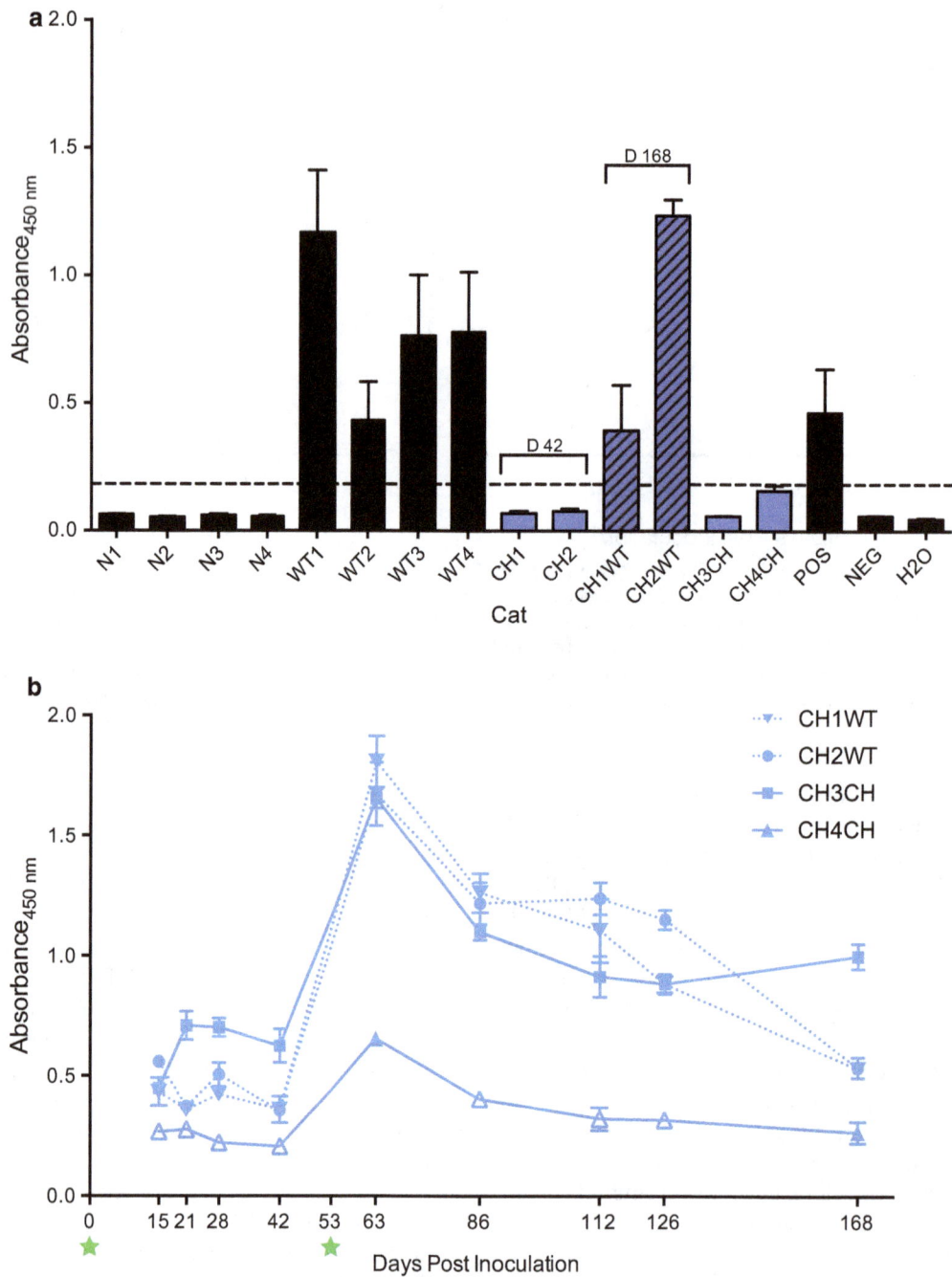

Fig. 8 Animals inoculated with wild-type FFV or FFV-Vif chimera seroconverted to FFV Bet or FIV Vif. Antibody response against FFV Bet and FIV Vif antigens were measured by antibody capture ELISAs as described in the "Methods" section. **a** Anti-Bet antigen reactivity for each animal at final time points unless specified. WT cats (red bars), and cats that received chimera and then wild-type FFV (CH×WT, black and blue striped bars) seroconverted against Bet. Animals exposed to only FFV-Vif W/*1 (cats CH1 and CH2 prior to day 53, and CH3CH and CH4CH, solid blue bars) were negative for anti-Bet antibodies as expected. Black bars show naïve cats, and positive and negative control samples. **b** Three out of 4 animals inoculated with chimeric virus developed a detectable anti-Vif immune response as early as 15 days p.i. Antibody response increased following re-inoculation for all animals, causing a detectable response in the fourth animal (CH4CH), though sero-reactivity was low compared to other animals for this individual, and only rose above positive cutoff absorbance on days 63 and 168. Filled shapes indicate positive ELISA absorbance values compared to negative controls (> 2 standard deviation above the mean of duplicate negative samples), whereas open triangles for CH4CH indicate ELISA absorbance values below positive cutoff. Values reported represent mean of duplicate samples and bars indicate standard deviation

feA3 proteins as shown for the major restriction factor of FFV, feA3Z2b (see Fig. 3).

In line with the assumption that the original Bet^{tr}Vif fusion protein conferred suboptimal protection against feA3 restriction, both mutations leading to the adaptive W/* mutations occurred in a sequence context of the negative strand that is indicative of feA3 editing, suggesting the chimeric viruses did not confer robust protection against feA3. Both mutated C residues of the negative strand are preceded by C residues in the sequence 5'-TCCC-3' (deaminated C residues in bold face letters, see also Fig. 2c), and therefore should function as optimal feA3 substrates, however, alternative mutational pathways might have also played a role. The fact that suboptimal feA3 inhibition leads to adaptive changes induced by feA3 DNA deamination supports our proposed concept that the heterologous and functionally relevant transgene FIV *vif* is essential for efficient propagation of the replicating virus, and thus confers a strong selective advantage by protecting against feA3 restriction. Consequently, the transgene *vif* has to be stably maintained in the absence of *bet* during serial passages, as demonstrated in Fig. 2b. The importance of the *vif* transgene for FFV-Vif replication is further underscored by the fact that additional adaptive changes, such as unlinking from N-terminal Bet sequences, were required to restore full biological activity as an inhibitor of feA3 restriction.

The advantage of adapting this replication-competent FV vector system as a vaccine delivery vehicle is that the immunogen Vif is essential for replication, and should be thus stably maintained by the engineered vector. Further, LV Vif has been shown to elicit T and B cell reactivity in HIV-infected individuals [59–63]. A corresponding PFV-based replicating vector system carrying the HIV *vif* gene may therefore be an interesting vector for the development of anti-HIV immunotherapies.

The in vivo wild-type FFV inoculations confirm that experimental infection of outbred, immunocompetent cats with clone pCF-7-derived wild-type FFV leads to a persistent infection with consistent detection of FFV proviral DNA in PBMC and a strong sero-reactivity against Gag and Bet proteins, similar to other reports [12, 21]. In contrast, animals inoculated with FFV-Vif W/*1 remained either proviral DNA negative or indeterminate throughout the study based on nested and qPCR analysis of PBMC DNA (Fig. 5b, d). Surprisingly, despite the inability to unambiguously detect FFV provirus in cats exposed to FFV-Vif W/*1, clear sero-reactivity against FFV Gag and heterologous Vif protein were detected after primary inoculation (Figs. 5, 7). This observation is consistent with previous studies in different FVs that serology is much more sensitive for the identification of

exposed animals than PCR-based studies using PBMC [21, 55, 64, 65].

FFV in vivo infection experiments were conducted with wild-type FFV or chimeric FFV-Vif W/*1. This resulted in detectable, but low, proviral load in wild-type-infected animals and either undetectable or indeterminate proviral loads in cats infected with the FFV-Vif chimera. It is feasible that the exchange of Bet for Vif altered tissue tropism and site of viral replication in FFV-Vif W/*1 exposed cats, and this contributed to the inability of tracking viral infection via peripheral blood PCR. While initially either negative or indeterminate based on PCR results, cat CH2WT was superinfected with wild-type FFV on day 53 p.i. and showed a productive PBMC FFV infection on a similar timeline after inoculation as the wild-type-infected animals.

The animals in the chimeric cohort did not seroconvert against Bet as anticipated but they displayed clear anti-Vif antibody responses starting at day 15 p.i., demonstrating that substituting Bet by Vif elicited specific immune responses. Given that anti-Vif antibodies have not been widely reported during FIV infection, our findings may indicate replication is occurring in cells or cell compartments where it is more easily recognized as a foreign antigen. Antibody production against Vif was initially not robust, but following re-inoculation with both wild-type and FFV-Vif chimeric virus, anti-Vif antibody response markedly increased (Fig. 8b). Following re-inoculation of the FFV-Vif-infected animals with wild-type FFV virus, both cats initially infected with FFV-Vif W/*1 also produced anti-Bet antibodies, demonstrating that infection with the chimera did not protect against subsequent infection with wild-type FFV (Figs. 5c, 8a).

The data document that, despite a lack of consistent detection of FFV provirus DNA, FFV-Vif W/*1 is able to induce persistent antibody responses in domestic cats that were boosted by re-inoculation. As noted above, we were able to document superinfection with two highly related FFV variants. Clinical evaluations following exposure to wild-type FFV or chimera suggests that FFV produces an apathogenic infection during the study period. Further studies should be conducted to understand chronic FFV infection and potential associated pathologic changes as well as the possibility of worsened pathology following superinfection with other FFV serotypes or other viral infections [66]. It would also be important to challenge wild-type FFV-infected cats with chimeric virus to determine whether infection with wild-type FFV may induce neutralizing immunity thus preventing superinfection with an attenuated FFV vaccine construct.

It cannot be ruled out that the antibody response detected in FFV chimera-infected animals was related to exposure to viral inoculum versus actively replicating virus, since PCR results were indeterminate. However, anti-Vif antibody production in three out of four FFV-Vif chimera-inoculated cats detected throughout the monitoring period, and an anti-Gag response equivalent to wild-type antibody titers is supportive of the conclusion that low-level viral replication occurred [21, 55, 64, 65]. Whether or not FFV-Vif W/*1 replicated poorly or not at all, the fact that pCF7-Vif W/*1 was highly replication-competent in CrFK cells but strongly attenuated in vivo suggests that Bet may play a currently unknown critical role in viral replication competence in vivo in addition to antagonizing A3-mediated restriction. Here, inactivation of other components of the host's innate or intrinsic immunity as well as an essential co-factorial role for the replication in specific cell types in vivo are plausible reasons for the attenuated phenotype. Alternatively, other aspects of the manipulated pCF7-Vif W/*1 genome may impede replication in the native host. Further studies may elucidate additional complex host-virus restriction pathways that are relevant in vivo but are functionally masked or not relevant during in vitro infections.

Findings presented here illustrate a role for pCF7-Vif W/*1 to be used as a novel anti-LV vaccine delivery scaffold. This system would exploit a non-pathogenic vector that has to stably retain the Vif vaccine antigen and may be a therapeutic option to boost immunity towards an existing HIV infection in order to eliminate infected cells. The option to insert additional B and T cell epitopes at the terminus of the truncated Bet may be a means to extend and direct the host immune response towards additional epitopes (Slavkovic Lukic and Löchelt, unpublished observations). The ability to administer repeatedly or simultaneously the FV-based vaccine vector, directing expression of additional or newly acquired antigens, is an additional strength of our system as low level or absence of replication would hinder use of pCF7-Vif W/*1 as a vector delivery system that requires greater viral replication. Our results suggest that prior infection with wild-type FFV might not impair response to FFV-Vif, though superinfection studies will need to be conducted before this vector could be commercially developed. Experiments determining the viability of FV-LV Vif chimeric variants would also have to include assays to determine stability and functionality of inserted heterologous epitopes. Since we have documented that seroconversion occurs against Vif and Gag during FFV-Vif W/*1 exposure in the absence of intentional adjuvation, the attenuated replication does not impair its use as an antigen expression platform for eliciting antibodies against foreign antigens, and could even improve its biological safety.

Conclusions

Our in vitro and in vivo studies show the feasibility of constructing a replicative FFV-Vif vector that incorporates FIV Vif and replaces FFV Bet protein expression to counteract intrinsic feline A3 restriction factors. The FFV-Vif chimera inoculation of domestic cats induced a specific immune response against the heterologous Vif protein which under superinfection boosted antibody production against both FFV Gag and FIV Vif. Superinfection was also possible using wild-type FFV as evidenced by seroconversion against FFV Bet in animals initially inoculated with the chimeric construct, which provides plausibility of using this vector in domestic cat populations which may already be infected with wild-type virus. These findings demonstrate that this and additional FV vector systems may be further studied to develop potential therapeutic or preventive avenues against lentiviral infections including HIV.

Methods

Cells, culture conditions, and DNA transfection

Crandell feline kidney (CrFK) cells were used for FFV infection and propagation [34, 66, 67]. Human embryonic kidney (HEK) 293T cells used for plasmid transfection were propagated as described [68]. FeFAB cells (CrFK-derived cells that carry a ß-galactosidase gene under the control of the FFV LTR promoter that is activated via FFV infection and subsequent Tas expression) were used to determine viral titer as described previously [68]. PBMC were purified from feline blood using Histopaque gradients (Sigma Aldrich, St. Louis, MO). HEK 293T cells were transfected or co-transfected by using a modified calcium phosphate method described previously [68]. In serial passage experiments, wild-type pCF-7 and Vif-chimera pCF-Vif-4 were transfected into HEK 293T cells [13]. Supernatants were harvested 2 days post transfection and used to infect feA3-positive CrFK cells. Supernatants from these infections were serially passaged twice a week (every third or fourth day p.i.) to new, uninfected CrFK cells. A total of 20 serial passages were conducted.

FFV propagation and titration

For viral propagation of wild-type FFV and chimera (generated by transfection of HEK 293T cells), 10^6 CrFK cells/ml were seeded and infected at a multiplicity of infection (MOI) of 0.1. Supernatants were harvested and used for viral titer estimation and further viral propagation. FFV titers were determined using 5×10^4 FeFAB cells/well grown in 24-well plates and infected with serial 1:5 dilutions as described [13]. Titers were calculated by determining the highest dilution that contained blue-colored infected cells through light microscopy.

Wild-type and FFV-Vif chimera viral propagation and titration for cat infections

2 μg of FFV pCF-7 [25] or pCF7-Vif W/*1 plasmid were transfected into CrFK cells using Lipofectamine and supernatants were harvested for amplification in CrFK cells. Microscopic observation of cells was conducted daily and considered to be infected if they displayed cytopathic effects (CPE) of vacuolization, cytomegaly, and multinucleation [69–71]. Supernatants of infected cells were harvested and frozen on 2, 6, 9, and 13 days p.i. CPE end-point dilution titration was conducted on CrFK cells to determine $TCID_{50}$/ml. CrFK (3×10^4 cells/well) were incubated with 25 μl of virus-containing supernatants in five-fold dilutions from the aforementioned days and observed for CPE up to 17 days p.i. The number of CPE-positive wells was used to determine $TCID_{50}$/ml using the method of Reed and Muench [72]. Supernatants that yielded the highest titers were selected for animal inoculations.

FIV titration system and FFV LTR luc reporter assay

Production of FIV luc reporter viruses, normalization according to reverse transcriptase activity, and target cell infection and reporter readout were done as previously

described [44]. FFV reporter assays using co-transfection of HEK 293T cells with the full-length FFV LTR luc reporter plasmid pFeFV-LTR-luc and the different FFV chimeras generated in this study or the FFV Tas expression construct pFeFV-Bel1 were conducted as described previously [73].

Molecular cloning

Replacement of FFV *bet* coding sequences by a codon-optimized FIV *vif* gene in the FFV provirus vector pCF7-BetMCS, which carries a multiple cloning site directly downstream of *bet* without affecting *tas* [50], was done via fusion PCR cloning using the proof-reading *Pfu* polymerase as specified by the supplier (New England Biolabs, Frankfurt Germany) [13]. For PCR primer sequences, see Table 2. In brief, the codon-optimized *vif* gene was first amplified using a sense primer with upstream sequences encompassing a terminal *Nhe*I site, followed by a *Sac*II site and the sequence encoding the FFV protease (PR) cleavage sequence AAVHTVKA (see Fig. 1a, and Additional file 2) directly fused in-frame to the start codon of *vif* while the antisense primer was complementary to the terminal *vif* sequence followed by an *Age*I restriction site (Fig. 1a, bottom panel, pair of blue primers, # 1 and 2). The other amplicon was generated with a sense primer also containing an *Age*I site and annealed to FFV sequences about 120 nt upstream of the essential FFV

Table 2 Primers used for cloning and PCR detection

Primer name	Sequence (5′–3′)
pCF7-Vif cloning	
FFV-Vif #1	GCGGGCTAGCGCCGCGGTACACACCGTCAAAGCCATGAGCGAGGGGACTGGCAG
FFV-Vif #2	GTGCTCTCCAAAGACCGGTTATCACAGCTCGCCGCTCCACAGCAGATTCC
FFV-Vif #3	GGCGAGCTGTGATAACCGGTCTTTGGAGAGCACAAGCTGATG
FFV-Vif #4	CGCTCTGTTGCATGCCG
Mutagenesis of the upstream start codon	
FFV 9233-F	GCGGTCCGGAACACCCAAGACGGATCCTACTCG
M/T-R	CGGCGCTAGCTCTAGTTAGCGTAGTCAAATCCCTCTCCCCAC
M+-R	CGGCGCTAGCTCTAGTTACCATAGTGAAATCCCTCTCCCCAC
PCR amplification of in vitro-selected FFV-Vif variants	
FFV 9366-F	CCACTTCTGTTTGGACCTTACC
FFV-10288-R	CAGCTTGTGCTCTCCAAAGC
Nested FFV PCR	
FFVgag-F1	CTACAGCCGCTATTGAAGGAG
FFVgag-R1	CCCTGCTGTTGAGGATTACC
FFVgag-F2	TTACAGATGGAAACTGGTCCTTAGT
FFVgag-R2	CATCAGAGTGTTGCTGTTGTTG
Real-time quantitative PCR	
FFVgag -F	GGACGATCTCAACAAGGTCAACTAAA
FFVgag-R	TCCACGAGGAGGTTGCGA
FFVgag-TM	AGACCCCCTAGACAACAACAGCAACACT

poly-purine tract while the antisense primer was down-stream of a unique *Sph*I site in the U3 region of the FFV LTR (Fig. 1a, bottom panel, pair of violet primers, # 3 and 4). The amplicons generated were fused in a third PCR using only the sense primer of the first and the antisense primer of the second reaction (primers # 1 and 4). The amplicon was digested with *Nhe*I and *Sph*I and inserted into pCF7-BetMCS [50] digested with *Nhe*I and *Sph*I. The resulting clone pCF7-Vif was analyzed by DNA restriction analysis and DNA sequencing. Similarly, site-directed W/* mutagenesis in pCF7-Vif-4 and mutagene-sis of the methionine codon and its flanking sequences in pCF7-Vif W/*1 and -W/*2, were done using PCR primers shown in Table 2. The resulting fragments were inserted into the clones pCF7-Vif W/*1 and pCF7-Vif W/*2 via three component ligations using unique *Bsp*EI, *Nhe*I and *Xho*I restriction sites.

Cloning and sequencing of in vitro selected FFV-Vif variants

DNA from CrFK cells infected with in vitro selected vari-ants of pCF7-Vif-4 was harvested at passage 18 using the DNeasy extraction kit as specified by the supplier (Qia-gen, Hilden, Germany). Sense primer FFV 9366 and antisense primer 10288 (Table 2) were used to amplify a 923 nt fragment of the *bel1–vif* region. Amplicons were cloned into pCR-TOPO TA vectors (Invitrogen, Karlsruhe, Germany) and subjected to in-house Sanger DNA sequencing of both strands.

Animals and experimental design

Twelve specific-pathogen-free (SPF) cats, aged 6–8 months and negative for common feline pathogens including FFV and FIV, were obtained from the Colorado State University (CSU) SPF Colony and housed in an Association for Assessment and Accreditation of Labora-tory Animal Care International-accredited animal facility at CSU. All procedures were approved by the CSU Insti-tutional Animal Care and Use Committee prior to initia-tion of the study. Cats were separated into three groups (n = 4 per group) based on inoculation type: FFV-nega-tive CrFK culture media (naïve, N), wild-type FFV (WT), or chimeric FFV-Vif W/*1 (CH) (Fig. 4). Virus-inoculated animals received 10^5 $TCID_{50}$ in 2 ml under ketamine anesthesia, split into 1 ml intramuscularly (i.m.) and 1 ml intravenously (i.v.). Cats were monitored daily for clinical signs of disease, and body temperature and weight were measured weekly. Peripheral blood was collected via cephalic or jugular venipuncture and processed to obtain serum and PBMC. On day 53 p.i., all cats in the CH cohort were re-inoculated each with 5 ml of undiluted virus (wild-type virus 2.78×10^5 $TCID_{50}$/ml or chimeric virus 5.56×10^4 $TCID_{50}$/ml, split into 1 ml i.m., 2 ml i.v.,

and 2 ml subcutaneously). Two of these cats were re-inoculated with wild-type FFV virus (henceforth referred to as CH1WT and CH2WT) and the other two cats with FFV-Vif W/*1 (now referred to as CH3CH and CH4CH). Animals were humanely euthanized for necropsy on day 176 p.i. (Fig. 4).

Nested and real-time quantitative PCR assays

Nested FFV PCR (nPCR) was performed on PBMC DNA to screen for initial infection status. Proviral DNA was purified and amplified using 0.5 µM *gag*-specific forward and reverse primers listed in Table 2 under the following cycling conditions for the first round of nPCR: 94 °C for 2 min, 35 cycles of 94 °C for 30 s, 57 °C for 30 s, 72 °C for 1 min, and a final elongation step at 72 °C for 5 min. For the second round, 2 µl of first-round product was added to the reaction and amplified in these conditions: 94 °C for 2 min, 35 cycles of 94 °C for 30 s, 57 °C for 30 s, 72 °C for 30 s, and 72 °C for 5 min. Products were elec-trophoresed in 1.5% agarose gel in Tris-acetate buffer and stained with GelRed™ Nucleic Acid Gel Stain (Biotium, Hayward, CA) then visualized to look for the 333 base-pair PCR product. Real-time quantitative PCR (qPCR) was performed in triplicate on viral DNA as previously described [64] using 0.5 uM forward and reverse *Gag*-based primers and 0.1 uM probe (Table 2) with the fol-lowing modified conditions: 95 °C for 3 min, 45 cycles of 95 °C for 10 s, and 60 °C for 40 s. Viral copy number quan-tification was based on a plasmid standard curve pre-pared from plasmid pCF-7. FFV-Gag real time PCR assay sensitivity is 1–10 viral copies per reaction [64]. Infection status was divided into 3 categories: positive, negative, and indeterminate. Animals considered unequivocally "positive" had qPCR results with Cq values less than or equal to 37 in 2–3 out of the three reactions, consistent with viral load greater than 10 copies/reaction. Animals considered "negative" were negative for all triplicate tests (this included all naïve cats and "no template" controls at all defined times). Animals classified as "indeterminate" had qPCR replicates with Cq values > 37, equivalent to 0–10 copies per well. Indeterminate copy number calcu-lations were not used in Fig. 6 since values obtained were below the assay's lower limit of quantitation.

Gag, Bet and Vif immunoblotting

Cell lysate from FFV-infected CrFK cells or transfected HEK 293T cells were subjected to immunoblot analy-ses as described [13, 21]. Identical amounts of proteins were separated by SDS-PAGE, blotted, and reacted against different anti-FFV sera. FFV Gag and Bet pro-teins were detected by rabbit anti-Gag polyclonal serum (1:3000 dilution) and rabbit anti-Bet polyclonal serum (1:2500 dilution) [13]. FIV Vif was detected by a mouse anti-FIV-Vif antibody (NIH AIDS repository, Maryland, USA) at a 1:500 dilution. Membranes were incubated with secondary anti-rabbit polyclonal antibodies or anti-mouse IgG (Sigma, Munich, Germany) conjugated to horseradish peroxidase (1:5000 to 1:2000 dilution) and visualized by chemiluminescence (ECL Western Blot Kit, Amersham Buchler, Braunschweig, Germany). Blots were then probed against actin using mouse anti-actin antibody (1:8000 dilution, Sigma).

GST-capture ELISA for detection of Gag and Bet seroconversion

GST-capture ELISA was performed to detect anti-FFV Gag and anti-FFV Bet antibodies as previously described [55, 74]. Glutathione casein was used to coat 96-well plates (Thermo Fisher Scientific, Waltham, MA) overnight at 4 °C then plates were blocked with casein blocking buffer (0.2% (w/v) casein in PBS and Tween20, Thermo Fisher Scientific). Plates were incubated with BL21 *E. coli*-produced lysates containing GST-tag, GST-Gag-tag, or GST-Bet-tag recombinant proteins (0.25 μg/μl in casein blocking buffer). Cat sera were pre-adsorbed with GST-tag lysate (2 μg/μl) in a 1:50 dilution and then incubated in duplicate (Fig. 7a, b) or triplicate (Additional file 6) with each GST conjugate. The plates were incubated with anti-cat IgG Protein A peroxidase (1:50,000 dilution, Sigma Aldrich). For the substrate reaction, plates were incubated with TMB substrate before stopping the reaction with sulfuric acid. Absorption (optical density, OD) at 450 nm was measured and the mean reactivity for each was used. Detection cutoff values were determined from negative sera as $2 \times (\text{mean} + 3$ standard deviations). A significant number of reactions at the serum dilution used were out of the linear range of the assay. For anti-Gag antibody titrations, sera from days 28, 42, 70, and 168 p.i. were diluted at 1:100, 1:250, 1:500, 1:1000, 1:2500, and 1:5000. Titer was determined as the highest dilution the cat tested positive for anti-Gag antibodies, using the cutoff formula mentioned above.

FIV Vif antibody capture ELISA

Sera were subjected to an FIV Vif antibody capture ELISA to detect corresponding antibodies in chimeric FFV-Vif-inoculated cats. 96-well plates were coated with 2 ng/μl Vif antigen and incubated overnight at 4 °C. Mouse Vif monoclonal antibody (obtained from Dr. Chris Grant, Custom Monoclonals International, Sacramento, CA) was used as a positive control. After blocking, cat sera (1:100 dilution) or Vif monoclonal antibody (10 ng/μL) were applied in duplicates, then goat anti-cat (or anti-mouse) IgG-HRP (MP Biomedicals, Santa Ana, CA) was used as secondary antibody (1:1000 dilution). TMB reagent was used for

the substrate reaction then stopped with sulfuric acid before measuring absorption (450 nm). For detection cutoff, the mean negative sera absorbance readout was used in the following formula: $\text{mean} + (2 \times \text{standard deviation})$. A number of reactions at the serum dilution used were out of the linear range of the assay.

Additional files

Additional file 1. Rescue of Vif-deficient FIV and Bet-deficient FFV by FIV Vif and FFV Bet. **A** Vif-deficient FIV plasmid DNA was co-transfected with plasmids expressing FIV Vif or FFV Bet together with different feA3 restriction factors as given in the legend (left panel). Empty vector pcDNA3.1 served as control. Two days after transfection, cell-free supernatants were used to infect FIV reporter cells and luc activity induced by FIV infection was measured two days p.i. Titers are expressed as luc values of a representative experiment. **B** The Bet-deficient FFV genome pCF7-BBtr was co-transfected with plasmids expressing untagged and V5-tagged FFV Bet or two different amounts of FIV Vif expression plasmid together with the major FFV-restricting feA3Z2b-HA as shown below the bar diagram (right panel). Empty vector pcDNA3.1 served as control. Two days after transfection, cell-free supernatants were titrated in triplicate using FFV reporter cells as described in the "Methods" section and are expressed as focus-forming units (FFU) per ml inoculum of a representative experiment. Error bars represent the standard deviation.

Additional file 2. Partial genome sequences from pCF7-Vif-4 and the stop mutations of the in vitro-selected FFV-Vif variants. The Trp codon and the downstream G residue (TGGG) ~ 130 bp upstream of the *vif* coding sequence are in bold face letters and underlined. In pCF7-Vif W/*1 (in blue), the mutation is from TGG to TGA and for mutant W/*2 (in green) the mutation is from TGGG to TAGA, with both mutations resulting in a Trp (W) to Stop (*) mutation (W/*) as indicated. The *bet* nucleotide sequence is in black, the linker sequence in pink with recognition sites for *Nhe*I (in brown) and *Sac*II (in light violet). The *vif* gene is marked in blue with the authentic Met start codon in bold. The Bet^{tr}Vif fusion protein is highlighted in yellow with the amino acids color-coded as described above for the genes. The Met residue 14 amino acids upstream of the authentic *vif* start codon is highlighted in bold and underlining. The C-terminal amino acid sequence of *tas* is highlighted in red.

Additional file 3. Mutations in *Tas* generated during the analysis of the upstream ATG do not affect Tas-mediated LTR transactivation. The LTR promoter-based luc reporter construct pFeFV-LTR-luc [73] was cotransfected into HEK 293T cells together with a CMV-IE-driven FFV Tas expression construct, the empty control pcDNA3.1 and proviral genomes pCF-7, pCF7-Vif-4, pCF7-Vif W/*1, and pCF7-Vif W/*2, and their engineered M/T and M+ variants. Two days post transfection, luc activity induced by FFV Tas expression was measured in duplicates. Data from a representative experiment normalized to co-expressed β-gal are expressed in a logarithmic bar diagram.

Additional file 4. Titers of pCF-7, pCF7-Vif-4 and engineered pCF7-Vif W/*1 and pCF7-Vif W/*2 variants. Plasmid pCF-7, pCF7-Vif-4, pCF7-Vif W/*1, and pCF7-Vif W/*2 and their engineered M+ variants were transfected into HEK 293T cells and 2 days post-transfection, cell-free supernatants were inoculated on CrFK cells and serially passaged every **A** 60 and **B** 84 h p.i. FFV titers were determined in duplicate using FeFAB reporter cells and are shown as bar diagrams for the different passages. Error bars represent the standard deviation.

Additional file 5. Date FFV was first detected by PCR and ELISA in experimentally infected cats. Day of first detection of FFV genomic DNA by qPCR with indeterminate and clear positive results (two left columns) and nested PCR (nPCR, middle column) after experimental infection with either wild-type FFV (WT), FFV-Vif W/*1 chimera (CH), chimera then wild-type FFV (CH1WT and CH2WT), twice with FFV-Vif W/*1 chimera (CH3CH and CH4CH), or sham inoculation in naïve cats. In addition, first detection of FFV Gag and Bet, and FIV Vif antibodies by ELISA is displayed correspondingly (right columns). Hyphens (-) mark negative results due to absence of reactivity.

Additional file 6. All cats infected with wild-type FFV and FFV-Vif W/*1 developed FFV Gag-specific immunoreactivity. A GST-capture ELISA was performed to evaluate antibody response to FFV infection. Anti-Gag reactivity (1:50 dilution) at the final time point for each animal is shown. All animals exposed to wild-type FFV (red bars) or FFV-Vif W/*1 (blue bars) seroconverted against Gag antigen and for many of these samples, reactivity is out of the linear range. Naïve animals (black bars) remained below the cutoff for detection (black dotted line). Black and blue striped bars denote chimeric animals re-inoculated with wild-type virus (CHxWT). Error bars represent standard deviation. POS = positive control, NEG = negative control, H2O = absolute negative (water) control.

Abbreviations
FV: foamy virus(es); FFV: feline foamy virus; LV: lentivirus(es); FIV: feline immunodeficiency virus; HIV: human immunodeficiency virus; A3: APOBEC3 proteins; feA3: feline A3 proteins; WT: wild-type pCF-7 inoculated group; CH: chimeric pCF7-Vif W/*1 inoculated group; N: naïve control group; PBMC: peripheral blood mononuclear cell(s); W/*: Trp/stop mutation; p.i: post-infection; i.m: intramuscular(ly); i.v: intravenous(ly); Py: pyrimidine residue; CSU: Colorado State University; MOI: multiplicity of infection; luc: luciferase; PR: protease; CrFK: Crandell feline kidney cell(s); HEK: human embryonic kidney cell(s); FFU: focus-forming units; Thr: threonine; Trp: tryptophan; CPE: cytopathic effect; w/v: weight per volume; SPF: specific-pathogen free.

Authors' contributions
CLF, SH, GW, DSL, DM, JZ performed the experiments and designed the study together with SVW and ML. RT, EM, and XZ provided valuable information, methods and assisted in experiments and sample collection. CLF, SH, CM, SVW and ML analyzed the data and wrote the manuscript. All authors read and approved the final manuscript.

Author details
[1] Department of Microbiology, Immunology, and Pathology, College of Veterinary Medicine and Biomedical Sciences, Colorado State University, Fort Collins, CO, USA. [2] Department of Molecular Diagnostics of Oncogenic Infections, Research Program Infection, Inflammation and Cancer, German Cancer Research Center, (Deutsches Krebsforschungszentrum Heidelberg, DKFZ), Im Neuenheimer Feld 242, 69120 Heidelberg, Germany. [3] Clinic for Gastroenterology, Hepatology, and Infectiology, Medical Faculty, Heinrich-Heine-University Düsseldorf, Düsseldorf, Germany. [4] Present Address: Roche Glycart AG, Schlieren 8952, Switzerland. [5] Present Address: Department of Microbiology and Immunology, Western University, London, ON, Canada. [6] Present Address: University of Dar es Salaam, Dar es Salaam, Tanzania. [7] Present Address: Department of Internal Medicine II, Division of Hematology, University Hospital of Würzburg, Würzburg, Germany. [8] Present Address: Roche Pharma AG, Grenzach-Wyhlen, Germany. [9] Present Address: Division of Infectious Disease, University of Colorado, Anschutz Medical Campus, Aurora, USA.

Acknowledgements
We thank Lutz Gissmann (DKFZ) for his interest in this project and his generous support, Dr. Timo Kehl (DKZF) for the development of the FFV anti-gag PCR and providing training for the FFV capture ELISA, Dr. Chris Grant (Custom Monoclonals Intl, Sacramento, CA, USA) and Dr. John Elder (The Scripps Research Institute, La Jolla, CA, USA) for developing and providing mouse monoclonal Vif antigen for the Vif antibody capture ELISA, and Martha McMillan for cell culture training, animal care, and help with regulatory matters.

Competing interests
The authors declare they have no competing interests.

Funding
SH, DSL and A-MR were supported by DKFZ PhD stipends. GW was supported by a PhD stipend from the China Scholarship Council. CLF was funded by Morris Animal Foundation (Grant Number: D16FE-402) and The National Institutes of Health (NIH T32 Grant Number: 4T32OD010437-15). The funding bodies played no role in the study design, data collection or analysis, or writing of the manuscript.

References
1. Rethwilm A, Lindemann D. Foamy viruses. In: Knipe D, Howley P, editors. Field's virology. Volume II. 6th ed. Philadelphia: Lippincott Williams & Wilkins; 2013. p. 1613–32.
2. Delelis O, Lehmann-Che J, Saib A. Foamy viruses—a world apart. Curr Opin Microbiol. 2004;7:400–6.
3. Linial ML. Foamy viruses are unconventional retroviruses. J Virol. 1999;73:1747–55.
4. Kehl T, Tan J, Materniak M. Non-simian foamy viruses: molecular virology, tropism and prevalence and zoonotic/interspecies transmission. Viruses. 2013;5:2169–209.
5. Rethwilm A, Bodem J. Evolution of foamy viruses: the most ancient of all retroviruses. Viruses. 2013;5:2349–74.
6. German AC, Harbour DA, Helps CR, Gruffydd-Jones TJ. Is feline foamy virus really apathogenic? Vet Immunol Immunopathol. 2008;123:114–8.
7. Weikel J, Löchelt M, Truyen U. Demonstration of feline foamy virus in experimentally infected cats by immunohistochemistry. J Vet Med A Physiol Pathol Clin Med. 2003;50:415–7.
8. Mouinga-Ondeme A, Kazanji M. Simian foamy virus in non-human primates and cross-species transmission to humans in Gabon: an emerging zoonotic disease in central Africa? Viruses. 2013;5:1536–52.
9. Switzer WM, Bhullar V, Shanmugam V, Cong ME, Parekh B, Lerche NW, Yee JL, Ely JJ, Boneva R, Chapman LE, et al. Frequent simian foamy virus infection in persons occupationally exposed to nonhuman primates. J Virol. 2004;78:2780–9.
10. Burtner CR, Beard BC, Kennedy DR, Wohlfahrt ME, Adair JE, Trobridge GD, Scharenberg AM, Torgerson TR, Rawlings DJ, Felsburg PJ, Kiem HP. Intravenous injection of a foamy virus vector to correct canine SCID-X1. Blood. 2014;123:3578–84.
11. Trobridge GD, Allen J, Peterson L, Ironside C, Russell DW, Kiem HP. Foamy and lentiviral vectors transduce canine long-term repopulating cells at similar efficiency. Hum Gene Ther. 2009;20:519–23.
12. Schwantes A, Truyen U, Weikel J, Weiss C, Löchelt M. Application of chimeric feline foamy virus-based retroviral vectors for the induction of antiviral immunity in cats. J Virol. 2003;77:7830–42.
13. Lei J, Osen W, Gardyan A, Hotz-Wagenblatt A, Wei G, Gissmann L, Eichmuller S, Löchelt M. Replication-competent foamy virus vaccine vectors as novel epitope scaffolds for immunotherapy. PLoS ONE. 2015;10:e0138458.
14. Gupta S, Leutenegger CM, Dean GA, Steckbeck JD, Cole KS, Sparger EE. Vaccination of cats with attenuated feline immunodeficiency virus proviral DNA vaccine expressing gamma interferon. J Virol. 2007;81:465–73.
15. Maksaereekul S, Dubie RA, Shen X, Kieu H, Dean GA, Sparger EE. Vaccination with vif-deleted feline immunodeficiency virus provirus, GM-CSF, and TNF-alpha plasmids preserves global CD4 T lymphocyte function after challenge with FIV. Vaccine. 2009;27:3754–65.

16. Liu W, Lei J, Liu Y, Lukic DS, Rathe AM, Bao Q, Kehl T, Bleiholder A, Hechler T, Löchelt M. Feline foamy virus-based vectors: advantages of an authentic animal model. Viruses. 2013;5:1702–18.

17. Kiem HP, Wu RA, Sun G, von Laer D, Rossi JJ, Trobridge GD. Foamy combinatorial anti-HIV vectors with MGMTP140 K potently inhibit HIV-1 and SHIV replication and mediate selection in vivo. Gene Ther. 2010;17:37–49.

18. Yamamoto JK, Hansen H, Ho EW, Morishita TY, Okuda T, Sawa TR, Nakamura RM, Pedersen NC. Epidemiologic and clinical aspects of feline immunodeficiency virus infection in cats from the continental United States and Canada and possible mode of transmission. J Am Vet Med Assoc. 1989;194:213–20.

19. Yamamoto JK, Sparger E, Ho EW, Andersen PR, O'Connor TP, Mandell CP, Lowenstine L, Munn R, Pedersen NC. Pathogenesis of experimentally induced feline immunodeficiency virus infection in cats. Am J Vet Res. 1988;49:1246–58.

20. Pedersen NC, Yamamoto JK, Ishida T, Hansen H. Feline immunodeficiency virus infection. Vet Immunol Immunopathol. 1989;21:111–29.

21. Alke A, Schwantes A, Zemba M, Flugel RM, Löchelt M. Characterization of the humoral immune response and virus replication in cats experimentally infected with feline foamy virus. Virology. 2000;275:170–6.

22. Elder JH, Lin YC, Fink E, Grant CK. Feline immunodeficiency virus (FIV) as a model for study of lentivirus infections: parallels with HIV. Curr HIV Res. 2010;8:73–80.

23. Hartmann K. Clinical aspects of feline retroviruses: a review. Viruses. 2012;4:2684–710.

24. Liem BP, Dhand NK, Pepper AE, Barrs VR, Beatty JA. Clinical findings and survival in cats naturally infected with feline immunodeficiency virus. J Vet Intern Med. 2013;27:798–805.

25. Schwantes A, Ortlepp I, Löchelt M. Construction and functional characterization of feline foamy virus-based retroviral vectors. Virology. 2002;301:53–63.

26. Pedersen NC. Feline syncytium-forming virus infection. In: Holyworth J, editor. Diseases of the cat. Philadelphia: The W. B. Saunder Co.; 1986. p. 268–72.

27. Trobridge GD, Miller DG, Jacobs MA, Allen JM, Kiem HP, Kaul R, Russell DW. Foamy virus vector integration sites in normal human cells. Proc Natl Acad Sci USA. 2006;103:1498–503.

28. Trobridge GD. Foamy virus vectors for gene transfer. Expert Opin Biol Ther. 2009;9:1427–36.

29. Trobridge G, Josephson N, Vassilopoulos G, Mac J, Russell DW. Improved foamy virus vectors with minimal viral sequences. Mol Ther. 2002;6:321–8.

30. Bastone P, Löchelt M. Kinetics and characteristics of replication-competent revertants derived from self-inactivating foamy virus vectors. Gene Ther. 2004;11:465–73.

31. Bastone P, Romen F, Liu W, Wirtz R, Koch U, Josephson N, Langbein S, Löchelt M. Construction and characterization of efficient, stable and safe replication-deficient foamy virus vectors. Gene Ther. 2007;14:613–20.

32. Löchelt M. Foamy virus transactivation and gene expression. Foamy Viruses. 2003;277:27–61.

33. Chareza S, Slavkovic Lukic D, Liu Y, Räthe A-M, Münk C, Zabogli E, Pistello M, Löchelt M. Molecular and functional interactions of cat APOBEC3 and feline foamy and immunodeficiency virus proteins: different ways to counteract host-encoded restriction. Virology. 2012;424:138–46.

34. Löchelt M, Romen F, Bastone P, Muckenfuss H, Kirchner N, Kim YB, Truyen U, Rosler U, Battenberg M, Saib A, et al. The antiretroviral activity of APOBEC3 is inhibited by the foamy virus accessory Bet protein. PNAS. 2005;102:7982–7.

35. Perkovic M, Schmidt S, Marino D, Russell RA, Stauch B, Hofmann H, Kopietz F, Kloke B-P, Zielonka J, Ströver H, et al. Species-specific inhibition of APOBEC3C by the prototype foamy virus protein bet. J Biol Chem. 2009;284:5819–26.

36. Russell RA, Wiegand HL, Moore MD, Schafer A, McClure MO, Cullen BR. Foamy virus Bet proteins function as novel inhibitors of the APOBEC3 family of innate antiretroviral defense factors. J Virol. 2005;79:8724–31.

37. Jaguva Vasudevan AA, Perkovic M, Bulliard Y, Cichutek K, Trono D, Haussinger D, Münk C. Prototype foamy virus Bet impairs the dimerization and cytosolic solubility of human APOBEC3G. J Virol. 2013;87:9030–40.

38. Cullen BR. Role and mechanism of action of the APOBEC3 family of antiretroviral resistance factors. J Virol. 2006;80:1067–76.

39. Münk C, Hechler T, Chareza S, Löchelt M. Restriction of feline retroviruses: lessons from cat APOBEC3 cytidine deaminases and TRIM5alpha proteins. Vet Immunol Immunopathol. 2010;134:14–24.

40. Malim MH, Bieniasz PD. HIV restriction factors and mechanisms of evasion. Cold Spring Harb Perspect Med. 2012;2:a006940.

41. Moris A, Murray S, Cardinaud S. AID and APOBECs span the gap between innate and adaptive immunity. Front Microbiol. 2014;5:534.

42. Yan N, Chen ZJ. Intrinsic antiviral immunity. Nat Immunol. 2012;13:214–22.

43. Iwasaki A, Medzhitov R. Regulation of adaptive immunity by the innate immune system. Science. 2010;327:291–5.

44. Zielonka J, Marino D, Hofmann H, Yuhki N, Löchelt M, Münk C. Vif of feline immunodeficiency virus from domestic cats protects against APOBEC3 restriction factors from many felids. J Virol. 2010;84:7312–24.

45. Lukic DS, Hotz-Wagenblatt A, Lei J, Rathe AM, Muhle M, Denner J, Münk C, Löchelt M. Identification of the feline foamy virus Bet domain essential for APOBEC3 counteraction. Retrovirology. 2013;10:76.

46. Wang JW, Zhang WY, Lv MY, Zuo T, Kong W, Yu XH. Identification of a Cullin5-ElonginB-ElonginC E3 complex in degradation of feline immunodeficiency virus Vif-mediated feline APOBEC3 proteins. J Virol. 2011;85:12482–91.

47. Zhang ZL, Gu QY, Vasudevan AAJ, Hain A, Kloke BP, Hasheminasab S, Mulnaes D, Sato K, Cichutek K, Haussinger D, et al. Determinants of FIV and HIV Vif sensitivity of feline APOBEC3 restriction factors. Retrovirology. 2016;13:46.

48. Stern MA, Hu CL, Saenz DT, Fadel HJ, Sims O, Peretz M, Poeschla EM. Productive replication of vif-chimeric HIV-1 in feline cells. J Virol. 2010;84:7378–95.

49. Sato K, Izumi T, Misawa N, Kobayashi T, Yamashita Y, Ohmichi M, Ito M, Takaori-Kondo A, Koyanagi Y. Remarkable lethal G-to-A mutations in vif-proficient HIV-1 provirus by individual APOBEC3 proteins in humanized mice. J Virol. 2010;84:9546–56.

50. Alke A, Schwantes A, Kido K, Flotenmeyer M, Flugel RM, Löchelt M. The bet gene of feline foamy virus is required for virus replication. Virology. 2001;287:310–20.

51. Lockridge KM, Himathongkham S, Sawai ET, Chienand M, Sparger EE. The feline immunodeficiency virus vif gene is required for productive infection of feline peripheral blood mononuclear cells and monocyte-derived macrophages. Virology. 1999;261:25–30.

52. Münk C, Beck T, Zielonka J, Hotz-Wagenblatt A, Chareza S, Battenberg M, Thielebein J, Cichutek K, Bravo IG, O'Brien SJ, et al. Functions, structure, and read-through alternative splicing of feline APOBEC3 genes. Genome Biol. 2008;9:R48.

53. Holtz CM, Sadler HA, Mansky LM. APOBEC3G cytosine deamination hotspots are defined by both sequence context and single-stranded DNA secondary structure. Nucleic Acids Res. 2013;41:6139–48.

54. Kozak M. An analysis of 5'-noncoding sequences from 699 vertebrate messenger RNAs. Nucleic Acids Res. 1987;15:8125–48.

55. Romen F, Pawlita M, Sehr P, Bachmann S, Schröder J, Lutz H, Löchelt M. Antibodies against Gag are diagnostic markers for feline foamy virus infections while Env and Bet reactivity is undetectable in a substantial fraction of infected cats. Virology. 2006;345:502–8.

56. Romen F, Backes P, Materniak M, Sting R, Vahlenkamp TW, Riebe R, Pawlita M, Kuzmak J, Löchelt M. Serological detection systems for identification of cows shedding bovine foamy virus via milk. Virology. 2007;364:123–31.

57. O'Neil C, Lee D, Clewley G, Johnson MA, Emery VC. Prevalence of anti-vif antibodies in HIV-1 infected individuals assessed using recombinant baculovirus expressed vif protein. J Med Virol. 1997;51:139–44.

58. Wieland U, Kuhn JE, Jassoy C, Rubsamen-Waigmann H, Wolber V, Braun RW. Antibodies to recombinant HIV-1 vif, tat, and nef proteins in human sera. Med Microbiol Immunol. 1990;179:1–11.

59. Ayyavoo V, Nagashunmugam T, Boyer J, Mahalingam S, Fernandes LS, Le P, Lin J, Nguyen C, Chattargoon M, Goedert JJ, et al. Development of genetic vaccines for pathogenic genes: construction of attenuated vif DNA immunization cassettes. AIDS. 1997;11:1433–44.

60. Wieland U, Kratschmann H, Kehm R, Kuhn JE, Naher H, Kramer MD, Braun RW. Antigenic domains of the HIV-1 vif protein as recognized by human sera and murine monoclonal antibodies. AIDS Res Hum Retrovir. 1991;7:861–7.

61. Schwander S, Braun RW, Kuhn JE, Hufert FT, Kern P, Dietrich M, Wieland U. Prevalence of antibodies to recombinant virion infectivity factor in the sera of prospectively studied patients with HIV-1 infection. J Med Virol. 1992;36:142–6.

62. Pistello M. Should accessory proteins be structural components of lentiviral vaccines? Lessons learned from the accessory ORF-A protein of FIV. Vet Immunol Immunopathol. 2008;123:144–9.

63. Inoshima Y, Miyazawa T, Mikami T. In vivo functions of the auxiliary genes and regulatory elements of feline immunodeficiency virus. Vet Microbiol. 1998;60:141–53.

64. Lee JS, Mackie RS, Harrison T, Shariat B, Kind T, Kehl T, Löchelt M, Boucher C, VandeWoude S. Targeted enrichment for pathogen detection and characterization in three felid species. J Clin Microbiol. 2017;55:1658–70.

65. Winkler IG, Löchelt M, Flower RLP. Epidemiology of feline foamy virus and feline immunodeficiency virus infections in domestic and feral cats: a seroepidemiological study. J Clin Microbiol. 1999;37:2848–51.

66. Winkler IG, Flügel RM, Löchelt M, Flower RLP. Detection and molecular characterisation of feline foamy virus serotypes in naturally infected cats. Virology. 1998;247:144–51.

67. Flower RL, Wilcox GE, Cook RD, Ellis TM. Detection and prevalence of serotypes of feline syncytial spumaviruses. Adv Virol. 1985;83:53–63.

68. Zemba M, Alke A, Bodem J, Winkler IG, Flower RL, Pfrepper K, Delius H, Flügel RM, Löchelt M. Construction of infectious feline foamy virus genomes: cat antisera do not cross-neutralize feline foamy virus chimera with serotype-specific Env sequences. Virology. 2000;266:150–6.

69. Kasza L, Hayward AH, Betts AO. Isolation of a virus from a cat sarcoma in an established canine melanoma cell line. Res Vet Sci. 1969;10:216–8.

70. Riggs JL, Oshiro LS, Taylor DO, Lennette EH. Syncytium-forming agent isolated from domestic cats. Nature. 1969;222:1190–1.

71. Arzi B, Kol A, Murphy B, Walker NJ, Wood JA, Clark K, Verstraete FJM, Borjesson DL. Feline foamy virus adversely affects feline mesenchymal stem cell culture and expansion: implications for animal model development. Stem Cells Dev. 2014;24:814–23.

72. Reed LJ, Muench H. A simple method of estimating fifty per cent endpoints. Am J Hyg. 1938;27:493–7.

73. Winkler I, Bodem J, Haas L, Zemba M, Delius H, Flower R, Flügel RM, Löchelt M. Characterization of the genome of feline foamy virus and its proteins shows distinct features different from those of primate spumaviruses. J Virol. 1997;71:6727–41.

74. Sehr P, Zumbach K, Pawlita M. A generic capture ELISA for recombinant proteins fused to glutathione S-transferase: validation for HPV serology. J Immunol Methods. 2001;253:153–62.

16

Digital PCR as a tool to measure HIV persistence

Sofie Rutsaert[1†], Kobus Bosman[2†], Wim Trypsteen[1], Monique Nijhuis[2] and Linos Vandekerckhove[1*] (ID)

Abstract

Although antiretroviral therapy is able to suppress HIV replication in infected patients, the virus persists and rebounds when treatment is stopped. In order to find a cure that can eradicate the latent reservoir, one must be able to quantify the persisting virus. Traditionally, HIV persistence studies have used real-time PCR (qPCR) to measure the viral reservoir represented by HIV DNA and RNA. Most recently, digital PCR is gaining popularity as a novel approach to nucleic acid quantification as it allows for absolute target quantification. Various commercial digital PCR platforms are nowadays available that implement the principle of digital PCR, of which Bio-Rad's QX200 ddPCR is currently the most used platform in HIV research. Quantification of HIV by digital PCR is proving to be a valuable improvement over qPCR as it is argued to have a higher robustness to mismatches between the primers-probe set and heterogeneous HIV, and forfeits the need for a standard curve, both of which are known to complicate reliable quantification. However, currently available digital PCR platforms occasionally struggle with unexplained false-positive partitions, and reliable segregation between positive and negative droplets remains disputed. Future developments and advancements of the digital PCR technology are promising to aid in the accurate quantification and characterization of the persistent HIV reservoir.

Keywords: Digital PCR, HIV, ddPCR

Background

During antiretroviral therapy (ART), HIV can persist for decades in latently infected CD4 + T cells as proviral DNA integrated in the human genome. If ART is interrupted, the proviral reservoir fuels rebound viremia and is therefore considered a major obstacle to HIV cure [1]. HIV cure efforts aim to reduce the size and replication-competence of the reservoir by evaluating the success of HIV cure interventions, which is represented by an effect on the level of proviral DNA and/or cell-associated viral RNA. The standard tool to quantify HIV DNA and cell-associated viral RNA has been real-time PCR (qPCR). However, digital PCR has become a promising quantification strategy that combines absolute quantification with high sensitivity [2]. Digital PCR is based on the concept of limiting dilution where target molecules are randomly divided among a multitude of partitions. After PCR amplification, partitions that contain a target molecule accumulate fluorescence whereas partitions without target remain low in fluorescence (Fig. 1). A threshold is applied to the partitions, which divides the partitions into a positive and a negative population. The ratio between the number of positive and negative partitions is used to calculate the absolute number of target molecules, corrected for the chance that partitions are shared by multiple target molecules by the Poisson distribution law [2]. The first steps towards digital PCR were taken 30 years ago when the concept of limiting dilution and Poisson distribution were applied to detect rare targets [3–5]. In the field of HIV research, Simmonds et al. [6] combined PCR with limiting dilution to quantify the proviruses in HIV-infected cells. The term 'digital PCR' was introduced by Vogelstein in [7] to identify specific mutated sequences in a minor fraction of a cell population. Nowadays digital PCR is a widely accepted quantification tool and applied in many fields.

*Correspondence: Linos.Vandekerckhove@UGent.be
†Sofie Rutsaert and Kobus Bosman have contributed equally to this work
[1] HIV Cure Research Center, Department of Internal Medicine, Ghent University, Ghent, Belgium
Full list of author information is available at the end of the article

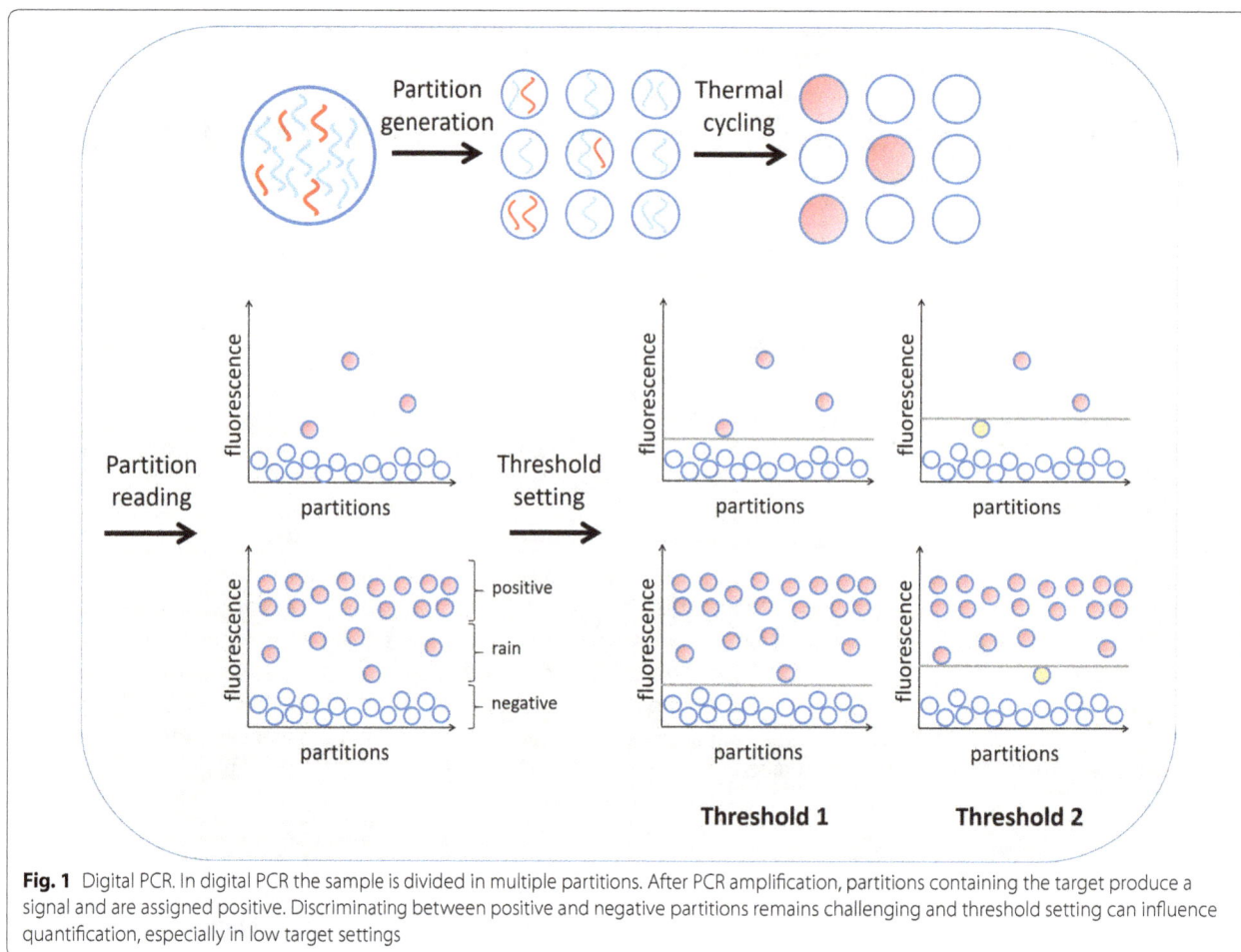

Fig. 1 Digital PCR. In digital PCR the sample is divided in multiple partitions. After PCR amplification, partitions containing the target produce a signal and are assigned positive. Discriminating between positive and negative partitions remains challenging and threshold setting can influence quantification, especially in low target settings

Digital PCR platforms

The key principle of digital PCR is the distribution of a sample among multiple partitions. Originally, partitions were created by manually distributing a sample over a number of wells [7]. Nowadays, manual partitioning is applied in case of complex protocols with a nested approach that cannot be adopted to an automated platform, such as the digital PCR described as a manual repetitive sampling protocol that is used to measure integrated HIV DNA [8, 9]. However, manually generating multiple partitions is very time-consuming and laborious. The past decade automated systems have emerged and different technologies and methods are being explored by various companies for digitizing PCR (for an overview, see Table 1). Currently available digital platforms differ in number of partitions, method of generating partitions or required specialized equipment. Partitions can be generated in a pre-manufactured array: BioMark™ HD System (Fluidigm) provides a wide range of specialized digital integrated fluidic circuits (IFCs) arrays where the sample is dispensed in a well and distributed over

multiple individual reaction chambers. QuantStudio 3D (Life Technologies/Applied Biosystems™) employs a silicon chip that consists of a single array of individual reaction wells onto which the sample is dispensed. CONSTELLATION® Digital PCR System (Formulatrix) utilizes a microplate where connecting channels are isolated into individual microfluidic chambers by a seal-compressing roller. In contrast to these array-based approaches, other digital PCR platforms such as the QX200™ Droplet Digital™ PCR (ddPCR) and RainDrop *plus*™ Digital PCR system (RainDance™ technologies) use water-in-oil emulsion chemistry to create partitions. The aqueous phase consisting of primers, probe and supermix, sample, and a mineral oil is loaded into a specifically designed holder. The droplet generator uses microfluidics to create a pressure that draws the aqueous and oil phase into the output channel, forming the droplets in the process. Each droplet is read one by one in a specialized droplet reader. Finally, Naica system from Stilla combines both the array and emulsion approaches.

Table 1 Characteristics of different digital PCR platforms. Information is extracted from companies' website unless cited otherwise

	Biomark	QuantStudio™ 3D	Naica	RainDrop plus™	QX200™ Droplet Digital™ PCR	CONSTELLATION® DPCR
Company	Fluidigm™	Applied Biosystems/Life technologies™	Stilla Technologies	RainDance™ Technologies	Bio-Rad	Formulatrix
Type	Integrated fluidic circuits (IFCS) arrays	Chip	Crystal droplets in an array	Picosized droplets	Nanosized droplets	Microfluidic chambers
Detection mode	Real-time and end-point	End-point	End-point	End-point	End-point	End-point
Chip/partitions consumables	qdPCR 37 K IFC, 48.770 and 12.765 Digital Array™ IFC	QuantStudio™ 3D Digital PCR Chip (v1/v2)	Sapphire chip	RainDance Source Chip	Microfluidic cartridge	CONSTELLATION® Digital PCR System microplate
Number of samples (max)						
Loading	48/12 samples per array	1 sample per chip	4 samples per chip	8 samples	96 samples	24/96 samples
Cycling	48/12 samples	24 samples	3 chips or 14 samples	96 samples	96 samples	24/96 samples
Reading	48/12 samples	1 sample per chip	3 chips or 14 samples	8 samples	96 samples	24/96 samples
Input volume per sample	4 µL/8 µL	14.5 µL	25 µL	25–50 µL	20 µL	10 µL
Reactions per sample	770/765	20,000	25,000-30,000	5–10 million	20,000	36,000/8000
Reaction volume per partition	0.85 nL/6 nL	0.755 nL (v2 chip) or 0.809 nL (v1 chip)	0.43 nL	5 pL	0.868 nL [10]	NA
Specialized equipment	IFC controller Biomark (thermal cycler and reader)	ProFlex™ 2 × Flat PCR System QuantStudio™ 3D Digital PCR Instrument	Naica Geode (thermal cycler) Naica Prism3 (reader)	RainDance Source/ThunderBolts™ System RainDrop® Sense Operator	QX200™ Droplet Generator QX200™ Droplet Digital™ PCR System	CONSTELLATION® Digital PCR System
Software	Digital PCR Analysis	QuantStudio™ 3D AnalysisSuite™	Crystal Miner	RainDrop Analyst II™	QuantaSoft™	CONSTELLATION®
Detection	Detection of up to 3 fluorescent dyes per assay	2 detection channels (FAM/VIC)	3 color detection (FAM/VIC/Cy5)	2 detection channels (FAM/VIC)	2 detection channels (FAM/VIC)	5 probe wavelengths per sample

In this system, a sample runs through the channels of a chip and droplets are created inside the chip.

Challenges and benefits of droplet digital PCR

There are multiple digital PCR platforms, but over the past years, the QX200 has steadily become the most widely used digital PCR platform across all research fields (Fig. 2). Therefore, in this review we will focus on the QX200 ddPCR from Bio-Rad to discuss challenges and benefits of digital PCR. It should however be noted that challenges with threshold determination and false-positives are not exclusively observed with the ddPCR from Bio-Rad but seem to be related to other digital platforms as well [11–15].

Threshold determination

In ddPCR generated droplets are identified as positive or negative based on a threshold at a certain fluorescence level and this ratio is used to calculate target abundance using Poisson-statistics. Therefore, determining a correct threshold is crucial for reliable quantification (Fig. 1). Defining a threshold is complicated by droplets with an intermediate fluorescence, termed as rain, which are puzzling to assign to the either positive or negative population. For the frequently used Bio-Rad ddPCR system, the QuantaSoft software offers an undisclosed method for automated threshold assignment and manual threshold setting by the end-user. The automated analysis often assigns thresholds so strict that a cloud of droplets is appointed positive that based on their low fluorescence is expected to be negative [16]. Alternatively, user-defined thresholds may be applied but these are generally not advised as they impair an unbiased interpretation of digital PCR data. Threshold setting can be challenging since the separation between positive and negative droplets may depend on many factors, such as the quality and

quantity of the input sample, melting temperature and length of primers and probe, mismatches between the assay and target sequences, time between droplet generation and readout, pipetting precision, type of fluorescent reporter and type of quencher. Several algorithms have been developed by end-users that aim to offer more data-driven approaches to set thresholds. First, clustering methods were developed by Strain et al. and Jones et al. based on k-nearest neighbor-joining [17, 18]. The method of Strain et al. defines the median and variance of the negative and positive clouds to assess the statistical likelihood that outliers should be included in either cloud ($p < 0.1$). Jones et al. developed "definetherain" that uses negative and positive control samples to identify the two clouds. Subsequently, the mean fluorescence minus or plus three times its standard deviation is used as thresholds that are applied to the samples. Both these clustering methods calculate a threshold for each cloud of droplets and exclude intermediate fluorescent droplets from further analysis. In contrast, Dreo et al. proposed a single threshold determination method since droplets with intermediate fluorescence intensity can hold true positive droplets [19, 20]. This global manual threshold is defined as the mean fluorescence signal in the NTCs (no template controls) plus a number of standard deviations until one positive droplet remains in the NTCs [19]. These described methods assume a normal (binomial) distribution of the negative and positive clouds and do not account for shifts in baseline fluorescence between droplet populations of different samples. However, distribution fitting experiments and normality testing shows that droplet clouds do not follow a normal distribution and cannot be described by a single family of distributions. Furthermore, baseline fluorescence of the negative cloud has been shown to vary between samples and influence quantification [16]. Therefore, an alternative

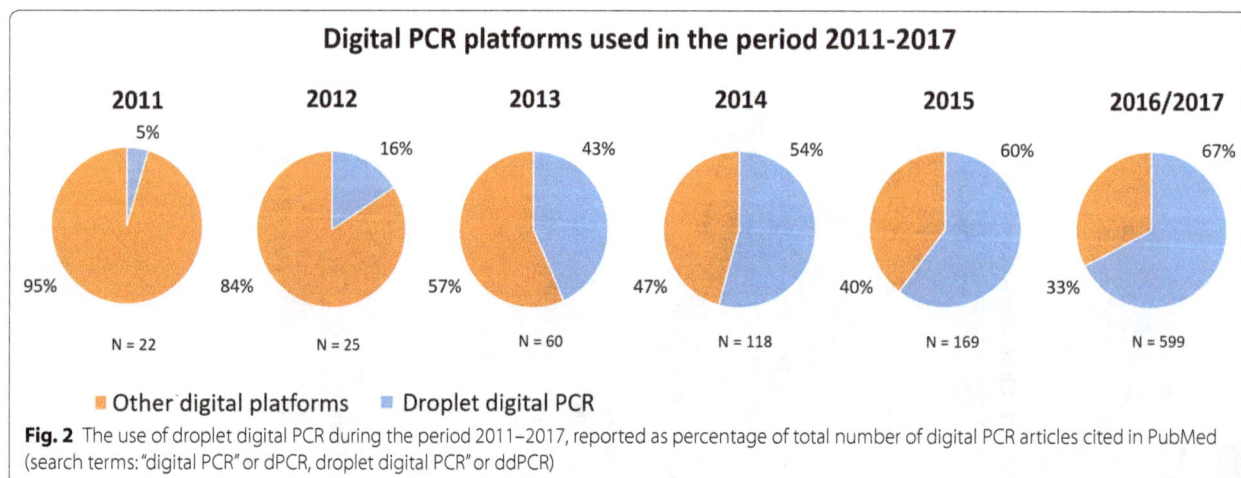

Fig. 2 The use of droplet digital PCR during the period 2011–2017, reported as percentage of total number of digital PCR articles cited in PubMed (search terms: "digital PCR" or dPCR, droplet digital PCR" or ddPCR)

thresholding method was devised by Trypsteen et al. [16] that assigns a threshold regardless of the many factors that may affect the intensity and distribution of droplet fluorescence. This method, ddpcRquant, feeds data from negative controls to a generalized extreme value model and applies this threshold to the samples. The algorithm does not make assumptions of the underlying distribution of the droplet populations and accounts for baseline shifts. Alternatively, Lievens et al. [20] determine the threshold based on the shape of the fluorescence density peaks but to account for the possibility that clouds are not normally distributed set the threshold above the uppermost limit of the negative cloud. Recently, a novel method, "Umbrella", was published that does not apply hard thresholding, but applies a model-based clustering and takes partition-specific classification probabilities into account to produce a final quantification result [21]. Threshold setting remains a challenging but crucial task. It is difficult to establish whether or not intermediate droplets represent true targets that should be used for analysis, since the current generation of ddPCR is not fitted with a fluorescence intensity sorter to allow for target confirmation by for example sequencing. Recent evidence however suggests that intermediate droplets should be considered to contain target molecules, as decreased amplification efficiency may arise from a suboptimal annealing temperature [22] or mismatches between the assay and the target sequence [16]. Furthermore, several studies that investigated ddPCR sensitivity have used a user-defined threshold that allocates rain to the positive fraction of droplets, and doing so have found results that are on par with the input reference and qPCR results [11, 20, 23, 24].

False-positives

Regardless of the method that is used to assign a threshold, currently available digital PCR platforms including the QX200 suffer from the observation of false-positive partitions and therefore false-positive results [11, 16, 18, 23–25]. One out of three wells of negative controls with no template had 2 or 3 positive droplets (0.16–0.22 copies/reaction) for HIV-1 RNA assay described by Kiselinova et al. [23]. These droplets had a similar fluorescence level as positive droplets in patients samples. The origin of these errors remains unclear and various hypotheses have been proposed. False-positive droplets can arise from contaminations or disturbed droplets that merge together, their joint fluorescence leading to a droplet with a higher baseline fluorescence that is miscalled as positive.

False-positive droplets can pose a threat to reliable HIV DNA quantification in settings with low HIV DNA concentrations such as mother-to-child transmission, early treatment initiation and allogeneic stem cell transplantation (alloSCT). AlloSCT is currently the only known approach by which the HIV reservoir can be drastically reduced. Following a successful stem cell transplantation, patients are kept on ART and are monitored for HIV DNA levels, but reliable ascertainment of remainder HIV DNA is a challenge, especially when the interpretation of true-positive droplets is obscured by false-positive ones. Same holds true for ART-treated children, which may have initiated ART early after birth based on the HIV-status of their mother whereas uncertainty may exist if the infection was transmitted from mother to child. In these seronegative children, HIV DNA is the only proof of HIV infection and therefore the only justification for treatment with ART. However, confirmation of the presence of HIV DNA is challenging since patients who initiated ART early after infection are known to have small reservoirs and sample volumes are restricted in case of young children, which reduces the statistical power to assess the presence of HIV DNA. Therefore, false-positives can unrightfully lead to confirmation of HIV infection and continuation of ART and it is not advised to use digital PCR if the question is to discriminate between presence or absence of HIV DNA [11]. Since only a minor fraction of all potential CD4 positive target cells carry HIV DNA, a large number of cells need to be tested in order to be able to reliably quantify HIV DNA concentrations. High concentrations of total DNA however affect the viscosity of the aqueous phase and complicate the formation of droplets. The amount of DNA that can be loaded into a single reaction is therefore restricted [18, 26]. Researchers who aim to report an HIV DNA concentration in a million CD4-cells are required to split the target DNA among a number of reactions, thereby increasing the risk of detecting false-positive droplets and influencing final HIV DNA concentration outcome. This effect is even greater when samples are used in which HIV DNA is even less abundant, such as PBMCs, whole blood, dried blood spots or tissue biopsies.

Advantages

Apart from the issue of false-positives, digital PCR has shown to be equal or superior to qPCR in several aspects. One major advantage is that digital PCR produces direct absolute quantification. The absolute quantification results produced by digital PCR eliminate the need for a standard curve in case of DNA quantifications and comparisons of RNA quantifications. Of note, RNA quantification represents cDNA molecules and should therefore be corrected for cDNA synthesis efficiency [27]. Accurate quantification by qPCR is based on the quality of the standard curve: instability of the standard curve can lead to inaccurate HIV DNA quantification

[28]. Additionally, Cq values in qPCR that arise from the standard and the samples are based on amplification efficiencies, and several factors may confound their correct interpretation. Amplification efficiency may be affected by inhibitors, amount of total DNA that is loaded as well as variation between the primer/probe and the patient's viral sequence, and these factors may unrightfully elevate the Cq values. In qPCR, such mismatches would increase the Cq and in turn present a target abundance that is lower than the actual input. In ddPCR however, a reduced amplification efficiency leads to less fluorescence at end-point. As long as end-point fluorescence remains above the assigned threshold and the ratio between positive and negative fraction of droplets is unaltered, mismatches between assay and target are allowed as they do not affect the quantification outcome [16, 29, 30]. Tolerance to target sequence variation is especially crucial for HIV quantification as a higher chance of mismatches with the primer–probe set is to be expected due to high heterogeneity of the virus [31]. Besides the robustness of ddPCR with respect to inhibition and reduced amplification efficiency, a higher precision and reproducibility was observed for ddPCR in comparison to qPCR [18, 32]. This is especially crucial in HIV cure efforts where the aim is to detect potential effects of the interventions on the HIV reservoir. However, it is important to note here that contradicting findings have been published that observed a higher sensitivity of the qPCR platform [23, 33]. In duplex digital PCR experiments on linked targets, a minority of partitions was observed in which only one out of two assays demonstrated amplification [34]. It remains however unclear whether this observation is artificial due to DNA shearing and physical separation of supposed linked targets, or genuine failure to amplify due to assay-specific inhibitors, DNA degradation or tertiary structures. Furthermore, in case of genuine failure to amplify it is currently unclear whether this potential mode of target underestimation pertains to digital PCR alone or if similar mechanisms are at play in case of (q) PCR.

Applicability and future perspectives

HIV reservoir measurement by digital PCR has been used to measure the effects of early treatment initiation [35–38], therapeutic vaccination [39–41], allogenic stem cell transplantation [42], structured treatment interruptions [40, 43], immunization by broadly neutralizing antibodies [44], latency reversing agents (LRA's) [41, 45–49], and other novel therapeutic agents [50–52]. The concept of digital PCR is well-established but automated platforms and implementations in HIV quantification are relatively recent and the field is looking forward to future

advancements. Where some platforms limit the number of specialized devices needed (CONSTELLATION® Digital PCR System microplate from Formulatrix), other companies are working on a multiplex system up to 6 colors (Naica system from Stilla) or enable the analysis of multiple samples in a single run (QX200 from Bio-Rad). The combination of these features combined in a single device with a high-throughput workflow and elaborate multiplex system is desired. In addition, data analysis and threshold setting should be further developed in order to keep up with advances in multiplexing. Considering the observed false-positive partitions in current digital PCR platforms, quality control of the partitions is crucial. Naica system from Stilla currently allows visual inspection of the size and geometry of a single crystal droplet and the exclusion of those that are aberrant. The QX200 digital PCR platform may benefit from an integrated fluorescence sorter for post-PCR analysis of droplets. Such a feature would improve our understanding of the nature of suspected false-positive droplets by allowing post-PCR sequencing to verify if fluorescence is the cause of PCR or rather through the acquisition of fluorescent dust or debris. In addition, post-PCR sorting of single-cell droplets may improve our understanding of the dynamics involved in latency [47]. Yucha et al. demonstrated that the QX200 cartridge can be used to create single-cell-droplets, after which HIV RNA was quantified using standard digital PCR protocol. Using a blunt needle, they manually selected positive droplets for post-PCR sequencing of HIV ENV and human CCR5, and future experiments may even investigate HIV integration site or viral protein production. This holistic approach to HIV latency research holds great promise, yet requires specialized equipment and trained personnel and would therefore benefit from a fluorescence sorter that is integrated into the QX200 reader. Although digital PCR allows the precise quantification of HIV DNA and RNA in patients, it does not enable researchers to gain information about the replication-competence of the reservoir. Whereas the cell culture based viral outgrowth assay is an underestimation of the true viral reservoir, HIV measured by PCR is an overestimation because it counts the non-replication competent viruses as well [53]. Multiplexed ddPCR may however improve our understanding of the gap between viral outgrowth and PCR-based assays. Anderson et al. [54] used a multiplexed ddPCR to observe an increase of the LTR:gag ratio during time on treatment, which can be explained by elimination of replication-competent viruses or clonal expansion of non-replication competent viruses. Additionally, multiplexed ddPCR could aid in determining the number of times an HIV sequence has been clonally expanded. Clonal expansion and its specific HIV integration site is an international focus point since it is linked to persistence of HIV-infected cells [55]. However, integration site analysis is laborious and expensive but designing a multiplex ddPCR that targets HIV and the human sequence adjacent to HIV, clonal expansion of that specific HIV sequence can be calculated based on the increase of double-positive droplets relative to expected number based on chance [56]. In summary, digital PCR has proven to be a valuable new technology and with additional improvements in prospect it is likely to mature into an indispensable tool in future HIV research.

Abbreviations
ART: antiretroviral therapy; ddPCR: droplet digital PCR; qPCR: real-time PCR; LRA: latency reversing agent.

Authors' contributions
SR, KB, MN and LV discussed and decided on the outline of the review. SR performed the digital platform investigations and subsequent table. SR and WT made the figures. KB focused on challenges of ddPCR under guidance of MN and WT. SR was responsible for the cohesiveness and final form under guidance of LV. All authors read and approved the final manuscript.

Author details
¹ HIV Cure Research Center, Department of Internal Medicine, Ghent University, Ghent, Belgium. ² Department of Medical Microbiology, Virology, UMC Utrecht, Utrecht, The Netherlands.

Acknowledgements
Not applicable.

Competing interests
The authors declare that they have no competing interests.

Funding
L. Vandekerckhove is funded by the Research Foundation Flanders (FWO 1.8.020.09.N.00). S. Rutsaert received a strategic basic research fund of the Research Foundation Flanders (FWO, 1S32916N). K. Bosman and M. Nijhuis received funding from Aidsfonds Project (P-2013034) and amfAR ARCHE (Grant-ID109552-61-RSRL) (IciStem). M. Nijhuis is funded by Aidsfonds Project (P-13204). The authors have no other relevant affiliations or financial involvement with any organization or entity with a financial interest in or financial conflict with the subject matter or materials discussed in the manuscript apart from those disclosed. No writing assistance was utilized in the production of this manuscript.

References
1. Chun T-W, Stuyver L, Mizell SB, Ehler LA, Mican JAM, Baseler M, et al. Presence of an inducible HIV-1 latent reservoir during highly active antiretroviral therapy. Proc Natl Acad Sci. 1997;94:13193–7.
2. Hindson BJ, Ness KD, Masquelier DA, Belgrader P, Heredia NJ, Makarewicz AJ, et al. High-throughput droplet digital PCR system for absolute quantitation of DNA copy number. Anal Chem. 2011;83:8604–10.
3. Ruano G, Kidd KK, Stephens JC. Haplotype of multiple polymorphisms resolved by enzymatic amplification of single DNA molecules. Proc Natl Acad Sci USA. 1990;87:6296–300.
4. Saiki RK, Gelfand DH, Stoffel S, Scharf SJ, Higuchi R, et al. Primer-directed enzymatic amplification of dna with a thermostable DNA polymerase. Sci Wash. 1988;239:487.
5. Sykes PJ, Neoh SH, Brisco MJ, Hughes E, Condon J, Morley AA. Quantitation of targets for PCR by use of limiting dilution. Biotechniques. 1992;13:444–9.
6. Simmonds P, Balfe P, Peutherer JF, Ludlam CA, Bishop JO, Brown AJ. Human immunodeficiency virus-infected individuals contain provirus in small numbers of peripheral mononuclear cells and at low copy numbers. J Virol. 1990;64:864–72.
7. Vogelstein B, Kinzler KW. Digital PCR. Proc Natl Acad Sci. 1999;96:9236–41.
8. Agosto LM, Yu JJ, Dai J, Kaletsky R, Monie D, O'Doherty U. HIV-1 integrates into resting CD4 + T cells even at low inoculums as demonstrated with an improved assay for HIV-1 integration. Virology. 2007;368:60–72.
9. Spiegelaere WD, Malatinkova E, Lynch L, Nieuwerburgh FV, Messiaen P, O'Doherty U, et al. Quantification of integrated HIV DNA by repetitive-sampling Alu-HIV PCR on the basis of poisson statistics. Clin Chem. 2014;60:886–95.
10. Pinheiro LB, Coleman VA, Hindson CM, Herrmann J, Hindson BJ, Bhat S, et al. Evaluation of a droplet digital polymerase chain reaction format for DNA copy number quantification. Anal Chem. 2012;84:1003–11.
11. Bosman KJ, Nijhuis M, van Ham PM, Wensing AMJ, Vervisch K, Vandekerckhove L, et al. Comparison of digital PCR platforms and semi-nested qPCR as a tool to determine the size of the HIV reservoir. Sci Rep. 2015;5:13811.
12. Lee H, Park Y-M, We Y-M, Han DJ, Seo J-W, Moon H, et al. Evaluation of digital PCR as a technique for monitoring acute rejection in kidney transplantation. Genom Inform. 2017;15:2–10.
13. Madic J, Zocevic A, Senlis V, Fradet E, Andre B, Muller S, et al. Three-color crystal digital PCR. Biomol Detect Quantif. 2016;10:34–46.
14. Papić B, Pate M, Henigman U, Zajc U, Gruntar I, Biasizzo M, et al. New approaches on quantification of Campylobacter jejuni in poultry samples: the use of digital PCR and real-time PCR against the ISO standard plate count method. Front Microbiol. 2017;8:331.
15. Wang Y, Tsang JYS, Cui Y, Cui J, Lin Y, Zhao S, et al. Robust and accurate digital measurement for HER2 amplification in HER2 equivocal breast cancer diagnosis. Sci Rep. 2017;7:6752.
16. Trypsteen W, Vynck M, Neve JD, Bonczkowski P, Kiselinova M, Malatinkova E, et al. ddpcRquant: threshold determination for single channel droplet digital PCR experiments. Anal Bioanal Chem. 2015;407:5827–34.
17. Jones M, Williams J, Gärtner K, Phillips R, Hurst J, Frater J. Low copy target detection by droplet digital PCR through application of a novel open access bioinformatic pipeline, 'definetherain'. J Virol Methods. 2014;202:46–53.
18. Strain MC, Lada SM, Luong T, Rought SE, Gianella S, Terry VH, et al. Highly precise measurement of HIV DNA by droplet digital PCR. PLoS ONE. 2013;8:e55943.
19. Dreo T, Pirc M, Ramšak Ž, Pavšič J, Milavec M, Žel J, et al. Optimising droplet digital PCR analysis approaches for detection and quantification of bacteria: a case study of fire blight and potato brown rot. Anal Bioanal Chem. 2014;406:6513–28.
20. Lievens A, Jacchia S, Kagkli D, Savini C, Querci M. Measuring digital PCR quality: performance parameters and their optimization. PLoS ONE. 2016;11:e0153317.
21. Jacobs BKM, Goetghebeur E, Vandesompele J, De Ganck A, Nijs N, Beckers A, et al. Model-based classification for digital PCR: your umbrella for rain. Anal Chem. 2017;89:4461–7.
22. Taylor SC, Carbonneau J, Shelton DN, Boivin G. Optimization of droplet digital PCR from RNA and DNA extracts with direct comparison to RT-qPCR: clinical implications for quantification of Oseltamivir-resistant subpopulations. J Virol Methods. 2015;224:58–66.

23. Kiselinova M, Pasternak AO, De Spiegelaere W, Vogelaers D, Berkhout B, Vandekerckhove L. Comparison of droplet digital PCR and seminested real-time PCR for quantification of cell-associated HIV-1 RNA. PLoS ONE. 2014;9:e85999.

24. Henrich TJ, Gallien S, Li JZ, Pereyra F, Kuritzkes DR. Low-level detection and quantitation of cellular HIV-1 DNA and 2-LTR circles using droplet digital PCR. J Virol Methods. 2012;186:68–72.

25. Vynck M, Trypsteen W, Thas O, Vandekerckhove L, De Spiegelaere W. The future of digital polymerase chain reaction in virology. Mol Diagn Ther. 2016;20:437–47.

26. Malatinkova E, Kiselinova M, Bonczkowski P, Trypsteen W, Messiaen P, Vermeire J, et al. Accurate quantification of episomal HIV-1 two-long terminal repeat circles by use of optimized DNA isolation and droplet digital PCR. J Clin Microbiol. 2015;53:699–701.

27. Sanders R, Mason DJ, Foy CA, Huggett JF. Evaluation of digital PCR for absolute RNA quantification. PLoS ONE. 2013;8:e75296.

28. Busby E, Whale AS, Ferns RB, Grant PR, Morley G, Campbell J, et al. Instability of 8E5 calibration standard revealed by digital PCR risks inaccurate quantification of HIV DNA in clinical samples by qPCR. Sci Rep. 2017;7:1209.

29. Dingle TC, Sedlak RH, Cook L, Jerome KR. Tolerance of droplet-digital PCR vs real-time quantitative PCR to inhibitory substances. Clin Chem. 2013;59:1670–2.

30. Taylor SC, Laperriere G, Germain H. Droplet Digital PCR versus qPCR for gene expression analysis with low abundant targets: from variable nonsense to publication quality data. Sci Rep. 2017;7:2409.

31. McNearney T, Hornickova Z, Markham R, Birdwell A, Arens M, Saah A, et al. Relationship of human immunodeficiency virus type 1 sequence heterogeneity to stage of disease. Proc Natl Acad Sci USA. 1992;89:10247–51.

32. Hindson CM, Chevillet JR, Briggs HA, Gallichotte EN, Ruf IK, Hindson BJ, et al. Absolute quantification by droplet digital PCR versus analog real-time PCR. Nat Methods. 2013;10:1003–5.

33. Hayden RT, Gu Z, Ingersoll J, Abdul-Ali D, Shi L, Pounds S, et al. Comparison of droplet digital PCR to real-time PCR for quantitative detection of cytomegalovirus. J Clin Microbiol. 2013;51:540–6.

34. Whale AS, Cowen S, Foy CA, Huggett JF. Methods for applying accurate digital PCR analysis on low copy DNA samples. PLoS ONE. 2013;8:e58177.

35. Malatinkova E, Spiegelaere WD, Bonczkowski P, Kiselinova M, Vervisch K, Trypsteen W, et al. Impact of a decade of successful antiretroviral therapy initiated at HIV-1 seroconversion on blood and rectal reservoirs. eLife. 2015;4:e09115.

36. Buzon MJ, Martin-Gayo E, Pereyra F, Ouyang Z, Sun H, Li JZ, et al. Long-term antiretroviral treatment initiated at primary HIV-1 infection affects the size, composition, and decay kinetics of the reservoir of HIV-1-infected CD4 T cells. J Virol. 2014;88:10056–65.

37. Henrich TJ, Hatano H, Bacon O, Hogan LE, Rutishauser R, Hill A, et al. HIV-1 persistence following extremely early initiation of antiretroviral therapy (ART) during acute HIV-1 infection: an observational study. PLOS Med. 2017;14:e1002417.

38. Oliveira MF, Chaillon A, Nakazawa M, Vargas M, Letendre SL, Strain MC, et al. Early antiretroviral therapy is associated with lower HIV DNA molecular diversity and lower inflammation in cerebrospinal fluid but does not prevent the establishment of compartmentalized HIV DNA populations. PLoS Pathog. 2017;13:e1006112.

39. Hancock G, Morón-López S, Kopycinski J, Puertas MC, Giannoulatou E, Rose A, et al. Evaluation of the immunogenicity and impact on the latent HIV-1 reservoir of a conserved region vaccine, MVA. HIVconsv, in antiretroviral therapy-treated subjects. J Int AIDS Soc. 2017;20:21171.

40. Rosás-Umbert M, Mothe B, Noguera-Julian M, Bellido R, Puertas MC, Carrillo J, et al. Virological and immunological outcome of treatment interruption in HIV-1-infected subjects vaccinated with MVA-B. PLoS ONE. 2017;12:e0184929.

41. Mothe B, Climent N, Plana M, Rosàs M, Jiménez JL, Muñoz-Fernández MÁ, et al. Safety and immunogenicity of a modified vaccinia Ankara-based HIV-1 vaccine (MVA-B) in HIV-1-infected patients alone or in combination with a drug to reactivate latent HIV-1. J Antimicrob Chemother. 2015;70:1833–42.

42. Cummins NW, Rizza S, Litzow MR, Hua S, Lee GQ, Einkauf K, et al. Extensive virologic and immunologic characterization in an HIV-infected individual following allogeneic stem cell transplant and analytic cessation of antiretroviral therapy: a case study. PLoS Med. 2017;14:e1002461.

43. ISALA. Analytical treatment interruption in HIV positive patients (ISALA). https://clinicaltrials.gov. NCT02590354.

44. Chun T-W, Murray D, Justement JS, Blazkova J, Hallahan CW, Fankuchen O, et al. Broadly neutralizing antibodies suppress HIV in the persistent viral reservoir. Proc Natl Acad Sci USA. 2014;111:13151–6.

45. Vibholm L, Schleimann MH, Højen JF, Benfield T, Offersen R, Rasmussen K, et al. Short-course toll-like receptor 9 agonist treatment impacts innate immunity and plasma viremia in individuals with human immunodeficiency virus infection. Clin Infect Dis. 2017;64:1686–95.

46. Rasmussen TA, Tolstrup M, Brinkmann CR, Olesen R, Erikstrup C, Solomon A, et al. Panobinostat, a histone deacetylase inhibitor, for latent-virus reactivation in HIV-infected patients on suppressive antiretroviral therapy: a phase 1/2, single group, clinical trial. Lancet HIV. 2014;1:e13–21.

47. Yucha RW, Hobbs KS, Hanhauser E, Hogan LE, Nieves W, Ozen MO, et al. High-throughput characterization of HIV-1 reservoir reactivation using a single-cell-in-droplet PCR assay. EBioMedicine. 2017;20:217–29.

48. Margolis DM, Archin NM. Proviral latency, persistent human immunodeficiency virus infection, and the development of latency reversing agents. J Infect Dis. 2017;215(suppl3):S111–8.

49. Søgaard OS, Graversen ME, Leth S, Olesen R, Brinkmann CR, Nissen SK, et al. The depsipeptide romidepsin reverses HIV-1 latency in vivo. PLoS Pathog. 2015;11:e1005142.

50. Paredes R, Vandekerkchove L, Clotet B, Moutchen M, De Wit S, Podzamczer D, et al. ABX464 decreases total HIV DNA in PBMC's when administered during 28 days to HIV-infected patients who are virologically suppressed. In: 9th IAS conference HIV Sci IAS 2017, Paris, France.

51. Bialek JK, Dunay GA, Voges M, Schäfer C, Spohn M, Stucka R, et al. Targeted HIV-1 latency reversal using CRISPR/Cas9-derived transcriptional activator systems. PLoS ONE. 2016;11:e0158294.

52. Tebas P, Stein D, Tang WW, Frank I, Wang SQ, Lee G, et al. Gene editing of CCR5 in autologous CD4 T cells of persons infected with HIV. N Engl J Med. 2014;370:901–10.

53. Ho Y-C, Shan L, Hosmane NN, Wang J, Laskey SB, Rosenbloom DIS, et al. Replication-competent non-induced proviruses in the latent reservoir increase barrier to HIV-1 cure. Cell. 2013;155:540–51.

54. Anderson E, Hill S, Bell J, Simonetti FR, Rehm C, Jones S, et al. Accumulation and persistence of deleted HIV proviruses following prolonged ART. In: 9th IAS Conference HIV Sci IAS 2017, MOAA0102 Paris, France.

55. Maldarelli F, Wu X, Su L, Simonetti FR, Shao W, Hill S, et al. Specific HIV integration sites are linked to clonal expansion and persistence of infected cells. Science. 2014;345:179–83.

56. Regan JF, Kamitaki N, Legler T, Cooper S, Klitgord N, Karlin-Neumann G, et al. A rapid molecular approach for chromosomal phasing. PLoS ONE. 2015;10:e0118270.

17

Potent suppression of HIV-1 cell attachment by Kudzu root extract

S. Mediouni[1†], J. A. Jablonski[1†], S. Tsuda[1], A. Richard[1], C. Kessing[1], M. V. Andrade[4], A. Biswas[1], Y. Even[3], T. Tellinghuisen[1,5], H. Choe[1], M. Cameron[2], M. Stevenson[4] and S. T. Valente[1*]

Abstract

There is a constant need to improve antiretrovirals against HIV since therapy is limited by cost, side effects and the emergence of drug resistance. Kudzu is a climbing vine from which the root extract (*Pueraria lobata*), rich in isoflavones and saponins, has long been used in traditional Chinese medicine for a variety of purposes, from weight loss to alcoholism prevention. Here we show that Kudzu root extract significantly inhibits HIV-1 entry into cell lines, primary human CD4$^+$T lymphocytes and macrophages, without cell-associated toxicity. Specifically, Kudzu inhibits the initial attachment of the viral particle to the cell surface, a mechanism that depends on the envelope glycoprotein gp120 but is independent from the HIV-1 cell receptor CD4 and co-receptors CXCR4/CCR5. This activity seems selective to lentiviruses since Kudzu inhibits HIV-2 and simian immunodeficiency virus, but does not interfere with Hepatitis C, Influenza, Zika Brazil and adenovirus infection. Importantly, depending on the dose, Kudzu can act synergistically or additively with the current antiretroviral cocktails against HIV-1 and can block viruses resistant to the fusion inhibitor Enfuvirtide. Together our results highlight Kudzu's root extract value as a supplement to current antiretroviral therapy against HIV.

Background

Current human immunodeficiency virus (HIV) antiretroviral therapy (ART) has dramatically benefited HIV-1 infected individuals, by reducing circulating virus to very low levels; however, it fails to completely eliminate infection and the emergence of drug resistance is an ongoing problem [1, 2]. It is highly desirable to develop additional anti-HIV-1 agents with superior efficacy and safety profiles.

HIV entry into target cells is a multistep process. The envelope glycoprotein is composed of the surface gp120 and the transmembrane gp41. The gp120 first attaches to the target cell through interactions with the negatively charged cell-surface heparan sulfate proteoglycans [3], α4β7 integrins [4, 5], the dendritic cell–specific intercellular adhesion molecular 3-grabbing non-integrin (DC-SIGN) [6] or the mannose binding C-type lectin receptors

(MCLR) [7]. These attachment receptors bring gp120/gp41 into close proximity with the virus receptor CD4 and the co-receptors CXCR4 or CCR5 on the cell surface, increasing infection efficiency. Following this initial contact, interaction of gp120 with CD4 induces a conformational change in gp120, exposing the co-receptor binding site to allow interaction with the co-receptors. This also leaves gp41 in an active form, resulting in fusion of virus and cell membranes and release of the nucleocapsid into the cytoplasm [8–10]. Soon after infection, the viral population is mainly composed of R5 strains, defined by their use of the CCR5 co-receptor. As the disease progresses, the R5 strains evolve to dual X4R5 or just X4 strains, defined by their use of the CXCR4 co-receptor.

Virus attachment and fusion (collectively termed "virus entry") have long been the target for drug development against HIV [11, 12]. Only three Food and Drug administration (FDA) approved drugs currently block the entry pathway. Enfuvirtide (Fuzeone) targets the HIV-1 envelope glycoprotein gp41 to prevent viral and host membrane fusion. It is mainly used as salvage therapy in multidrug resistance cases, given that it is dosed

*Correspondence: svalente@scripps.edu
†S. Mediouni and J. A. Jablonski have contributed equally to this work
[1] Department of Immunology and Microbiology, The Scripps Research Institute, 130 Scripps Way, 3C1, Jupiter, FL 33458, USA
Full list of author information is available at the end of the article

twice-daily by subcutaneous injection [13–15]. Maraviroc, is a selective and reversible CCR5 antagonist [16, 17], and genotypic tropism testing for co-receptor usage is usually recommended before administration. Finally, Ibalizumab is an antibody that targets the CD4 receptor. It is administrated intravenously every 2 weeks, approved for multidrug resistant cases [18]. The gp120 is critical for viral entry, but unfortunately drug discovery against this protein has remained unsuccessful so far, possibly due to the incredible ability of this protein of mutating and evading drug-selective pressure.

Natural products have always been a valuable resource for the pharmaceutical industry and have been of great benefit in virtually all-clinical therapeutic areas. Kudzu (also named *Pueraria lobata*, Kudzu vine, foot-a-night vine, vine-that-ate-the-South, and Ko-hemp) belonging to the genus Pueraria, is a fast-growing evergreen vine originating from China. Kudzu was introduced in the United States from Japan at the Philadelphia Centennial Exposition in 1876. Initially it was used as forage crop and ornamental plant, but later in the 1930s, many Southern farmers were encouraged to plant Kudzu for erosion control. Kudzu quickly became invasive, and today an estimated 2 million acres of forestland in the southern United States are covered with Kudzu.

Kudzu's root extract (or radix Pueariae or Gegen) has been traditionally used in Asian countries (since at least 200 BC) as an herbal remedy to treat colds, headaches and diarrhea. The entire plant is edible, however the health supporting benefits of Kudzu comes from its flowers and roots, which contain many natural products including isoflavones and saponins. In Asia, Kudzu root extract is often found in food products, beverages, as well as soaps and lotions as an antimicrobial agent [19, 20]. Recently, in a clinical trial, Kudzu has been found to reduce alcoholism [21]. The chemical composition of Kudzu differs depending on geographic origin and extraction method (Additional file 1: Table 1S) [20, 22, 23]. Chemical analysis of Kudzu root extract revealed several chemical entities including Daidzein (antimicrobial and anti-inflammatory agent), Daidzin (prevents development of cancer), Genistein (anti-bacterial and anti-leukemic agent), and is also a distinct source of the isoflavone puerarin (Additional file 1: Table 1S). Kudzu root extract has also been linked to improvements in glucose metabolism, neuron regeneration, stroke prevention, inflammation, oxidative stress reduction, migraines and cluster headaches reduction [24, 25].

Given the known general antimicrobial activity of Kudzu, we investigated its activity against HIV-1 replication. Here we demonstrate that Kudzu root extract significantly inhibits HIV-1 entry into target cells. Kudzu inhibits both R5 and X4 tropic strains of HIV-1, HIV-2 and simian immunodeficiency virus (SIV). This activity

seems selective since Kudzu has no activity against viruses from other families. Kudzu root extract specifically blocks the attachment of HIV gp120 to the target cell. Importantly, Kudzu acts synergistically or additively depending on the dose, with current cocktails of antiretrovirals (ARVs), and can block viruses resistant to the commercial entry inhibitor, Enfuvirtide. Overall, these results define Kudzu root extract as a potential HIV-1 inhibitor that, combined to ART, could improve therapy outcomes by acting at a novel target site of the viral replication cycle.

Results and discussion
Kudzu extract inhibits HIV-1 replication
HIV-1 susceptibility to Kudzu root extract was assayed using a reporter cell line that stably expresses the β-galactosidase (β-Gal) gene (LacZ) [HeLa-CD4-LTR-LacZ cells]; LacZ expression is driven by the 5′LTR promoter of HIV-1 and responds to Tat expressed by an incoming virus. HeLa-CD4-LTR-LacZ cells were infected with HIV-1 isolate NL4-3 (clade B, X4 tropic), in the presence of increasing dilutions of Kudzu, and β-Gal activity was measured 72 h later (Fig. 1a). The inhibition of Tat-dependent transcription of LacZ was dose-dependent, presenting an IC_{50} of 1:5263 $\pm$ 6 $\times$ 10^{-5} dilution of the Kudzu extract. More than 90% inhibition was observed at dilution 1:1600, a concentration that does not impact HeLa-CD4-LTR-LacZ cells viability (Additional file 1: Fig. 1SA). The IC_{50} of currently used ARVs was included for comparison (Additional file 1: Fig. 2SA).

Kudzu root extract is a tincture comprised of 33% of dried kudzu root and 66% of solvent (a mix of ethanol and glycerol). To verify that Kudzu activity was not aspecifically linked to these solvents, both solutions, at different percentages, were tested in infectivity assays (Additional file 1: Fig. 2SB and C). No viral inhibition was observed at the highest and effective dilution of Kudzu (1:200), which corresponds to 0.3% glycerol or ethanol.

The activity of Kudzu was also assessed by measuring p24 capsid in the supernatant by p24 ELISA, revealing an IC_{50} of 1:1556 (Fig. 1b). The differences in IC_{50} between the β-Gal and p24 ELISA assays most likely reflect the ability of p24 ELISA to detect all p24 production, whether the protein is incorporated into virions or not. Similar results were obtained with Kudzu purchased from another company (data not shown), suggesting that Kudzu's activity is consistent between brands.

Kudzu extract blocks the first steps of HIV-1 entry into target cells
To investigate the mechanism by which Kudzu suppresses HIV-1, we first monitored the integration of proviral DNA into the genome of HeLa-CD4-LTR-LacZ cells 24 h post-infection by Alu-PCR, followed by

quantitative real time PCR (qPCR). Kudzu (1:200) significantly inhibited the integration of proviral HIV DNA, similar to Efavirenz (a reverse transcriptase inhibitor, 200 nM), Raltegravir (an integrase inhibitor, 200 nM) and AMD3100 (a CXCR4 antagonist, 10 nM), used as positive controls. As expected, Saquinavir, a protease inhibitor (200 nM) did not inhibit HIV integration during this 24 h assay (Fig. 1c). Dimethyl sulfoxide (DMSO) was used as negative control since the ARVs are solubilized in 0.001 or 0.002% DMSO. Furthermore, ethanol and glycerol, at the highest concentrations of Kudzu, did not interfere with HIV replication (Additional file 1: Fig. 2SB and C).

To insure Kudzu's activity was not cell line dependent, we also assessed the activity of Kudzu on primary human CD4$^+$T cells isolated from blood of 3 individuals. Cells were infected for 24 h with NL4-3 in the presence of the most potent but non-toxic dilutions of Kudzu (1:400 and 1:200; Additional file 1: Fig. 1SB), or a cocktail of ARVs (Raltegravir 200 nM, Efavirenz 100 nM and AZT 180 nM) or Enfuvirtide (1 μg/ml). Total viral DNA was measured by qPCR (Fig. 1d). Kudzu inhibited the infection of primary human CD4$^+$T cells equally well as Enfuvirtide or a cocktail of ARVs. Together these results suggest that Kudzu activity is not cell type dependent and targets an early event of the HIV-1 life cycle.

We next measured the early and late HIV-1 reverse transcription (RT) products by qPCR 10 h post-infection of HeLa-CD4-LTR-LacZ cells (Fig. 1e). Efavirenz and AMD3100 (200 nM and 10 nM respectively) used as controls, inhibited early RT products by approximately 40% and 60% respectively, while the late RT products were decreased by approximately 84%, consistent with the literature [26]. Treatment of the cells with Kudzu resulted in a similar reduction of early and late RT products to controls (60% and 75% respectively). Saquinavir (200 nM), as expected, did not impact the production of late RT products. Altogether these results suggest that Kudzu inhibits an early event occurring before or at the reverse transcription step.

To further understand which step was blocked by Kudzu, we performed time-of-addition assays as previously described [27], using entry and RT inhibitors as controls. We infected HeLa-CD4-LTR-LacZ cells with NL4-3, then added Kudzu at different time points post-infection (from 1 to 6 h), and measured β-Gal activity 72 h later (Fig. 1f). Both dilutions of Kudzu (1:800 and 1:400) displayed similar inhibitory kinetics to the entry inhibitor AMD3100 (4 nM). When Kudzu or AMD3100 were added 3 h post infection, their inhibitory activity started to decline, showing almost no activity if added 6 h later. As expected, Efavirenz (10 nM) displayed stronger inhibition when added at later time points. These results suggest that Kudzu inhibits the entry step of HIV-1 into the target cell.

Kudzu extract inhibits HIV-1 infection independently of tropism

The interaction between gp120 and CD4, followed by interaction with CXCR4 or CCR5 is determinant for HIV-1 entry into the target cell. To determine if the coreceptors usage is determinant for Kudzu-mediated inhibition of HIV-1, we tested the susceptibility of R5 tropic viruses. We infected GHOST-CCR5 cells with JRCSF or YU2 viruses, in the presence of Kudzu concentrations that did not impact cell viability (1:400 and 1:200; Additional file 1: Fig. 1SC), and assessed p24 in the supernatant 72 h post infection (Fig. 2a). Raltegravir (100 nM) and Emtricitabine (a reverse transcriptase inhibitor, 100 nM) were used as positive controls. We observed a dose-dependent inhibition of both R5 viruses, suggesting that Kudzu inhibits HIV-1 entry independently of coreceptor usage.

(See figure on next page.)

Fig. 1 Kudzu inhibits HIV-1 replication of X4 tropic viruses. **a, b** Activity of Kudzu in acute infection of HeLa-CD4-LTR-LacZ cells with NL4-3. HeLa-CD4-LTR-LacZ cells were infected with HIV-1 NL4-3 strain in the presence of different dilutions of Kudzu. **a** β-Gal activity was measured 72 h later. Untreat.: untreated. The mean ± SD of 5 independent experiments is represented. **b** Viral supernatants recovered 72 h post infection were assayed for their p24 antigen content using a sandwich ELISA kit. Untreat.: untreated. Data is a mean ± SD of 2 independent experiments. **c** Impact of Kudzu on HIV-1 integration. HeLa-CD4-LTR-LacZ were infected with NL4-3 in presence of compounds for 24 h. Next day, DNA was extracted and provirus integration was quantified by Alu-PCR followed by qPCR. Saquinavir (Saq., a protease inhibitor, 200 nM), Efavirenz (Efav., a reverse transcriptase inhibitor, 200 nM), Raltegravir (Ralt., an integrase inhibitor, 200 nM), and AMD3100 (an entry inhibitor, 10 nM) were used as controls. Kudzu was used at 1:200. The mean ± SD of 5 independent experiments is represented. **d** Impact of Kudzu on HIV-1 integration in primary CD4$^+$T cells 24 h post-infection and treatment. A cocktail of antiretrovirals (ARVS: 180 nM AZT, a reverse transcriptase inhibitor, 100 nM Efavirenz and 200 nM Raltegravir) and Enfuvirtide (1 μg/ml) were used as controls. Shown is the mean ± SD of 3 independent experiments. **e** Activity of Kudzu on reverse-transcription products of HIV-1 10 h post-infection. HeLa-CD4-LTR-LacZ were infected with NL4-3 in presence of compounds for 10 h. Next, DNA was extracted and early and late RT products were measured by qPCR. Kudzu was used at 1:200. Error Bars from qPCR (n = 3) ± SD from 2 independent experiments for early products. The mean ± SD of 4 independent experiments is represented for late products. **f** Time-of-addition experiment of kudzu in HeLa-CD4-LTR-LacZ infected with NL4-3 strain. Kudzu or control compounds (4 nM AMD3100 and 10 nM Efavirenz) were added at 1, 2, 3, 4, 5 and 6 h postinfection. β-Gal activity was measured 72 h later. Data shown is representative of 2 independent experiments. The two-tailed paired *t* test was used for statistical comparisons. *: *p* value < 0.05, ***: *p* value < 0.0005

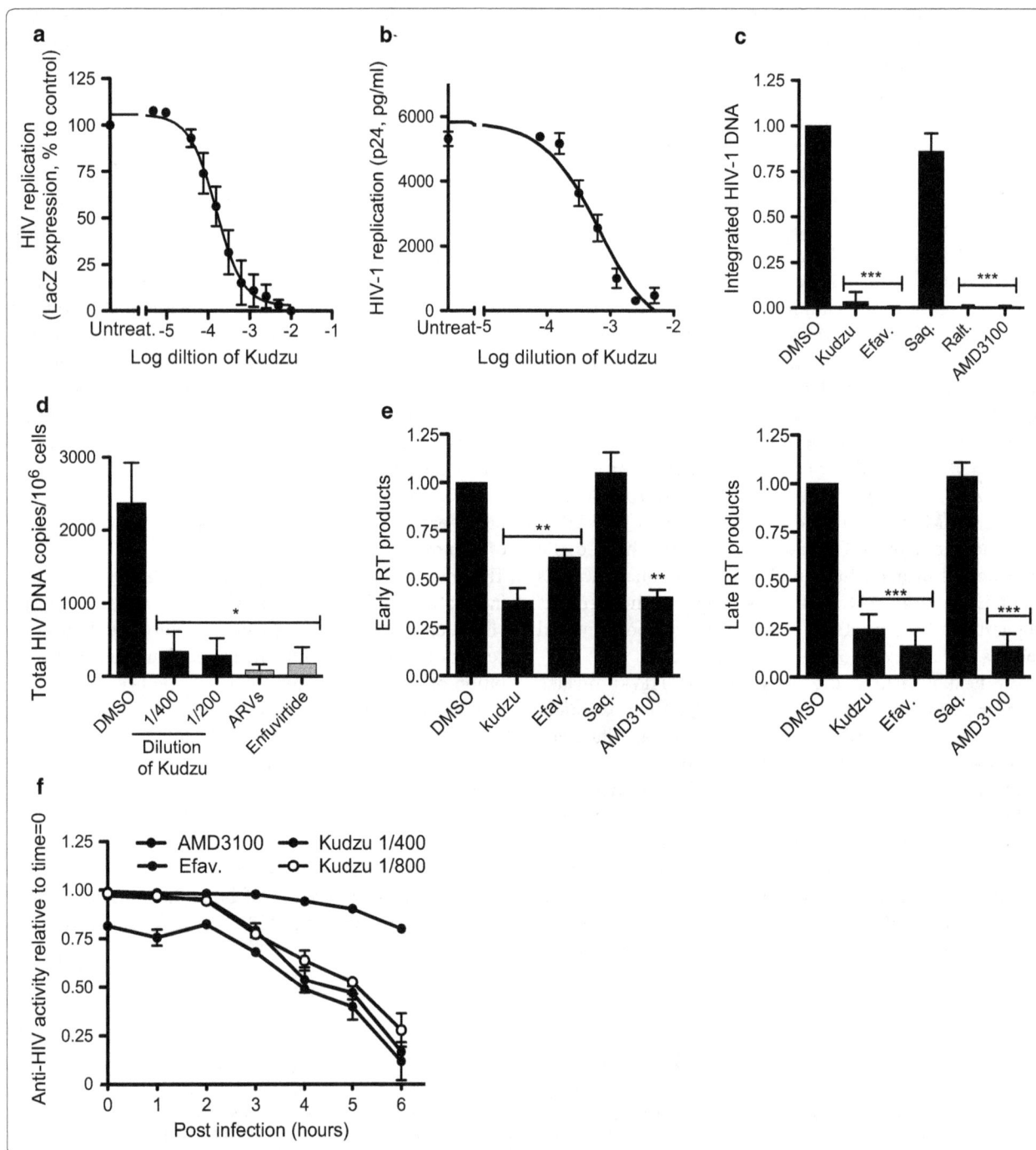

(See figure on next page.)
Fig. 2 Kudzu blocks HIV-1 replication of R5 tropic viruses. **a** Activity of Kudzu on acute replication of GHOST-CCR5 cells with JRCSF and YU2 viruses. Cells were infected with both viruses in presence of 2 potent dilutions of Kudzu. Viral supernatants recovered 72 h post-infection from cells were assayed for their p24 antigen content. Raltegravir (Ralt, an integrase inhibitor, 100 nM) and Emtricitabine (Emt., a reverse transcriptase inhibitor, 100 nM) were used as controls. The mean ± SD of 2 independent experiments is shown. **b** Impact of Kudzu on acute replication of primary Human macrophages infected with macrophage-tropic stains ADA and 5002 M. Cells were infected with both viruses in presence of 1:100 dilution of Kudzu or 5 µg/ml of Enfurvirtide (a fusion inhibitor). Viral supernatants recovered at different times post-infection were assayed for their p24 antigen content

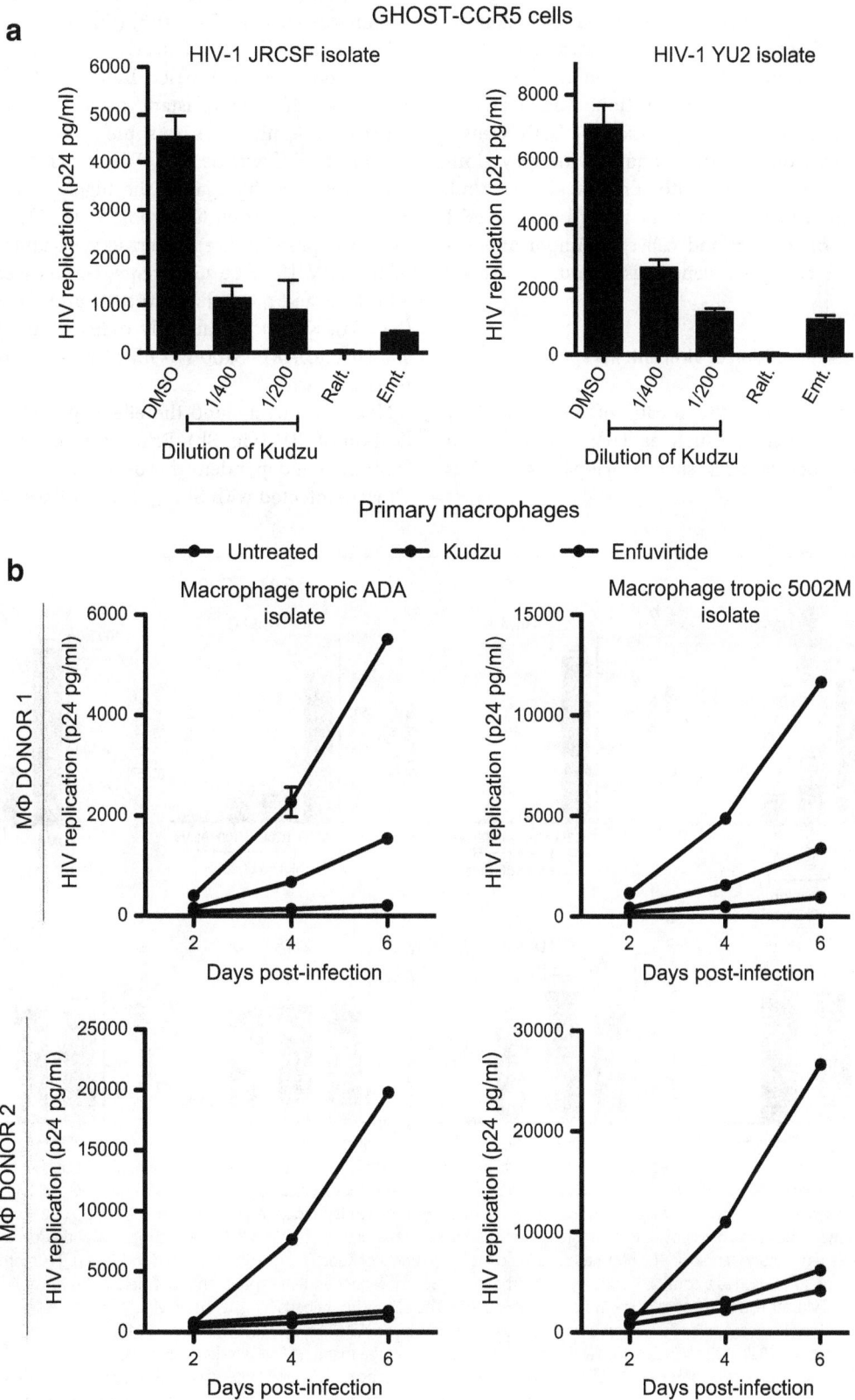

Next, we assessed the susceptibility of Kudzu against infection of primary macrophages from two donors, using two R5 macrophages tropic viruses (ADA and 5002 M). We measured p24 production in the supernatant at different times post-infection. Kudzu (1:100) drastically inhibited HIV-1 replication of both viruses in macrophages from the two donors, with very similar kinetics as the fusion inhibitor Enfuvirtide (5 µg/ml, Fig. 2b). In sum, Kudzu seems to be able to block HIV-1 independently of tropism and cell type, important features as HIV-1 changes receptor usage during disease progression.

Kudzu-mediated inhibition of viral entry is specific to lentiviruses

We set out to evaluate the breath of Kudzu activity against other lentiviruses such as HIV-2 and SIV or viruses from other families such as Hepatitis C virus

(HCV), Influenza A (H1N1), Zika virus (Zika Brazil) and adenovirus serotype 5 (ADV5) (Fig. 3).

HIV-2, initially found in West Africa, has spread to Europe, other parts of Africa, India and the United States. HIV-2 is naturally resistant to nonnucleoside reverse transcriptase inhibitors, to some protease inhibitors [28, 29] and to Enfuvirtide [30]. We assessed Kudzu's (1:300 and 1:150) activity against the highly cytopathic isolate HIV-2 CBL-20 strain (X4 tropic virus) [31], using TZM-bl cells expressing the luciferase gene under the control of the HIV LTR. Luminescence counts were quantified 48 h later and normalized to total protein concentration (Fig. 3a). Kudzu significantly reduced HIV-2 replication similarly to AMD3100 (10 nM) or Raltegravir (100 nM) used as controls.

Next, we investigated the effect of Kudzu on the replication of SIV (Fig. 3b). Primary macaque CD4[+]T cells from three independent rhesus macaques (RhM A, B and C) were infected with $SIV_{mac}239$. Six days post-infection,

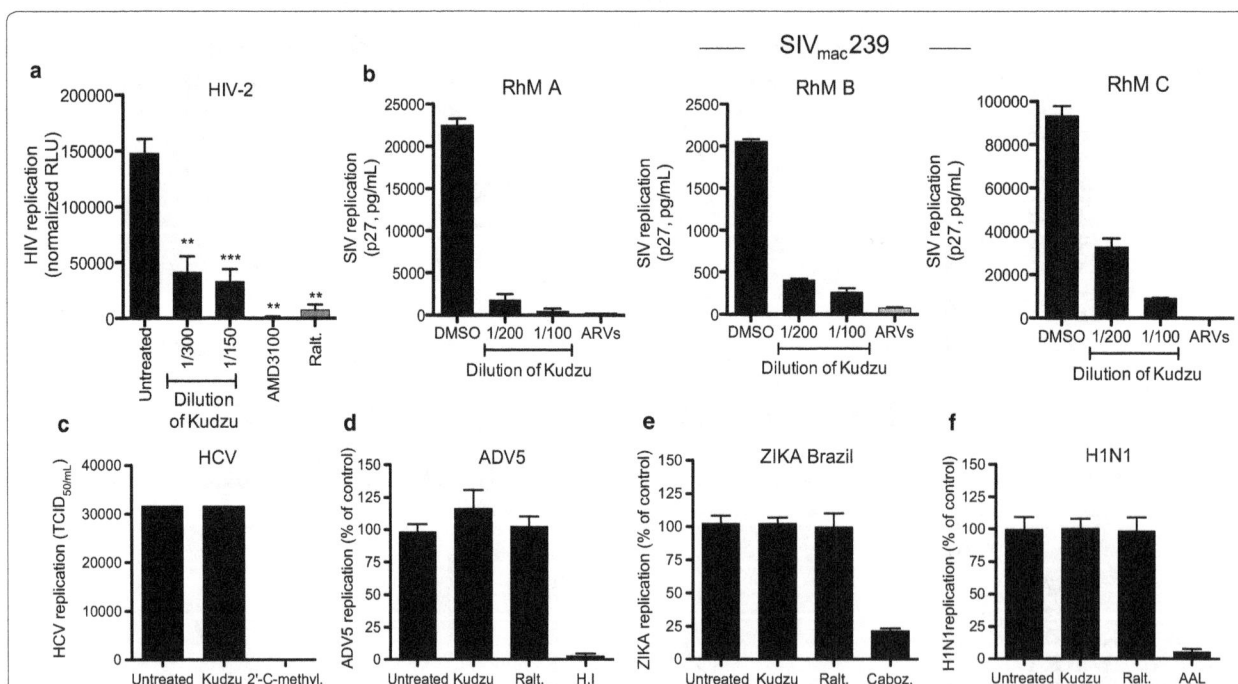

Fig. 3 Activity of Kudzu on diverse viruses. **a** Activity of Kudzu in acute infection of TZM-bl with HIV-2 CBL-20 strain. TZM-bl cells were infected with HIV-2 in presence of different concentrations of Kudzu for 24 h. Luminescence normalized to total protein was measured 48 h later. AMD3100 and Raltegravir used at 10 nM and 100 nM respectively. Data is the mean ± SD of 3 independent experiments. **b** Activity of Kudzu on SIV-infected primary rhesus macaque cells 6 days post-infection. Virus in the supernatant measured by capsid p27 ELISA. A cocktail of antiretrovirals (ARVs, Emtracitabine, Raltegravir and Tenofovir, 200 nM) was used as control. **c** No effect of Kudzu on HCV infection in Huh 7.5 cells. 2′-Cmethyladenosine (2′-C-methyl., 10 µM) was used as a control. Results represent the mean ± SD of 2 independent experiments. **d–f** Hela-CD4-LTR-LacZ were infected with the indicated viruses in the presence of the indicated compounds. The cells were stained 24 h later using virus-specific antibodies to assess the levels of infection and analyzed by flow cytometry. **d** Kudzu has no activity on ADV5 virus infection of HeLa-CD4-LTR-LacZ cells. Heat inactivated virus (H.I) and Raltegravir (Ralt., 100 nM) were used as controls. Results represent the mean ± SD of 3 independent experiments. **e** No activity of Kudzu on ZIKA Brazil virus infection of HeLa-CD4-LTR-LacZ cells. Cabozantinib (Caboz., 1 µM) and Raltegravir (Ralt., 100 nM) were used as controls. Results represent the mean ± SD of 3 independent experiments. **f** No impact of Kudzu on H1N1 virus infection of HeLa-CD4-LTR-LacZ cells. Aleuria Aurantia Lectin (AAL, 100 nM) and Raltegravir (Ralt., 100 nM) were used as controls. Results represent the mean ± SD of 3 independent experiments. Kudzu was used at the dilution 1:200 in **c–f**. The two-tailed paired t test was used for statistical analysis. **: p value < 0.005, ***: p value < 0.0005

p27 capsid in the supernatant was measured by ELISA. A cocktail of ARVs (Emtricitabine, Tenofovir and Raltegravir, 200 nM) was used as control. Kudzu extract inhibited $SIV_{mac}239$ replication in a dose-dependent manner at concentrations (1:200 and 1:100) that did not alter cell viability (Additional file 1: Fig. 1SE). Altogether, these results suggest that Kudzu has a broad activity against lentiviruses, likely because these share similar target cell entry mechanisms.

HCV replication was investigated using Huh-7.5 cells in the presence of either Kudzu (1:200) or 2'-C-methyladenosine (10 μM), an RNA-dependent RNA polymerase inhibitor known to suppress HCV replication. Unlike the latter, Kudzu had no effect on HCV infection (Fig. 3c). The replication of H1N1, Zika or ADV5 was also assessed in HeLa-CD4-LTR-LacZ cells in the presence of Kudzu or known inhibitors of each virus. The Aleuria Aurantia lectin (100 nM) binds the envelope hemagglutinin glycoprotein of H1N1 and blocks its entry [32]. Cabozantinib (1 μM), a tyrosine-kinase inhibitor, suppresses Zika infection [33]. ADV5 infection was controlled by heat inactivation. While all our positive controls proved able to inhibit these viruses, Kudzu (1:200) showed no activity (Fig. 3d–f).

Collectively, these results suggest that Kudzu is specific to lentiviruses, HIV-1, HIV-2 and SIV. This large breath of activity suggests Kudzu targets an aspect of viral entry that is very conserved across lentiviruses, which may potentially limit resistance development.

The anti-HIV-1 activity of Kudzu depends on gp120

The interaction between gp120 and CD4, followed by interaction with CXCR4 or CCR5 is determinant for HIV-1 entry into the target cell. After determining that Kudzu does not affect CD4, CXCR4 and CCR5 cell surface expression (Additional file 1: Fig. 3S), we investigated whether Kudzu affects the virus or the cells. As such, we either pre-incubated Kudzu with HeLa-CD4-LTR-LacZ cells for 6 h, then washed the cells and added NL4-3 virus; or, incubated kudzu and NL4-3 at the same time with HeLa-CD4-LTR-LacZ cells. β-Gal activity was measured 72 h later (Fig. 4a). Kudzu (1:400) was significantly active only when added to the cells simultaneously with the virus. Similar result was obtained with the negative control Raltegravir (100 nM). These results suggest that Kudzu mainly affects the virus, and is not the result of an activity on the target cell.

Given the key role of gp120 and gp41 proteins in the entry process, we assessed whether gp160 (precursor of gp120 and gp41) was necessary for Kudzu's activity by comparing susceptibility of HIV virus-like particles pseudotyped with either the vesicular stomatitis virus G (VSV-G) envelope protein or the X4 gp160 envelope from HXB2 strain. We infected HeLa-CD4-LTR-LacZ cells with VSV-G-NL4-3 or HXB2 gp160-NL4-3 in the presence of Kudzu or a series of control compounds, and measured p24 production in the supernatant 72 h later (Fig. 4b and c). Efavirenz (200 nM) and Raltegravir (200 nM), which inhibit HIV-1 post-entry events, decreased both VSV-G-NL4-3 and HXB2 gp160-NL4-3

(See figure on next page.)

Fig. 4 Kudzu blocks HIV-1 attachment. **a** Kudzu specifically affect the virus and not the cells. Kudzu (1:400) was either preincubated for 6 h with the HeLa-CD4-LTR-LacZ cells then washed and NL4-3 virus was added to the cells ("preincubation with compound/washed") or simultaneously added with the virus to the cells ("virus + compound together"). β-Gal activity was measured 72 h later. Ralt.: Raltegravir, 100 nM. Results represent the mean ± SD of 3 independent experiments. **b** Absence of activity of Kudzu on infected HeLa-CD4-LTR-LacZ cells with VSV-G-NL4-3 pseudovirus. Efavirenz (Efav., 200 nM), Raltegravir (Ralt., 200 nM), AMD3100 (10 nM) and Enfuvirtide (1 μg/ml) were used as controls. Kudzu: 1:400 dilution. Viral supernatants recovered 72 h postinfection from cells were assayed for their p24 antigen content. The mean ± SD of 4 experiments is represented. **c** Activity of Kudzu on infected HeLa-CD4-LTR-LacZ cells with HXB2 gp160 pseudotyped NL4-3 env-. Same controls and Kudzu dilution as in **b**. Viral supernatants recovered 72 h post-infection from cells were assayed for their p24 antigen content. The mean ± SD of 4 independent experiments is presented. **d** No impact of Kudzu on interaction of monomeric YU2 gp120 and CD4-Ig receptor in ELISA. s: soluble. Emtricitabine (Emt., 500 nM) and soluble gp120 or CD4 were used as controls. The mean ± SD of 4 independent experiments is represented. **e** Kudzu does not affect fusion of HeLa-CD4-LTR-LacZ and HL2/3 cells. Emtricitabine (Emt., 100 nM), Enfuvirtide (1 μg/ml), cells only and untreated cells were used as controls. β-Gal activity was measured 48 h later. Data is the mean ± SD of 3 independent experiments. **f** No activity of Kudzu on shedding of transfected JRCSF gp160 in HEK293T cells, revealed by western blot. Data is representative of 3 independent experiments. CD4-Ig (45 μg) was used as a control. **g** No activity of Kudzu on shedding of NL4-3 gp120 from NL4-3 virus. HIV-1 directly loaded on gel (HIV-1+) was used as positive control of the gp120 protein. The other samples were filtered through a column and a fraction of the flow-through was analyzed by western blot. CD4 (30 μg) was used as control of the shedding. Data is representative of 2 independent experiments and quantification of the 2 independent experiments is shown below the blot. **h–j** Kudzu significantly reduces the attachment of HIV-1 and HIV-2 to TZM-bl cells. **h** Schematic of the attachment assay. The attachment assay is performed by adding virus to cells in presence of the different compounds for 3 h at 4 °C. After this period of incubation at 4 °C, the cells are washed with cold PBS and then allowed to incubate at 37 °C for 72 h before luciferase is quantified. **i** Kudzu inhibits HIV-1 attachment. Enfuvirtide (a fusion inhibitor, 1 μg/ml) and Heparin (competes with Heparan sulfate proteoglycans binding to gp120, 1 mg/ml) were used as controls. The data is the mean ± SD of 3 independent experiments. **j** Kudzu inhibits HIV-2 CBL-20 attachment. AMD3100 (10 nM) and Heparin were used as controls. The data is the mean ± SD of 4 independent experiments. The two-tailed paired t test was used for statistical comparisons. **: p value < 0.005, ***: p value < 0.0005

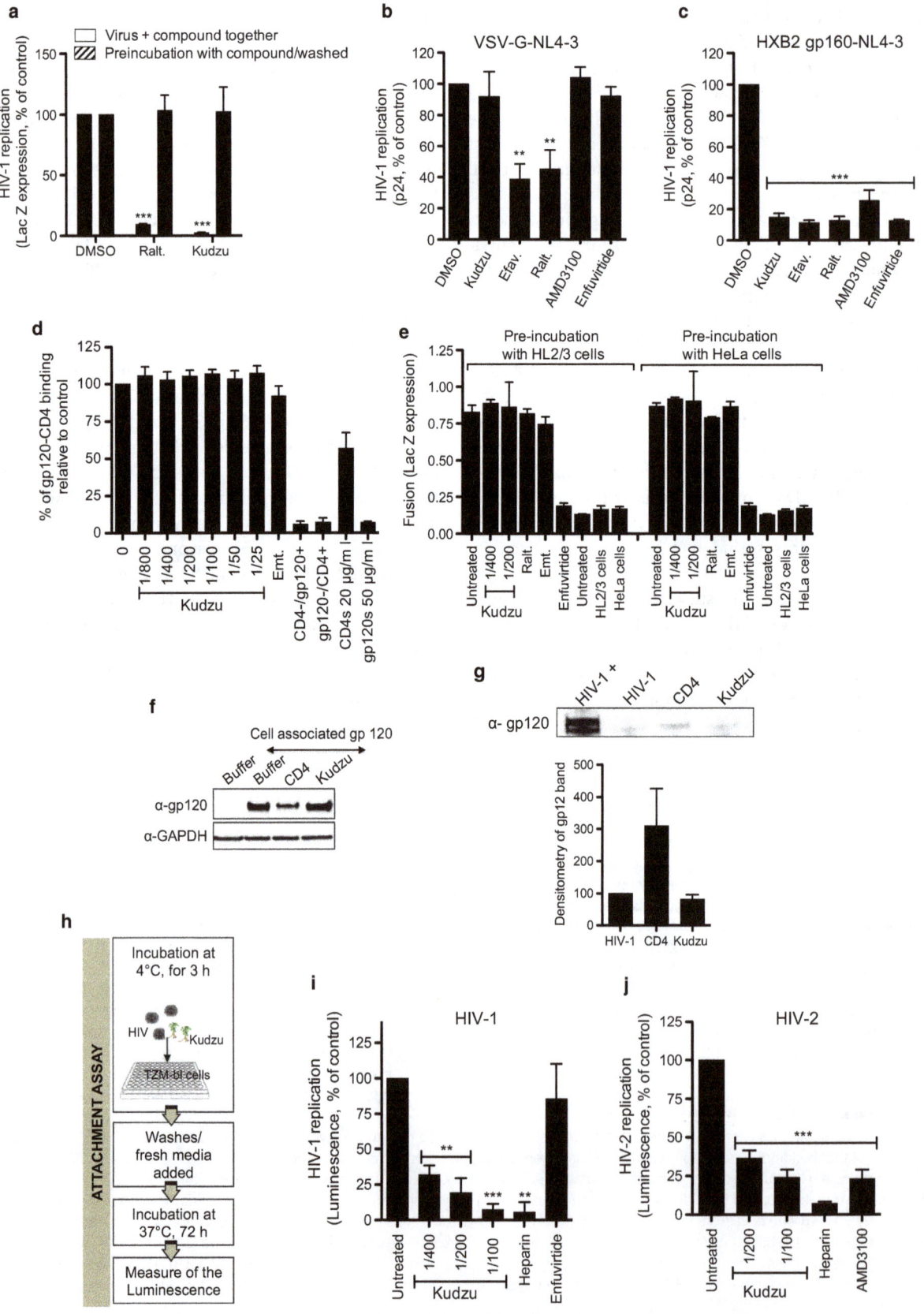

infection. However, the entry inhibitor AMD3100 (10 nM), the fusion inhibitor Enfuvirtide (1 µg/ml) and Kudzu (1:400) significantly inhibited HXB2 gp160-, but not VSV-G-driven infection of the cells. Collectively, these data suggest that Kudzu targets HIV entry, and is dependent on virus-target cell entry mechanisms mediated by gp120 and/or gp41.

To investigate whether Kudzu was targeting gp120 directly, we first assessed its ability to interfere with the interaction between gp120 and CD4. For this, we coated monomeric recombinant gp120 on an ELISA plate and measured its interaction with CD4-Ig (as in [34]), in the presence of increasing concentrations of Kudzu (Fig. 4d). The intensity of the absorbance is directly proportional to the binding of gp120 to CD4-Ig. Kudzu did not interfere with the gp120-CD4-Ig interaction, while soluble gp120 and soluble CD4 both acted as competitors. Emtricitabine (500 nM) was used as a negative control. The background of the assay was evaluated by measuring the signal generated in buffer-coated wells (instead of gp120), as well as buffer-treated wells (instead of CD4-Ig). Together these results suggest that Kudzu does not interfere with gp120 interaction with CD4.

We further investigated whether Kudzu could interfere with the fusion between gp160-expressing cells and target cells that express both CD4 and CXCR4 (Fig. 4e). HL2/3 cells express viral Gag, Env, Tat, Rev, and Nef proteins. Their co-culture with HeLa-CD4-LTR-LacZ cells results in cell fusion, and subsequent activation of 5′-LTR-driven LacZ expression by HL2/3-produced Tat protein. In this assay, we individually pre-incubated HL2/3 cells or HeLa-CD4-LTR-LacZ cells with compounds for 2 h before co-culture for another 48 h, followed by measurement of β-Gal activity. As shown in Fig. 4e, while Enfuvirtide (1 µg/ml) inhibited cell fusion, Kudzu (1:400 and 1: 200) had no inhibitory activity. Raltegravir (100 nM), Emtracitabine (100 nM), untreated and cells alone were used as negative controls. Together these results suggest that Kudzu does not interfere with the fusion between virus and cell membranes, especially with gp120 interaction with CXCR4 and gp41mediated fusion.

We then evaluated the effect of Kudzu on the shedding of gp120 (Fig. 4f), as previously described [35]. The gp120 was ectopically expressed in HEK293T cells after transfection of JR-FL gp160Δtail constructs. After 48 h, cells were incubated for 4 h with Kudzu (1:400), or soluble CD4-Ig (45 µg) used as a positive control. Cells were washed, lysed, and the remaining gp120 attached to the cell surface was detected by immunoblotting using anti-gp120 serum. As shown in Fig. 4f, the amount of gp120 remaining after Kudzu treatment was similar to the control, while soluble CD4-Ig decreased the presence of gp120 on the cell surface. To confirm this result,

we exposed concentrated NL4-3 virus to Kudzu (1:200) or CD4-Ig (30 µg) for 6 h, and then passed the solution through a 300-kDa filter, to recover shedded gp120 in the flow-through. A fraction of the flow-through was then analyzed by immunoblotting with an anti-gp120 serum. The gp120 bands and corresponding densitometry are shown in Fig. 4g. Kudzu did not increase shedding of gp120 from the virus surface as opposed to CD4. Altogether these results suggest that the inhibition of HIV-1 entry by Kudzu is not mediated by gp120 shedding.

Kudzu inhibits HIV attachment to the target cell

As we mentioned above, gp120 first attaches to the target cell by interacting with cell-surface heparan sulfate proteoglycans, α4β7 integrins, DC-SIGN or MCLR. These attachment receptors bring gp120/gp41 into close proximity to CD4 and CXCR4 or CCR5, increasing infection efficiency. As such, we monitored the involvement of Kudzu in HIV-1 attachment to the target cell, as previously described [36, 37]. Pre-chilled TZM-bl cells were incubated with NL4-3 and increasing concentrations of Kudzu for 3 h at 4 °C (Fig. 4h). This allows only attachment of the virus to the cell, but not fusion and entry of the virus. After washing with cold PBS to remove unattached virions and/or drugs bound to virions, fresh medium (without compounds) was added. The cells were then further incubated at 37 °C for 72 h, before luciferase activity was measured. The peptide fusion inhibitor Enfuvirtide (1 µg/ml), which binds to gp41, was used as a negative control, while soluble heparin (1 mg/ml), which reduces attachment of the virus to the target cell by competing with the cell surface heparan sulfate proteoglycans [38], was used as a positive control. We observed a dose-dependent inhibition of virus attachment in the presence of Kudzu compared to the untreated control (Fig. 4i). We also verified that Kudzu did not affect TZM-bl cell viability at the indicated concentrations (Additional file 1: Fig. 1SD left). Similar results were obtained with HIV-2 (Fig. 4j). Kudzu inhibited HIV-2 attachment to the same extent as the entry inhibitor AM3100, which tightly binds to CXCR4 on the cell surface. Taken together our results suggest that Kudzu root extract blocks attachment of gp120 to the cell surface, a process independent of CD4, thus inhibiting the first step of the HIV entry life cycle.

Kudzu does not inhibit HIV-1 late replication events

We also investigated the ability of Kudzu to inhibit late replication events, i.e., after integration of the viral DNA into the host cell genome. First, we tested the activity of Kudzu on viral transcription by analyzing the viral production from chronically-infected HeLa-CD4 cells for a period of 72 h (Fig. 5a). We used the Tat inhibitor didehydro-Cortistatin A (dCA) as a control [39]. While dCA

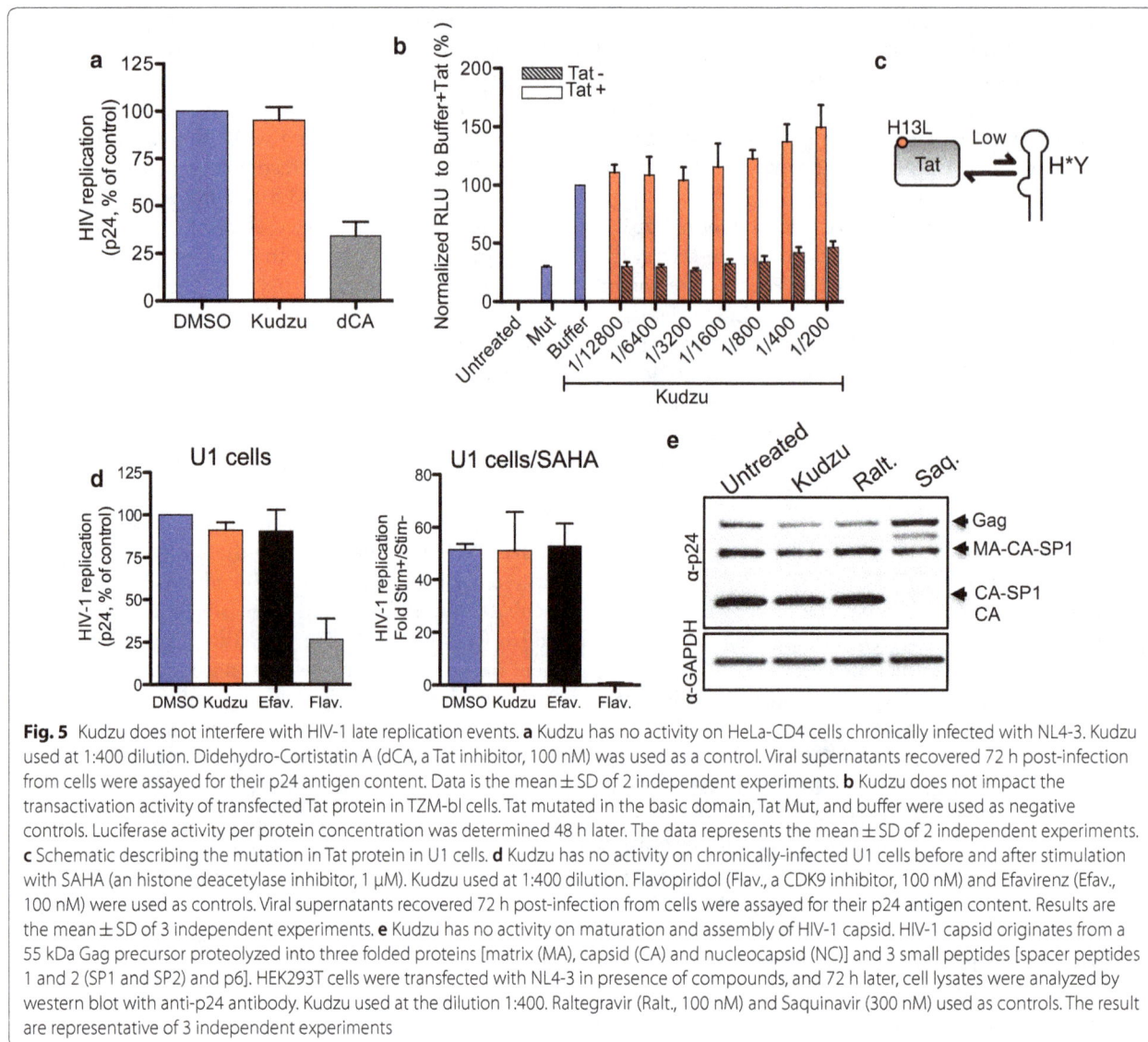

Fig. 5 Kudzu does not interfere with HIV-1 late replication events. **a** Kudzu has no activity on HeLa-CD4 cells chronically infected with NL4-3. Kudzu used at 1:400 dilution. Didehydro-Cortistatin A (dCA, a Tat inhibitor, 100 nM) was used as a control. Viral supernatants recovered 72 h post-infection from cells were assayed for their p24 antigen content. Data is the mean ± SD of 2 independent experiments. **b** Kudzu does not impact the transactivation activity of transfected Tat protein in TZM-bl cells. Tat mutated in the basic domain, Tat Mut, and buffer were used as negative controls. Luciferase activity per protein concentration was determined 48 h later. The data represents the mean ± SD of 2 independent experiments. **c** Schematic describing the mutation in Tat protein in U1 cells. **d** Kudzu has no activity on chronically-infected U1 cells before and after stimulation with SAHA (an histone deacetylase inhibitor, 1 μM). Kudzu used at 1:400 dilution. Flavopiridol (Flav., a CDK9 inhibitor, 100 nM) and Efavirenz (Efav., 100 nM) were used as controls. Viral supernatants recovered 72 h post-infection from cells were assayed for their p24 antigen content. Results are the mean ± SD of 3 independent experiments. **e** Kudzu has no activity on maturation and assembly of HIV-1 capsid. HIV-1 capsid originates from a 55 kDa Gag precursor proteolyzed into three folded proteins [matrix (MA), capsid (CA) and nucleocapsid (NC)] and 3 small peptides [spacer peptides 1 and 2 (SP1 and SP2) and p6]. HEK293T cells were transfected with NL4-3 in presence of compounds, and 72 h later, cell lysates were analyzed by western blot with anti-p24 antibody. Kudzu used at the dilution 1:400. Raltegravir (Ralt., 100 nM) and Saquinavir (300 nM) used as controls. The result are representative of 3 independent experiments

inhibited viral production from these cells, Kudzu (1:400) showed no activity. We further confirmed this result by measuring the activity of Kudzu during Tat transactivation of the HIV-1 promoter in TZM-bl cells (Fig. 5b). A dominant negative variant of Tat mutated in the basic domain ("Tat Mut"), and unable to transactivate HIV-1 promoter, was used as a negative control. We confirmed that Kudzu had no impact on Tat-mediated transcription of HIV-1 while not altering the viability of TZM-bl cells (Additional file 1: Fig. 2SD right). We also investigated the activity of Kudzu on basal transcription using U1 cells, a model of HIV-1 latency where a H13L mutation in Tat abolishes the activity of the protein (Fig. 5c and d). The controls performed as expected, with a CDK9 inhibitor, Flavopiridol, inhibiting basal transcription, but not

Efavirenz (Fig. 5d left). In this case again, Kudzu (1:400) did not alter basal transcription. We observed the same results after stimulating the cells with Suberoylanilide Hydroxamic acid (SAHA) for 24 h, a histone deacetylase inhibitor (Fig. 5d right). Collectively, these data suggest that Kudzu does not interfere with the transcription of HIV-1 genome.

To investigate whether Kudzu could interfere with late events of the viral life cycle, such as Gag expression and maturation, we transfected HEK293T cells with NL4-3 molecular clone in the presence of Kudzu or controls, and measured Gag expression in cell lysates by immunoblot, using an anti-p24 antibody (Fig. 5e). The expression of Gag protein and its maturation were similar in Kudzu (1:400), Raltegravir (100 nM), and untreated samples, while the protease inhibitor, Saquinavir (300 nM), blocked the maturation of Gag into Matrix (MA) and Capsid (CA) proteins. Taken together, our results strongly suggest that Kudzu does not impact the late events of HIV-1 life cycle.

Individual antiviral activity of the chemical components of Kudzu

The geographic origin, as well as the methods of culture and root extraction, dictate the chemical composition of Kudzu extract. Several reports ascribe more than 40 chemical entities to Kudzu root extract (Additional file 1: Table 1S). In an effort to identify the compound responsible for Kudzu's activity, we tested its main components and as many as of the commercially available less abundant ones (Fig. 6a). To our surprise, none of the most abundant components presented antiviral activity, including Puerarin (60% of the total isoflavones in Kudzu), Daidzein and Daidzin, which have been previously reported to have anti-microbial activity [25]. In addition, the combination of the highly represented compounds still did not display antiviral activity (data not shown). Moreover, we assessed whether the activity of Kudzu was potentially due to protein traces in the extract. For this, we denatured Kudzu by boiling and tested its activity in infectivity assays using HeLa-CD4-LTR-LacZ cells. Figure 6b shows that the denaturation did not affect the activity of Kudzu. Furthermore, the denatured Kudzu was ran on a denatured electrophoresis gel, transferred to a nitrocellulose membrane, and no proteins were observed after Coomassie blue staining (data not shown). Altogether, these results suggest that Kudzu antiviral activity most likely derives from a component present at a very low concentration or it results from an additive/synergistic effect of several compounds.

Activity of Kudzu in combination with current ART and activity against viruses resistant to Enfuvirtide

We assessed the activity of Kudzu in combination with two different cocktails: ATRIPLA® (Efavirenz, Tenofovir and Emtricitabine) as a single tablet regime, and ALE, Combivir (AZT and Lamivudine) combined with Sustiva (Efavirenz). We first determined the IC_{50} of each ARV cocktail and Kudzu alone. Next, Kudzu and the cocktail at their IC_{50} were mixed together at different ratios (Kudzu: cocktail, 1:1, 4:1, 8:1) to obtain an IC_{50} of the mix. The data was plotted as concentration of ARVs cocktails per Kudzu dilution (Fig. 7a). The mixes of Kudzu with ATRIPLA® at the different ratios presented IC_{50} concentrations lower than the trend line (dotted line between Individual IC_{50}), which is associated with synergistic activity [40]. With the ALE cocktail, the activity of

Kudzu was additive when used at ratio of 1:1, and synergistic when used at doses higher than 1:1.

A number of characterized HIV-1 isolates are resistant to the entry inhibitor Enfuvirtide. We evaluated the susceptibility to Kudzu of three of these viral isolates, which carry mutations in gp41 (gp41 D36G V38E N42S, gp41 D36G V38A and gp41 D36G V38A N42D) [41]. As expected, these viruses were resistant to Enfuvirtide (150 ng/ml). The inhibition by Kudzu was as potent as Raltegravir (100 nM) and AMD3100 (10 nM).

Collectively these results suggest that Kudzu does not compete with current ART, but acts additively/synergistically with ART, rationalizing its use as a complement to current HIV-1 therapy. Kudzu may also be helpful in cases of Enfuvirtide resistance, highlighting its potential to complement HIV-1 salvage therapy.

Importantly, we did not observe development of resistance after passaging the NL4-3 strain every 4 days, onto naïve HeLa-CD4 cells in the presence of sub IC_{50} concentrations over a 54 days period.

Conclusion

Only a few agents are currently used in the clinic that target the HIV-1 entry process (Enfuvirtide, Maraviroc and Ibalizumab). There is a continuing need for development of novel antiretroviral drugs and regimens in order to address tolerability, long-term safety concerns, the immune dysfunction mediated by HIV and the emergency of drug resistance. The cost of current treatment and accessibility is also a concern to a significant portion of the HIV affected population. Traditional medicine is very popular in many countries, and it has been used to replace ARVs or off-set side effects from antiretroviral medication. Such medicinal plants have not been properly identified and documented probably due to the lack of collaborations between scientists and traditional healers. Kudzu is a safe and very well-known natural product that has been used for hundreds of years. Here we demonstrated its potent activity against the attachment of HIV-1 gp120 to receptors on the host cell membrane, blocking HIV entry into cell lines, primary CD4+T cells and macrophages. To date, no small molecule compound has been described that targets this step of the life cycle. Kudzu's efficacy against HIV-2 is further appreciated given that HIV-2 is naturally resistant to Enfuvirtide, nonnucleoside reverse transcriptase inhibitors, and to some protease inhibitors. Moreover, Kudzu has also been shown to reduce inflammation and oxidative stress, an affliction that is often identified in HIV infected individuals. So far, we have not been able to identify the chemical entity of Kudzu extract that is responsible for the antiretroviral activity. In future studies, we will use a combination of HPLC fractionation and 1H-NMR to identify

a

Compounds	Structure	IC$_{50}$ (µM)	CC$_{50}$ (µM)
Daidzin		> 500 ± 0.0	> 500 ± 0.0
Daidzein		81.6 ± 4.3	151.6 ± 25.5
Genistein		100.9 ± 15.2	135.4 ± 22.8
Puerarin		> 500 ± 0.0	> 500 ± 0.0
Lupeol		> 56.3 ± 3.9	56.3 ± 3.9
Ononin		> 500 ± 0.0	> 500 ± 0.0
β- Sitosterol		> 500 ± 0.0	> 500 ± 0.0
Lupenone		> 500 ± 0.0	> 500 ± 0.0
Allantoin		> 500 ± 0.0	> 500 ± 0.0
Formononetin		> 500 ± 0.0	> 500 ± 0.0
Coumestrol		> 182.4 ± 5.6	182.4 ± 5.6
Diisobutyl phthalate		> 500 ± 0.0	> 500 ± 0.0
Bis 2-(ethylhexyl) phthalate		> 500 ± 0.0	> 500 ± 0.0
Sissotrin		> 500 ± 0.0	> 500 ± 0.0

b

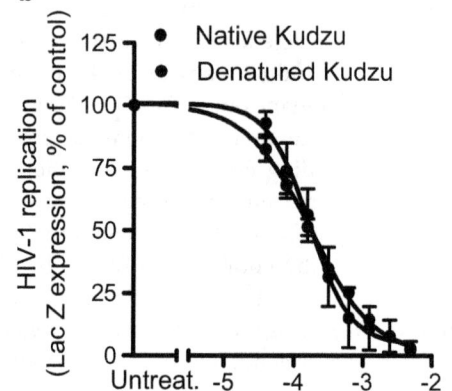

Fig. 6 Activity of the different components of Kudzu on acute replication of HIV-1 of X4 tropic virus in HeLa-CD4-LTR-LacZ cells. **a** HeLa-CD4-LTR-LacZ cells were infected with HIV-1 NL4-3 strain in presence of different concentrations of the indicated compounds. β-Gal activity and viability assays were performed 72 h later. Results represent the mean ± SD of 3 independent experiments. **b** The activity of Kudzu does not involve proteins. HeLa-CD4-LTR-LacZ cells were infected with HIV-1 NL4-3 strain in presence of denatured Kudzu by heat or native Kudzu. β-Gal activity was measured 72 h later. Data is the mean ± SD of 4 independent experiments. Untreat.: untreated

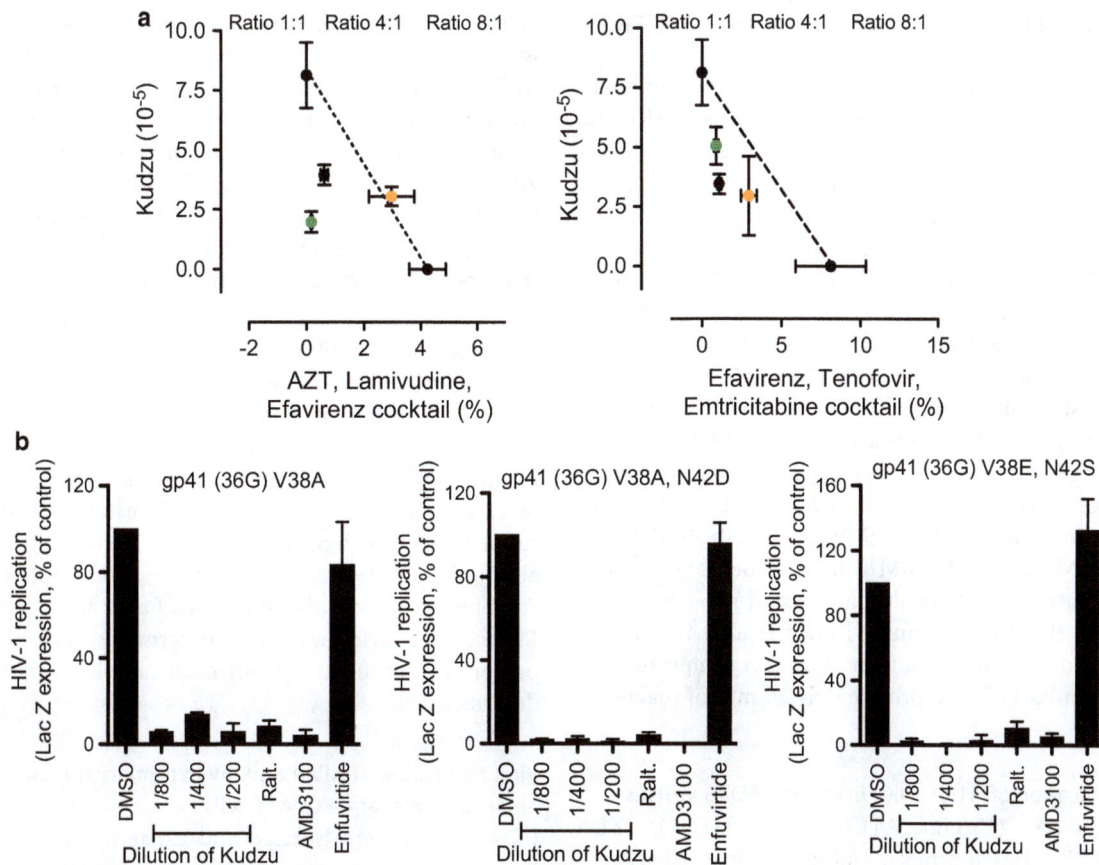

Fig. 7 Activity of Kudzu in combination with antiretrovirals. **a** Combination of Kudzu with different cocktails of antiretrovirals prescribed to HIV-1 patients. HeLa-CD4-LTR-LacZ cells were infected with HIV-1 NL4-3 strain in presence of different amounts of Kudzu or the indicated antiretrovirals. β-Gal activity was measured 72 h later. The IC_{50} of the cocktails or Kudzu alone (black) or the mix of both at different ratios (orange, green, and blue) are represented. Results represent the mean ± SD of 3 independent experiments. **b** Activity of Kudzu in HeLa-CD4-LTR-LacZ cells infected with viruses resistant to Enfuvirtide. HeLa-CD4-LTR-LacZ cells were infected in presence of different dilutions of Kudzu. β-Gal activity was measured 72 h later. AMD3100 and Enfuvirtide used at 10 nM and 0.15 µg/ml respectively. Data is the mean ± SD of 2 independent experiments

active compounds. In sum, given Kudzu's low cost, safety, oral bioavailability, tissue distribution, activity with ART and potent activity against HIV gp120 attachment to host cell, it should be considered as a promising supplement to current HIV therapeutic strategies.

Methods

Kudzu

Kudzu (Hawaii pharm LLC), was used in all experiments. Its activity was confirmed with Kudzu from Secrets of the Tribe (Nevada pharm LLC). Both Kudzus are a tincture solution with 33% of Kudzu and 66% of ethanol-glycerol-water.

Viral replication of HIV-1 in cell lines detected by p24 ELISA

HeLa-CD4-LTR-LacZ cells (5×10^3/well in a 96-well-plate) were first incubated with Kudzu or the indicated

controls (Raltegravir: 100 nM, Efavirenz: 100 nM, AMD3100: 10 nM, Enfuvirtide: 1 µg/ml,) then infected overnight (ON) with wild-type HIV-1 isolate NL4-3 (3.2 ng/well). Cells were washed and further cultured in fresh media (DMEM supplemented with 5% Fetal bovine serum (FBS), L-glutamine (292 µg/ml) and antibiotics (100 units/ml penicillin and streptomycin)) containing compounds for another 72 h. HIV-1 replication was assessed by measuring the viral capsid in the supernatant with a p24 ELISA kit (Advances Bioscience Laboratories). Similar protocol was used for the infection of GHOST-CCR5 cells (gift from Dr. Michael Farzan) with JRCSF (21.3 ng/well, NIH AIDS Reagent Program, cat# 394) or YU2 (2.32 ng, NIH AIDS Reagent Program, cat# 1350) viruses. The amount of virus was chosen to obtain similar p24 capsid outputs between the different cell lines.

Viral replication of HIV-1 in cell lines, revealed by chlorophenol red-β-d-galactopyranoside assay (CPRG assay)

HeLa-CD4-LTR-LacZ cells (5×10^3/well in a 96-well-plate) were first incubated with compounds (Kudzu, Kudzu's components, indicated ARVs controls, Glycerol, Ethanol, or denatured Kudzu boiled for 10 min at 90 °C). NL4-3 virus (6.6 ng/well) or viruses resistant to Enfuvirtide (gifts from NIH AIDS Reagent Program, cat# 9490 (5.4 ng/well), cat# 9488 (2 ng/well), cat# 9496 (0.6 ng/ml)) were then added for 72 h. Cells were disrupted with lysis buffer (60 mM Na2HPO4, 40 mM NaH2PO4, 10 mM KCl, 10 mM MgSO4, 2.5 mM EDTA, 50 mM ß-mercaptoethanol, 0.125% Nonidet P-40) for 1 h at 4 °C and a quantitative CPRG-based (Boehringer Mannheim) assay was performed per manufacturer's instructions. The cell extracts were incubated in reaction buffer (0.9 M phosphate buffer [pH 7.4], 9 mM MgCl2, 11 mM ß-mercaptoethanol, 7 mM CPRG) until a red color developed and measured with an LP400 (Becton–Dickinson) plate reader at 572 nm. The amount of virus used for infection aimed to produce a similar OD at approximately 20 min of reaction.

Viral replication of H1N1, ZIKV Brazil and ADV5 viruses

Influenza A (Virginia/ATCC1/2009 H1N1), Zika virus (PB81, Brazil strain), and adenovirus serotype 5 (ADV5) were produced in MDCK, Vero and HEK293T cells, respectively. Each virus was mixed with the indicated compounds, and added to Hela-CD4-LTR-LacZ cells. Aleuria Aurantia lectin (100 nM), an inhibitor of H1N1 entry, cabozantinib (1 µM), a tyrosine kinase inhibitor known to suppress Zika infection, and heat inactivation of ADV5 for 30 min at 70 °C, were used as positive controls. After 1 h at 37 °C, the inoculum was removed, and the cells further grown in DMEM containing 10% FBS and the indicated compounds. Twenty-four hours after the inoculation, the cells were collected, fixed with PBS containing 2% of paraformaldehyde, permeabilized using PBS containing 2% of saponin, and stained with either the monoclonal mouse anti-H1N1/H2N2 antibody clone C179 (H1N1), or the monoclonal mouse pan anti-flavivirus antibody clone 4G2 (Zika), or the mouse monoclonal anti-adenovirus antibody clone 2/6 (ADV5), followed with an Alexa647-conjugated, anti-mIgG antibody (Jackson ImmunoResearch). The cells were then washed, fixed, and analyzed using flow cytometry (BD Biosciences C6 Accuri and IntelliCyt HyperCyt sampler powered by FlowCyt software). Infection levels were normalized to those of cells infected in the absence of any compound.

Viral replication of pseudotyped viruses

Hela-CD4-LTR-LacZ cells (1×10^5/in a 6-well-plate) were infected ON with VSV-G-NL4-3 (70.2 ng or 5.6 ng/well) or with HXB2 gp160-NL4-3 (25.4 ng/well) pseudotyped viruses (constructs gifted by Dr. Michael Farzan), in the presence of Kudzu (1:400) or controls (Raltegravir: 200 nM, Efavirenz: 200 nM, AMD3100: 10 nM, Enfuvirtide: 1 µg/ml). Cells were washed and fresh media containing compounds was added for 72 h. The capsid p24 in the supernatant was assessed by ELISA.

Viral replication of HIV2 CBL-20 strain

TZM-bl cells (4×10^4/well in a 6-well-plate) were incubated with different concentrations of Kudzu or the indicated controls, then infected ON with HIV-2 CBL-20 virus (NIH AIDS Reagent Program, cat# 600, 0.2 ng/well). Media was then removed and fresh media (DMEM supplemented with 5% FBS, L-glutamine (292 µg/ml) and antibiotics (100 units/ml penicillin and streptomycin)) containing compounds were added for an additional 48 h. Luciferase activity was then determined and reported per protein concentration of each sample as previously described [39].

Viral replication of HIV-1 and SIV in primary human and rhesus macaque CD4+T cells

CD4+T cells were isolated and expanded as previously described [42]. Briefly, PBMCs were extracted from 3 healthy human donors (purchased from One Blood-Florida) and 3 healthy rhesus macaques (obtained from the Wisconsin National Primate Research Center). Total CD4+T cells were isolated using positive selection kit (StemCell Technologies). Cells were expanded with 1 µg/ml of PHA (Sigma Aldrich), 100 U/ml of IL-2 (Roche) and irradiated feeder PBMCs (OneBlood) and cultured in RPMI and human serum for 3 days. Primary human CD4+ T cells were treated with DMSO, kudzu or a cocktail of ARVs (AZT: 180 nM, Efavirenz: 100 nM, Raltegravir: 200 nM) then infected with NL4-3 (100 ng). After 24 h, cells were pelleted, DNA extracted, followed by PCR (see below). Primary macaque CD4+T cells were treated with DMSO, Kudzu or a cocktail of ARVs (Emtracitabine, Raltegravir and Tenofovir, 200 nM) then infected with $SIV_{mac}239$ (100 ng). SIV replication was assessed 6 days later, by measuring the viral capsid in the supernatant with p27 ELISA (Advances Bioscience Laboratories).

Viral replication of ADA and 5002M viruses in primary macrophages

Human monocyte-derived macrophages were isolated from elutriated blood PBMCs by Ficoll-Hypaque density gradient centrifugation (GE Healthcare). Monocytes were negatively selected using magnetic particles from EasySep™ Human Monocyte CD14+without CD16 depletion Enrichment kit (Stem Cell Technologies). Monocytes were differentiated in DMEM (Gibco) supplemented with 10% heat inactivated human serum (Sera Care Life Sciences), 2 mM L–glutamine (Gibco), 10 μg/ml gentamicin (Sigma–Aldrich) and 10 ng/ml MCSF (R&D System) and cultured for 7 days at 37°C with 5% CO_2. Macrophages were then seeded onto 48-well plate (1×10^5 cells/well), infected with 1×10^6 CPMs of macrophage-tropic strains ADA or 5002M in the presence of kudzu (1:100) or Enfuvirtide (5 μg/ml). Viral inoculum was removed, and media replaced with fresh compounds 24 h post-infection. Compounds were added every day to the media, and half media was replaced every 2 days. An aliquot of the supernatant was harvested every day for 6 days, for capsid p24 quantification (ClonTech).

Viral replication of HCV, assessed by immunohistochemistry

Huh 7.5 cells were infected with HCV JC1 virus and Kudzu (at the dilution 1:200) was subsequently added. A blank (without compounds, "untreated") or 2′-C-methyladenosine (10 μM) [43] was used as control. After 48 h, cell supernatants/lysates were harvested, cell lysates prepared with 2 cycles of freeze thawing, and stored (− 80 °C) for infection of naïve cells for titration. Naïve Huh-7.5 cells (cultured in 96-well plates) were inoculated with the supernatant/lysates for limiting dilution virus titration assay. After 48 h, cells were washed, fixed in methanol, and then probed for NS5A expression using the 9E10 monoclonal antibody. $TCID_{50}$ was calculated as previously described [44].

Latently infected cells

NL4-3 latently infected HeLa-CD4 cells (2.5×10^5/well) and U1 cells (5×10^5/well) were treated with compounds for 72 h, and p24 in the supernatant was assessed by ELISA. HeLa-CD4 cells were treated with 1:400 dilution of Kudzu or 100 nM of dCA. U1 cells were treated with 1:400 dilution of Kudzu, 100 nM of Efavirenz or 100 nM of Flavopiridol. U1 cells reactivation was performed with 1 μM of SAHA for 24 h.

Time-of-addition experiment

HeLa-CD4-LTR-LacZ cells (5×10^3/well in a 96-well-plate) were infected with NL4-3 (6.6 ng/well). Kudzu and ARVs controls were added to the infected cells, at the indicated concentrations, at time 0, 1, 2, 3, 4, 5, and 6 h post-infection. β-Gal activity was measured 72 h later.

Attachment assay in TZM-bl cells

TZM-bl cells (2×10^4) were seeded in a 96-well plate. Next day, cells were incubated for 1 h at 4 °C. In parallel, compounds (Kudzu: 1:400–1:100, Heparin: 1 mg/ml, Enfuvirtide: 1 μg/ml and AMD3100: 10 nM) were mixed with NL4-3 (16.6 ng/well) or HIV-2 CBL-20 (0.8 ng/well) for 1 h at 4 °C. Compounds with virus were then added to the cells and incubated at 4 °C for 3 h. Cells were washed twice with ice cold PBS and incubated with fresh media for 72 h at 37 °C, 5% CO_2. The infection was assessed by measuring the luminescence with Bright Glo (Promega) according to the manufacturer's protocol.

Transactivation assay in TZM-bl cells

Cells were seeded at 2×10^6 in a 10 cm^2 tissue culture dish and transfected with 5 μg of the constructs expressing Tat (PGK-Flag-Tat) or Tat Mut (PGK-Flag-Tat Mut) driven by the murine phosphoglycerate kinase-1 (PGK) promoter, with TransIT-LT1 transfection reagent (Mirus Bio LLC) according to the manufacturer's protocol. The cells were split 24 h post transfection and treated with Kudzu at different concentrations. Luciferase activity per protein concentration of each sample was determined 48 h later as previously described [39].

Quantification of early and late reverse transcription product and provirus integration

In HeLa-CD4-LTR-LacZ cells

Cells were plated at 1×10^5 cells per well in a six-well plate. Twenty-four hours later, cells were infected with NL4-3 virus (66 ng) in the presence of DMSO, Kudzu (1:200), Efavirenz (200 nM), Saquinavir (200 nM), Raltegravir (200 nM) and AMD3100 (10 nM). At 10 h and 24 h post-infection, genomic DNA was prepared and early and late viral DNA products and the integrated proviruses were quantified as previously described [45].

In primary CD4+T lymphocyte cells

Cell pellets were digested at 133 μl/million cells with lysis buffer (10 mM Tris–HCL, 50 nM KCl, 400 μg/ml proteinase K (Invitrogen) to extract DNA. Total HIV or SIV DNA content was quantified by PCR amplification with Taq polymerase, 1X Taq Buffer (Invitrogen), $MgCl_2$, dNTPs, HIV/SIV and CD3 primers for 12 cycles. The second amplification involved a nested PCR using 1:10 dilution of amplification product, HIV/SIV and CD3 primers, SsoAdvanced Universal Probe Supermix (Bio-rad) using qPCR. A standard curve was established using ACH2 cell lysates (ATCC) that contain a single copy of

HIV per cell or SIV$_{mac}$239 plasmid. Primers used are listed in Additional file 1: Table S2.

gp120-CD4 interaction by ELISA
Recombinant YU2 gp120 protein (Immune Tech, cat# IT-001-0027p, 1.5 μg/ml) was coated onto a 96-well ELISA plate ON at 4 °C. Next day, wells were washed twice with 150 μl of PBS supplemented with Tween 0.05%, and saturated with 5% milk for 1 h at 37 °C. CD4-Ig (gift from Dr. Michael Farzan, 5 μg/ml) in presence or not of increasing concentrations of Kudzu was then added and the plate was incubated at 37 °C for 1 h. Secondary anti-human antibodies were then added at the dilution 1:5000 for 1 h at 37 °C. Then, 50 μl of TMB (Immunochemistry) was added at room temperature and the reaction was stopped with TMB stop solution. The absorbance was read at 450 nm. Several washes were performed after each step except after saturation. Emtracitabine (500 μM), soluble recombinant YU2 gp120 protein (Immune Tech, cat# IT-001-0027p) and soluble mouse CD4 (gift from Dr. Michael Farzan) were used as controls in the assay.

Expression of CD4 and CXCR4 in HeLa-CD4-LTR-LacZ cells analyzed by flow cytometry
Cells were seeded at 1×10^6 in a 6-well plate. The next day, compounds (Kudzu 1:400, PMA 100 nM or buffer) were added. Cells were then collected at different time points, stained with PE/Cy7 anti-human CD184 (for CXCR4, Biolegend) or PE antihuman CD4 (Biolegend) and fixed with 2% formaldehyde in PBS. Cells were analyzed on a LSRII flow cytometer (BD Bioscience).

Expression of CCR5 in Ghost-CCR5 cells analyzed by flow cytometry
Cells were seeded at 1×10^6 per 6-well plate. The following day, compounds (Kudzu 1:400 and 1:200) were added. Cells were then collected at 6 h post treatment, stained with PE anti-human CD195 (Biolegend) or PE control (Biolegend). Flow cytometry was afterwards performed (BD Biosciences C6 Accuri and IntelliCyt HyperCyt sampler powered by FlowCyt software).

Fusion of HeLa-CD4-LTR-LacZ cells with HL2/3 cells
Similar protocol to [27] was performed. Briefly, HL2/3 cells (gift from AIDSreagent program), expressing the HXB2 envelope, Tat, Gag, Rev, and Nef proteins, were co-cultured with HeLa-CD4-LTR-LacZ cells at 1:1 density ratio (2.5×10^4 cells/well in a 96-well-plate) for 48 h in presence of different compounds (Kudzu: 1:400 and 1:200, Raltegravir: 100 nM, Emtricitabine: 100 nM, Enfuvirtide: 1 μg/ml). Upon fusion of the two cell lines, Tat protein from HL2/3 cells activates β-gal expression, measured by a CPRG assay.

Shedding of gp120 from transfected gp160
Performed as previously reported [35]. Briefly, HEK293T cells were transfected with the constructs JR-FL gp160Δtail (1.5 μg) and pCMV Rev (0.5 μg) (gifts from Dr. Michael Farzan) for 48 h with TransIT-2020 transfection reagent (Mirus Bio LLC) according to the manufacturer's protocol. JR-FL gp160Δtail was used to achieve higher envelope trimer expression [46]. CD4-Ig (45 μg, a gift from Dr. Michael Farzan) or Kudzu (1:400 dilution) were incubated with cells for 4 h. Cells were then washed several times with PBS 10 mM EDTA and lysed with RIPA buffer supplemented with a cocktail of protease inhibitor (Roche). Protein concentration was determined by Bradford assay. The cell lysates were analyzed on a reducing gel 4–20% gradient gel (Biorad) and subsequently blotted onto a nitrocellulose membrane (Biorad). gp120 content was determined by immunoblotting using a gp120 serum at 1:500 dilution (a gift from Dr. Michael Farzan) and goat anti-human antibody (1:5000, Santa Cruz).

Shedding of gp120 from NL4-3 virus
Kudzu and CD4-Ig (gift from Dr. Michael Farzan, 30 μg) were incubated with NL4-3 (44.8 ng) for 6 h. Samples were then filtered through 300 kDa column (Vivaspin, Sartorius). A fraction of the flow trough was analyzed by immunoblot as described above.

Maturation of HIV-1 capsid
HEK293T cells were transfected with pNL4-3 encoding plasmid (12.5 μg) with TransIT-2020 transfection reagent (Mirus Bio LLC) according to the manufacturer's protocol. Six hours later, cells were washed, trypsinized and split between the conditions tested. Cells were treated with either buffer, Kudzu (1:400), Raltegravir (100 nM), Saquinavir (300 nM) and incubated at 37 °C for 72 h. Next, cells were lysed in RIPA buffer supplemented with a cocktail of protease inhibitors (Roche) and analyzed by immunoblotting with anti-p24 antibody (1:2500, NIH AIDS Reagent Program cat# 3537). Anti-GAPDH antibody (1:500, Santa cruz) was used as loading control.

Assessment of Kudzu's cytotoxicity
MTT (3-[4,5-dimethylthiazol-2-yl]-2,5-diphenyltetrazolium bromide) assay (ATCC) or cell titer Glo luminescent cell viability (Promega) was performed in the presence of increasing concentrations of Kudzu or Kudzu components according to the manufacturer's protocol.

Authors' contributions

AM, JJA, STV and YE involved in conceptualization. SM, JJA, ST, AR, CK, AB, MC performed experiments and analyzed data. TT, CH, MC, STV responsible for methodology, supervision, validation and in funding acquisition. All authors read and approved the final manuscript.

Author details

[1] Department of Immunology and Microbiology, The Scripps Research Institute, 130 Scripps Way, 3C1, Jupiter, FL 33458, USA. [2] Department of Molecular Therapeutics, The Scripps Research Institute, Jupiter, FL, USA. [3] The Botanist's Beach Farm, Jupiter, FL, USA. [4] University of Miami Miller School of Medicine, Miami, FL, USA. [5] Present Address: Roche, Basel, Switzerland.

Acknowledgements

This work was supported by The Scripps Research institute. We thank the NIH AIDS Reagent Program for reagents and Dr. Michael Farzan, Dr. Guillaume Mousseau, Dr. Travis Grim for advice and helpful discussions.

Competing interests

The authors declare that they have no competing interests.

Funding

This work was supported with funding from The Scripps Research Institute.

References

1. Clavel F, Hance AJ. HIV drug resistance. N Engl J Med. 2004;350:1023–35.
2. Wainberg MA, Zaharatos GJ, Brenner BG. Development of antiretroviral drug resistance. N Engl J Med. 2011;365:637–46.
3. Saphire AC, Bobardt MD, Zhang Z, David G, Gallay PA. Syndecans serve as attachment receptors for human immunodeficiency virus type 1 on macrophages. J Virol. 2001;75:9187–200.
4. Arthos J, Cicala C, Martinelli E, Macleod K, Van Ryk D, Wei D, Xiao Z, Veenstra TD, Conrad TP, Lempicki RA, McLaughlin S, Pascuccio M, Gopaul R, McNally J, Cruz CC, Censoplano N, Chung E, Reitano KN, Kottilil S, Goode DJ, Fauci AS. HIV-1 envelope protein binds to and signals through integrin alpha4beta7, the gut mucosal homing receptor for peripheral T cells. Nat Immunol. 2008;9:301–9.
5. Cicala C, Martinelli E, McNally JP, Goode DJ, Gopaul R, Hiatt J, Jelicic K, Kottilil S, Macleod K, O'Shea A, Patel N, Van Ryk D, Wei D, Pascuccio M, Yi L, McKinnon L, Izulla P, Kimani J, Kaul R, Fauci AS, Arthos J. The integrin alpha4beta7 forms a complex with cell-surface CD4 and defines a T-cell subset that is highly susceptible to infection by HIV-1. Proc Natl Acad Sci USA. 2009;106:20877–82.
6. Geijtenbeek TB, Kwon DS, Torensma R, van Vliet SJ, van Duijnhoven GC, Middel J, Cornelissen IL, Nottet HS, KewalRamani VN, Littman DR, Figdor CG, van Kooyk Y. DC-SIGN, a dendritic cell-specific HIV-1-binding protein that enhances trans-infection of T cells. Cell. 2000;100:587–97 (see comments).
7. Gummuluru S, Rogel M, Stamatatos L, Emerman M. Binding of human immunodeficiency virus type 1 to immature dendritic cells can occur independently of DC-SIGN and mannose binding C-type lectin receptors via a cholesterol-dependent pathway. J Virol. 2003;77:12865–74.
8. Clapham PR, Reeves JD, Simmons G, Dejucq N, Hibbitts S, McKnight A. HIV coreceptors, cell tropism and inhibition by chemokine receptor ligands. Mol Membr Biol. 1999;16:49–55.
9. Kwong PD, Wyatt R, Sattentau QJ, Sodroski J, Hendrickson WA. Oligomeric modeling and electrostatic analysis of the gp120 envelope glycoprotein of human immunodeficiency virus. J Virol. 2000;74:1961–72.
10. Moore JP, Binley J. HIV. Envelope's letters boxed into shape. Nature. 1998;393:630–1 (news; comment).
11. Caffrey M. HIV envelope: challenges and opportunities for development of entry inhibitors. Trends Microbiol. 2011;19:191–7.
12. Didigu CA, Doms RW. Novel approaches to inhibit HIV entry. Viruses. 2012;4:309–24.
13. Hardy H, Skolnik PR. Enfuvirtide, a new fusion inhibitor for therapy of human immunodeficiency virus infection. Pharmacotherapy. 2004;24:198–211.
14. Duffalo ML, James CW. Enfuvirtide: a novel agent for the treatment of HIV-1 infection. Ann Pharmacother. 2003;37:1448–56.
15. Tang MW, Shafer RW. HIV-1 antiretroviral resistance: scientific principles and clinical applications. Drugs. 2012;72:e1–25.

16. Dorr P, Westby M, Dobbs S, Griffin P, Irvine B, Macartney M, Mori J, Rickett G, Smith-Burchnell C, Napier C, Webster R, Armour D, Price D, Stammen B, Wood A, Perros M. Maraviroc (UK-427,857), a potent, orally bioavailable, and selective small-molecule inhibitor of chemokine receptor CCR5 with broad-spectrum anti-human immunodeficiency virus type 1 activity. Antimicrob Agents Chemother. 2005;49:4721–32.
17. Hunt JS, Romanelli F. Maraviroc, a CCR5 coreceptor antagonist that blocks entry of human immunodeficiency virus type 1. Pharmacotherapy. 2009;29:295–304.
18. Fessel WJ, Anderson B, Follansbee SE, Winters MA, Lewis ST, Weinheimer SP, Petropoulos CJ, Shafer RW. The efficacy of an anti-CD4 monoclonal antibody for HIV-1 treatment. Antiviral Res. 2011;92:484–7.
19. Zhong Y, Li Y, Zhao Y. Physicochemical, microstructural, and antibacterial properties of beta-chitosan and kudzu starch composite films. J Food Sci. 2012;77:E280–6.
20. Li G, Zhang Q, Wang Y. Chemical constituents from roots of *Pueraria lobata*. Zhongguo Zhong Yao Za Zhi. 2010;35:3156–60.
21. Penetar DM, Toto LH, Lee DY, Lukas SE. A single dose of kudzu extract reduces alcohol consumption in a binge drinking paradigm. Drug Alcohol Depend. 2015;153:194–200.
22. Liu B, Kongstad KT, Qinglei S, Nyberg NT, Jager AK, Staerk D. Dual high-resolution alpha-glucosidase and radical scavenging profiling combined with HPLC-HRMS-SPE-NMR for identification of minor and major constituents directly from the crude extract of *Pueraria lobata*. J Nat Prod. 2015;78:294–300.
23. Du G, Zhao HY, Zhang QW, Li GH, Yang FQ, Wang Y, Li YC, Wang YT. A rapid method for simultaneous determination of 14 phenolic compounds in *Radix puerariae* using microwave-assisted extraction and ultra high performance liquid chromatography coupled with diode array detection and time-of-flight mass spectrometry. J Chromatogr A. 2010;1217:705–14.
24. Zhou YX, Zhang H, Peng C. Puerarin: a review of pharmacological effects. Phytother Res. 2014;28:961–75.
25. Zhang Z, Lam TN, Zuo Z. *Radix puerariae*: an overview of its chemistry, pharmacology, pharmacokinetics, and clinical use. J Clin Pharmacol. 2013;53:787–811.
26. Abram ME, Ferris AL, Das K, Quinones O, Shao W, Tuske S, Alvord WG, Arnold E, Hughes SH. Mutations in HIV-1 reverse transcriptase affect the errors made in a single cycle of viral replication. J Virol. 2014;88:7589–601.
27. Lara HH, Ayala-Nunez NV, Ixtepan-Turrent L, Rodriguez-Padilla C. Mode of antiviral action of silver nanoparticles against HIV-1. J Nanobiotechnology. 2010;8:1.
28. Ren J, Bird LE, Chamberlain PP, Stewart-Jones GB, Stuart DI, Stammers DK. Structure of HIV-2 reverse transcriptase at 2.35-A resolution and the mechanism of resistance to non-nucleoside inhibitors. Proc Natl Acad Sci USA. 2002;99:14410–5.
29. Witvrouw M, Pannecouque C, Switzer WM, Folks TM, De Clercq E, Heneine W. Susceptibility of HIV-2, SIV and SHIV to various anti-HIV-1 compounds: implications for treatment and postexposure prophylaxis. Antivir Ther. 2004;9:57–65.
30. Poveda E, Briz V, Soriano V. Enfuvirtide, the first fusion inhibitor to treat HIV infection. AIDS Rev. 2005;7:139–47.
31. Schulz TF, Whitby D, Hoad JG, Corrah T, Whittle H, Weiss RA. Biological and molecular variability of human immunodeficiency virus type 2 isolates from the Gambia. J Virol. 1990;64:5177–82.
32. Sato Y, Morimoto K, Kubo T, Sakaguchi T, Nishizono A, Hirayama M, Hori K. Entry inhibition of influenza viruses with high mannose binding lectin ESA-2 from the red alga *Eucheuma serra* through the recognition of viral hemagglutinin. Mar Drugs. 2015;13:3454–65.
33. Rausch K, Hackett BA, Weinbren NL, Reeder SM, Sadovsky Y, Hunter CA, Schultz DC, Coyne CB, Cherry S. Screening bioactives reveals nanchangmycin as a broad spectrum antiviral active against zika virus. Cell Rep. 2017;18:804–15.
34. Fellinger CH, Gardner MR, Bailey CC, Farzan M. Simian immunodeficiency virus SIVmac239, but not SIVmac316, binds and utilizes Human CD4 more efficiently than rhesus CD4. J Virol. 2017;91(18):e00847.
35. Ruprecht CR, Krarup A, Reynell L, Mann AM, Brandenberg OF, Berlinger L, Abela IA, Regoes RR, Gunthard HF, Rusert P, Trkola A. MPER-specific antibodies induce gp120 shedding and irreversibly neutralize HIV-1. J Exp Med. 2011;208:439–54.

36. Rapista A, Ding J, Benito B, Lo YT, Neiditch MB, Lu W, Chang TL. Human defensins 5 and 6 enhance HIV-1 infectivity through promoting HIV attachment. Retrovirology. 2011;8:45.

37. Saphire AC, Bobardt MD, Gallay PA. Host cyclophilin A mediates HIV-1 attachment to target cells via heparans. EMBO J. 1999;18:6771–85.

38. Vives RR, Imberty A, Sattentau QJ, Lortat-Jacob H. Heparan sulfate targets the HIV-1 envelope glycoprotein gp120 coreceptor binding site. J Biol Chem. 2005;280:21353–7.

39. Mousseau G, Clementz MA, Bakeman WN, Nagarsheth N, Cameron M, Shi J, Baran P, Fromentin R, Chomont N, Valente ST. An analog of the natural steroidal alkaloid cortistatin A potently suppresses Tat-dependent HIV transcription. Cell Host Microbe. 2012;12(1):97–108.

40. Tallarida RJ. Drug combinations: tests and analysis with isoboles. Curr Protoc Pharmacol. 2016;72:9.19.1–19.19.

41. Pan C, Cai L, Lu H, Qi Z, Jiang S. Combinations of the first and next generations of human immunodeficiency virus (HIV) fusion inhibitors exhibit a highly potent synergistic effect against enfuvirtide- sensitive and -resistant HIV type 1 strains. J Virol. 2009;83:7862–72.

42. Mousseau G, Kessing CF, Fromentin R, Trautmann L, Chomont N, Valente ST. The tat inhibitor didehydro-Cortistatin A prevents HIV-1 reactivation from latency. MBio. 2015;6:e00465.

43. Carroll SS, Tomassini JE, Bosserman M, Getty K, Stahlhut MW, Eldrup AB, Bhat B, Hall D, Simcoe AL, LaFemina R, Rutkowski CA, Wolanski B, Yang Z, Migliaccio G, De Francesco R, Kuo LC, MacCoss M, Olsen DB. Inhibition of hepatitis C virus RNA replication by 2′-modified nucleoside analogs. J Biol Chem. 2003;278:11979–84.

44. Lindenbach BD, Evans MJ, Syder AJ, Wolk B, Tellinghuisen TL, Liu CC, Maruyama T, Hynes RO, Burton DR, McKeating JA, Rice CM. Complete replication of hepatitis C virus in cell culture. Science. 2005;309:623–6.

45. Thenin-Houssier S, de Vera IM, Pedro-Rosa L, Brady A, Richard A, Konnick B, Opp S, Buffone C, Fuhrmann J, Kota S, Billack B, Pietka-Ottlik M, Tellinghuisen T, Choe H, Spicer T, Scampavia L, Diaz-Griffero F, Kojetin DJ, Valente ST. Ebselen, a small-molecule capsid inhibitor of HIV-1 replication. Antimicrob Agents Chemother. 2016;60:2195–208.

46. Binley JM, Cayanan CS, Wiley C, Schulke N, Olson WC, Burton DR. Redox-triggered infection by disulfide-shackled human immunodeficiency virus type 1 pseudovirions. J Virol. 2003;77:5678–84.

18

Adeno-associated virus gene delivery of broadly neutralizing antibodies as prevention and therapy against HIV-1

Allen Lin[1,2] and Alejandro B. Balazs[1]*

Abstract

Vectored gene delivery of HIV-1 broadly neutralizing antibodies (bNAbs) using recombinant adeno-associated virus (rAAV) is a promising alternative to conventional vaccines for preventing new HIV-1 infections and for therapeutically suppressing established HIV-1 infections. Passive infusion of single bNAbs has already shown promise in initial clinical trials to temporarily decrease HIV-1 load in viremic patients, and to delay viral rebound from latent reservoirs in suppressed patients during analytical treatment interruptions of antiretroviral therapy. Long-term, continuous, systemic expression of such bNAbs could be achieved with a single injection of rAAV encoding antibody genes into muscle tissue, which would bypass the challenges of eliciting such bNAbs through traditional vaccination in naïve patients, and of life-long repeated passive transfers of such biologics for therapy. rAAV delivery of single bNAbs has already demonstrated protection from repeated HIV-1 vaginal challenge in humanized mouse models, and phase I clinical trials of this approach are underway. Selection of which individual, or combination of, bNAbs to deliver to counter pre-existing resistance and the rise of escape mutations in the virus remains a challenge, and such choices may differ depending on use of this technology for prevention versus therapy.

Keywords: Vectored delivery, Antibody gene transfer, AAV, HIV-1, bNAb, Clinical trials, Animal models

Background

HIV-1 remains a significant contributor to the global burden of disease. In 2016, 1.8 million individuals were newly infected with HIV-1, and more than 36 million individuals were living with HIV-1, of whom only 44% were virally suppressed with antiretroviral therapy (ART) [1]. The need for daily dosing of ARTs remains a challenge for their effective use for both viral suppression as well as pre-exposure prophylaxis of HIV-1. Whether due to lack of drug access, stigma, inability, or drug-drug interactions, failure to maintain drug pressure in the body can result in breakthrough infection or drug-resistant viral rebound. Long-term, continuous, systemic expression of anti-HIV-1 antibodies by a single administration of recombinant adeno-associated viruses (rAAV) may be an alternative to ARTs.

This review will summarize advances in using recombinant AAV (rAAV) for gene transfer, and describe broadly neutralizing antibodies (bNAbs) against HIV-1 and the results of recently completed clinical trials that passively transfer these bNAbs into individuals living with HIV-1. It also describes recent progress of vectored delivery of bNAbs for long-lasting expression in humanized mouse models, macaque models, and in ongoing clinical trials, and concludes with the challenges faced in deciding which bNAbs to deliver.

Main text

Recombinant adeno-associated viruses (rAAV) for gene transfer

AAVs have long been contemplated as attractive vectors for use in gene transfer [2]. AAV is a replication-defective 20–25 nm *Parvoviridae* virus consisting of a non-enveloped, icosahedral protein shell (capsid) surrounding one copy of a linear single-stranded DNA genome. Initially

*Correspondence: abalazs@mgh.harvard.edu
[1] Ragon Institute of MGH, MIT and Harvard, Cambridge, MA 02139, USA
Full list of author information is available at the end of the article

found in 1965 as a contaminant of adenovirus preparations [3], AAV can only replicate within cells in the presence of helper functions provided by viruses such as adenovirus or herpesvirus. The 4.7 kb AAV genome encodes for *rep* and *cap* in between two palindromic 145 bp inverted terminal repeats (ITRs). These ITRs self-anneal into T-shaped hairpin structures [4]. *rep* is translated into four non-structural proteins for packaging and replication and *cap* into three structural capsid proteins that protect the genome and modulate cell binding and trafficking. In addition, a recently discovered alternative open-reading frame in *cap* encodes for assembly-activating protein, which is necessary for capsid assembly in certain AAV serotypes [5]. Thirteen serotypes of AAV (named AAV1-13) have been discovered to date, and these serotypes differ in tissue tropisms, transduction efficiencies, and expression levels dependent on their viral capsid sequence [6]. Screening in humans and non-human primates and ancestral sequence reconstruction have identified numerous additional infectious capsids that are variants of the 13 representative serotypes [7–9].

The ITRs are the only sequence elements required *in cis* for packing of the genome into the capsid and for replication. Thus, recombinant AAV (rAAV) vectors used for gene transfer need only consist of an expression cassette encoding a promoter and transgene placed between the ITRs, in lieu of *rep* and *cap*. Helper functions of *rep* and *cap* are supplied *in trans* via a separate plasmid, co-transfected during production, and thus no viral genes are encoded by rAAV. The serotype choice for *cap* provided *in trans* dictates the identity of the capsid shell of the recombinant vector and thus which tissues are preferentially infected by rAAV. Given the importance of *cap* in modulating tissue tropism and possibly immunogenicity [10, 11], numerous efforts are underway to engineer *cap* for greater specificity and desirable activities [12].

AAVs have no apparent pathogenicity, as they are not known to be associated with any human disease [13]. Natural AAV infection occuring without helper virus functions can enter a latent phase and integrate site-specifically into the AAVS1 site on the 19th chromosome in humans, in a process that requires proteins encoded by *rep* [14–16]. Because rAAV vectors do not encode *rep*, their genomes persist as extrachromosomal episomal concatemers that rarely integrate into the chromosome [17–19]. Despite the episomal nature of rAAV, a single intramuscular injection of rAAV has been shown to maintain transgene expression for a number of years in a variety of animal models including humans [20–23], in one case enabling detection of rAAV transgene expression in a patient over 10 years after administration [24].

There are several general considerations to using rAAV as a gene transfer vector. First, rAAV has a limited transgene carrying capacity. AAV has a genome of 4.7 kb, and rAAVs that are produced with transgenes of more than approximately 5 kb result in substantially reduced transduction efficiencies [25]. Second, transgene expression upon transduction of target tissues with single-stranded rAAV is not immediate, as the cell must first synthesize the second strand using the single-stranded DNA genomic template [26, 27]. Lastly, pre-existing immunity of individuals to AAV from natural exposure may limit the efficiency of transduction. Global seroprevalences of different AAV serotypes range from 30 to 60% [28, 29]. Even if transduction is able to occur, adaptive immune responses can severely limit transgene expression. In early gene therapy trials using AAV2 to deliver factor IX to patients with hemophilia B, factor IX expression was limited to only several months, likely due to transduced cells presenting AAV capsid peptides, which reactivated memory T cells targeting those transduced cells [30]. Subsequent trials using AAV8 were successful in stable expression of factor IX when they excluded patients with detectable anti-AAV antibodies and used the lowest dose of rAAV8 that still provided therapeutic benefit [23, 31]. Efforts to discover rare and ancestral AAV capsids and to create new capsids for which humans do not yet have an immune response are underway [9]. Since a patient who receives rAAV will likely develop immunity against the capsid upon injection, subsequently giving the same patient another rAAV with the same capsid serotype is unlikely to result in additional transgene expression.

Only two rAAV gene therapy products have been licensed to date, but many more are in clinical trials [32]. Glybera (alipogene tiparvovec) for lipoprotein lipase deficiency was the first gene therapy product licensed in Europe in 2012, in which the human lipoprotein lipase gene in an AAV1 capsid is administered via intramuscular injection. Luxturna (voretigene neparvovec) for inherited retinal dystrophy was the first gene therapy product approved by the FDA in 2017, in which the RPE65 gene in an rAAV2 vector is injected subretinally to treat blindness [33, 34]. Affordability and patient accessibility of gene therapy products remain to be determined. Priced at 1 million dollars per treatment, Glybera was withdrawn from the market by its manufacturer after 5 years [35]. Due to difficulty of convincing national reimbursers to pay for the treatment, it was only used in one patient. Luxtura has been similarly priced at $425,000 per eye [36]. To increase its acceptability, its manufacturer is seeking reimbursement only with positive outcomes. The prices of future gene therapy products will depend on the commercial outcomes of these initial products and further maturation and widespread adoption of these technologies.

Anti-HIV-1 broadly neutralizing antibodies (bNAbs)

Gene transfer of anti-HIV-1 broadly neutralizing antibodies (bNAbs) with rAAV may be an effective method to prevent and suppress HIV-1 infection. Approximately half of chronically infected HIV-1 individuals naturally develop sera capable of neutralizing half of the diversity of HIV-1 at low to moderate titers [37]. However, only a small proportion of individuals develop bNAbs of great potency and breadth that cross-clade neutralize diverse HIV-1 strains, by binding to conserved regions of the HIV-1 envelope spike. These rare bNAbs are heavily somatically hypermutated from years of coevolution with the virus [38]. Several properties of HIV-1 envelope impede the development of such antibodies. First, a single HIV-1 virion displays only ~14 envelope spikes on its surface [39]. Such low-density surface protein limits the potential for avidity effects and thus may result in less BCR cross-linking for B cell activation. Second, the envelope surface is covered by shifting glycosylation sites and flexible variable loops that sterically hinder access to conserved epitopes buried deep inside the protein, and thus antibodies against HIV-1 are more likely to be strain-specific than broad [40, 41].

Nevertheless, improvements in antibody discovery techniques have resulted in the identification of new bNAbs each year [42]. Antibodies appear to bind to several preferential target regions on the HIV-1 envelope: the V1/V2 site at the trimer apex, the N332 glycan supersite near the V3 loop, the CD4 binding site, the gp120–gp41 interface, and the membrane-proximal external region (MPER) [43]. The CD4 binding site is of particular interest as it is well conserved due to the need for HIV-1 to bind to its primary receptor for infection. bNAbs that target the CD4 binding site include b12 [44], VRC01 [45, 46], 3BNC117 [47], N6 [48], and N49P7 [49]. These latter antibodies possess great breath and potency, as N49P7 neutralized 86% of a 117 multi-clade pseudovirus panel at an $IC_{50} < 1$ µg/ml [49], and N6 neutralized 96% of another 181 multi-clade pseudovirus panel at an $IC_{50} < 1$ µg/ml [48].

However, eliciting bNAbs in individuals through vaccination is likely to be difficult as a consequence of the extensive somatic hypermutation and unusually long sequence complementarity determining regions observed in many bNAb lineages. Thus, novel sequential administration of different immunogens may be needed to elicit bNAbs in patients [50]. Multiple immunogen design strategies have emerged to first stimulate bNAb germline precursors and then drive affinity maturation against bNAb target epitopes [51]. In lineage-based immunogen design, immunogens mimic natural viral evolution found in a patient who develops a bNAb, starting with the founder strain [52]. In germline-targeting immunogen design, the first immunogen seeks to engage bNAb germline precursors. For instance, eOD-GT8 is a multivalent nanoparticle, presenting a structure-based design of gp120 outer domain molecule selected through iterative random mutagenesis and yeast cell surface display [53]. Priming with this immunogen followed by more native Env-like boosts in a VRC01 germline knock-in model resulted in antibodies of intermediate VRC01 maturity [54]. Results of these approaches are promising, but guiding such maturation in diverse patient populations may be difficult due to allelic diversity at immunoglobulin loci. Given the likely difficulty of eliciting bNAbs via traditional vaccines, alternative approaches using existing bNAbs either through passive transfer or gene transfer are being explored.

Passive transfer of bNAbs in clinical trials

Given the challenges of eliciting highly somatically mutated bNAbs in naïve individuals, direct administration of mature bNAbs for prevention or therapy is currently being tested in humans. Experimental designs for these clinical trials are shown in Fig. 1. Six phase I or IIa trials of passive infusion of single bNAbs (VRC01 [55, 56], 3BNC117 [57, 58], and 10-1074 [59]) into HIV-1 infected individuals have been published to date (Table 1), with many more underway or planned [60]. These studies use one of two therapy trial protocols. The first consists of administration of antibody into viremic individuals and observing the decline in viral load and time until viral rebound (Fig. 1e). The second is an analytic treatment interruption (ATI), where ART-suppressed HIV-infected individuals are given multiple sequential antibody infusions and taken off ART shortly after the first infusion (Fig. 1c). The delay in latent viral rebound is then observed. Overall, these studies have shown that the examined bNAbs have a therapeutic effect and exert selection pressure on the virus. The degree of suppression varied across antibodies and patients, depending on antibody potency and the presence of pre-existing resistance mutations in a patient. Interestingly, despite theoretical concerns over the degree of somatic hypermutation these antibodies exhibit, these bNAbs have not been found to be particularly immunogenic in humans, as anti-drug antibody (ADA) responses have not been observed in these trials. Across all of these trials, bNAb half-life was consistently shorter in HIV-1 infected individuals than in uninfected individuals, perhaps due to increased clearance of antibody-antigen immune complexes.

The first clinical trials in HIV-1 infected individuals examined CD4 binding site bNAbs. In a phase I trial, Caskey et al. [57] administered a single infusion of 3BNC117 to eight HIV-1 infected, viremic individuals, which significantly reduced mean viremia from baseline

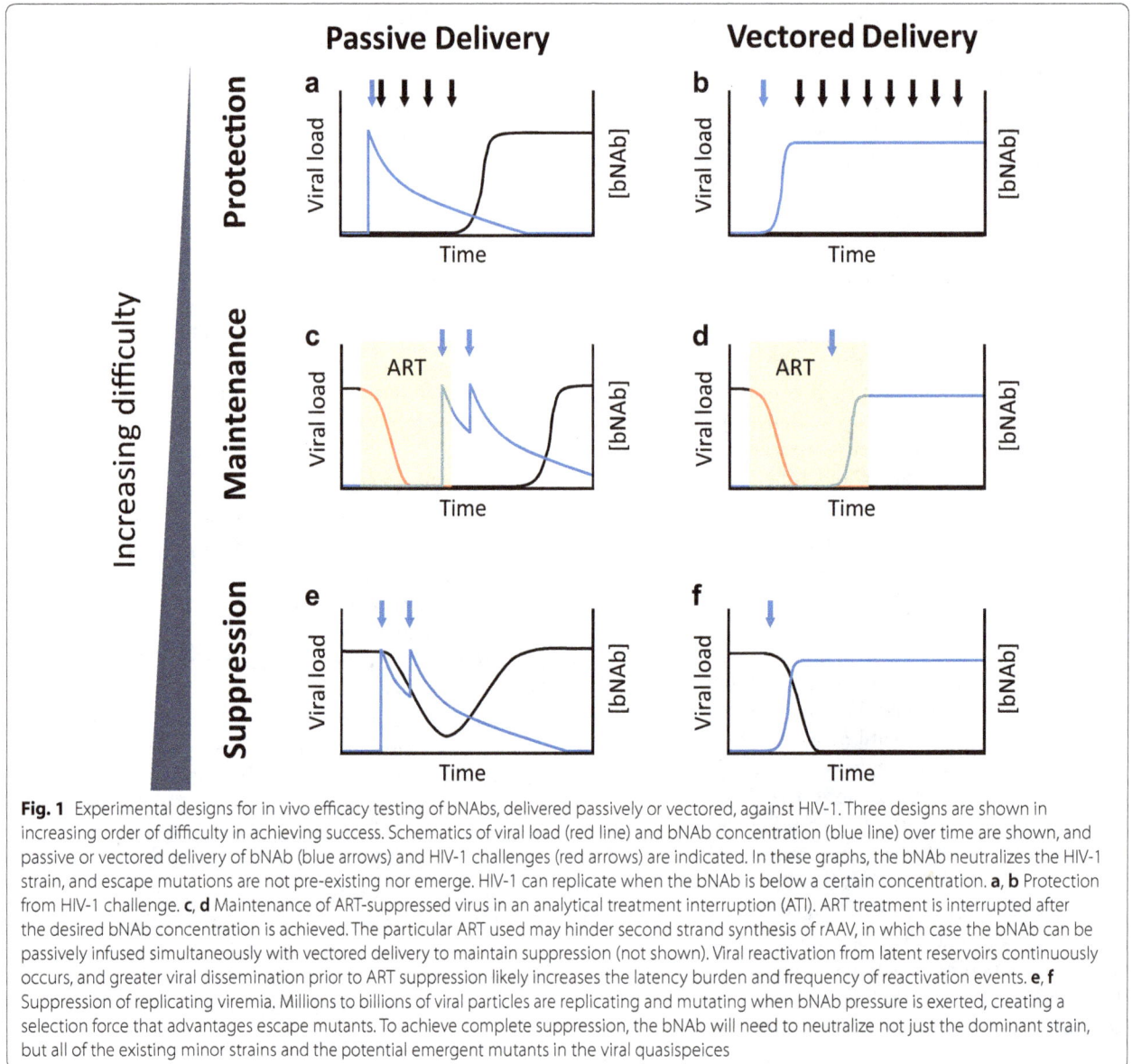

Fig. 1 Experimental designs for in vivo efficacy testing of bNAbs, delivered passively or vectored, against HIV-1. Three designs are shown in increasing order of difficulty in achieving success. Schematics of viral load (red line) and bNAb concentration (blue line) over time are shown, and passive or vectored delivery of bNAb (blue arrows) and HIV-1 challenges (red arrows) are indicated. In these graphs, the bNAb neutralizes the HIV-1 strain, and escape mutations are not pre-existing nor emerge. HIV-1 can replicate when the bNAb is below a certain concentration. **a, b** Protection from HIV-1 challenge. **c, d** Maintenance of ART-suppressed virus in an analytical treatment interruption (ATI). ART treatment is interrupted after the desired bNAb concentration is achieved. The particular ART used may hinder second strand synthesis of rAAV, in which case the bNAb can be passively infused simultaneously with vectored delivery to maintain suppression (not shown). Viral reactivation from latent reservoirs continuously occurs, and greater viral dissemination prior to ART suppression likely increases the latency burden and frequency of reactivation events. **e, f** Suppression of replicating viremia. Millions to billions of viral particles are replicating and mutating when bNAb pressure is exerted, creating a selection force that advantages escape mutants. To achieve complete suppression, the bNAb will need to neutralize not just the dominant strain, but all of the existing minor strains and the potential emergent mutants in the viral quasispeices

for 4 weeks by up to 1.5 $\log_{10}$ copies/ml. A subsequent 3BNC117 ATI phase IIa trial gave multiple infusions in 13 HIV-1 infected individuals [58]. Individuals were pre-screened for PMBC viral outgrowth cultures with 3BNC117 sensitivity (IC$_{50}$ ≤ 2.0 μg/ml). Viral rebound was significantly delayed by a mean of 6.7 weeks in individuals with 2 infusions, or by a mean of 9.9 weeks in individuals with 4 infusions, compared to historical controls of 2.6 weeks. 3BNC117 levels at viral rebound ranged from 6 to 168 μg/ml, and these values correlated with the IC$_{80}$ of recrudescent viruses.

Two findings from these 3BNC117 trials suggested that 3BNC117 imposed a high barrier to viral escape. First, in

a majority of participants of the second ATI trial (8/13), the recrudescent viruses were at least threefold more resistant by IC$_{80}$. In 5 out of these 8, the rebounded virus appeared to have emerged from a single resistant provirus. In contrast, virus rebound after standard analytical treatment interruption without additional treatment is typically polyclonal, as multiple latent viruses are reactivated [61]. The restriction of recrudescent viruses suggests that 3BNC117 was preventing the rise of most latent clones. The virus that rebounded would have pre-existed at low frequencies such as not to have decreased bulk pre-infusion virus neutralizability. The first trial similarly found that recrudescent viruses with a reduction in

Table 1 Clinical trials of bNAbs in HIV-1 infected individuals with published results

Clinical trial	Trial design	Delivery	bNAb	Highest dose given (mg/kg)	HIV-1 infected individuals given highest dose	Dosing schedule	bNAb sensitivity prescreening	Viral response	References
NCT02018510	Suppression	Passive	3BNC117	30	8 viremic individuals	One dose	Some	Viral load was reduced by mean of 1.5 log_{10} copies/ml (range of 0.8–2.5), and significant for 28 days	[57]
NCT02446847	Maintenance	Passive	3BNC117	30	13 suppressed individuals	2 doses 3 weeks apart, or 4 doses 2 weeks apart; ART discontinued 2 days after first dose	All	2 infusions delayed rebound by mean of 6.7 weeks (range of 5–9) after ATI, and 4 infusions by mean of 9.9 weeks (range 3–19)	[58]
NCT01950325 (VRC 601)	Suppression	Passive	VRC01	40	8 viremic individuals	One dose	None	Amongst responders (6/8), viral load was reduced by 1.1–1.8 log_{10} copies/ml, and significant for 21 days	[55]
NCT02463227 (ACTG A5340)	Maintenance	Passive	VRC01	40	14 suppressed individuals	Dose 1 week before and 2 and 5 weeks after ART discontinuation	None	Rebound was delayed by 4 weeks (IQR 3–5) after ATI	[56]
NCT02471326 (NIH 15-I-0140)	Maintenance	Passive	VRC01	40	10 suppressed individuals	Dose 3 days before, 2 weeks after, and each subsequent month after ART discontinuation	None	Rebound was delayed by 5.6 weeks (IQR 4.1–5.6) after ATI	[56]
NCT02511990	Suppression	Passive	10-1074	30	13 viremic individuals	One dose	None	Amongst responders (11/13), viral load was reduced by mean of 1.5 log_{10} copies/ml (range 0.9–2.1), and significant for 27 days	[59]

3BNC117 sensitivity tended to cluster in low-diversity lineages. Second, in the ATI trial, of the four individuals who were suppressed until antibody concentration fell below 20 µg/ml, three appeared to not have gained 3BNC117 resistance. Thus, a resistant mutant failed to emerge in the presence of the antibody, demonstrating antibody potency.

Three phase I trials of VRC01 passive infusion found that VRC01 could similarly suppress HIV-1, although suppression seemed to be less than that of 3BNC117. In Lynch et al. [55], in the 8 viremic patients given the highest dose, mean viral load was lower than baseline for 3 weeks. Individuals appeared to follow one of three patterns. Two individuals with mostly pre-existing resistant viruses did not respond, and two individuals with baseline viral loads less than 1000 copies/ml were briefly undetectable and then remained below baseline for at least 6 weeks. The last four individuals had sensitive viruses with a 14 to 59-fold reduction in viral load, but their virus started rebounding after 10 days. Except in the first two individuals with already completely resistant viruses, rebounded viruses had decreased sensitivity to VRC01 after infusion. These rebounded viruses were polyclonal except in one individual, where a pre-existing resistant minor lineage expanded to dominate the population.

In the two other VRC01 ATI trials, viral rebound was delayed by 4 or 5.6 weeks [56]. In a majority of individuals, the rebounded virus was polyclonal. Individuals with detected pre-existing resistant viruses had earlier viral rebounds, and individuals with pre-existing resistance throughout their viral diversity were more likely to have a polyclonal rebound. VRC01 resistance increased in most participants after infusion.

The 10-1074 trial tested a bNAb with an epitope outside of the CD4 binding site [59]. In this trial, 11 out of the 13 individuals who received the highest dose responded with a mean decrease of 1.5 $\log_{10}$ copies/ml, and the decrease was significant for almost four weeks. The two other individuals harbored pre-existing resistance and did not respond. Mean serum concentration was 77 µg/ml at rebound.

Across all VRC01 and 3BNC117 trials, mutations were observed occurring in or near the V5 loop, the D loop, and the CD4 binding site, epitopes common to CD4 binding site antibodies. In contrast, escape mutations in the 10-1074 trial were concentrated to the well-defined potential N-linked glycosylation N332 sequon (PNGS) and a ^{324}G(D/N)IR^{327} motif. Resistance to 10-1074 was highly polyclonal in individual patients, suggesting that there were multiple ways the virus could escape antibody neutralization without greatly sacrificing viral infectivity and replicative fitness. Interestingly, the authors also

found that baseline codon composition at these sites influenced the observed escaped mutations. Specifically, one individual, who in pre-treatment harbored a TCT serine codon instead of the more common AGT serine codon at the S334 PNGS, exhibited single point mutations at that codon to a different set of amino acids than other individuals after 10-1074 infusion. Lastly, in 5 out of 6 individuals sequenced after 10-1074 was no longer detectable, the N332 sequon and ^{324}G(D/N)IR^{327} motif re-emerged, suggesting these escape mutations have sufficient in vivo fitness cost to necessitate reversion when antibody levels diminished.

Overall, these bNAbs are at least transiently efficacious in the therapeutic setting of suppressing viremia or preventing the emergence of latent viruses. In the case of 3BNC117 and VRC01, in patients where rebound virus emerged with reduced sensitivity to the infused bNAb, the rebound strains were often nearly identical and clustered together in low-diversity lineages in phylogenetic trees, distinct from the pre-existing quasispecies. This suggests that the bNAb bottlenecked the rebound virus—one or only a few strains escaped antibody pressure and subsequently expanded. These strains may have either been pre-existing at low-frequencies, or they represent chance emergence of resistant mutants during antibody therapy. In contrast, the rebound virus from 10-1074 was consistently polyclonal, suggesting that the barrier to escape may be lower for this bNAb. Whether this is because the 10-1074 epitope faces less selection pressure to remain as conserved as the CD4 binding site is unclear.

These clinical trials also found evidence that bNAbs have additional advantages over ARTs against HIV-1. In particular, 3BNC117 was found to have in vivo functionality beyond neutralization. 3BNC117 improved the anti-HIV-1 neutralization activity of autologous antibody responses and also increased clearance of infected cells through Fcγ receptor engagement [62, 63]. Further investigation of how these antibodies may engage additional innate immune functions such as antibody-dependent cellular cytotoxicity and phagocytosis in vivo is needed [64, 65]. This is particularly important in the context of HIV-1 cure as antibodies may target cells within the latent viral reservoir that have been reactivated to produce virus [66].

In contrast to clinical trials for therapy, clinical trials for prevention are harder to conduct, as many more patients need to be repeatedly reinfused to detect treatment significance. The ongoing Antibody Mediated Prevention (AMP) study (HVTN 703/HPTN 081, https://clinicaltrials.gov/ct2/show/NCT02568215 and HVTN 704/HPTN 085, https://clinicaltrials.gov/ct2/show/NCT02716675) seeks to passively infuse VRC01 into thousands of trial participants every other month over the course of 10 infusions (Fig. 1a). Results from these trials are eagerly anticipated, as they are poised to be the first to show that bNAbs can actually prevent HIV infection in humans. Regardless of the outcomes of these trials, implementing continuous passive infusion globally, which requires repeated hospital visits from patients and cold chain transport, is infeasible. Steady-state antibody concentrations from passive transfer may also decline below prophylactic levels if the infusion schedule is delayed. Thus, vectored antibody delivery represents an attractive alternative for sustained bNAb production as a means of prevention. Sustained antibody levels, potentially achievable with gene transfer, may also result in long-term viral suppression, as suggested in the few 3BNC117 patients in whom viral rebound occurred only after antibody concentration greatly diminished and without increased resistance.

Efficacy of vectored delivery of bNAbs in animal models

Gene delivery of bNAbs may result in the sustained, systemic expression of such antibodies with as little as one rAAV intramuscular injection, in contrast to passive transfer (Fig. 1). In this approach, antibodies are endogenously produced in muscle cells, targeted for export with secretion peptides, and passively circulated around the body. Table 2 summarizes the studies of vectored delivery of bNAbs covered in this review, and Table 3 lists considerations in using different animal models.

Lewis et al. [67] first demonstrated sustained expression of a bNAb in mice in 2002. They delivered b12, a CD4 binding site bNAb, using an rAAV2 vector encoding both CMV and EF1-α promoters separately expressing the heavy and light chain genes. Injection into Rag1-immunodeficient mice resulted in peak serum levels of 4–9 μg/ml after 12 weeks, and the extracted serum was biologically active when measured by in vitro neutralization assays against HIV-1.

Johnson et al. [68] in 2009 subsequently delivered anti-SIV immunoadhesins via AAV in macaques. These immunoadhesins were based on anti-SIV Fabs obtained from PCR amplification of bone marrow cells of SIV-infected macaques and selected using phage display [69]. The variable light and heavy chains of these Fabs were joined by a linker to make a single chain variable fragment (scFv), which was then fused to a rhesus IgG2 Fc fragment. The authors constructed two such immunoadhesins, 4L6 and 5L7, as well as N4 that contained domains 1 and 2 of rhesus CD4. rAAVs encoding each of these constructs were intramuscularly injected into three macaques using an AAV1 capsid. N4 was constructed as a single-stranded genome, and 4L6 and 5L7 as self-complementary genomes, where two halves of an inverted repeat genome fold into a double-stranded DNA

upon transduction, thereby bypassing the rate-limiting second-strand synthesis step. After 4 weeks, 4L6 or 5L7 immunoadhesin levels were 40–190 μg/ml, except for one macaque, in which 5L7 expression was eliminated due to the development of anti-5L7 antibodies. N4 levels were lower at 3–10 μg/ml. When these macaques were challenged intravenously with SIVmac316 a month after transduction, six out of nine animals were protected, but three were infected. Upon investigation, these three infected macaques had developed endogenous immunogenic responses against the immunoadhesins prior to challenge, thereby limiting the effectiveness of prevention.

In 2005, Fang et al. [70] first demonstrated the long-lasting delivery of full-length antibodies at therapeutic levels using single-stranded rAAV vectors. They achieved this by expressing a single open reading frame encoding the antibody heavy and light chains, linked by a 24-amino acid 2A self-processing sequence derived from picornavirus. Separation of these chains occurs between the last two residues of the 2A sequence through a ribosomal skip mechanism which prevents the formation of the peptide bond during translation [71]. A 4-amino acid furin cleavage sequence was added after the heavy chain and before the 2A sequence, which resulted in the removal of the residual 2A peptide in the Golgi. The single 2A amino acid at the N-terminus of the light chain is located prior to the signal peptide, and thus was not present in the mature antibody. Using this system, the authors demonstrated that injection of an rAAV8 vector carrying a VEGFR2-neutralizing antibody gene into mice resulted in > 1 mg/ml expression of the antibody for over 4 months with in vivo therapeutic efficacy. In a follow-up study, Fang et al. [72] optimized the furin cleavage site to achieve more complete and uniform cleavage.

Our lab used these developments to demonstrate that full-length bNAbs identical to those found in humans could be continuously produced at therapeutic levels via AAV gene transfer and that such vectored immunoprophylaxis (VIP) can prevent intravenous HIV transmission [73]. In addition to using codon-optimized 2A and furin sequences in the expression cassette, we also developed a muscle-optimized promoter (CASI), made from combining a CMV enhancer, a chicken β-actin promoter, and a ubiquitin enhancer embedded within a synthetic intron. A woodchuck hepatitis virus posttranscriptional regulatory element (WPRE) was included downstream of the antibody transgene to increase expression. For the vector, rAAV8 was used as it efficiently transduces non-dividing, post-mitotic muscle tissues, which have limited turnover, and human seroprevalence against AAV8 is lower than against AAV1 or AAV2 [74]. In addition, unlike AAV2, AAV8 does not activate capsid-specific T

Table 2 Evaluation of vectored delivery of bNAbs against HIV-1 in animal models

Experimental design	Model	Delivery	Antibody	Highest rAAV genome copies given	Challenge virus	Challenge route	Week of 1st challenge post vectored delivery	[Antibody] in serum at challenge	Viremia in experimental arm	Viremia in control arm	References
Expression	Rag1 KO mice	rAAV2	b12	5×10^{11}	HIV-1 IIIB	N/A (in vitro neutralization with serum)	20	2–6 µg/ml	1/6 not neutralize	No control	[67]
Protection	Macaques	rAAV1	4L6, 5L7, or N4 immunoadhesins	2×10^{13}	SIVmac316	Intravenous	4	0–190 µg/ml (1/9 developed ADA)	3/9 after 1 challenge	6/6 after 1 challenge	[68]
Protection	HuPMBC-NSG mice	rAAV8	b12 or VRC01	1×10^{11}	HIV NL4-3	Intravenous	4	198–313 µg/ml	0/8 after 1 challenge	8/8 after 1 challenge	[73]
Protection	BLT mice	rAAV8	VRC01	1×10^{11}	HIV JR-CSF	Intravaginal	4	45–151 µg/ml	2/10 after 15 challenges	9/9, after mean 4.25 challenges	[77]
Protection	BLT mice	rAAV8	VRC07-G54W	1×10^{11}	HIV REJO.c	Intravaginal	4	56–118 µg/ml	0/13 after 21 challenges	12/12, after mean 7.45 challenges	[77]
Maintenance	Hu-CD34-NSG mice	rAAV2	10-1074	2.5×10^{11}	HIVYU-2-NL4-3	N/A	N/A	~200 µg/ml	1/7 rebounded	No control	[80]
Protection	Macaques	rAAV1	IgG1 versions of 4L6 or 5L7	1.6×10^{13}	SIVmac239	Intravenous	14 or 44	0–270 µg/ml (9/12 developed ADA)	11/12 after 6 challenges	6/6 after 6 challenges	[106]
Protection	Macaques, with cyclosporine administration (CsA) for 4 weeks	rAAV8	Simianized VRC07	1×10^{13}	SHIV-BaLP4	Intrarectal	5.5	0–39 µg/ml (1/6 developed ADA during CsA, 2/5 after CsA)	2/6 after 1 challenge	5/5 after 1 challenge	[107]
Protection	Macaques	rAAV1/2	Rhesus eCD4-Ig with rhesus tyrosine-protein sulfotransferase 2	2.5×10^{13}	SHIV-AD8	Intravenous	8	17–77 µg/ml	0/4 after 6 challenges	4/4 after 6 challenges	[108]

Table 3 Considerations in model choice for evaluating vectored delivery of bNAbs against HIV-1

Characteristics	Hu-PBMC-NSG mice	Hu-CD34-NSG mice	Bone marrow-liver-thymus (BLT) mice	Macaques
Construction	Injection of expanded human PBMCs into NSG mice	Injection of fetal hu-CD34+ hematopoietic stem cells into newborn irradiated NSG mice	Injection of fetal hu-CD34+ hematopoietic stem cells into newborn irradiated NSG mice, along with surgical implantation of autologous thymus and liver tissue	Not needed
Antibody immunogenicity	(+) No strong anti-drug antibody response, permitting sustained antibody expression	(+) No strong anti-drug antibody response, permitting sustained antibody expression	(+) No strong anti-drug antibody response, permitting sustained antibody expression	(−) Strong anti-drug antibody responses, which is not fully resolved with antibody simianization
Immune functionality	(−) Activated human T-cell engraftment, but largely lacking other lineages, no hematopoietic regenerative source, no HLA-restriction, and no primary immune response	(-) Multi-lineage hematopoiesis with functional human T cell compartment that is mouse H2-restricted, but inconsistent humoral and Fc receptor effector responses	(+/−) Multi-lineage hematopoiesis with functional human T cell compartment that is HLA-restricted, but inconsistent humoral and Fc receptor effector responses	(+/−) Functional immune system, but is simian
Model longevity	(−) Up to 8 weeks due to GvHD	(+) Up to a year	(+) Up to a year	(+) Many years
HIV replication	(+) Supports HIV replication	(+) Supports HIV replication	(+) Supports HIV replication	(−) Does not support HIV replication (have to use either SIV or SHIV)
Challenge routes	(−) Intravenous only	(−) Intravenous only	(+) Intravenous, Intravaginal, Intrarectal	(+) Intravenous, Intravaginal, Intrarectal
Genetic homogeneity	(+) Genetic homogeneity within cohort with same graft, increasing reproducibility	(+) Genetic homogeneity within cohort with same graft, increasing reproducibility	(+) Genetic homogeneity within cohort with same graft, increasing reproducibility	(+/−) Genetic diversity, which can complicate analysis with small numbers
Similarity to human physiology and size	(−) Less	(−) Less	(−) Less	(+) More
Costs	(+) Lowest cost	(+) Low cost	(+/−) Moderate cost, but requires surgery	(−) High cost

cells, due to lack of heparin binding which likely leads to uptake by dendritic cells [75], and may induce immune tolerance [10, 76]. In a first experiment, rAAV8-b12 was transduced into huPMBC-NSG humanized mice. Antibody levels were sustained at levels greater than 100 µg/ml a month after transduction. Transduced mice were fully protected from a challenge dose of NL4-3 HIV-1 that was 100-fold higher than needed to infect 7 out of 8 control mice. In a second dose-response experiment, the minimum amounts of rAAV-b12 or rAAV-VRC01 to fully protect mice from NL4-3 HIV-1 infection were found to be 1.25×10^{10} genome copies in both cases, corresponding to a mean concentration of 34 µg/ml for b12 and 8 µg/ml for VRC01.

Subsequently, our lab demonstrated that VIP can also protect humanized mice from low-dose repetitive intravaginal challenge [77]. To better model mucosal transmission of HIV-1, we used a more advanced bone marrow-liver-thymus (BLT) humanized mouse model, as described later in this review. In a first experiment, humanized mice transduced with rAAV8-VRC01 were challenged weekly with JR-CSF, a clade B, R5-tropic virus, starting a month after transduction. Upon transduction, VRC01 was detected at 100 µg/ml in the serum and a minimum of 100 ng/ml in the cervicovaginal lavage fluid, which represented an underestimate of the actual mucosal concentration as antibody was diluted by the vaginal wash procedure. Control mice were infected after a mean of 4.25 exposures, whereas only two of ten transduced mice were infected after 13 and 15 exposures. In a second experiment, VRC07-G54W was delivered via rAAV8 to humanized mice a month before beginning weekly challenges with a transmitted founder clade B, R5-tropic virus, REJO.c. VRC07 was created by pairing the original VRC01 light chain with a newly discovered heavy chain from the VRC01 patient [78], and the G54W mutation increased the antibody potency via mimicry of Phe43 in CD4 [79]. In this experiment, control mice were infected after a mean of 7.45 exposures, whereas none of the mice given VRC07-G54W antibody were infected after 21 exposures. These works demonstrated the protective effect of bNAbs delivered via rAAV against intravaginal HIV-1 challenge in a humanized mouse model.

Other labs have shown that rAAV-delivered bNAbs can also be used for therapeutic purposes. Horwitz et al. [80] in 2013 demonstrated that suppression of HIV-1 can be maintained with rAAV gene transfer of bNAbs in the NSG-CD34+ humanized mouse model. Because they found that ART interfered with AAV transduction, they first suppressed the virus with ART, then passively infused a bNAb while withdrawing ART, and subsequently maintained suppression with rAAV delivery of the same bNAb. They found that rAAV2-10-1074

sustained antibody concentrations of approximately 200 µg/ml and maintained suppression of YU-2-NL4-3 HIV-1 in 6 out of 7 mice. Future work could explore the use of other ART combinations to eliminate the need for a passive infusion bridge.

These studies demonstrate that rAAV delivery can sustain expression of anti-HIV-1 bNAbs in humanized mouse models. Similar VIP approaches have also been shown to protect mouse models against other infectious diseases, such as influenza [81], malaria [82], HCV [83], and Ebola [84].

Evaluating vectored delivery in humanized mouse models

The natural immune response to HIV-1 is reflected to different degrees amongst the various humanized mouse models. The simplest mouse model infuses adult human T-cells derived from PBMCs into immunodeficient mice [85]. These mice support HIV-1 infection and ongoing viral replication, but the graft quickly depletes after several weeks as there is no regenerative source of T-cells. Furthermore, these mice develop graft-versus-host disease (GvHD) within 6–8 weeks as the graft is not tolerant of the foreign environment [73]. Another model involves the transplantation of human CD34+ stem cells into newborn immunodeficient mice [80, 86, 87]. This allows for the development of a regenerating T-cell compartment and improved longevity as a consequence of T-cell tolerance, which may be a consequence of human T-cell progenitors being educated in mouse thymus tissue. However, the lack of human thymus results in an immune system that is unable to recognize peptides presented in the context of human HLA molecules and thus a largely incompetent adaptive immune response to infection. The most complete humanized mouse model is the bone marrow-liver-thymus (BLT) mouse model, in which newborn immunodeficient mice are surgically implanted with tissue fragments from human fetal liver and thymus, followed by intravenous injection of purified autologous fetal human CD34+ hematopoietic stem cells derived from the remainder of unimplanted liver [88–90]. The T cell compartment of the BLT mice reconstitutes over several months and T cells mature in the transplanted human thymus and are largely tolerant to mouse antigens. The BLT mouse can model multiple aspects of HIV-1 infection, such as prevention, viral evolution in response to T-cell pressure, mucosal transmission, CTL responses, and viral latency [77, 91–94].

Humanized mouse models have the benefit of genetic homogeneity when engrafted with tissue from the same donor. Isogenic cohorts can be as large as tens to over one hundred and fifty mice, allowing for the observation of chance behaviors in response to HIV-1 infection. These humanized mouse models are also significantly less expensive than macaque models. Importantly, natural human bNAbs with specificity against HIV can be tested in humanized mice without eliciting strong ADA responses that confound experiments in other systems.

However, the existing BLT mouse model does not yet faithfully replicate all aspects of a fully-functional human immune system. Our lab and others have observed inconsistent humoral responses against viral proteins in BLT mice during HIV-1 infection. This could be due to previous observations of disorganized germinal centers, and defects in antigen presentation. In addition, the BLT model does not fully capture the pharmacokinetics and pharmacodynamics of human bNAbs given the murine origin of the neonatal Fc receptor (FcRn) recycling receptors [95]. Fc-mediated behaviors beyond neutralization, such as antibody-dependent cell-mediated cytotoxicity (ADCC) may not be well supported in this model due to a paucity of natural killer cells. Furthermore, complement-dependent cytotoxicity (CDC) is not supported in this model due to genetic defects in the underlying NSG mouse strain complement cascade [96].

Evaluating vectored delivery of bNAbs in macaques

Evaluating the effectiveness of rAAV gene transfer of anti-HIV-1 bNAbs in nonhuman primates has proven to be challenging, due to a lack of naturally-existing, effective antibodies against SIV and the propensity of macaques to develop strong immunogenic responses against human bNAbs. However, macaques are better models of human physiology, have fully functional immune systems that are analogous to that of humans, and are of more comparable size. Importantly, HIV-1 does not replicate in macaques and thus a closely related virus, SIVmac, is used to model HIV-1 infection and the corresponding AIDS-like symptoms that develop [97]. However, while functionally similar, SIV and HIV-1 share only about 50% sequence homology, and SIV encodes an additional accessory protein (Vpx), not found in HIV-1, that induces degradation of host restriction factor SAMHD1 [98, 99].

Given that human bNAbs do not recognize SIVmac, a chimeric virus (SHIV) is often used for antibody-mediated protection experiments in which the SIVmac envelope is replaced with an HIV-1 envelope [100]. However, this chimeric virus is not fully adapted and may be of lower fitness than natural SIV strains, as unlike HIV-1 in humans or in BLT humanized mice, some SHIV strains are occasionally controlled in untreated macaques [101, 102]. Interestingly, not all HIV-1 envelopes can be made into functional SHIV, although substantial progress has been made in doing so [103]. In addition, unlike mice, macaques are not inbred, and genetic diversity in a cohort may lead to disparate immunological responses to infection that can complicate analysis of divergent

behavior within a group. Most importantly, as reviewed in this section, human bNAbs appear to elicit significant immunogenic responses in macaques [104, 105], and these responses are not seen when passively transferring bNAbs in humans.

Fuchs et al. [106] in 2015 constructed full-length rhesus IgG1 counterparts of the 4L6 or 5L7 immunoadhesins used in Johnson et al. [68] and delivered them via rAAV1 to macaques. Although antibody concentrations reached 20–300 µg/ml, endogenous ADA responses were detected within a month in three of the six macaques given 5L7, and in all six macaques given 4L6. These ADA responses limited continual expression of the antibody, as antibody concentrations fell below 10 µg/ml in macaques that developed ADA responses. The authors then repeatedly challenged the macaques with SIVmac239, a strain more difficult to neutralize than SIVmac319 used by Johnson et al. Although neither gene transfer appeared to be more effective at preventing infection than the negative control, 5L7 delayed time to peak viral load, and lowered peak and set viral loads. It was later found that the variable regions of these antibodies were immunogenic, which contributed to their xenogeneic elimination [105].

Other works have sought to simianize bNAbs to reduce cross-species immunogenicity with mixed results. Saunders et al. [104] in 2015 found that a single infusion of human VRC01 resulted in detectable anti-VRC01 plasma IgG eight weeks after infusion, but not for simianized VRC01. They subsequently infused simianized simVRC01 or simVRC01-LS four times over 8 months into eight macaques, and found that the bNAb could persist for more than 2 or 3.5 months, respectively, after the last infusion. However, in two of the eight macaques, ADA response was nonetheless detected against the simianized antibody. The six other macaques were intrarectally challenged with SHIV-BaLP4 2 months after last the passive infusion, of which five were protected.

In a parallel study, Saunders et al. [107] evaluated whether administering immunosuppressant cyclosporine before rAAV injection reduced immunogenicity against bNAbs. The authors first delivered simianized VRC07 via rAAV8 to macaques. Serum concentrations peaked at 2.5–7.7 µg/ml at weeks 2–4, and substantial ADA response was detected. The same constructs given at a lower dose to immunodeficient mice resulted in levels greater than 100 µg/ml. In a second study, six macaques were given cyclosporine starting 9 days prior to, and until 4 weeks after, rAAV8-simVRC07 administration. Peak mean concentration of simVRC07 was 38 µg/ml. Three of six macaques retained simVRC07 expression for 16 weeks without developing ADA, whereas the others exhibited ADA, including one that completely eliminated simVRC07 expression. Macaques were intrarectally challenged with SHIV-BaLP4 5.5 weeks after transduction, and the two of the six macaques with the lowest simVRC07 concentrations became infected. Overall, ADA response was inversely correlated with simVRC07 concentration, and transient immunosuppression did increase transgene expression.

Since bNAbs, even simianized, were still immunogenic after long-term expression in macaques, Gardner et al. [108] in 2015 took an alternative approach and delivered rh-eCD4-Ig, which is rhesus CD4-Ig fused at its carboxyl terminus to a 15-amino acid CCR5-mimetic sulfopeptide, in an rAAV1/2 vector into macaques. Rhesus tyrosine-protein sulfotransferase 2 was also co-administered in a second rAAV at a 1:4 ratio to increase rh-CD4-Ig sulfation, as this is required for its neutralizing activity. rh-eCD4-Ig was expressed at 17-77 µg/ml for more than 40 weeks and protected four macaques from four increasingly stringent challenges with SHIV-AD8. Less anti-transgene response was detected against rh-eCD4-Ig than against simianized 3BNC117, NIH45-46, 10-1074, PGT121, and no antibody response against the sulfopeptide was detected.

In summary, there are substantial challenges associated with evaluating the long-term expression of bNAbs in nonhuman primates, through both repeated passive infusions and rAAV gene delivery. Although simianization, in which human variable regions are engrafted onto a rhesus antibody, reduces bNAb immunogenicity in passive transfer studies, it does not fully eliminate ADA responses as those variable regions are descended from the human germline and not from their simian counterparts. Thus, it may be inherently difficult to evaluate the anti-HIV-1 efficacy of sustained human bNAb expression in macaques with confounding xenogenic responses. Immunosuppressants such as cyclosporine reduce but do not completely eliminate the immunogenicity of bNAbs [107]. Future studies aiming to deliver fully simian antibodies against SIV or HIV, cloned in a manner analogous to methods used to isolate human bNAbs, may more accurately predict the potential for translation of this approach in humans.

Vectored delivery of bNAbs in clinical trials

There are currently only two bNAb AAV gene transfer studies. The first trial (IAVI A003/CHOP HVDDT 001, https://clinicaltrials.gov/ct2/show/NCT0193745 5) is a phase I trial in 21 healthy males without HIV-1 or HIV-2 infection and uses an rAAV1 vector encoding PG9 heavy and light chain under two separate promoters. Either 4×10^{12}, 4×10^{13}, 8×10^{13}, or 1.2×10^{14} viral genomes regardless of weight or placebo were given in a single intramuscular administration to participants without evidence of pre-existing anti-AAV1 antibodies.

These participants were then followed for a year, with the option of enrolling into a follow-up study. This trial was completed in February 2018, but results have not yet been reported in the literature. The second trial (VRC 603, https://clinicaltrials.gov/ct2/show/NCT0337420 2) is a phase I trial in an estimated 25 adults living with suppressed HIV-1 infection and uses an rAAV8 vector encoding a CASI-promoter driven VRC07 transgene in a nearly identical configuration to those used in our previously published studies [73, 77]. Participants in VRC603 must have controlled viremia, have been on stable ART for at least 3 months, and not have evidence of pre-existing anti-AAV8 antibodies. Either 5×10^{10}, 5×10^{11}, or 2.5×10^{12} viral genomes per kg will be given in a single intramuscular administration to the upper arm or thigh, with a study goal of achieving 50 µg/ml 4 weeks post-injection and a set point of 5 µg/ml 12 weeks post-injection. Participants will be followed intensely for a year, and then every 6 months for another 4 years. This trial has an estimated primary completion date of March 2019. Longer-term follow up of patients in these trials, past these primary study completion dates, is desirable to evaluate the duration of sustained bNAb expression and the potential immunogenic responses from chronic bNAb exposure.

Selection of bNAbs for vectored delivery

Since the characterization of PG9 in 2009 [109], over 90 bNAbs have been described, exhibiting a wide range of breadth and potency as determined by neutralization assays on large global panels of HIV-1 isolates [42, 110]. Given that most infections are initiated by a single transmitted founder virus [111, 112], low in vivo bNAb concentrations that reduce the probability of the establishment of infection may be sufficient to provide a benefit in the context of prevention. As more potent antibodies are discovered, the prophylactic dose of bNAb necessary to yield protective concentrations is likely to be reduced.

In contrast, suppressing actively replicating virus with bNAb is more challenging given the millions to billions of virions that must be neutralized. In addition, instead of a single viral genotype, the bNAb is faced with neutralizing a quasispecies of closely related HIV-1 strains [113]. Since the virus mutates as it replicates, the quasispecies may harbor a variant that evades antibody neutralization, thereby allowing for escape. Such variants that escape bNAb pressure may face a replicative fitness penalty, particularly if conserved sites such as those involved in interacting with CD4 are mutated. It may be useful to consider the fitness costs of escaping each bNAb, and use antibodies that impose a high escape cost when optimizing bNAb delivery, particularly in a therapeutic setting [114, 115].

Another feature specific to rAAV delivery is that bNAb expression may take several weeks to achieve steady state levels [73, 77], as second strand synthesis of the rAAV genome is necessary for expression to occur [26, 27]. From the viral perspective, this steadily rising concentration of antibody represents a gradually increasing selective force which may more readily select for escape mutants. Use of a stronger promoter or of a more efficient AAV serotype may result in faster expression. Alternatively, co-adminstration of both an adenovirus vector and an AAV vector can result in immediate and sustained antibody expression, as previously shown for a monoclonal antibody against anthrax [116].

Similar to existing HAART regimens, which employ a combination of antiretroviral drugs to control HIV-1, the use of antibody combinations to suppress HIV-1 has been long proposed and may be necessary, particularly in the context of therapy [117, 118]. Klein et al. [119] repeatedly passively infused either a tri-mix or penta-mix of bNAbs into YU-2-NL4-3 HIV-1 infected humanized mice. The tri-mix (which neutralized >98% of clades with IC_{80} of 0.121 µg/ml) led to complete suppression in 3 of 12 mice, and the penta-mix (which neutralized >98% of clades with IC_{80} of 0.046 µg/ml) led to complete suppression in 11 of 13 mice. This and other work suggests that antibodies which bind to different epitopes and with very low IC_{50} across diverse HIV-1 strains should be chosen [119–121]. Bispecific monoclonal antibodies, where each arm of the antibody binds to a different epitope, may also have greater breath and potency than each constituent antibody alone or mixed [122, 123]. rAAV delivery of bispecifics may require two separate rAAVs injected into the same site, due to the carrying capacity of the vector, but this has not yet been reported in the literature. Another approach is to study viral mutants that arise after administration of a single bNAb and then design variants of that bNAb that neutralize those mutants. In particular, Diskin et al. [124] rationally designed NIH45-46 variants by increasing the buried surface area of the antibody with escape variants and avoiding steric clashes. However, when NIH45-46 and its variants were passively infused as a combination into infected humanized mice, mutants escaped in a previously unseen path by shifting an N-linked glycosylation site by three residues, highlighting the magnitude of the challenge of designing antibody combinations to suppress actively evolving viremia.

Conclusion

Phase I and IIa trials of passive transfer of bNAbs have thus far demonstrated the safety of bNAbs in humans and shown that bNAbs can both transiently lower viral loads and delay viral rebound. In some patients, viral rebound happened only after the bNAb concentration fell to low concentrations and occurred without escape mutations, suggesting that continuous bNAb expression might result in sustained suppression. Given the difficulty of eliciting bNAbs through sequential vaccination and the complexity of life-long passive transfer of bNAbs, using a single intramuscular administration of rAAV to attain continuous, systemic, long-term expression of bNAbs is an exciting possibility.

rAAVs have a favorable safety profile and can stably express transgenes in humans for many years. However, pre-existing immunity in individuals against AAV due to natural exposure may limit successful vectored delivery. To avoid this, immunosuppressants may be temporarily administered, or novel AAV capsids with little cross-reactivity to circulating AAVs may be used [125]. In humanized mouse models, vectored delivery resulted in the long-term expression of bNAbs, protected against intravenous and intravaginal HIV-1 challenges, and maintained suppression of previously ART-suppressed HIV-1. However, pre-existing and emergent viral resistance to bNAbs may limit their effectiveness in patients. Whereas bNAbs may be able to neutralize a few slightly resistant virions in the context of prevention, using bNAbs to suppress replicating HIV-1 may require additional innovations to prevent the evolution and selection of viral mutants. Prevention studies in macaques with AAV-delivered simianized bNAbs elicited strong anti-bNAb responses, although it seems likely that the immunogenicity of the human antibody variable regions in macaques complicates this model. Most importantly, Phase I clinical trials of vectored delivery of bNAbs are currently underway and should provide critically important information to determine the feasibility of this approach. Irrespective of their outcome, we believe that whatever challenges may be encountered will ultimately be overcome and that vectored delivery of broadly neutralizing antibodies will become an important new approach towards ending the HIV-1 epidemic.

Abbreviations

AAV: adeno-associated virus; ADA: anti-drug antibody; ART: antiretroviral therapy; ATI: analytical treatment interruption; BCR: B-cell receptor; BLT: bone marrow-liver-thymus; bNAb: broadly neutralizing antibody; HIV: human immunodeficiency virus; ITR: inverted terminal repeat; PNGS: potential N-linked glycosylation sequon; rAAV: recombinant adeno-associated virus; SIV: simian immunodeficiency virus; VIP: vectored immunoprophylaxis.

Authors' contributions

AL and ABB conceived of the review together. AL wrote the review. AL and ABB edited the review together. Both authors read and approved the final manuscript.

Author details
[1] Ragon Institute of MGH, MIT and Harvard, Cambridge, MA 02139, USA.
[2] Department of Systems Biology, Harvard University, Boston, MA 02115, USA.

Acknowledgements
Not applicable.

Competing interests
The authors declare that they have no competing interests.

Funding
A.B.B. is supported by the National Institutes for Drug Abuse (NIDA) Avenir New Innovator Award DP2DA040254, the MGH Transformative Scholars Program as well as funding from a contract from the NIH. This independent research was supported by the Gilead Sciences Research Scholars Program in HIV. A.L. is supported by the Paul and Daisy Soros Fellowship for New Americans and the NSF Graduate Research Fellowship Program.

References
1. UNAIDS. Global AIDS Update. Sep 2017.
2. Hermonat PL, Muzyczka N. Use of adeno-associated virus as a mammalian DNA cloning vector: transduction of neomycin resistance into mammalian tissue culture cells. Proc Natl Acad Sci USA. 1984;81:6466–70.
3. Casto BC, Hammon WM, Atchison RW. Adenovirus-associated defective virus particles. Science. 1965;149:754–6.
4. Lusby E, Fife KH, Berns KI. Nucleotide sequence of the inverted terminal repetition in adeno-associated virus DNA. J Virol. 1980;34:402–9.
5. Sonntag F, Schmidt K, Kleinschmidt JA. A viral assembly factor promotes AAV2 capsid formation in the nucleolus. Proc Natl Acad Sci USA. 2010;107:10220–5.
6. Zincarelli C, Soltys S, Rengo G, Rabinowitz JE. Analysis of AAV serotypes 1–9 mediated gene expression and tropism in mice after systemic injection. Mol Ther. 2008;16:1073–80.
7. Gao G, Alvira MR, Somanathan S, Lu Y, Vandenberghe LH, Rux JJ, et al. Adeno-associated viruses undergo substantial evolution in primates during natural infections. Proc Natl Acad Sci USA. 2003;100:6081–6.
8. Gao G, Vandenberghe LH, Alvira MR, Lu Y, Calcedo R, Zhou X, et al. Clades of adeno-associated viruses are widely disseminated in human tissues. J Virol. 2004;78:6381–8.
9. Zinn E, Pacouret S, Khaychuk V, Turunen HT, Carvalho LS, Andres-Mateos E, et al. In silico reconstruction of the viral evolutionary lineage yields a potent gene therapy vector. Cell Rep. 2015;12:1056–68.
10. Mays LE, Vandenberghe LH, Xiao R, Bell P, Nam H-J, Agbandje-McKenna M, et al. Adeno-associated virus capsid structure drives CD4-dependent CD8+ T cell response to vector encoded proteins. J Immunol. 2009;182:6051–60.
11. Mays LE, Wang L, Tenney R, Bell P, Nam H-J, Lin J, et al. Mapping the structural determinants responsible for enhanced T cell activation to the immunogenic adeno-associated virus capsid from isolate rhesus 32.33. J Virol. 2013;87:9473–85.
12. Kotterman MA, Schaffer DV. Engineering adeno-associated viruses for clinical gene therapy. Nat Rev Genet. 2014;15:445–51.
13. Berns KI, Parrish CR. Parvoviridae. In: Knipe DM, Howley PM, Cohen JI, Griffin DE, Lamb RA, Martin MA, et al., editors. Fields virology. 6th ed. Philadelphia: Lippincott Williams & Wilkins; 2013.
14. Kotin RM, Siniscalco M, Samulski RJ, Zhu XD, Hunter L, Laughlin CA, et al. Site-specific integration by adeno-associated virus. Proc Natl Acad Sci USA. 1990;87:2211–5.
15. Samulski RJ, Zhu X, Xiao X, Brook JD, Housman DE, Epstein N, et al. Targeted integration of adeno-associated virus (AAV) into human chromosome 19. EMBO J. 1991;10:3941–50.
16. Surosky RT, Urabe M, Godwin SG, McQuiston SA, Kurtzman GJ, Ozawa K, et al. Adeno-associated virus Rep proteins target DNA sequences to a unique locus in the human genome. J Virol. 1997;71:7951–9.
17. Schnepp BC, Chulay JD, Ye G-J, Flotte TR, Trapnell BC, Johnson PR. Recombinant adeno-associated virus vector genomes take the form of long-lived, transcriptionally competent episomes in human muscle. Hum Gene Ther. 2016;27:32–42.
18. Schnepp BC, Clark KR, Klemanski DL, Pacak CA, Johnson PR. Genetic fate of recombinant adeno-associated virus vector genomes in muscle. J Virol. 2003;77:3495–504.
19. Nowrouzi A, Penaud-Budloo M, Kaeppel C, Appelt U, Le Guiner C, Moullier P, et al. Integration frequency and intermolecular recombination of rAAV vectors in non-human primate skeletal muscle and liver. Mol Ther. 2012;20:1177–86.
20. Herzog RW, Yang EY, Couto LB, Hagstrom JN, Elwell D, Fields PA, et al. Long-term correction of canine hemophilia B by gene transfer of blood coagulation factor IX mediated by adeno-associated viral vector. Nat Med. 1999;5:56–63.
21. Xiao X, Li J, Samulski RJ. Efficient long-term gene transfer into muscle tissue of immunocompetent mice by adeno-associated virus vector. J Virol. 1996;70:8098–108.
22. Rivera VM, Gao G-P, Grant RL, Schnell MA, Zoltick PW, Rozamus LW, et al. Long-term pharmacologically regulated expression of erythropoietin in primates following AAV-mediated gene transfer. Blood. 2005;105:1424–30.
23. Nathwani AC, Reiss UM, Tuddenham EGD, Rosales C, Chowdary P, McIntosh J, et al. Long-term safety and efficacy of factor IX gene therapy in hemophilia B. N Engl J Med. 2014;371:1994–2004.
24. Buchlis G, Podsakoff GM, Radu A, Hawk SM, Flake AW, Mingozzi F, et al. Factor IX expression in skeletal muscle of a severe hemophilia B patient 10 years after AAV-mediated gene transfer. Blood. 2012;119:3038–41.
25. Dong JY, Fan PD, Frizzell RA. Quantitative analysis of the packaging capacity of recombinant adeno-associated virus. Hum Gene Ther. 1996;7:2101–12.
26. Ferrari FK, Samulski T, Shenk T, Samulski RJ. Second-strand synthesis is a rate-limiting step for efficient transduction by recombinant adeno-associated virus vectors. J Virol. 1996;70:3227–34.
27. Fisher KJ, Gao GP, Weitzman MD, DeMatteo R, Burda JF, Wilson JM. Transduction with recombinant adeno-associated virus for gene therapy is limited by leading-strand synthesis. J Virol. 1996;70:520–32.
28. Boutin S, Monteilhet V, Veron P, Leborgne C, Benveniste O, Montus MF, et al. Prevalence of serum IgG and neutralizing factors against adeno-associated virus (AAV) types 1, 2, 5, 6, 8, and 9 in the healthy population: implications for gene therapy using AAV vectors. Hum Gene Ther. 2010;21:704–12.
29. Calcedo R, Vandenberghe LH, Gao G, Lin J, Wilson JM. Worldwide epidemiology of neutralizing antibodies to adeno-associated viruses. J Infect Dis. 2009;199:381–90.
30. Manno CS, Pierce GF, Arruda VR, Glader B, Ragni M, Rasko JJ, et al. Successful transduction of liver in hemophilia by AAV-Factor IX and limitations imposed by the host immune response. Nat Med. 2006;12:342–7.
31. George LA, Sullivan SK, Giermasz A, Rasko JEJ, Samelson-Jones BJ, Ducore J, et al. Hemophilia B gene therapy with a high-specific-activity factor IX variant. N Engl J Med. 2017;377:2215–27.
32. Naso MF, Tomkowicz B, Perry WL, Strohl WR. Adeno-associated virus (AAV) as a vector for gene therapy. BioDrugs. 2017;31:317–34.
33. Maguire AM, Simonelli F, Pierce EA, Pugh EN, Mingozzi F, Bennicelli J, et al. Safety and efficacy of gene transfer for Leber's congenital amaurosis. N Engl J Med. 2008;358:2240–8.
34. Bainbridge JWB, Smith AJ, Barker SS, Robbie S, Henderson R, Balaggan K, et al. Effect of gene therapy on visual function in Leber's congenital amaurosis. N Engl J Med. 2008;358:2231–9.
35. Senior M. After Glybera's withdrawal, what's next for gene therapy? Nat Biotechnol. 2017;35:491–2.

36. Spark's gene therapy price tag: $850,000. Nat Biotechnol. 2018;36:122–2. https://doi.org/10.1038/nbt0218-122.

37. Hraber P, Seaman MS, Bailer RT, Mascola JR, Montefiori DC, Korber BT. Prevalence of broadly neutralizing antibody responses during chronic HIV-1 infection. AIDS. 2014;28:163–9.

38. Liao H-X, Lynch R, Zhou T, Gao F, Alam SM, Boyd SD, et al. Co-evolution of a broadly neutralizing HIV-1 antibody and founder virus. Nature. 2013;496:469–76.

39. Zhu P, Liu J, Bess J, Chertova E, Lifson JD, Grisé H, et al. Distribution and three-dimensional structure of AIDS virus envelope spikes. Nature. 2006;441:847–52.

40. Wei X, Decker JM, Wang S, Hui H, Kappes JC, Wu X, et al. Antibody neutralization and escape by HIV-1. Nature. 2003;422:307–12.

41. Rusert P, Krarup A, Magnus C, Brandenberg OF, Weber J, Ehlert A-K, et al. Interaction of the gp120 V1V2 loop with a neighboring gp120 unit shields the HIV envelope trimer against cross-neutralizing antibodies. J Exp Med. 2011;208:1419–33.

42. Eroshkin AM, LeBlanc A, Weekes D, Post K, Li Z, Rajput A, et al. bNAber: database of broadly neutralizing HIV antibodies. Nucleic Acids Res. 2013;42:D1133–9.

43. Wibmer CK, Moore PL, Morris L. HIV broadly neutralizing antibody targets. Curr Opin HIV AIDS. 2015;10:135–43.

44. Burton DR, Pyati J, Koduri R, Sharp SJ, Thornton GB, Parren PW, et al. Efficient neutralization of primary isolates of HIV-1 by a recombinant human monoclonal antibody. Science. 1994;266:1024–7.

45. Wu X, Yang Z-Y, Li Y, Hogerkorp C-M, Schief WR, Seaman MS, et al. Rational design of envelope identifies broadly neutralizing human monoclonal antibodies to HIV-1. Science. 2010;329:856–61.

46. Zhou T, Georgiev I, Wu X, Yang Z-Y, Dai K, Finzi A, et al. Structural basis for broad and potent neutralization of HIV-1 by antibody VRC01. Science. 2010;329:811–7.

47. Scheid JF, Mouquet H, Ueberheide B, Diskin R, Klein F, Oliveira TYK, et al. Sequence and structural convergence of broad and potent HIV antibodies that mimic CD4 binding. Science. 2011;333:1633–7.

48. Huang J, Kang BH, Ishida E, Zhou T, Griesman T, Sheng Z, et al. Identification of a CD4-binding-site antibody to HIV that evolved near-pan neutralization breadth. Immunity. 2016;45:1108–21.

49. Sajadi MM, Dashti A, Rikhtegaran Tehrani Z, Tolbert WD, Seaman MS, Ouyang X, et al. Identification of near-pan-neutralizing antibodies against HIV-1 by deconvolution of plasma humoral responses. Cell. 2018;173:1783–95.e14.

50. Wang S, Mata-Fink J, Kriegsman B, Hanson M, Irvine DJ, Eisen HN, et al. Manipulating the selection forces during affinity maturation to generate cross-reactive HIV antibodies. Cell. 2015;160:785–97.

51. Andrabi R, Bhiman JN, Burton DR. Strategies for a multi-stage neutralizing antibody-based HIV vaccine. Curr Opin Immunol. 2018;53:143–51.

52. Williams WB, Zhang J, Jiang C, Nicely NI, Fera D, Luo K, et al. Initiation of HIV neutralizing B cell lineages with sequential envelope immunizations. Nat Commun. 2017;8:1732.

53. Jardine JG, Kulp DW, Havenar-Daughton C, Sarkar A, Briney B, Sok D, et al. HIV-1 broadly neutralizing antibody precursor B cells revealed by germline-targeting immunogen. Science. 2016;351:1458–63.

54. Briney B, Sok D, Jardine JG, Kulp DW, Skog P, Menis S, et al. Tailored immunogens direct affinity maturation toward HIV neutralizing antibodies. Cell. 2016;166(1459–1470):e11.

55. Lynch RM, Boritz E, Tressler R, Coates EE, DeZure A, Bailer RT, et al. Virologic effects of broadly neutralizing antibody VRC01 administration during chronic HIV-1 infection. Sci Transl Med. 2015;7:319ra206.

56. Bar KJ, Sneller MC, Harrison LJ, Justement JS, Overton ET, Petrone ME, et al. Effect of HIV antibody VRC01 on viral rebound after treatment interruption. N Engl J Med. 2016;375:2037–50.

57. Caskey M, Klein F, Lorenzi JCC, Seaman MS, West AP, Buckley N, et al. Viraemia suppressed in HIV-1-infected humans by broadly neutralizing antibody 3BNC117. Nature. 2015;522:487–91.

58. Scheid JF, Horwitz JA, Bar-On Y, Kreider EF, Lu C-L, Lorenzi JCC, et al. HIV-1 antibody 3BNC117 suppresses viral rebound in humans during treatment interruption. Nature. 2016;535:556–60.

59. Caskey M, Schoofs T, Gruell H, Settler A, Karagounis T, Kreider EF, et al. Antibody 10-1074 suppresses viremia in HIV-1-infected individuals. Nat Med. 2017;23:185–91.

60. Cohen YZ, Caskey M. Broadly neutralizing antibodies for treatment and prevention of HIV-1 infection. Curr Opin HIV AIDS. 2018;13:366–73.

61. Rothenberger MK, Keele BF, Wietgrefe SW, Fletcher CV, Beilman GJ, Chipman JG, et al. Large number of rebounding/founder HIV variants emerge from multifocal infection in lymphatic tissues after treatment interruption. Proc Natl Acad Sci USA. 2015;112:E1126–34.

62. Schoofs T, Klein F, Braunschweig M, Kreider EF, Feldmann A, Nogueira L, et al. HIV-1 therapy with monoclonal antibody 3BNC117 elicits host immune responses against HIV-1. Science. 2016;352:997–1001.

63. Lu C-L, Murakowski DK, Bournazos S, Schoofs T, Sarkar D, Halper-Stromberg A, et al. Enhanced clearance of HIV-1-infected cells by broadly neutralizing antibodies against HIV-1 in vivo. Science. 2016;352:1001–4.

64. Burton DR, Mascola JR. Antibody responses to envelope glycoproteins in HIV-1 infection. Nat Immunol. 2015;16:571–6.

65. Bruel T, Guivel-Benhassine F, Amraoui S, Malbec M, Richard L, Bourdic K, et al. Elimination of HIV-1-infected cells by broadly neutralizing antibodies. Nat Commun. 2016;7:10844.

66. Halper-Stromberg A, Lu C-L, Klein F, Horwitz JA, Bournazos S, Nogueira L, et al. Broadly neutralizing antibodies and viral inducers decrease rebound from HIV-1 latent reservoirs in humanized mice. Cell. 2014;158:989–99.

67. Lewis AD, Chen R, Montefiori DC, Johnson PR, Clark KR. Generation of neutralizing activity against human immunodeficiency virus type 1 in serum by antibody gene transfer. J Virol. 2002;76:8769–75.

68. Johnson PR, Schnepp BC, Zhang J, Connell MJ, Greene SM, Yuste E, et al. Vector-mediated gene transfer engenders long-lived neutralizing activity and protection against SIV infection in monkeys. Nat Med. 2009;15:901–6.

69. Johnson WE, Sanford H, Schwall L, Burton DR, Parren PWHI, Robinson JE, et al. Assorted mutations in the envelope gene of simian immunodeficiency virus lead to loss of neutralization resistance against antibodies representing a broad spectrum of specificities. J Virol. 2003;77:9993–10003.

70. Fang J, Qian J-J, Yi S, Harding TC, Tu GH, VanRoey M, et al. Stable antibody expression at therapeutic levels using the 2A peptide. Nat Biotechnol. 2005;23:584–90.

71. Donnelly ML, Luke G, Mehrotra A, Li X, Hughes LE, Gani D, et al. Analysis of the aphthovirus 2A/2B polyprotein 'cleavage' mechanism indicates not a proteolytic reaction, but a novel translational effect: a putative ribosomal 'skip'. J Gen Virol. 2001;82:1013–25.

72. Fang J, Yi S, Simmons A, Tu GH, Nguyen M, Harding TC, et al. An antibody delivery system for regulated expression of therapeutic levels of monoclonal antibodies in vivo. Mol Ther. 2007;15:1153–9.

73. Balazs AB, Chen J, Hong CM, Rao DS, Yang L, Baltimore D. Antibody-based protection against HIV infection by vectored immunoprophylaxis. Nature. 2011;481:81–4.

74. Gao G-P, Alvira MR, Wang L, Calcedo R, Johnston J, Wilson JM. Novel adeno-associated viruses from rhesus monkeys as vectors for human gene therapy. Proc Natl Acad Sci USA. 2002;99:11854–9.

75. Vandenberghe LH, Wang L, Somanathan S, Zhi Y, Figueredo J, Calcedo R, et al. Heparin binding directs activation of T cells against adeno-associated virus serotype 2 capsid. Nat Med. 2006;12:967–71.

76. Mays LE, Wang L, Lin J, Bell P, Crawford A, Wherry EJ, et al. AAV8 induces tolerance in murine muscle as a result of poor APC transduction, T cell exhaustion, and minimal MHCI upregulation on target cells. Mol Ther. 2014;22:28–41.

77. Balazs AB, Ouyang Y, Hong CM, Chen J, Nguyen SM, Rao DS, et al. Vectored immunoprophylaxis protects humanized mice from mucosal HIV transmission. Nat Med. 2014;20:296–300.

78. Rudicell RS, Kwon YD, Ko S-Y, Pegu A, Louder MK, Georgiev IS, et al. Enhanced potency of a broadly neutralizing HIV-1 antibody in vitro improves protection against lentiviral infection in vivo. J Virol. 2014;88:12669–82.

79. Diskin R, Scheid JF, Marcovecchio PM, West AP, Klein F, Gao H, et al. Increasing the potency and breadth of an HIV antibody by using structure-based rational design. Science. 2011;334:1289–93.

80. Horwitz JA, Halper-Stromberg A, Mouquet H, Gitlin AD, Tretiakova A, Eisenreich TR, et al. HIV-1 suppression and durable control by combining single broadly neutralizing antibodies and antiretroviral drugs in humanized mice. Proc Natl Acad Sci USA. 2013;110:16538–43.

81. Balazs AB, Bloom JD, Hong CM, Rao DS, Baltimore D. Broad protection against influenza infection by vectored immunoprophylaxis in mice. Nat Biotechnol. 2013;31:647–52.

82. Deal C, Balazs AB, Espinosa DA, Zavala F, Baltimore D, Ketner G. Vectored antibody gene delivery protects against Plasmodium falciparum sporozoite challenge in mice. Proc Natl Acad Sci USA. 2014;111:12528–32.

83. de Jong YP, Dorner M, Mommersteeg MC, Xiao JW, Balazs AB, Robbins JB, et al. Broadly neutralizing antibodies abrogate established hepatitis C virus infection. Sci Transl Med. 2014;6:254ra129-9.

84. van Lieshout LP, Soule G, Sorensen D, Frost KL, He S, Tierney K, et al. Intramuscular adeno-associated virus-mediated expression of monoclonal antibodies provides 100% protection against Ebola virus infection in mice. J Infect Dis. 2018;217:916–25.

85. Mosier DE, Gulizia RJ, Baird SM, Wilson DB, Spector DH, Spector SA. Human immunodeficiency virus infection of human-PBL-SCID mice. Science. 1991;251:791–4.

86. Traggiai E, Chicha L, Mazzucchelli L, Bronz L, Piffaretti J-C, Lanzavecchia A, et al. Development of a human adaptive immune system in cord blood cell-transplanted mice. Science. 2004;304:104–7.

87. Ishikawa F, Yasukawa M, Lyons B, Yoshida S, Miyamoto T, Yoshimoto G, et al. Development of functional human blood and immune systems in NOD/SCID/IL2 receptor γ chain[null] mice. Blood. 2005;106:1565–73.

88. Lan P, Tonomura N, Shimizu A, Wang S, Yang Y-G. Reconstitution of a functional human immune system in immunodeficient mice through combined human fetal thymus/liver and CD34+ cell transplantation. Blood. 2006;108:487–92.

89. Melkus MW, Estes JD, Padgett-Thomas A, Gatlin J, Denton PW, Othieno FA, et al. Humanized mice mount specific adaptive and innate immune responses to EBV and TSST-1. Nat Med. 2006;12:1316–22.

90. Karpel ME, Boutwell CL, Allen TM. BLT humanized mice as a small animal model of HIV infection. Curr Opin Virol. 2015;13:75–80.

91. Dudek TE, No DC, Seung E, Vrbanac VD, Fadda L, Bhoumik P, et al. Rapid evolution of HIV-1 to functional CD8+ T cell responses in humanized BLT mice. Sci Transl Med. 2012;4:143ra98.

92. Denton PW, Olesen R, Choudhary SK, Archin NM, Wahl A, Swanson MD, et al. Generation of HIV latency in humanized BLT mice. J Virol. 2012;86:630–4.

93. Marsden MD, Kovochich M, Suree N, Shimizu S, Mehta R, Cortado R, et al. HIV latency in the humanized BLT mouse. J Virol. 2012;86:339–47.

94. Denton PW, Estes JD, Sun Z, Othieno FA, Wei BL, Wege AK, et al. Antiretroviral pre-exposure prophylaxis prevents vaginal transmission of HIV-1 in humanized BLT mice. PLoS Med. 2008;5:e16.

95. Petkova SB, Akilesh S, Sproule TJ, Christianson GJ, Khabbaz Al H, Brown AC, et al. Enhanced half-life of genetically engineered human IgG1 antibodies in a humanized FcRn mouse model: potential application in humorally mediated autoimmune disease. Int Immunol. 2006;18:1759–69.

96. Baxter AG, Cooke A. Complement lytic activity has no role in the pathogenesis of autoimmune diabetes in NOD mice. Diabetes. 1993;42:1574–8.

97. Simon MA, Brodie SJ, Sasseville VG, Chalifoux LV, Desrosiers RC, Ringler DJ. Immunopathogenesis of SIVmac. Virus Res. 1994;32:227–51.

98. Pollom E, Dang KK, Potter EL, Gorelick RJ, Burch CL, Weeks KM, et al. Comparison of SIV and HIV-1 genomic RNA structures reveals impact of sequence evolution on conserved and non-conserved structural motifs. PLoS Pathog. 2013;9:e1003294.

99. Laguette N, Sobhian B, Casartelli N, Ringeard M, Chable-Bessia C, Ségéral E, et al. SAMHD1 is the dendritic- and myeloid-cell-specific HIV-1 restriction factor counteracted by Vpx. Nature. 2011;474:654–7.

100. Reimann KA, Li JT, Voss G, Lekutis C, Tenner-Racz K, Racz P, et al. An env gene derived from a primary human immunodeficiency virus type 1 isolate confers high in vivo replicative capacity to a chimeric simian/human immunodeficiency virus in rhesus monkeys. J Virol. 1996;70:3198–206.

101. Shingai M, Donau OK, Plishka RJ, Buckler-White A, Mascola JR, Nabel GJ, et al. Passive transfer of modest titers of potent and broadly neutralizing anti-HIV monoclonal antibodies block SHIV infection in macaques. J Exp Med. 2014;211:2061–74.

102. Julg B, Pegu A, Abbink P, Liu J, Brinkman A, Molloy K, et al. Virological control by the CD4-binding site antibody N6 in simian-human immunodeficiency virus-infected rhesus monkeys. J Virol. 2017;91:e00498-17.

103. Li H, Wang S, Kong R, Ding W, Lee F-H, Parker Z, et al. Envelope residue 375 substitutions in simian-human immunodeficiency viruses enhance CD4 binding and replication in rhesus macaques. Proc Natl Acad Sci USA. 2016;113:E3413–22.

104. Saunders KO, Pegu A, Georgiev IS, Zeng M, Joyce MG, Yang Z-Y, et al. Sustained delivery of a broadly neutralizing antibody in nonhuman primates confers long-term protection against simian/human immunodeficiency virus infection. J Virol. 2015;89:5895–903.

105. Martinez-Navio JM, Fuchs SP, Pedreño-López S, Rakasz EG, Gao G, Desrosiers RC. Host anti-antibody responses following adeno-associated virus-mediated delivery of antibodies against hiv and siv in rhesus monkeys. Mol Ther. 2016;24:76–86.

106. Fuchs SP, Martinez-Navio JM, Piatak M, Lifson JD, Gao G, Desrosiers RC. AAV-delivered antibody mediates significant protective effects against SIVmac239 challenge in the absence of neutralizing activity. PLoS Pathog. 2015;11:e1005090.

107. Saunders KO, Wang L, Joyce MG, Yang Z-Y, Balazs AB, Cheng C, et al. Broadly neutralizing human immunodeficiency virus type 1 antibody gene transfer protects nonhuman primates from mucosal simian-human immunodeficiency virus infection. J Virol. 2015;89:8334–45.

108. Gardner MR, Kattenhorn LM, Kondur HR, von Schaewen M, Dorfman T, Chiang JJ, et al. AAV-expressed eCD4-Ig provides durable protection from multiple SHIV challenges. Nature. 2015;519:87–91.

109. Walker LM, Phogat SK, Chan-Hui P-Y, Wagner D, Phung P, Goss JL, et al. Broad and potent neutralizing antibodies from an African donor reveal a new HIV-1 vaccine target. Science. 2009;326:285–9.

110. Seaman MS, Janes H, Hawkins N, Grandpre LE, Devoy C, Giri A, et al. Tiered categorization of a diverse panel of HIV-1 Env pseudoviruses for assessment of neutralizing antibodies. J Virol. 2010;84:1439–52.

111. Keele BF, Giorgi EE, Salazar-Gonzalez JF, Decker JM, Pham KT, Salazar MG, et al. Identification and characterization of transmitted and early founder virus envelopes in primary HIV-1 infection. Proc Natl Acad Sci USA. 2008;105:7552–7.

112. Salazar-Gonzalez JF, Bailes E, Pham KT, Salazar MG, Guffey MB, Keele BF, et al. Deciphering human immunodeficiency virus type 1 transmission and early envelope diversification by single-genome amplification and sequencing. J Virol. 2008;82:3952–70.

113. Eigen M. Selforganization of matter and the evolution of biological macromolecules. Naturwissenschaften. 1971;58:465–523.

114. Lynch RM, Wong P, Tran L, O'Dell S, Nason MC, Li Y, et al. HIV-1 fitness cost associated with escape from the VRC01 class of CD4 binding site neutralizing antibodies. J Virol. 2015;89:4201–13.

115. Louie RHY, Kaczorowski KJ, Barton JP, Chakraborty AK, McKay MR. Fitness landscape of the human immunodeficiency virus envelope protein that is targeted by antibodies. Proc Natl Acad Sci USA. 2018;115:E564–73.

116. De BP, Hackett NR, Crystal RG, Boyer JL. Rapid/sustained anti-anthrax passive immunity mediated by co-administration of Ad/AAV. Mol Ther. 2008;16:203–9.

117. Trkola A, Kuster H, Rusert P, Joos B, Fischer M, Leemann C, et al. Delay of HIV-1 rebound after cessation of antiretroviral therapy through passive transfer of human neutralizing antibodies. Nat Med. 2005;11:615–22.

118. Mehandru S, Vcelar B, Wrin T, Stiegler G, Joos B, Mohri H, et al. Adjunctive passive immunotherapy in human immunodeficiency virus type 1-infected individuals treated with antiviral therapy during acute and early infection. J Virol. 2007;81:11016–31.

119. Klein F, Halper-Stromberg A, Horwitz JA, Gruell H, Scheid JF, Bournazos S, et al. HIV therapy by a combination of broadly neutralizing antibodies in humanized mice. Nature. 2012;492:118–22.

120. Kong R, Louder MK, Wagh K, Bailer RT, deCamp A, Greene K, et al. Improving neutralization potency and breadth by combining broadly reactive HIV-1 antibodies targeting major neutralization epitopes. J Virol. 2014;89:2659–71.

121. Wagh K, Bhattacharya T, Williamson C, Robles A, Bayne M, Garrity J, et al. Optimal combinations of broadly neutralizing antibodies for prevention and treatment of HIV-1 Clade C infection. PLoS Pathog. 2016;12:e1005520.

122. Huang Y, Yu J, Lanzi A, Yao X, Andrews CD, Tsai L, et al. Engineered bispecific antibodies with exquisite HIV-1-neutralizing activity. Cell. 2016;165:1621–31.

123. Bournazos S, Gazumyan A, Seaman MS, Nussenzweig MC, Ravetch JV. Bispecific anti-HIV-1 antibodies with enhanced breadth and potency. Cell. 2016;165:1609–20.

124. Diskin R, Klein F, Horwitz JA, Halper-Stromberg A, Sather DN, Marcovecchio PM, et al. Restricting HIV-1 pathways for escape using rationally designed anti-HIV-1 antibodies. J Exp Med. 2013;210:1235–49.

125. Mingozzi F, High KA. Immune responses to AAV vectors: overcoming barriers to successful gene therapy. Blood. 2013;122:23–36.

Permissions

All chapters in this book were first published in RETROVIROLOGY, by BioMed Central; hereby published with permission under the Creative Commons Attribution License or equivalent. Every chapter published in this book has been scrutinized by our experts. Their significance has been extensively debated. The topics covered herein carry significant findings which will fuel the growth of the discipline. They may even be implemented as practical applications or may be referred to as a beginning point for another development.

The contributors of this book come from diverse backgrounds, making this book a truly international effort. This book will bring forth new frontiers with its revolutionizing research information and detailed analysis of the nascent developments around the world.

We would like to thank all the contributing authors for lending their expertise to make the book truly unique. They have played a crucial role in the development of this book. Without their invaluable contributions this book wouldn't have been possible. They have made vital efforts to compile up to date information on the varied aspects of this subject to make this book a valuable addition to the collection of many professionals and students.

This book was conceptualized with the vision of imparting up-to-date information and advanced data in this field. To ensure the same, a matchless editorial board was set up. Every individual on the board went through rigorous rounds of assessment to prove their worth. After which they invested a large part of their time researching and compiling the most relevant data for our readers.

The editorial board has been involved in producing this book since its inception. They have spent rigorous hours researching and exploring the diverse topics which have resulted in the successful publishing of this book. They have passed on their knowledge of decades through this book. To expedite this challenging task, the publisher supported the team at every step. A small team of assistant editors was also appointed to further simplify the editing procedure and attain best results for the readers.

Apart from the editorial board, the designing team has also invested a significant amount of their time in understanding the subject and creating the most relevant covers. They scrutinized every image to scout for the most suitable representation of the subject and create an appropriate cover for the book.

The publishing team has been an ardent support to the editorial, designing and production team. Their endless efforts to recruit the best for this project, has resulted in the accomplishment of this book. They are a veteran in the field of academics and their pool of knowledge is as vast as their experience in printing. Their expertise and guidance has proved useful at every step. Their uncompromising quality standards have made this book an exceptional effort. Their encouragement from time to time has been an inspiration for everyone.

The publisher and the editorial board hope that this book will prove to be a valuable piece of knowledge for researchers, students, practitioners and scholars across the globe.

List of Contributors

Xiaocao Ma, Qifei Hu, Feng Huang, Junsong Zhang, Ting Pan, Chao Liu and Hui Zhang
Institute of Human Virology, Zhongshan School of Medicine, Sun Yat-sen University, Guangzhou 510080, China
Key Laboratory of Tropical Disease Control of Ministry of Education, Zhongshan School of Medicine, Sun Yatsen University, Guangzhou 510080, China

Cancan Chen
Institute of Human Virology, Zhongshan School of Medicine, Sun Yat-sen University, Guangzhou 510080, China
Key Laboratory of Tropical Disease Control of Ministry of Education, Zhongshan School of Medicine, Sun Yatsen University, Guangzhou 510080, China
Department of Pathology, The First Affiliated Hospital, Sun Yat-sen University, Guangzhou 510080, China

Xinghua Li and Jinyu Xia
Department of Infectious Diseases, The Fifth Affiliated Hospital, Sun Yat-sen University, Zhuhai 519000, China

Danica D. Wiredja, Caroline O.Tabler, Daniela M.Schlatzer, Mark R. Chance and John C. Tilton
Department of Nutrition, Center for Proteomics and Bioinformatics, School of Medicine, Case Western Reserve University, Cleveland, OH 44106, USA

Ming Li
Department of Population and Quantitative Health Sciences, School of Medicine, Case Western Reserve University, Cleveland, OH 44106, USA

Hiroshi Yotsuyanagi
Division of Infectious Diseases and Applied Immunology, Research Hospital, The Institute of Medical Science, The University of Tokyo, Tokyo, Japan

Masato Ogishi
Division of Infectious Diseases and Applied Immunology, Research Hospital, The Institute of Medical Science, The University of Tokyo, Tokyo, Japan
National Center for Global Health and Medicine, Tokyo, Japan

Yoshio Koyanagi
Laboratory of Systems Virology, Institute for Frontier Life and Medical Sciences, Kyoto University, Kyoto, Japan

Yoriyuki Konno and Shumpei Nagaoka
Laboratory of Systems Virology, Institute for Frontier Life and Medical Sciences, Kyoto University, Kyoto, Japan
Graduate School of Biostudies, Kyoto University, Kyoto, Japan

Izumi Kimura
Laboratory of Systems Virology, Institute for Frontier Life and Medical Sciences, Kyoto University, Kyoto, Japan
Graduate School of Pharmaceutical Sciences, Kyoto University, Kyoto, Japan

Hirofumi Aso
Laboratory of Systems Virology, Institute for Frontier Life and Medical Sciences, Kyoto University, Kyoto, Japan
Graduate School of Pharmaceutical Sciences, Kyoto University, Kyoto, Japan
Faculty of Pharmaceutical Sciences, Kyoto University, Kyoto, Japan

Keisuke Yamamoto
Laboratory of Systems Virology, Institute for Frontier Life and Medical Sciences, Kyoto University, Kyoto, Japan
Graduate School of Medicine, Kyoto University, Kyoto, Japan

Yumiko Kagawa
Laboratory of Systems Virology, Institute for Frontier Life and Medical Sciences, Kyoto University, Kyoto, Japan
Faculty of Medicine, Kyoto University, Kyoto, Japan

Ryuichi Kumata
Laboratory of Systems Virology, Institute for Frontier Life and Medical Sciences, Kyoto University, Kyoto, Japan
Faculty of Science, Kyoto University, Kyoto, Japan

Kei Sato
Laboratory of Systems Virology, Institute for Frontier Life and Medical Sciences, Kyoto University, Kyoto, Japan
CREST, Japan Science and Technology Agency, Saitama, Japan
Division of Systems Virology, Department of Infectious Disease Control, International Research Center for Infectious Diseases, Institute of Medical Science, The University of Tokyo, 4-6-1 Shirokanedai, Minato-ku, Tokyo 1088639, Japan

Mahoko Takahashi Ueda
Micro/Nano Technology Center, Tokai University, Kanagawa, Japan

So Nakagawa
Micro/Nano Technology Center, Tokai University, Kanagawa, Japan
Department of Molecular Life Science, Tokai University School of Medicine, Tokai University, Kanagawa, Japan

Tomoko Kobayashi
Department of Animal Science, Faculty of Agriculture, Tokyo University of Agriculture, Kanagawa, Japan

Paul D. Bieniasz
Howard Hughes Medical Institute and Laboratory of Retrovirology, The Rockefeller University, New York, NY 10065, USA

Sebla B. Kutluay
Department of Molecular Microbiology, Washington University School of Medicine, Saint Louis, MO 63110, USA

Kenta Iijima and Yukihito Ishizaka
Department of Intractable Diseases, National Center for Global Health and Medicine, 1-21-1 Toyama, Shinjuku-ku, Tokyo 162-8655, Japan

Junya Kobayashi
Department of Genome Repair Dynamics, Radiation Biology Center, Kyoto University, Yoshidakonoe-cho, Sakyo-ku, Kyoto 606-8501, Japan

Jakub Chojnacki
MRC Human Immunology Unit, Weatherall Institute of Molecular Medicine, University of Oxford, Oxford OX3 9DS, UK

Christian Eggeling
MRC Human Immunology Unit, Weatherall Institute of Molecular Medicine, University of Oxford, Oxford OX3 9DS, UK
Institute of Applied Optics, Friedrich-Schiller-University Jena, Max-Wien Platz 4, 07743 Jena, Germany
Leibniz Institute of Photonic Technology e.V., Albert-Einstein-Straße 9, 07745 Jena, Germany

Paul D. Bieniasz
Laboratory of Retrovirology and Howard Hughes Medical Institute, The Rockefeller University, New York, NY, USA

Daniel Blanco-Melo
Laboratory of Retrovirology and Howard Hughes Medical Institute, The Rockefeller University, New York, NY, USA

Present Address: Department of Microbiology, Icahn School of Medicine at Mount Sinai, New York, NY, USA

Robert J.Gifford
MRC-University of Glasgow Centre for Virus Research, Glasgow, UK

Jérémy Dufloo
Virus and Immunity Unit, Department of Virology, Institut Pasteur, Paris, France
CNRS-UMR3569, Paris, France

Timothée Bruel and Olivier Schwartz
Virus and Immunity Unit, Department of Virology, Institut Pasteur, Paris, France
CNRS-UMR3569, Paris, France
Vaccine Research Institute, Créteil, France

Xu Zhang, Xiancai Ma, Shuliang Jing and Hui Zhang
Institute of Human Virology, Zhongshan School of Medicine, Sun Yat-Sen University, Guangzhou 510080, China
Key Laboratory of Tropical Disease Control of Ministry of Education, Zhongshan School of Medicine, Sun Yat-Sen University, Guangzhou 510080, China
Guangdong Engineering Research Center for Antimicrobial Agent and Immunotechnology, Zhongshan School of Medicine, Sun Yat-Sen University, Guangzhou 510080, China

Yijun Zhang
Section of Infectious Diseases, Department of Internal Medicine, Yale University School of Medicine, New Haven, CT 06520, USA

Jolien Blokken, Stéphanie De Houwer, Lieve Dirix, Frauke Christ and Zeger Debyser
Laboratory for Molecular Virology and Gene Therapy, Department of Pharmaceutical and Pharmacological Sciences, KU Leuven, Kapucijnenvoer 33, VCTB +5, Bus 7001, 3000 Leuven, Flanders, Belgium

Jonas Demeulemeester
Laboratory for Molecular Virology and Gene Therapy, Department of Pharmaceutical and Pharmacological Sciences, KU Leuven, Kapucijnenvoer 33, VCTB +5, Bus 7001, 3000 Leuven, Flanders, Belgium
The Francis Crick Institute, London, UK

Hugo Klaassen and Arnaud Marchand
Center for Innovation and Stimulation of Drug Discovery (CISTIM), Leuven, Belgium

Patrick Chaltin
Center for Innovation and Stimulation of Drug Discovery (CISTIM), Leuven, Belgium

Center for Drug Design and Development (CD3), KU Leuven R&D, Leuven, Belgium

Alba Torrents de la Peña
Department of Medical Microbiology, Academic Medical Center, University of Amsterdam, 1105 AZ Amsterdam, The Netherlands

Rogier W. Sanders
Department of Medical Microbiology, Academic Medical Center, University of Amsterdam, 1105 AZ Amsterdam, The Netherlands
Department of Microbiology and Immunology, Weill Medical College of Cornell University, New York, NY 10021, USA

Johnson Mak
Institute for Glycomics, Griffith University Gold Coast, Southport, QLD, Australia

Alex de Marco
Department of Biochemistry and Molecular Biology, Monash University, Clayton, VIC, Australia

Gert van Zyl
Division of Medical Virology, Stellenbosch University and NHLS Tygerberg, Cape Town, South Africa

Michael J. Bale and Mary F. Kearney
HIV Dynamic and Replication Program, Center for Cancer Research, National Cancer Institute at Frederick, 1050 Boyles Street, Building 535, Room 109, Frederick, MD 21702-1201, USA

Carmen Ledesma-Feliciano Xin Zheng, Esther Musselman and Sue VandeWoude
Department of Microbiology, Immunology, and Pathology, College of Veterinary Medicine and Biomedical Sciences, Colorado State University, Fort Collins, CO, USA

Ryan Troyer
Department of Microbiology, Immunology, and Pathology, College of Veterinary Medicine and Biomedical Sciences, Colorado State University, Fort Collins, CO, USA
Department of Microbiology and Immunology, Western University, London, ON, Canada

Sarah Hagen and Martin Löchelt
Department of Molecular Diagnostics of Oncogenic Infections, Research Program Infection, Inflammation and Cancer, German Cancer Research Center, (Deutsches Krebsforschungszentrum Heidelberg, DKFZ), Im Neuenheimer Feld 242, 69120 Heidelberg, Germany

Daniel Maeda
Department of Molecular Diagnostics of Oncogenic Infections, Research Program Infection, Inflammation and Cancer, German Cancer Research Center, (Deutsches Krebsforschungszentrum Heidelberg, DKFZ), Im Neuenheimer Feld 242, 69120 Heidelberg, Germany
University of Dar es Salaam, Dar es Salaam, Tanzania

Dragana Slavkovic Lukic
Department of Molecular Diagnostics of Oncogenic Infections, Research Program Infection, Inflammation and Cancer, German Cancer Research Center, (Deutsches Krebsforschungszentrum Heidelberg, DKFZ), Im Neuenheimer Feld 242, 69120 Heidelberg, Germany
Department of Internal Medicine II, Division of Hematology, University Hospital of Würzburg, Würzburg, Germany

Ann-Mareen Franke
Department of Molecular Diagnostics of Oncogenic Infections, Research Program Infection, Inflammation and Cancer, German Cancer Research Center, (Deutsches Krebsforschungszentrum Heidelberg, DKFZ), Im Neuenheimer Feld 242, 69120 Heidelberg, Germany
Roche Pharma AG, Grenzach-Wyhlen, Germany

Guochao Wei
Department of Molecular Diagnostics of Oncogenic Infections, Research Program Infection, Inflammation and Cancer, German Cancer Research Center, (Deutsches Krebsforschungszentrum Heidelberg, DKFZ), Im Neuenheimer Feld 242, 69120 Heidelberg, Germany
Division of Infectious Disease, University of Colorado, Anschutz Medical Campus, Aurora, USA

Carsten Münk
Clinic for Gastroenterology, Hepatology, and Infectiology, Medical Faculty, Heinrich-Heine-University Düsseldorf, Düsseldorf, Germany

Jörg Zielonka
Clinic for Gastroenterology, Hepatology, and Infectiology, Medical Faculty, Heinrich-Heine-University Düsseldorf, Düsseldorf, Germany
Roche Glycart AG, Schlieren 8952, Switzerland

Sofie Rutsaert, Wim Trypsteen and Linos Vandekerckhove
HIV Cure Research Center, Department of Internal Medicine, Ghent University, Ghent, Belgium

Kobus Bosman and Monique Nijhuis
Department of Medical Microbiology, Virology, UMC Utrecht, Utrecht, The Netherlands

S. Mediouni, J.A.Jablonski, S.Tsuda, A.Richard, C. Kessing, A. Biswas, H. Choe and S.T.Valente
Department of Immunology and Microbiology, The Scripps Research Institute, 130 Scripps Way, 3C1, Jupiter, FL 33458, USA
Department of Molecular Therapeutics, The Scripps Research Institute, Jupiter, FL, USA

T. Tellinghuisen
Department of Immunology and Microbiology, The Scripps Research Institute, 130 Scripps Way, 3C1, Jupiter, FL 33458, USA
Roche, Basel, Switzerland

M. Cameron
Department of Molecular Therapeutics, The Scripps Research Institute, Jupiter, FL, USA

Y. Even
The Botanist's Beach Farm, Jupiter, FL, USA

M. V. Andrade and M. Stevenson
University of Miami Miller School of Medicine, Miami, FL, USA

Alejandro B. Balazs
Ragon Institute of MGH, MIT and Harvard, Cambridge, MA 02139, USA

Allen Lin
Ragon Institute of MGH, MIT and Harvard, Cambridge, MA 02139, USA
Department of Systems Biology, Harvard University, Boston, MA 02115, USA

Index

www.ingramcontent.com/pod-product-compliance
Lightning Source LLC
Chambersburg PA
CBHW080455200326
41458CB00012B/3978

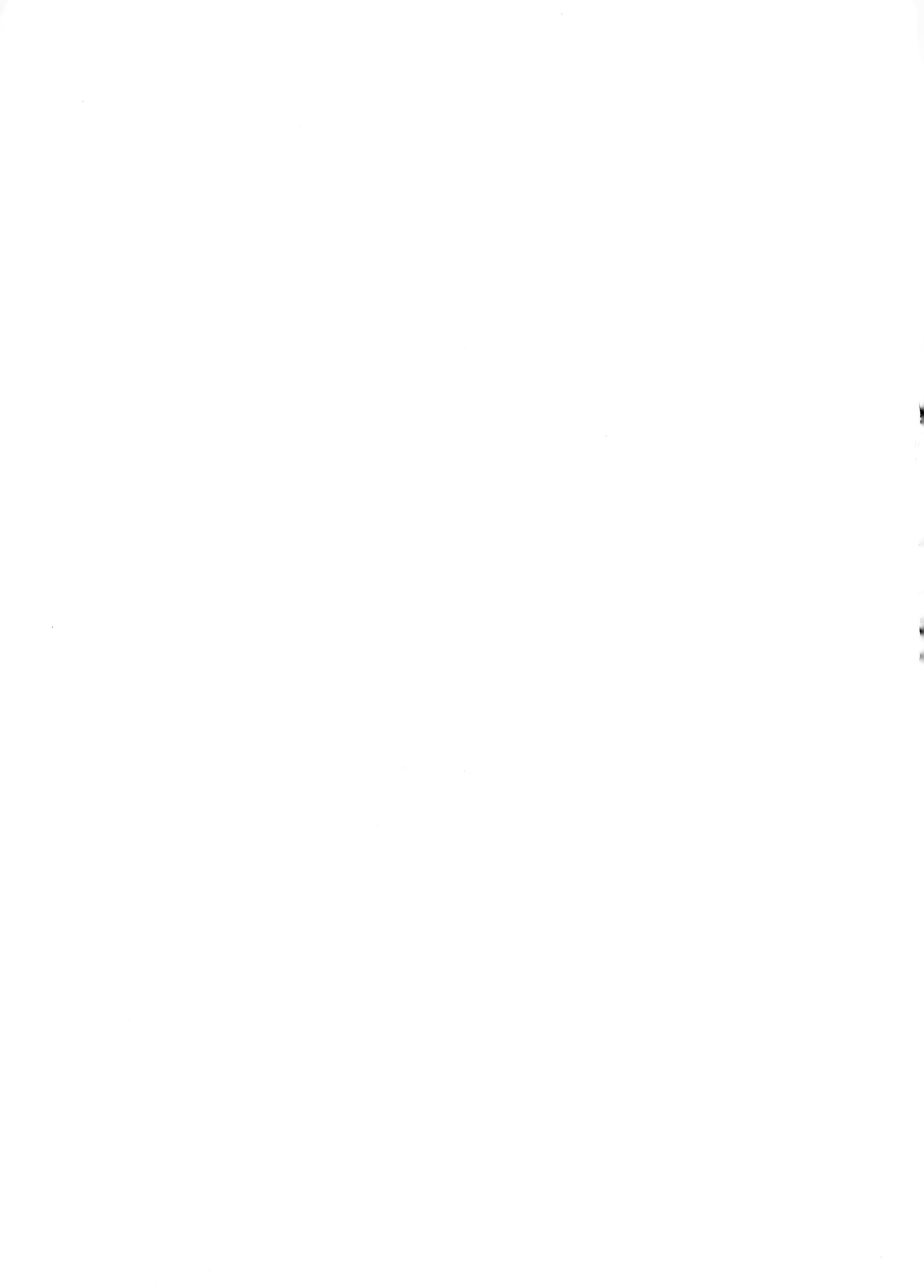